Pediatric Nuclear Medicine

S. T. Treves

Pediatric Nuclear Medicine

With 370 Figures in 735 Parts

Springer-Verlag
New York Berlin Heidelberg Tokyo

S. T. Treves, M.D.
Division of Nuclear Medicine
The Children's Hospital Medical Center
300 Longwood Avenue
Boston, Massachusetts 02115 USA

Library of Congress Cataloging in Publication Data
Treves, S.T. (Salvador T.)
Pediatric nuclear medicine.
Includes bibliographies and index.
1. Radioisotopes in pediatrics. 2. Radioisotope scanning. 3. Nuclear medicine. I. Title.
RJ51.R33T74 1985 618.92′007′575 84-22189

Typeset by University Graphics, Inc., Atlantic Highlands, New Jersey.
Printed and bound by Halliday Lithographers, West Hanover, Massachusetts.
Printed in the United States of America.

9 8 7 6 5 4 3 2 1

ISBN 0-387-96001-5 Springer-Verlag New York Berlin Heidelberg Tokyo
ISBN 3-540-96001-5 Springer-Verlag Berlin Heidelberg New York Tokyo

To Isa, Erik, and Alex

Foreword

This book comes at a good time. The differentiation of pediatric nuclear medicine from the general practice of nuclear medicine has developed over the past 15 years and is now a reality. Dr. Treves has been one of a small band of pediatric specialists who have made this happen. He recounts the reasons for this in his introduction—the development of technetium-99m-labeled radiopharmaceuticals making possible the use of these procedures in nonmalignant diseases, the appreciation that infants and children require special techniques and adapted technology, the availability of computer methods for handling the dynamic data of pediatric cardiology and urology, and the difference in the spectrum of disease seen in the pediatric versus the adult nuclear medicine clinic.

The book is a compendium of a single-person's experience, rather than the amalgam generally found in a multiauthored work. In a sense this is atavistic, but it provides the old-fashioned comfort of a coherent and personal approach. Its success is due largely to Dr. Treves' broad experience and his special talent for describing each test in relation to this experience. It is probably aided by the relatively recent emergence of pediatric nuclear medicine as a special activity and follows in the footsteps of other volumes on the pediatric subspecialties that have taken off from general adult practice in the past.

The book also points out that nuclear medicine is part of general diagnostic medicine, in this case pediatric medicine, and can never exist in isolation. It makes clear the role of nuclear medicine tests in the overall approach to common, and not so common, hospital problems. It reminds us that diagnostic methods must be integrated to provide maximum information with a minimum of harm.

S. J. Adelstein, M.D.
Harvard Medical School
1984

Preface

At a time when radiology is characterized as an amalgam of "imaging techniques," it becomes important to have at hand a reference on available modalities for all who are involved in pediatric medicine. One hopes that any reference is up-to-date and that it contains material that is well documented by the experience of the author or authors. To the radiologist, the need for consultation with clinicians regarding a particular disorder becomes increasingly significant, as does the need for clinicians to communicate with the radiologist. There is the need for the most efficacious diagnostic approach that embodies concern for, and realization of, the opportunity for obtaining the most helpful information while remaining mindful of radiation exposure and cost. Thus this book becomes a valuable asset.

The areas that Dr. Treves has included emphasize appropriate pharmaceuticals and the dose of each; imaging techniques; and a review of common conditions for which scintigraphy can be diagnostically applied. The elucidation of dose is very important for those whose practice is not primarily concerned with infants and children. Further, it is significant that differential diagnosis is stressed as well as the appearance of benign and aggressive lesions and those that are acquired. Of course, scintigraphy has the great advantage of providing functional data from relatively noninvasive techniques. The disorders discussed in the 17 chapters encompass those that are common as well as those that are infrequently encountered but figure in daily differential diagnosis. The nature of the scintigraphic information, anatomic and functional, is discussed with emphasis on new instrumentation, the application of computers, and the generation of appropriate pharmaceutical agents.

I feel confident that this volume will put a diagnostically significant specialty into perspective for all of us who deal with the pediatric patient.

John A. Kirkpatrick, M.D.
Harvard Medical School
The Children's Hospital
1984

Contents

Foreword *S. J. Adelstein* vii

Preface *John A. Kirkpatrick* ix

Contributors xiii

Introduction *S. T. Treves, Royal T. Davis, James B. Conway, Carolyn S. Turner* xv

1 Bone *S. T. Treves, John A. Kirkpatrick* 1

2 Skeletal Scintigraphy for Assessment of Mandibular Growth and Asymmetry *Leonard B. Kaban, S. T. Treves* 49

3 Bone Marrow *S. T. Treves* 59

4 Kidneys *S. T. Treves, Robert L. Lebowitz, Alvin Kuruc, Sydney Heyman, Paul Rosen* 63

5 Radionuclide Voiding Cystography *U. V. Willi, S. T. Treves* 105

6 Scrotal Scintigraphy *George Taylor, S. T. Treves* 121

7 Liver *S. T. Treves, John A. Markisz* 129

8 Spleen *S. T. Treves* 141

9 Hepatobiliary Scintigraphy *S. T. Treves, Alun Jones* 157

10 Gastroesophageal Reflux and Gastric Emptying *Paul Rosen, S. T. Treves* 171

11 Meckel's Diverticulum *S. T. Treves, Richard Grand* 179

12 Thyroid *S. T. Treves, Reed Larsen, Roger Pezzuti* 191

13 Brain *S. T. Treves, Roy L. Strand, Robert K. Crone, Annalise Lipp* 205

14 Cerebrospinal Fluid *S. T. Treves, Keasley Welch, Alvin Kuruc* 223

15 Dacryoscintigraphy *Sydney Heyman, James A. Katowitz* 233

16 Heart *S. T. Treves, Roger Hurwitz, Alvin Kuruc, H. W. Strauss* 245

17 Lung *S. T. Treves, G. B. C. Harris* 289

Index 331

Contributors

S. J. Adelstein, M.D. Dean of Academic Programs, Professor of Radiology, Harvard Medical School, Boston, Massachusetts USA

James B. Conway Administrator, Department of Radiology, The Children's Hospital, Boston, Massachusetts USA

Robert K. Crone, M.D. Director of the Multidisciplinary, Intensive Care Unit, Children's Hospital, Assistant Professor of Anesthesia (Pediatrics), Harvard Medical School, Boston, Massachusetts USA

Royal T. Davis, CNMT Technical Director, Division of Nuclear Medicine, The Children's Hospital, Boston, Massachusetts USA

Richard Grand, M.D. Chief, Division of Pediatric Gastroenterology and Nutrition, New England Medical Center, Professor of Pediatrics, Tufts University School of Medicine, Boston, Massachusetts USA

G. B. C. Harris, M.D. Associate Radiologist-in-Chief, The Children's Hospital, Associate Professor of Radiology, Harvard Medical School, Boston, Massachusetts USA

Sydney Heyman, M.D. Director, Division of Nuclear Medicine, Children's Hospital of Pennsylvania, Clinical Assistant Professor of Radiology and Pediatrics, University of Pennsylvania, Philadelphia, Pennsylvania USA

Roger Hurwitz, M.D. Professor of Pediatrics, Section of Cardiology, Riley Research, Indiana University Medical Center, Indianapolis, Indiana USA

Alun Jones, Ph.D. Associate in Radiology (Nuclear Medicine), Brigham and Women's Hospital, Associate Professor of Radiology, Harvard Medical School, Boston, Massachusetts USA

Leonard B. Kaban, D.M.D., M.D. Associate in Surgery, The Children's Hospital, Surgeon, Brigham and Women's Hospital, Associate Professor of Oral and Maxillofacial Surgery, Harvard Medical School, Boston, Massachusetts USA

James A. Katowitz, M.D. Director of Ophthalmic, Plastic, Reconstructive Surgery, Children's Hospital of Philadelphia and Schei Eye Institute, Associate Professor, Department of Ophthalmology, University of Pennsylvania School of Medicine, Philadelphia, Pennsylvania USA

John A. Kirkpatrick, M.D. Radiologist-in-Chief, The Children's Hospital, Professor of Radiology, Harvard Medical School, Boston, Massachusetts USA

Alvin Kuruc, M.D. Research Associate, Division of Nuclear Medicine, The Children's Hospital, Boston, Massachusetts USA

Reed Larsen, M.D. Director of Thyroid Diagnostic Center, Brigham and Women's Hospital, Investigator, Howard Hughes Medical Institute, Professor of Medicine, Harvard Medical School, Boston, Massachusetts USA

Robert L. Lebowitz, M.D. Radiologist, Director of Uroradiology, Associate Professor of Radiology, Harvard Medical School, Boston, Massachusetts USA

Annalise Lipp, M.D. Research Fellow in Radiology (Nuclear Medicine), The Children's Hospital, Boston, Massachusetts, Assistant Professor of the Neurodevelopmental Unit, Children's Hospital of Zurich, Switzerland

John A. Markisz, Ph.D., M.D. Assistant Professor of Radiology, Cornell University Medical Center—The New York Hospital, New York, New York USA

Roger Pezzuti, M.D. Fellow in Nuclear Medicine, New England Deaconess Hospital—The Children's Hospital, Boston, Massachusetts USA

Paul Rosen, M.D. Division of Nuclear Medicine, The Children's Hospital, Assistant Professor of Radiology, Harvard Medical School, Boston, Massachusetts USA

Roy L. Strand, M.D. Neuroradiologist, The Children's Hospital, Associate Professor of Radiology, Harvard Medical School, Boston, Massachusetts USA

H. W. Strauss, M.D. Director, Division of Nuclear Medicine, Radiologist, Massachusetts General Hospital, Professor of Radiology, Harvard Medical School, Boston, Massachusetts USA

George Taylor, M.D. Research Fellow in Radiology, The Children's Hospital, Boston, Massachusetts USA

S. T. Treves, M.D. Director, Division of Nuclear Medicine, The Children's Hospital, Associate Professor of Radiology, Harvard Medical School, Boston, Massachusetts USA

Carolyn S. Turner, Ph.D. Child Development Unit, The Children's Hospital, Boston, Massachusetts USA

Keasley Welch, M.D. Neurosurgeon-in-Chief, The Children's Hospital, Chief, Division of Neurosurgery, Brigham and Women's Hospital, Francis D. Ingraham Professor of Neurosurgery, Harvard Medical School, Boston, Massachusetts USA

U. V. Willi, M.D. Pediatric Radiologist, Department of Radiology, Children's Hospital, Assistant Professor of Radiology, University of Zurich, Switzerland

Introduction

S.T. Treves
Royal T. Davis
James B. Conway
Carolyn S. Turner

What makes pediatric nuclear medicine unique is its subject, the child with his unique physiology and pathophysiology. Pediatric nuclear medicine has experienced rapid development during the past decade and a half. Its growth is due in great part from the need for information about many pediatric disorders that could not be obtained, or could not be obtained easily, with other diagnostic methods. Nuclear medicine diagnostic procedures are safe, minimally invasive, sensitive, and provide morphologic as well as accurate quantitative information of function of organs and systems in the body.

During the mid-1960s the majority of nuclear medicine studies in children were indicated in those patients who were severely ill, or were known to have cancer. Most of those patients were hospitalized. Radiopharmaceuticals available then were tagged with radioisotopes with relatively long physical half-lives, which resulted in significant radiation exposure to patients. At the Children's Hospital in Boston during 1971 more than 75% of all nuclear medicine studies were performed on inpatients. Most of the early studies in pediatric patients were obtained for anatomic information only. For example, detection of tumors of the brain and liver accounted for the vast majority of studies performed in the 1960s. Major current thrusts of nuclear medicine, including its potential for early diagnosis of disease and the measurement of function, were not being realized.

The introduction of computed tomography together with refinements in ultrasonography, two modalities that provide excellent anatomic information, have not resulted, as originally anticipated, in a significant reduction in the overall activity in nuclear medicine. Advances in the clinical applications of these two modalities have encouraged investigators in nuclear medicine to focus less on the anatomic definition of disease and more on its functional aspects. This is reflected by the reductions in radionuclide brain imaging and static hepatic scintigraphy with a concomitant increase in radionuclide angiography, hepatobiliary scintigraphy, renal scintigraphy, radionuclide voiding cystography, ventilation-perfusion studies, studies to evaluate gastroesophageal reflux and gastric emptying, scrotal scintigraphy, and those to aid in the diagnosis of a variety of inflammatory disorders.

The growth of the pediatric applications of nuclear medicine has been made possible largely by its increased capacity to achieve earlier and improved diagnosis, and by advances in the fields of radiopharmaceuticals and instrumentation.

In radiopharmaceutical research, major improvements have occurred including the introduction of a variety of radiopharmaceuticals labelled with radionuclides with short physical half-lives (technetium-99m, iodine-123, thallium-201, iridium-191m). These radiopharmaceuticals result in acceptably low patient radiation exposure. Radiopharmaceuticals are physiologically innocuous and can be given safely even to severely ill patients. These substances contain materials in trace amounts, do not produce toxic or pharmacologic effects, do not produce allergic reactions, and do not result in hemodynamic or osmotic overload.

Newer gamma cameras have been developed

that are capable of higher spatial resolution, better field uniformity, and improved spatial and count linearity. Improvements in spatial resolution along with magnification techniques (pinhole, converging collimator) facilitate the evaluation of small children.

Digital computers are now essential components of gamma cameras. At present, more than 75% of nuclear medicine studies in our institution are computer-assisted, and it is expected that within the next few years, all studies will be in digital format. These instruments permit recording and sophisticated qualitative and quantitative analysis of studies. Computers have permitted the use in routine pediatric nuclear medicine of studies for the evaluation of function of organs and systems in a rather unique way. For example, quantitation of left-to-right shunting, evaluation of regional and total renal function, evaluation of regional pulmonary function, measurement of ventricular ejection fraction, vesicoureteric reflux, gastroesophageal reflux, etc., can all be done rapidly, accurately, and conveniently with digital computers. Also, storage of studies on magnetic media (i.e., diskettes) allows rapid retrieval, review, and comparison of multiple studies.

Computerized, mobile gamma cameras extend the capabilities of nuclear medicine as they permit evaluation of severely ill children in intensive care units, neonatal care units, recovery rooms, and operating rooms.

Changes in Type and Distribution of Pediatric Nuclear Medicine Examinations

From 1971 to 1983 there has been an almost five-fold increase in the number of pediatric nuclear medicine examinations at The Children's Hospital in Boston (Fig. I-1).

There has been a dramatic increase in the number of studies for the diagnosis of benign disorders and in the evaluation of function. Although evaluation of pediatric oncologic disorders is still an important part of nuclear medicine, less than 20% of the patients studied at present belong to this group. In addition, the emphasis of nuclear medicine studies in pediatric oncology now is greater in the area of early diagnosis and evaluation of tumors, not just in the diagnosis of metastatic disease.

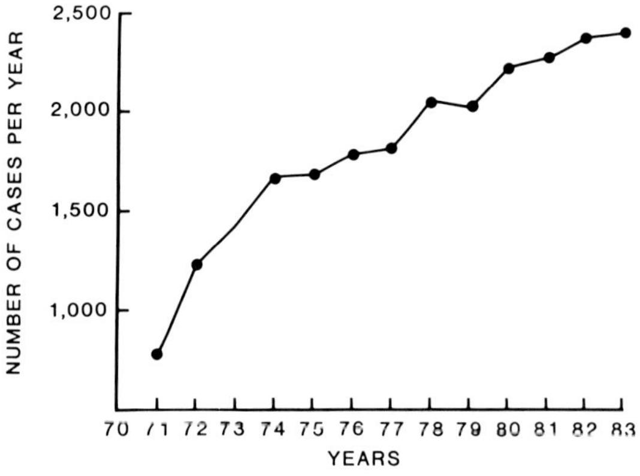

Figure I-1.

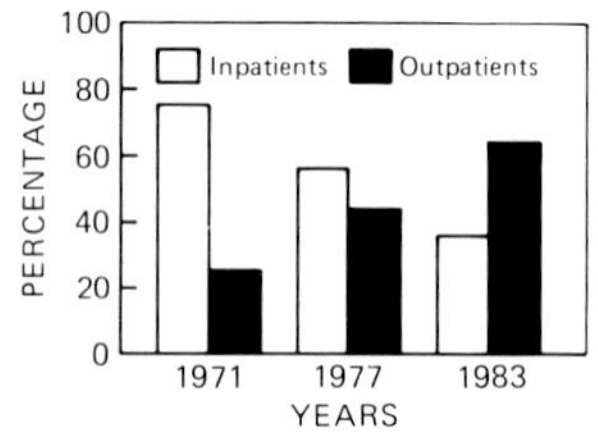

Figure I-2.

The majority of patients undergoing nuclear medicine examinations in our institution at present are outpatients. These patients account for about 65% of the total (Fig. I-2). A larger number of outpatients necessitates more orderly and precise scheduling in order to reduce patient wait and to achieve a more effective utilization of personnel and resources.

Some specific examples of the change in character and distribution of pediatric nuclear medicine examinations during the past decade in our hospital is presented in Table I-1.

Radionuclide brain scanning, which was the most frequent examination in 1973, due to the successful introduction of computed tomography and advances in ultrasonography, had decreased by a factor of 10 in 1983. Similarly, the number of hepatic and splenic scintigrams has decreased by almost 30%.

Skeletal scintigraphy with the increased use of this method in the evaluation of benign disorders (osteomyelitis, stress fractures, aseptic necrosis) has increased by about 300%.

Radionuclide studies of the cardiovascular system have increased by almost 60% in the past 10 years. The indications for these studies include

Table I-1. Number and Distribution of Examinations, 1973–1983, Division of Nuclear Medicine, The Children's Hospital, Boston

	1973		1983	
Examination	Total	Percentage	Total	Percentage
Brain	557	38	54	2
Bone	163	11	645	27
Liver-Spleen	212	15	152	6
Kidneys	207	14	323	14
Voiding Cystography	0	0	458	20
Heart	106	7	167	7
Lungs	65	4	109	5
Abdomen (Meckel's)	66	4	56	2
Gastroesophageal Reflux	0	0	220	9
Gallium	0	0	81	4
Scrotal Scintigraphy	0	0	46	2
Thyroid	58	4	39	2
Others	20	3	0	0

quantitation of shunts, evaluation of myocardial perfusion, and quantitation of cardiac function.

With advances in radiopharmaceuticals and methods of analysis, there is a renewed interest on the part of pediatric urologists and nephrologists in the radionuclide evaluation of the kidneys. Renal studies exhibited an increase of about 55%.

Radionuclide voiding cystography, which in our hospital was introduced in the mid-1970s, has gained wide acceptance, with 458 studies performed in 1983. This represented about 20% of all studies during that year.

Similarly, radionuclide evaluation of gastroesophageal reflux, gastric emptying, and pulmonary aspiration have shown a rapid increase.

Other studies introduced during the past decade that have shown a significant increase included scrotal scintigraphy for the diagnosis of testicular torsion, and gallium-67 scintigraphy for the detection of inflammatory disease.

Studies that have not changed significantly in number include thyroid and abdominal (Meckel's) scintigraphy.

The Consult

Most pediatric patients are referred to nuclear medicine by a variety of pediatric specialists including pediatricians, urologists, nephrologists, general surgeons, orthopedic surgeons, cardiologists, pneumonologists, oncologists, neonatologists, endocrinologists, neurosurgeons, and neurologists.

Although there is a "routine" for many pediatric nuclear medicine examinations, studies frequently need to be adapted to permit evaluation of a particular clinical problem. The nuclear medicine consult is usually scheduled by a physician, a nurse, a medical student, or, frequently, by a clerk. During this initial communication, sufficient information about the patient and his condition should be obtained so as to permit appropriate scheduling, and in order to facilitate tailoring of the study to the specific problem being evaluated. A consultation form must be completed by the referring physician providing appropriate information about the problem being investigated and the type of examination desired. Of prime importance is a clear statement of the clinical question being asked. Useful information to the pediatric nuclear medicine consultant includes patient's age, sex, a succinct clinical history, results of other imaging procedures and laboratory tests, and information about previous therapy or surgery. It is useful to know in advance if the patient may require sedation and if there are any special precautions. Knowledge of potentially conflicting imaging tests already scheduled is essential in planning the studies.

Once the patient arrives in the nuclear medicine department a physician or assistant should interview the patient and/or the parents in order to gain additional information about the patient's condition that may help with the examination. Upon arrival, every patient must be properly identified (i.e., hospital I.D. badge). The patient's medical record must always accompany the patient to the department of nuclear medicine. If the nuclear medicine consultant determines that the examination requested is not appropriate to the problem in question, or that another type of examination is indicated, he or she should communicate such concern to the referring physician in order to avoid unnecessary examinations.

A limited physical examination of the patient is not necessary in all cases, but is crucial in many patients. Examples when physical examination is important in the evaluation of nuclear medical information include patients with questions of osteomyelitis, cellulitis, urinary diversion, testicular torsion, trauma, sports injuries, fractures, pulmonary disorders, nodules of the neck, abdominal masses, and tumors. Also, patients should be examined for metallic objects that will shield gamma radiation (keys, belt buckles, coins, jewelry, etc.). Diapers, clothing, or gauze contaminated with radionuclides should be removed. Contaminated skin should be thoroughly washed and monitored.

After the pediatric nuclear medicine physician reviews and approves the consult, the study is discussed with the technologist in charge of performing the examination.

After the examination is performed, the physician should review and evaluate the quality and adequacy of the study with the technologist, and order additional examination(s) if necessary. The physician may need to reexamine the patient and the clinical data, in order to interpret the results.

Failure to obtain pertinent information may result in incomplete examinations, the wrong examination being performed, excessive or unnecessary examinations, and erroneous interpretation of results.

The results of nuclear medicine examinations should be reported promptly to the referring physician. In abnormal studies it is useful to telephone the results as soon as possible. A written report should follow in all cases. The report should be clear, concise, and should address the question(s) being asked.

Administered Doses and Absorbed Doses

Administered doses in pediatric nuclear medicine have been developed by experience, taking into account absorbed radiation dose, photon flux, instrumentation, and examination time. Administered dose of radionuclides in pediatric nuclear medicine should be determined by that minimal amount necessary to permit a satisfactory examination. Higher or lower doses represent unnecessary radiation exposure. There is not a perfect formula that applies to the calculation of administered dose in children. Estimation of dose for pediatric patients based on adult dose corrected for body weight or body surface area generally provides a good guide for most children above the age of about 1 year. In premature and newborn infants the concept of minimal dose should be introduced. The minimal administered dose in pediatric nuclear medicine does not relate to body surface area or weight. It relates more to the minimal amount of radioactivity below which the study will be inadequate. This minimal dosage is dictated also by the type of study, dynamic or static, and by limitations in the sensitivity of the recording equipment. For example, the usual pediatric dose of technetium-99m (Tc-99m) pertechnetate for radionuclide angiography is 200 μCi/kg of body weight. However, a radionuclide angiogram on a premature baby who weighs 900 g requires a minimum total dose of 2 mCi. In small children, dynamic studies require a higher dose of tracer than do static studies.

Accurate data on absorbed doses in pediatric patients are not available at present due to a general lack of detailed information on the biodistribution and kinetics of radiopharmaceuticals in children, particularly in premature and newborn infants.

Lack of information on pediatric absorbed doses, the desire of some physicians and/or technologists to obtain a study in the shortest possible time, and lack of experience in handling pediatric patients are factors that frequently contribute to radiopharmaceutical overdosage in children.

Most biodistribution data used for the estimation of absorbed radiation dose in children have been extrapolated from adult human and animal studies. These studies have generally been carried out on healthy individuals. Information on biodistribution of radiopharmaceuticals in disease, however, is not generally available even for adult patients.

Absorbed doses in pediatric nuclear medicine vary with the age and weight of the patient, as well as with the physiologic or pathologic condition of the patient. For example, the whole-body radiation absorbed dose with Tc-99m diethylenetriamine pentaacetic acid (DTPA) is greater in a patient in renal failure than in a patient with normal renal function.

The biokinetics of radiotracers in the neonate are often different from those in the older child or the adult. For example, compared with adults and older children, in newborns there is a lower renal blood flow and glomerular filtration rate, faster washout of radioactive gases from the lungs, faster circulation times, and greater skeletal deposition of bone-seeking radiotracers. As maturation takes place, physiologic processes in children become more like those in adults.

The distribution of radiotracers in children in many instances is different than in adults. For example, in children the concentration of Tc-99m methylenediphosponate (MDP) in growth centers

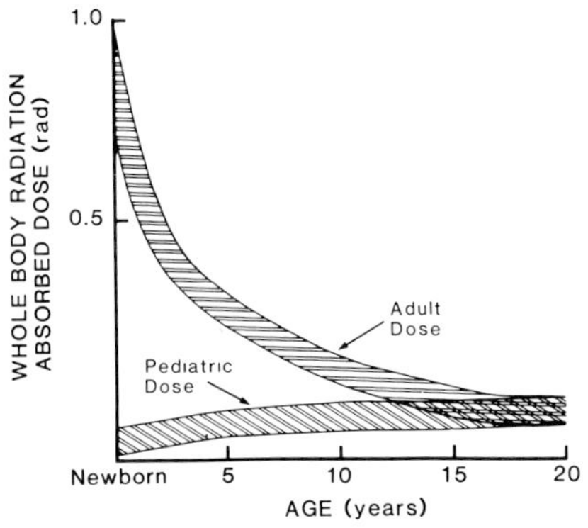

Figure I-3.

is high, resulting in a relatively higher local dose than that of the rest of the skeleton. When the growth centers are closed, the distribution of Tc-99m MDP will be more uniform throughout the skeleton and so will be the absorbed dose of radiation.

In spite of the current scarcity of biodistribution and kinetic data for children, estimates of absorbed dose have been calculated. The Radiopharmaceutical Internal Dose Information Center at the Oak Ridge Associated Universities has graciously provided much of the pediatric radiation dose estimates in this volume.

On a millicurie per millicurie basis, whole body radiation absorbed doses in newborn infants are about 10 times greater than in older children or adults. When administered doses are adjusted for body weight or body surface area, however, a comparable absorbed dose is achieved over a wide range of ages (Fig. I-3).

In recent years a new system of units has been adopted, the Systeme International d'Unités (SI). The transition from the units currently employed, rad and curie, to the SI units is going to take some time. The SI unit names are gray (Gy) for unit of absorbed dose and becquerel (Bq) for unit of activity (see Table I-2). To convert from one set of units to the other, see Table I-3.

Risk vs. Benefit

To date, there has been no indication or reports of any deleterious effect secondary to the administration of diagnostic amounts of radiopharmaceuticals in children. In addition, administration of radiotracers does not result in toxic, pharmacologic, or osmotic effect.

Table I-2.

	Activity	Absorbed Dose	Dose Equivalent
Units	dps	J/kg	J/kg
Old	curie (Ci)	radiation absorbed dose (rad)	roentgen equivalent (in) man (rem)
New	Becquerel (Bq)	Gray (Gy)	Sievert (Sv)

Table I-3.

To Convert From	To	Multiply by
Millicuries (mCi)	Megabecquerels (Mbq)	37
Millirads (mrad)	Centigray (cGy)	10^{-3}
Millirems (mrem)	Microsieverts (μSv)	10

This does not mean that radionuclide techniques should be employed indiscriminately. As with any diagnostic or therapeutic procedure in pediatric nuclear medicine, one should in every case weigh the potential benefit associated with such procedure against any potential risk, even if such risk is minimal or unmeasurable.

Therapy

Therapy with internal administration of radionuclides is an exception in children. During the past 13 years only two such treatments were performed at Children's Hospital in Boston. Both treatments were with iodine-131. One was on a young female patient with widespread papillary carcinoma of the thyroid. The other treatment was on a female in her late teens with hyperthyroidism refractory to medical treatment, and who refused surgery.

Personnel

Physicians and technologists in pediatric nuclear medicine should be familiar with children, their varied behavior, and the disorders that affect them. Every pediatric patient must be treated as an individual with individual emotional needs.

The offices of pediatric nuclear medicine physicians and technologists should be adjacent to the clinic. A physician should always be available on the premises.

Pediatric nuclear medicine examinations are "people intensive" procedures. Certain procedures that may necessitate one technologist in the examination of an adult patient may require two in the case of a pediatric patient. More time and patience is necessary in dealing with children than with adults. In spite of the best efforts of personnel, nuclear medicine procedures in children take generally about twice as long as in adults. Therefore, nuclear medicine studies in children are more expensive than in adults.

Training programs in nuclear medicine for physicians and certain schools of nuclear medicine technology include some training in pediatric nuclear medicine; however, additional practical experience with children is recommended.

The Examining Room

As more pediatric institutions are opening or are in the process of opening new departments of nuclear medicine, it seems appropriate to discuss desirable characteristics of examining and waiting rooms.

Examining rooms should be designed so that they are attractive and sufficiently spacious to contain the equipment, permit proper examination, allow sufficient privacy, and permit the presence of the patient's parents in the room. Examining rooms should be flexible in design and adaptable to the changing technology in nuclear medicine. The room should have the following attributes:

Quiet, pleasant and attractive
Sufficiently general ambient light (In addition, dimmers should be available in order to be able to provide a soothing effect. Some children fall asleep during the examination.)
A ceiling-mounted spotlight for illuminating the field of injection or catheterization
Several ceiling-mounted hangers to hold bottles for intravenous infusion
Ceiling-mounted heating lamps
A complete set of emergency medicines and resuscitation equipment
Stethoscopes and sphygmomanometers for all ages
A telephone with a cancellable bell. Emergency numbers must be posted clearly on the telephone
An intercom unit
Oxygen and vacuum outlets, preferably wall-mounted
Facilities for safe disposal of radioactive gases
Air conditioning for patient comfort and for proper functioning of the electronic equipment and computers
An adjustable imaging table
A small television set mounted over the examining table within easy view of the patient. A video player to be able to select appropriate programming for the patient
Sufficient space to store collimators of the gamma camera so that they are not in the way when not in use
Sufficient space to house the gamma camera, console, computers, and other associated electronic equipment such as electrocardiographs, external detectors
Easy access to the radiopharmacy or radiopharmaceutical dispensing area
Doors must be wide enough to permit the access of regular and special patient beds.
The room should be designed in order to permit the safe maneuvering of the patient's bed in relation to the examining equipment.
Provisions must be made for all cables necessary for the camera, computer, television, transmission, etc.
Sufficient number of electrical wall outlets with the proper power requirements for the gamma camera, computer, and additional electronic equipment in nuclear medicine, plus equipment that arrives with patients such as respirators, monitors, bassinets, etc.
Sufficient space for the storage of supplies such as bedding, pillows, absorbent paper, towels, tape, sand bags, gauze, etc.
A scale

The Waiting Room

Careful scheduling of studies tends to reduce waiting time for patient and parents. However, in practice there is almost always some variable waiting time before, during, and after an examination.

Certain nuclear medicine examinations require that the patient wait in the department for a few minutes after the administration of the radiopharmaceutical, before imaging; e.g., liver-spleen scanning and brain scanning.

Other examinations require in addition that the patient return to nuclear medicine one or more times after initial imaging, e.g., scintigraphy of the bone, kidney, gastroesophageal reflux, thyroid, myocardium, hepatobiliary system, and brain.

Also parents, siblings, other family, and/or friends who may accompany the patient may wait for 15 min to 2 h while the patient is undergoing an examination. Consequently many people may be waiting at one time outside the examining room.

A waiting room should be spacious, attractively decorated, well lit, and if possible provide some privacy. Seating should be sufficient and comfortable. Toys, reading material, and a blackboard are useful items to have in the waiting area. A television set may also serve to help "the time go faster," although some people find it irritating.

Busy pediatric nuclear medicine departments should have a room for administration of radiopharmaceuticals, so that examining rooms may be used more effectively. This facility will also reduce patients' and parents' waiting time. Such room should be immediately adjacent to the radiopharmacy or radiopharmaceutical dispensing area.

Informing Patients

Patients (whenever possible) and parents should be well informed about the nuclear medicine examination, before the patient is directed to the examination room. The fewer surprises there are, the better it is for all involved. Children need to know what is expected of them, and they need reassurance and positive verbal reinforcement as well. Children have highly developed imaginations that raise their anxiety about the examination.

Parents are very concerned about what is going to happen to their child. The word *nuclear* in nuclear medicine creates much concern, as it is frequently associated with radiation therapy and cancer. Unfortunately this concept is quite misleading since it does not reflect the low radiation exposures of nuclear medicine examinations, and the chemical and physiologic nature of this field. The first contact, whether by phone or in person, is very important and everything about the nuclear medicine examination should be explained clearly and honestly. Radiation exposure should be explained. If the mother of the patient having an examination is pregnant she should be cautioned and instructed on how to avoid or reduce her radiation exposure.

If the patient is an outpatient it is useful to mail information about the nuclear medicine examination to the patient's home in advance. It is important, particularly in the case of outpatients, to let parents know approximately how long the examination will take and if it will be necessary to return later the same day, or the next day so that they can make necessary arrangements. Also, brochures with information about nuclear medicine and its various tests should be available in the waiting room.

Physicians and technologists should make a concerted effort to inform patients personally about the examination that they are going to undergo. For example, they should be informed if there is going to be an injection, if it will cause pain, the injection site, and any other appropriate explanations, which in most cases will tend to reduce anxiety. The procedure should be explained to the child at least twice, first in the waiting area and then in the examination room. Patients should be given a brief orientation of the department, pointing out equipment and toys. Under appropriate circumstances, if another patient is being imaged one may allow the new patient to talk to the patient being examined to show the child that the examination is not that threatening. A child should be allowed to hold a toy during the examination as long as it does not interfere with the test.

Should the Patient's Family Be Allowed in Examining Rooms?

Children from about 8 months to about 3 years of age may suffer from separation anxiety and will generally fare better with the parent(s) in the room. In most instances it is a good idea to allow the patient's parents, a relative, or a friend in the examining room. This tends to have a calming effect on the patient and facilitates examination. In some instances the presence of parents in the examining room has the opposite effect, in which instance they should be asked to leave. Some children can cope better with the examination being alone rather than with their parents.

Sedation and Immobilization

In our experience, children undergoing nuclear medicine examinations require sedation only exceptionally. Patience, time, and understanding work wonders with most children. Only about 1% of our patients have needed sedation. If necessary, its side effects, such as aspiration and respiratory arrest, should be anticipated and appropriate means of treatment be available.

In addition, the most commonly used sedatives frequently produce the opposite effect in young children. Although a few minutes after the administration of the sedative they appear sleepy, attempts to move them and to give them injections will cause them to awaken and react irritably. Also sedation can affect quantitative measurements such as shunt flow, renal function, gastric emptying, etc. In order to avoid sedation it is necessary to have personnel experienced in handling pediatric patients.

In some cases it is necessary to use physical restraints to help maintain the patient in a relatively fixed position. Sand bags and tape, a papoose wrap with blanket, Velcro straps, and contoured pillows can be used depending on the size and activity of the patient. Newborns usually find wrapping of a sheet around their body comforting. Older children may need restraint with tape to help avoid motion.

We find that a television set mounted within easy view is useful in distracting and entertaining most pediatric patients while they are being examined. A video player in order to be able to select appropriate programming for individual patients would be an additional advantage.

Patients must never be left alone in the examining room. One should anticipate that children may fall off the examination table, choke on a small toy, or remove an intravenous line or a nasogastric tube.

Technique of Injection

Many nuclear medicine examinations require the intravenous administration of a radiopharmaceutical. The technique of intravenous injection is very important.

A tray lined with absorbent paper should be prepared for each patient. This tray should have disposable gloves, skin antiseptic, needles, gauze, the dose of radiopharmaceutical in a shielded syringe, adhesive tape, and a tourniquet. The syringe with the radiopharmaceutical should be clearly labelled with the name of the patient, name of the tracer, dose, time, and volume.

The injection technique for static studies, such as hepatic, splenic, renal, myocardial, pulmonary, and skeletal scintigraphy is usually easier than for dynamic studies.

In most cases, the patients are supine for the injection. The site of injection should not overlap the area of interest being examined in case of partial contamination with the tracer. Once an appropriate site is identified, a tourniquet is applied, and the skin is cleaned with an antiseptic. We recommend the use of butterfly type needles of a 25–23 gauge. The tubing is filled with sterile saline. The extremity is held by an aide if necessary, and the vein is entered. Free flow of venous blood should occur. The tourniquet is then released. If there is no free retrograde venous flow into the tube, no attempt should be made to inject the radiopharmaceutical. Another site for the injection should be identified. After successful venous entry the needle is held in place with one or two pieces of adhesive tape. One should check again to make sure that there is still free retrograde flow of blood. It is good practice to flush the tubing with a few milliliters (1–3 ml) of normal saline before injecting the tracer. The radiopharmaceutical should then be injected, and the tubing flushed again with sterile saline. The volume of radiopharmaceutical solution and the speed of injection are not critical for static studies.

In dynamic qualitative studies such as cerebral radionuclide angiography, renal angiography, hepatic angiography, and peripheral angiography, the volume, speed, and site of injection are important. These studies require good temporal resolution so that a rapid and compact bolus of the tracer should be given. The radiopharmaceutical should be in a small volume (0.2–1.0 ml). Premature and newborn infants require smaller volumes (0.2–0.4 ml), while in older children, a volume of 1.0 ml is tolerable. A large proximal vein such as an antecubital vein should be adequate to permit the rapid administration of the radiopharmaceutical and the saline flush. A 25–23 gauge needle of the butterfly type is used. A disposable "T" type connector with a one-way valve permits the rapid injection of the tracer and the saline flush without interruption.

Dynamic quantitative studies such as in left-to-right shunt quantitation and estimation of ventricular ejection fraction require an even more meticulous technique. A rapid ($>$ 2 sec), small, and unique bolus of radiotracer should be administered as closely to the heart as possible. Injections given in antecubital veins frequently (15–25%) result in fragmentation of the bolus and consequently in inadequate studies. We employ and recommend as the first choice the use of one external jugular vein. For this technique two aides are necessary to immobilize the patient's head and neck and to handle the instruments while the physician introduces the needle and injects. Again we use a 25–23 gauge needle of the butterfly type. The patient lies supine on the table. With the patient's head slightly extended and turned to the side, the vein is entered. Free retrograde flow should be present. The needle is secured to the skin with adhesive tape and the tubing flushed with saline. The patient is positioned within the field of view of the camera, and the injection is given. More than ninety-five percent of jugular injections result in a satisfactory bolus.

With the development and implementation of techniques of deconvolution analysis, many studies, which in the past were rejected due to prolonged or fragmented injections, can now be analyzed with a high degree of confidence. These techniques, however, have their limits so that one should still aim for a good intravenous bolus. Further details on injection technique and deconvolution analysis are discussed in Chapter 16.

Instrumentation in Pediatric Nuclear Medicine

A gamma camera with a large field of view is desirable for most purposes in pediatric nuclear medicine. Such a camera is quite versatile, as it permits examination of babies and teenagers. The use of pinhole collimators in conjunction with such a camera permits improved spatial resolution with reasonable sensitivity due to a relatively large solid angle. Magnification as discussed below is essential in the evaluation of premature and newborn infants. Newer cameras have much better spatial resolution and field uniformity than older models and are preferred for pediatric applications.

Disadvantages of cameras with a large field of view are that they are too large to permit comfortable examination of small children, and that they are not mobile.

Small, mobile cameras are necessary for the evaluation of patients in intensive care units, recovery rooms, catheterization laboratories, and operating rooms. These cameras, which can also be used as fixed instruments within the department of nuclear medicine, are easier to position for the examination of premature or newborn infants than are the larger models. These smaller cameras are very useful for cardiovascular studies. They are not as practical for whole-body imaging in children, particularly older children and adolescents, as those with a large field of view.

Each camera must have its own dedicated or integrated digital computer system. Such systems should be able to record, store, display, and analyze all nuclear medicine studies. Computer systems within a nuclear medicine department should be compatible via magnetic media or by direct link. All programs for analysis of routine nuclear medicine studies should be standardized, and easy to use by most physicians and technologists. Analysis should be immediate so that the results can be reported within a clinically useful time. The digital output should be in a format that is easily understood by most physicians. Most of the studies should be available on-line for at least 1 month. Long-term storage of digital studies is still a problem due to technologic limitations. Magnetic tape is currently the least expensive medium; however, replay time is long and cumbersome. Selective storage of digital studies on magnetic diskettes, which may be kept within the nuclear medicine folder or on a separate file library, appears at present to be a viable alternative. Sequential studies on the same patient can be reviewed rapidly and relatively conveniently. Future technology may improve the long-term storage problem.

Magnification

Magnification is a useful, and often indispensable, technique in pediatric nuclear medicine. Magnification may be achieved using two different collimators: the pinhole collimator and the converging multihold collimator. The characteristics of these collimators are quite different.

The pinhole collimator provides the best spatial resolution practicable with conventional gamma camera systems. The pinhole collimator is useful for static imaging in the evaluation of disorders of the hips, kidneys, myocardium, thyroid, spleen, liver, and the posterior fossa. Characteristics of pinhole collimators include the following:

1. The smaller the diameter of the pinhole, the better the spatial resolution. Using a 2-mm pin-

hole on a gamma camera with large field of view achieves good magnification.
2. The closer the object-pinhole distance, the greater the spatial resolution; however, the greater the distortion.
3. Pinhole collimators have a nonuniform flood response with higher count response at the center and lower at the edges of the field of view. Also, these collimators exhibit spherical distortion.
4. Pinhole collimators have lower count sensitivity than multihole collimators so that imaging time is relatively long.

Converging collimators are useful for dynamic studies because they provide magnification without loss of count sensitivity. They do not achieve as good resolution as the pinhole collimators. Converging collimators are useful for dynamic studies in small children, in whom sensitivity is more critical than is spatial resolution. Characteristics of converging collimators are as follows:

1. The more pronounced the angle of convergence of the holes, the greater the magnification; however, the greater the distortion.
2. The closer the distance from the collimator to the object the less magnification.
3. Count sensitivity is comparable or higher than parallel multihole collimators. Therefore, imaging time is similar, or depending on the design, frequently shorter than with parallel-hole collimators.

This book reflects in great part the pediatric applications of nuclear medicine at the Children's Hospital in Boston during the past 12 years. Therefore it is not intended to present an exhaustive review of the world literature on the subject. It is directed to the professionals who are engaged in the care of children, and we hope that physicians, fellows, residents, interns, students, and technologists may find here useful information.

This work is divided according to organs and systems. Each chapter contains an introduction in which principles, indications, and general considerations are discussed. Next, a section on methods is presented including radiopharmaceuticals, administered doses, absorbed doses, examination technique, and analysis. Finally, clinical applications of pediatric nuclear medicine are discussed and many examples of pediatric disorders are illustrated.

Pediatric nuclear medicine has a bright future indeed, and within the next few years, many further advances in this field should be anticipated.

Chapter 1 Bone

S. T. Treves
John A. Kirkpatrick

Radiopharmaceuticals, Dosimetry, and Imaging Method

Technetium-99m Phosphate Compounds

Mechanism of Uptake: General Considerations

Since the introduction of phosphates labelled with technetium-99m (Tc-99m) by Subramanian and coworkers in 1971, skeletal scintigraphy has become one of the most common examinations in Pediatric Nuclear Medicine.[144] These bone-seeking radiopharmaceuticals offer high photon flux for imaging with an acceptable radiation dose to the patient.

Skeletal scintigraphy provides a functional image of the skeleton with concentrations of Tc-99m phosphate in those regions of bone which relate to blood flow and growth. This normally irregular distribution of radionuclide in the sekeleton is even more pronounced in children, whose growth centers are active. Accordingly, the absorbed radiation dose to the skeleton is not uniform: it varies with the irregular distribution of radiopharmaceutical

The technetium-99m compounds with affinity for the bone include polyphosphate, pyrophosphate, ethane-1-hydroxy-1,1-diphosphonate (EHDP), and methylene diphosphonate (MDP). Practitioners in Pediatric Nuclear Medicine seem to favor Tc-99m MDP because it exhibits a more rapid blood disappearance and greater bony accretion rate than the other technetium-labelled bone-seeking radiopharmaceuticals.

In tissue radioassay experiments in rodents, Subramanian et al.[144] found that skeletal concentrations of MDP and EHDP were higher than those of pyrophosphate. These authors also showed that the total body retention of MDP was higher than that of polyphosphate. In humans, the blood clearance of Tc-99m MDP was faster than that of Tc-99m EHDP, pyrophosphate, and polyphosphate, in that order. These authors found that blood levels of Tc-99m MDP fell to 4–10% of the injected dose by 2 h and to 3–5% by 3 h. Less than 2% of the dose was present in the blood at 24 h after injection. About 30% of the MDP plasma activity was protein-bound in the first hour, increasing to 45% at 3 h and 100% at 24 h.[144]

The urinary excretion of diphosphonate at 24 h after injection was more complete than that of pyrophosphate or polyphosphate. About 40% of injected activity appeared in the urine within the first hour after injection of Tc-99m MDP. This increased to 60% and 70% at 4 and 24 h, respectively.[144]

Administered Dose and Absorbed Radiation Dose Estimates

An intravenous injection of Tc-99m MDP is given 2–4 h prior to imaging. A usual dose is 200 μCi/kg of body weight with a minimal total dose of 500 μCi. The radiation absorbed doses for Tc-99m MDP in various age groups are listed on Table 1-1.

Imaging Technique

Good patient hydration and frequent voiding before imaging help to reduce the gonadal radiation dose and also allow a better evaluation of the pelvic bones.

The so-called three-phased skeletal scintigraphy

Table 1-1. Estimated Absorbed Doses (rad) from Intravenous Injection of Tc-99m MDP

Age (years)	Newborn	1	5	10	15
Body weight (kg)	3.5	9.4	19.1	32.1	54.5
Administered dose (mCi)	0.7	1.9	3.8	6.42	10.9
Bladder wall	1.5	1.4	1.5	1.7	2.0
Bone surfaces	—	2.5	2.1	2.1	2.2
Kidneys	0.09	0.13	0.14	0.16	0.19
Red marrow	—	0.32	0.33	0.33	0.36
Ovaries	0.05	0.10	0.12	0.13	0.15
Testes	0.04	0.09	0.10	0.11	0.12
Total body	0.05	0.07	0.08	0.10	0.10

includes a radionuclide angiogram of the area of interest at one frame/sec for 60 sec, an early image (improperly called blood-pool image), and delayed images obtained 2–4 h after injection. In most patients, the entire skeleton should be scanned with a large field-of-view gamma camera fitted with a high-resolution collimator. The patient should void before imaging. Positioning during scanning may be supine or prone. An initial image of 500,000 counts is taken of the anterior chest. The rest of the skeleton (anterior and posterior) is imaged for the same length of time so that the relative intensities of radiopharmaceutical concentration in the various regions of the skeleton can be compared. Additional views of regions of interest (ROIs) or suspicious areas of the bone are obtained as needed, making images of high count density with a high-resolution collimator and/or a pinhole collimator.

For scanning the hips, the following protocol is suggested: anterior and frog leg projections using the high-resolution and pinhole collimators (300,000 and 150,000 counts, respectively). The smallest available (1.5–3 mm) insert for the pinhole should be used in order to attain high spatial resolution.

Gallium-67 Citrate

Mechanism of Uptake: General Considerations

In some disorders involving the skeleton, Tc-99m MDP scans appear to be less sensitive and specific than originally believed. One of the problems in detecting early inflammation in bone with Tc-99m phosphates is that increased intramedullary pressure may result in tamponade of the intraosseous vessels and prevent an increase in bone blood flow. Uptake of gallium (Ga-67) citrate is less dependent on blood flow and seems capable of accumulating in inflammatory lesions in spite of the vascular tamponade. The high sensitivity of the Ga-67 should not result in an abandonment of the Tc-99m phosphate bone scan for this purpose. Because the phosphate bone scan can be done relatively quickly, gives a low radiation dose to the patient, and has an 80–90% sensitivity, it is the preferred initial study. An abnormal bone scan in the proper clinical setting establishes the diagnosis, but a normal study does not exclude osteomyelitis.

When an infection is suspected and the technetium phosphate scan is normal, a Ga-67 citrate scan may be indicated. When osteomyelitis is suspected as a result of spread from an adjacent area of cellulitis, the gallium scan may be difficult to interpret due to inability to distinguish activity in the bone from that in the soft tissues. The Ga-67 scan is rarely abnormal when chronic noninflammatory disease is present; thus a normal phosphate scan and an abnormal gallium study strongly suggest an active inflammatory process. Areas of chronic osteomyelitis may take up Ga-67.[62]

Administered Dose and Absorbed Dose Estimates

The usual dose of Ga-67 citrate is 0.25–3.0 mCi. Suggested administered activity and absorbed ra-

Table 1-2. Estimated Absorbed Dose from Intravenous Injection of Ga-67 Citrate (rad)

Age (years)	Newborn	1	5	10	15
Body weight (kg)	3.5	9.4	19.1	32.1	54.5
Administered dose (mCi)	0.25	0.38	0.76	1.3	2.2
Small intestine	0.6	0.72	0.76	0.87	0.92
Wall of upper intestine	1.5	1.2	1.	1.3	1.4
Wall of lower large intestine	3.0	2.1	2.2	2.2	2.2
Kidneys	1.1	0.91	1.1	1.2	1.3
Liver	1.3	1.1	1.2	1.4	1.6
Red marrow	—	2.2	2.2	2.2	2.4
Bone surface	—	18.0	15.0	16.0	16.0
Spleen	2.1	1.4	1.6	1.7	1.9
Ovaries	0.63	0.61	0.66	0.75	0.9
Testes	0.5	0.42	0.43	0.47	0.51
Total body	0.7	0.53	0.59	0.64	0.68

diation dose estimates from this radioisotope are shown in Table 1-2.

Imaging Technique

When searching for an acute infection imaging is sometimes done at 4–6 h after injection. A better lesion-to-background ratio is obtained after 24 h.[62] Bowel preparation is needed for imaging at 24 h, but some patients may be too ill for this. Imaging at 72 h is recommended when bowel preparation cannot or should not be done. A whole body scan (posterior and anterior) should be obtained.

Technetium-99m Sulfur Colloid

Mechanism of Uptake: General Considerations

Tc-99m sulfur colloid, which is used widely for imaging the reticuloendothelial system of the liver and spleen, also concentrates 5–10% of the intravenously injected dose in the bone marrow. This low concentration can be used for imaging most of the bone marrow with the exception of the marrow of the thoracic and lumbar spine, which is obscured by overwhelming hepatic and splenic activity.

The normal pattern of radiocolloid distribution in various age groups has been established by Oseas et al.[119] There is progressive loss of uptake with increasing age from < 2 years to > 10 years of age. The distribution of Tc-99m sulfur colloid in normal children older than 10 years of age appears similar to that in adults.[119,135] Normal children under the age of 10 years show more extensive uptake of the colloid toward the extremities.

After radiation therapy, the bone marrow activity extends to peripheral sites with diminution of colloidal uptake in the areas receiving radiation therapy. Tumor involvement in the marrow is accompanied by decreased or absent colloidal uptake, but decreased bone marrow uptake in patients bearing tumors may also be due to fibrosis.

Current radiopharmaceuticals for bone marrow imaging have shortcomings. The uptake of Tc-99m sulfur colloid in the bone marrow is poor. Indium-111 (In-111) chloride clears slowly from the bloodstream and delivers a relatively high radiation dose to the marrow.

Use of particles of smaller size has been proposed in order to increase the bone marrow uptake. Martindale et al.[95] report on a Tc-99m antimony colloid with particles smaller than 50 nm (1–13 nm). Their experiments on rabbits and rats indicate that this agent concentrates in the bone marrow in a greater amount than Tc-99m sulfur colloid.

McAffee et al.[101] compared the biodistributions of five Tc-99m colloids, iron-59 (Fe-59), and In-111 in dogs by direct radioassay. These authors found that one formulation of Tc-99m minimicroaggregated albumin with a particle size of 30–100 nm produced the highest marrow concentration, approximately six times that of Tc-99m sulfur colloid, with similar blood and liver concentrations and a lower splenic uptake. This was lower than the

24-h concentration of In-111, however, and much lower than the Fe-59 concentration at 24 h.

Several factors affect the rate of blood disappearance and distribution of colloids: particle size, number of particles, presence of stabilizers, surface-active agents, competing colloids, opsonins,[129] charge of the particles, chemical nature of colloid surface, and electrophoretic mobility.[3,29,100] Smaller particles are cleared from the blood at a slower rate than the larger ones.[30] Greenberg et al.[50] reported that the fractional distribution of sulfur colloid in the skeleton was almost identical to the distribution of Fe-59 as ferrous citrate.

In our laboratory, Heyman et al.[59] estimated the marrow uptake of different Tc-99m colloids using camera-and-computer techniques on the baboon. Compared with Tc-99m sulfur colloid, marrow uptake with minimicroaggregated albumin was increased by a factor of 3. With Tc-99m antimony sulfate of microaggregated albumin, there was a factor of 2 increase over the colloid concentration in bone marrow.

Administered Dose and Absorbed Dose Estimates

Tc-99m sulfur colloid is given in a dose of 100 μCi/kg of body weight. A minimum total dose of 500 μCi is suggested for newborns. Absorbed radiation doses for this agent are shown in Table 9-1 in Chapter 9.

Imaging Technique

Imaging is begun 15–30 min after injection of the radiotracer. A high-resolution collimator is used, and 300,000 counts are taken over the pelvic area while shielding the liver and spleen from the field-of-view. The rest of the body is imaged using the same exposure time used for the first image.

Indium-111 (Chloride)

Mechanism of Uptake: General Considerations

Intravenously administered In-111 chloride binds to transferrin[64] and has been mentioned as a hematologic imaging agent.[88,142] There are still controversial reports, however, as to whether In-111 chloride should be used for the evaluation of hematologic diseases.[108,142]

A number of important differences between the in vivo and in vitro behaviors of indium and iron cast doubt on the comparability of red cell information and In-111 activity accumulation. The most striking of these differences are:

1. In-111- and Fe-59-labelled transferrin show different labelling yields to reticulocytes.[6]
2. The reduction of radionuclide uptake in irradiated marrow is significantly larger for iron than for indium.[103]
3. Several patients with pure red cell aplasia have reportedly shown normal In-111 chloride bone marrow images.[108]

The clinical applications of In-111 chloride scintigraphy have been studied in a few human hematologic disorders, such as pure red cell aplasia, myelofibrosis, aplastic anemia, and malignant lymphoma.[12,106,115,122,125] Further, animal experiments support the idea that both Fe-59 and In-111 transferrin are bound to erythroid precursors, in which case In-111 chloride could be an effective in vivo marker for early erythropoietic stages.[75]

In addition, some attention has been paid to the fact that In-111 chloride may be stored in bone marrow by reticuloendothelial uptake alone or in combination with the erythropoietic accumulation.[107] At present, no distinction can be made between these two processes. We should realize, however, that the bone marrow of patients suffering from aplastic anemia contains considerable amounts of macrophages and that phagocytosis alone would lead to high bone marrow uptake in every patient. In view of the varying results obtained in different clinical conditions of aplastic anemia, however, perhaps these macrophages do not play a major role in In-111 concentration in bone marrow.[122]

Like Horn et al.,[63] we incubate the indium with the patient's plasma rather than directly injecting the radionuclide intravenously. They report more satisfactory scans with this approach. We have not had the opportunity to evaluate this effect in our patients as our technique has been uniformly the same.

Administered Dose and Dosimetry

In-111 chloride is given in a dose of approximately 15 μCi/kg of body weight (Table 1-3).

Table 1-3. Estimated Absorbed Radiation Dose from Intravenous Injection of Indium-111 Chloride (rad)

Age (years)	Newborn	1	5	10	15
Body weight (Kg)	3.5	9.4	19.1	32.1	54.5
Administered dose (mCi)	0.52	0.141	0.286	0.481	0.817
Liver	2.6	2.80	3.23	3.84	4.49
Red marrow	2.6	2.76	2.80	2.79	3.10
Ovaries	0.32	0.34	0.43	0.48	0.59
Testes	0.15	0.17	0.20	0.22	0.24
Total body	0.39	0.42	0.49	0.53	0.59

Imaging Technique

Imaging is performed at 24 or 48 h after injection of the tracer. Images of the whole body are obtained with a medium-energy parallel-hole or diverging collimator. An anterior or posterior view of the chest is taken for 100,000 counts while shielding the liver. The rest of the body is imaged for the same exposure time used for the first image. Anterior and posterior whole-body images are obtained.

Skeletal Scintigraphy: Clinical Applications

In children, the distribution patterns of bone-seeking radiotracers are quite different than in adults. Their skeletons undergo constant and rapid osteoblastic and osteoclastic activity. The skeletal scintiscan in a normal child shows heterogeneous radiotracer distribution with higher concentration around growth centers. Because blood flow is the major determinant of radiopharmaceutical access to the target tissue, hyper- and hypovascular lesions are those most clearly perceived on scintigrams of bone.

Abnormal findings on the bone scintiscan are rarely specific by themselves and must be evaluated in light of historic, clinical, laboratory, and radiographic data. If radiographs are not available, it is important to obtain them, particularly if abnormalities are found on the scan. Once a bone lesion is at a stage at which it can be defined radiologically, the use of skeletal scintigraphy is limited to evaluation of the activity and extent of the lesion and to identification of distant lesions.

The major value of bone scanning is in early diagnosis of bone disease rather than definition of precise etiology (Table 1-4). The scan may show increased concentration of radionuclide in primary or secondary tumors of bone, inflammatory disorders, fractures, metabolic diseases, or arthritides. Decreased radiopharmaceutical uptake may be seen in bone cysts, avascular necrosis, infarcts, radiotherapy fields, osteonecrosis, and histiocytosis.

Osteomyelitis

Osteomyelitis, particularly when hematogenous in origin, is a rather common problem in pediatric medicine. Early diagnosis and treatment frequently lead to complete recovery, but early diagnosis is difficult to achieve because the clinical signs and symptoms as well as conventional laboratory

Table 1-4. Indications for Skeletal Scintigraphy in Children

Early diagnosis of osteomyelitis
Evaluation of unexplained bone pain
Diagnosis of avascular necrosis and revasularization
Diagnosis of stress reaction and fracture
Diagnosis, localization and evaluation of the extent of primary and metastatic bone tumors (osteosarcoma, Ewing's sarcoma, rhabdomyosarcoma, neuroblastoma, parosteal osteosarcoma, leukemia, lymphoma, and others)
Diagnosis and localization of osteoid osteoma

and radiologic findings are often nonspecific, subtle, or simply absent.

Taking into consideration the difficulty in establishing time zero for onset of the disease, the available information indicates that skeletal scintigraphy speeds diagnosis of osteomyelitis by 1–2 days to almost a week. When used as part of the initial evaluation for suspected osteomyelitis, scintigraphy can establish an early diagnosis in many cases and can thus lead to therapy before much bone destruction occurs (Figs. 1-1–1-13). The experience with bone scintigraphy thus far supports a recommendation that it be used in the initial evaluation of children with signs and symptoms of osteomyelitis.

Radiographs remain an integral part of the diagnostic process in osteomyelitis together with clinical assessment, laboratory studies, and scintigraphy. Trying to interpret a bone scintiscan without the benefit of a radiograph is not advisable. What scintigraphically appears to be osteomyelitis may be revealed on a radiograph to be a fracture or a traumatized bone cyst. The anatomic information provided by the radiograph complements the functional information on the scan and vice versa.

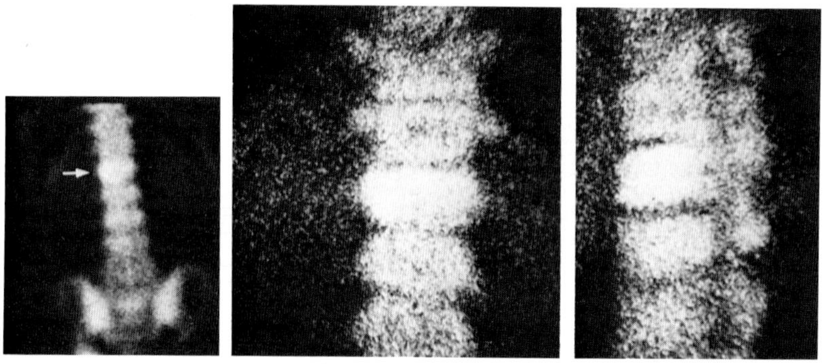

Figure 1-1. Acute osteomyelitis of the spine. This 9-year-old boy with left flank pain had jumped off a swing 3 weeks previously and had fallen on his left side. He developed pain in the lumbosacral area. Radiographs of the lumbosacral spine were normal. The white blood cell count was 13,200/mm^3 and the erythrocyte sedimentation rate was 30 mm/h with a temperature of 101°F. He subsequently had spike temperatures up to 103°F for several nights. Tc-99m-MDP bone scan is abnormal with increased uptake in the body of the first lumbar vertebra on the left. These findings are compatible with infection or trauma. Tomograms of the same vertebra were normal. *Left and center:* posterior view; *right:* left posterior oblique view.

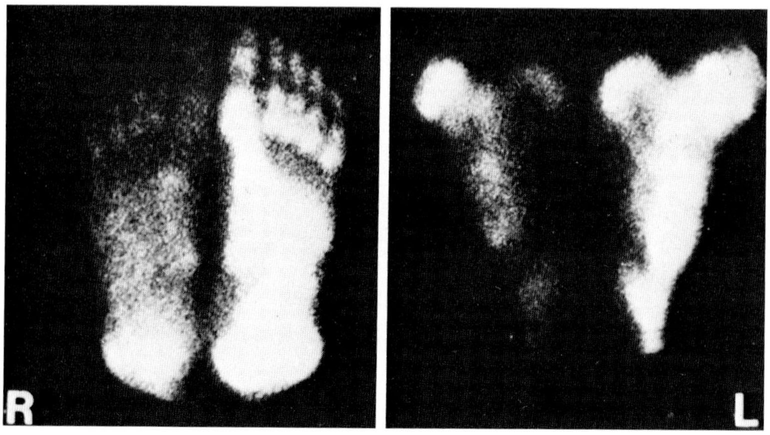

Figure 1-2. Acute osteomyelitis of the left foot. This 11-year-old boy had insidious onset of pain in the left foot for 5 days and 2 days of temperature of 102°F. He was unable to walk comfortably due to the pain. His erythrocyte sedimentation rate was 20 mm/h and his white blood cell count was 7200/mm^3. Radiographs were normal. His scintiscan shows increased uptake of Tc-99m MDP through the left foot, particularly in the proximal metaphysis of the left great toe. Blood cultures were positive for *S. aureus*. Incision and drainage of the proximal metaphysis of the first metatarsal revealed osteomyelitis of the left foot. R, Right side; L, left side.

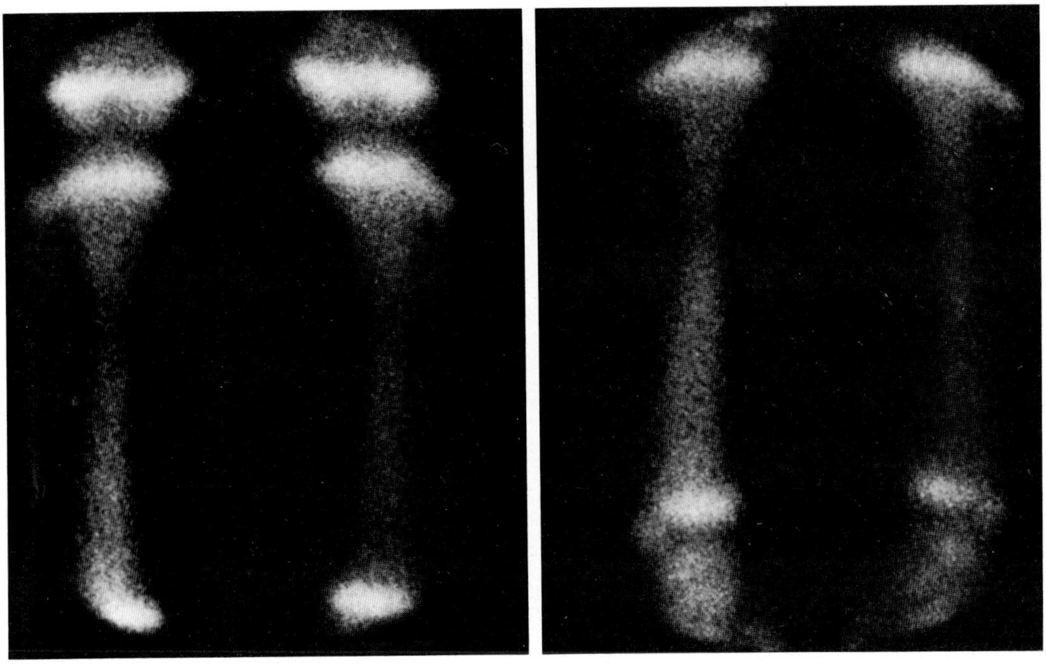

Figure 1-3. Acute osteomyelitis of the right tibia. After minor trauma, this 3-year-old boy presented with right leg pain, an inability to walk for 3 days, and a temperature of 103°F. He had tenderness over the distal right tibia and fibula, with increased local temperature. The white blood cell count was $13{,}200/mm^3$ and the erythrocyte sedimentation rate was 26 mm/h. Radiographs of the right leg were normal. The bone scan on admission *(left)* shows increased uptake of Tc-99m MDP in the right lower tibia. After treatment with antibiotics, the fever recurred. The white blood cell count rose to $16{,}000/mm^3$ and the erythrocyte sedimentation rate was 50 mm/h. A repeat bone scan *(right)* again shows increased uptake of Tc-99m MDP in the right distal tibia. Repeated radiographs showed no signs of osteomyelitis. The patient improved on antibiotics and was discharged.

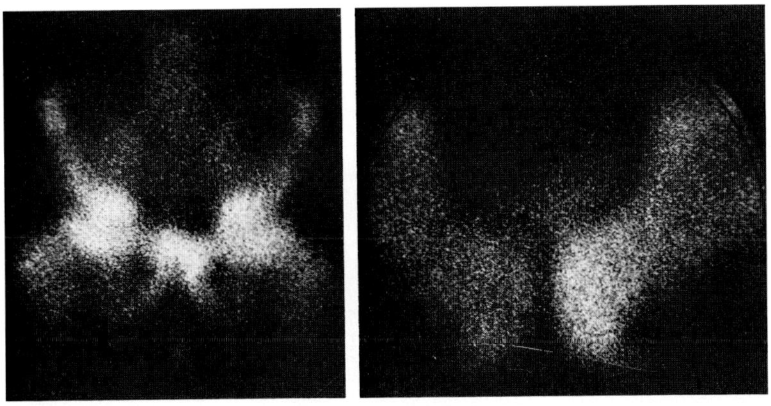

Figure 1-4. Acute osteomyelitis of the left pubis. A 13-year-old boy entered the hospital with fever and thigh pain for 4 days. He was unable to walk to admission. By the third hospital day the pain had localized to the symphysis pubis. Blood cultures were negative, and radiographs of the pelvis showed normal bones and soft tissues. Retrospectively after the scan was seen, a slight irregularity at the left margin of the symphysis could be observed on the radiograph. There was persistent pain in this region, and the bone scan shows increased uptake of Tc-99m MDP in the left pubis. The findings at biopsy revealed focal areas of osteostreptococcus. The patient was treated intravenously with oxacillin and subsequently penicillin. The fever abated quickly, and the patient had no further complaints of pain. R, right side. *Left:* parallel hole collimator; *right:* pinhole collimator. (Reproduced with permission from Treves et al. Pediatrics 1976; 57:173–86.)

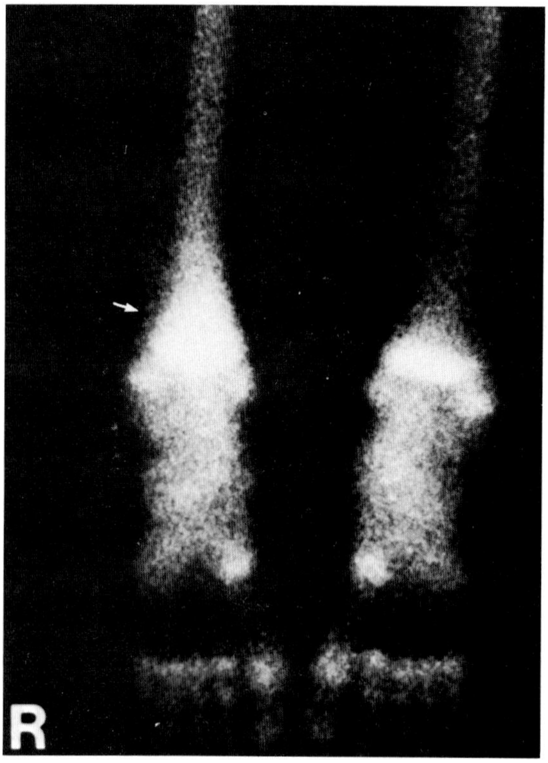

Figure 1-5. Acute osteomyelitis of the right distal tibia. A 10-year-old boy was seen after acute onset of right ankle pain, fever, chills, fatigue, stiff neck, sore throat, cough, running nose, vomiting, diarrhea, and headache. At physical examination, he had exquisite tenderness and warmth over the distal right leg. Radiographs of the area were normal. The bone scan shows intense uptake of Tc-99m MDP in the right lower tibia. Biopsy drainage of the site yielded *S. aureus*. R, Right side.

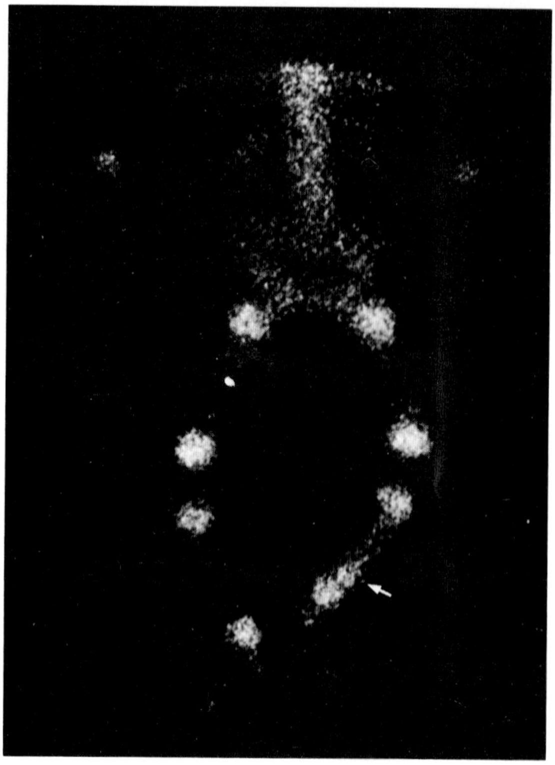

Figure 1-6. Osteomyelitis in a premature infant. This 1300 g baby girl had hyaline membrane disease, physiologic jaundice, and patent ductus arteriosus. The baby was noted to have a swollen left ankle and was treated with oxacillin. Blood cultures and cultures of the local site were negative, but the Tc-99m bone scan is abnormal over the left distal fibula. The patient improved on treatment.

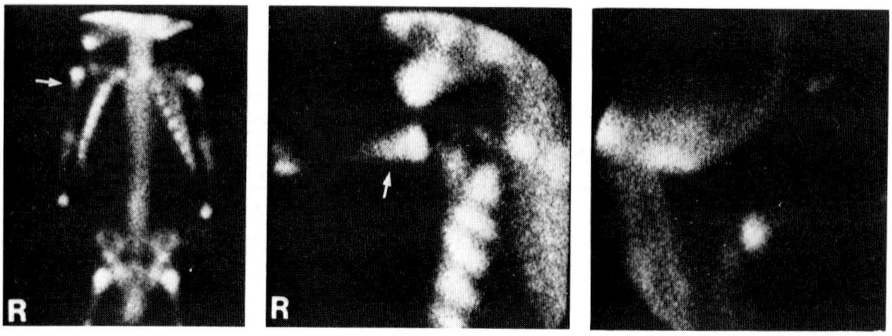

Figure 1-7. Osteomyelitis of the right humerus. This 20-day-old female had fever (101°F) and decreased movement of her right arm. The white blood cell count was 16,400/mm^3. Radiographs *(left)* of the right shoulder, elbow, and chest were within normal limits. The Tc-99m bone scan is normal. Blood and cerebrospinal fluid cultures grew group B streptococcus. The repeat bone scan 4 days later *(center and right)* reveals increased uptake in the right proximal humerus suggestive of osteomyelitis. R, Right side.

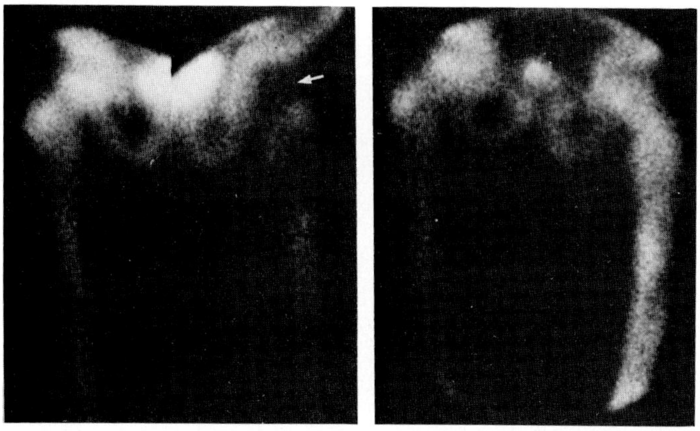

Figure 1-8. Osteomyelitis with decreased Tc-99m MDP uptake. This 7-year-old boy had left leg pain for several months and a temperature of 103°F. The radiographs were normal. The initial bone scan *(left)* shows no uptake of Tc-99m MDP in the left femoral head, neck, and midshaft. Subsequent incision and drainage of the left femur yielded pus. Although treated with antibiotics, the patient did not improve. At a second operation, multiple windows were drilled along the left femoral diaphysis and abundant pus was again obtained. A bone scan *(right)* following surgery shows increased uptake throughout the femur. The patient improved and was discharged.

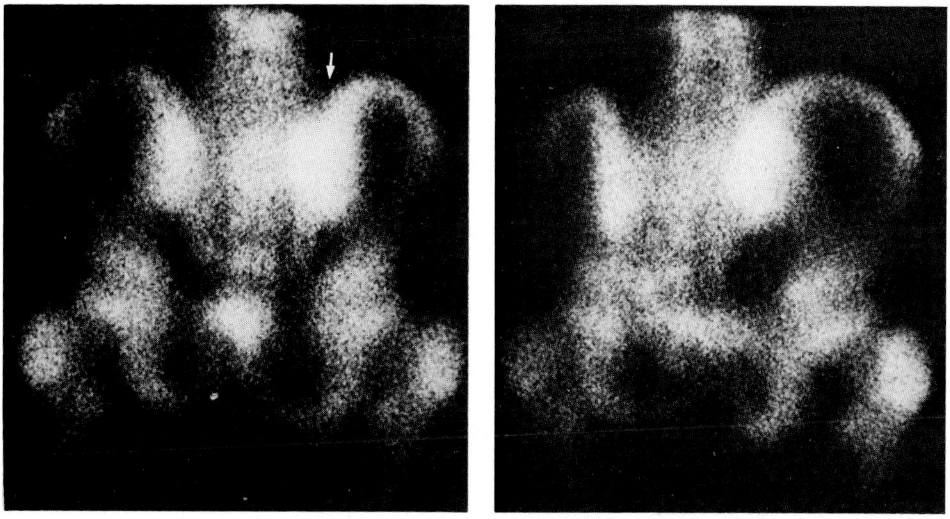

Figure 1-9. Sacroiliac osteomyelitis. This 15-year-old male was admitted for severe pain in the right buttock with radiation to the thigh and knee. Approximately 1 month prior to admission, the patient had first developed the pain but it improved in several days with conservative treatment. The pain returned 5 days prior to admission. At admission, the pain and fever (101.4°F) had increased and the patient was unable to walk without crutches. The pain would decrease at rest. There was no local tenderness over the right sacroiliac joint, hip, or thigh. When the iliac crests were squeezed together, there was a marked increase in pain. The laboratory results were: erythrocyte sedimentation rate, 54 mm/h; white blood cell count 8100/mm^3; antinuclear antibody, negative; latex, negative. Radiographs of the lumbosacral spine, pelvis, and knee were all normal. The bone scan on admission shows increased Tc-99m MDP activity in the right iliac bone at the sacroiliac joint. The remainder of skeletal structure had uniform and symmetric distribution of the radionuclide. Needle aspiration of the sacroiliac joint space was negative for organisms by culture and gram stain. The patient improved on treatment for osteomyelitis with intravenous antibiotics. *Left:* posterior view; *right:* right posterior oblique view.

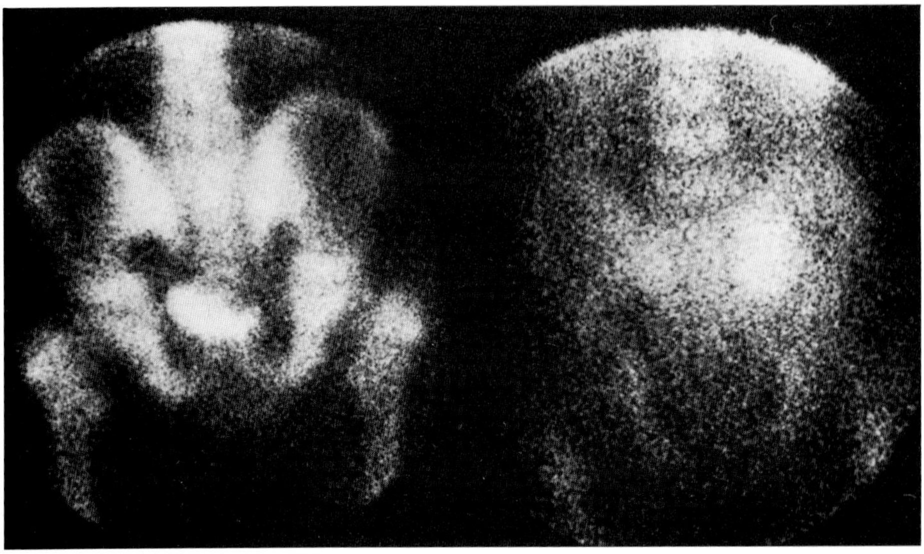

Figure 1-10. Infection of the sacroiliac joint. A 14-year-old male had acute onset of pain in his right buttock and thigh with fever (103°F) for 24 h. The Tc-99m MDP scan *(left)* is normal, but the Ga-67 scan *(right)* shows an area of intense uptake in the right iliac bone posteriorly. White blood cell count was 19,700/mm^3, and the erythrocyte sedimentation rate was 50 mm/h. The patient improved on antibiotics.

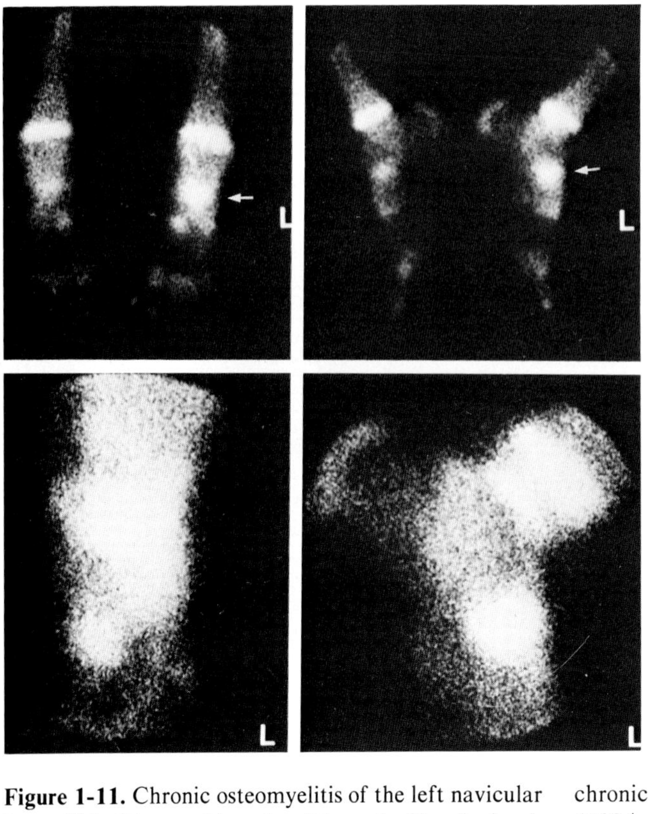

Figure 1-11. Chronic osteomyelitis of the left navicular bone. This 17-year-old male with cystic fibrosis developed an insidious pain in the dorsum of the left foot a month and a half before admission. Three days before admission, there was dorsal swelling of the foot. The radiographs demonstrated a navicular lesion suggestive of chronic osteomyelitis. The white blood cell count was 4100/mm^3 and erythrocyte sedimentation rate was 27 mm/h. The bone scan shows obvious increased uptake of Tc-99m MDP in the left navicular bone, consistent with osteomyelitis. Surgical exploration of the left navicular bone confirmed the osteomyelitis. L, Left side.

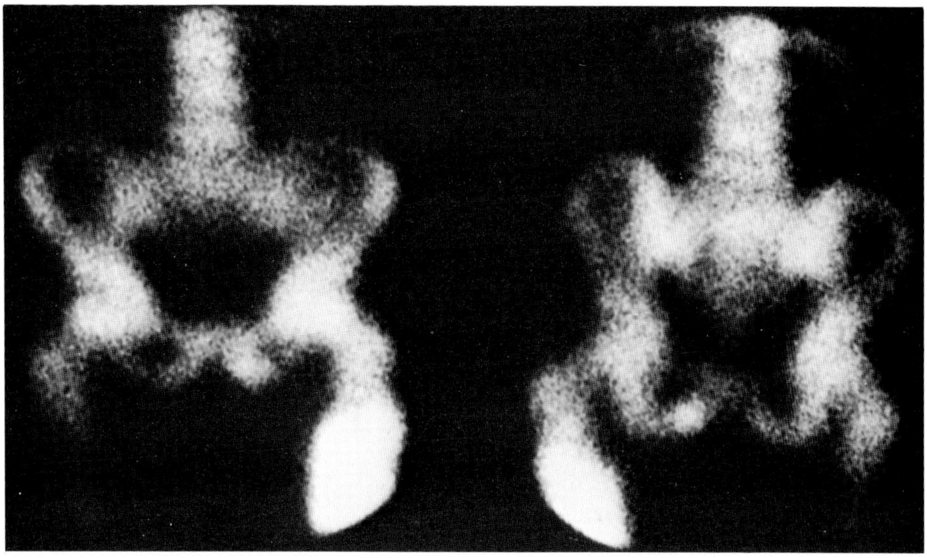

Figure 1-12. Chronic osteomyelitis. This 13-year-old boy developed a painful destructive lesion of the proximal left femur that was initially thought to be Ewing's sarcoma. The bone scan shows increased uptake of Tc-99m MDP in the left upper femur and the left pubic ramus. *Left:* anterior view; *right:* posterior view.

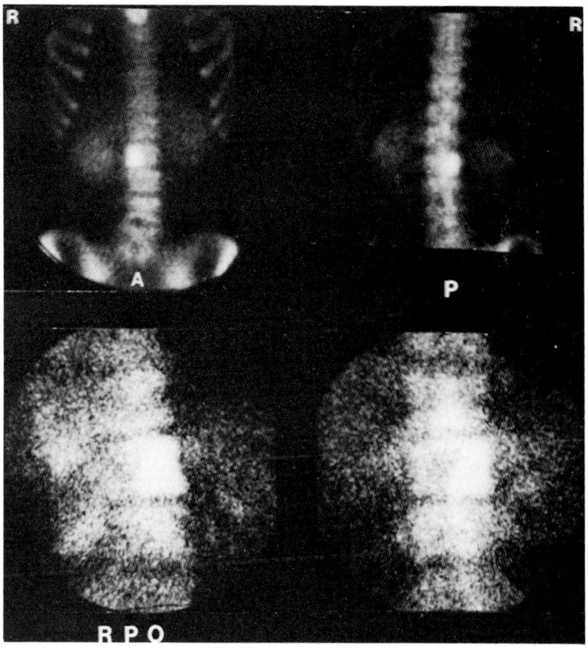

Figure 1-13. Chronic osteomyelitis of the spine. This 19-year-old female had a 9-month history of low back pain. She was active in sports and had spondylosis bilaterally at the fourth and fifth lumbar vertebrae on recent radiographs. The bone scan shows an intense increase in uptake of Tc-99m MDP at the level of the second lumbar vertebra. The abnormality involves the vertebral body and is located anteriorly and to the right. Review of radiographs as well as tomography of the lumbar spine confirmed the presence of a sclerotic lesion at the second lumbar vertebra. The patient was afebrile with a normal white blood cell count. Her erythrocyte sedimentation rate was 43 mm/h. One week after the scan was performed, biopsy of the second lumbar vertebra revealed findings consistent with chronic osteitis and low-grade osteomyelitis. Stains and cultures were negative. The patient was treated with antibiotics. No causative organism was found. R, Right side; A, anterior view; P, posterior view; RPO, right posterior oblique view.

Pathology

Acute hematogenous osteomyelitis most often involves rapidly growing bone and characteristically localizes in the metaphysis of long bones (especially the femur or tibia). Trauma has been invoked to explain this predilection for long bones. The absence of functional phagocytic cells in regional capillaries and sluggish regional blood flow have been cited as factors favoring localization in the metaphysis. In infants less than a year old, blood vessels that temporarily link metaphyseal and epiphyseal regions allow any primary infection of either the metaphysis or joint to spread across the growth plate and involve both sites. The most common organism responsible for hematogenous osteomyelitis is *Staphylococcus aureus*.

Clinical Features

Patients with acute osteomyelitis present with localized bone pain, swelling, tenderness, and fever. In children, however, atypical presentations occur frequently, particularly with respect to reported symptoms. Sometimes the initial findings may be only one or more of the following: fever of unknown origin, swelling, limping, guarding, or limitation of motion. Laboratory findings typically include an elevated white blood cell count and an increased sedimentation rate, but absence of these findings does not rule out osteomyelitis. Blood cultures may or may not grow bacteria and repeat culturing may be necessary.

Radiologic Appearance

The earliest changes on radiographs of patients with osteomyelitis involve the surrounding soft tissue and not the bone itself. The radiologic changes developing by about 3 days after the onset of symptoms have been described as: deep swelling adjacent to the metaphysis with displacement of fat lines; increased swelling with obliteration of lucent planes between muscles; and subcutaneous edema. In general, these changes are easier to identify in the extremeties than in the trunk or pelvis.

In the untreated patient by 7–10 days after the onset of symptoms, periosteal new bone and bone lysis become apparent radiologically.

Biopsy

Many physicians stress that the diagnosis of osteomyelitis is facilitated when material from the lesion is recovered by biopsy and cultured. Drainage of the pus relieves pain from pressure and offers precise identification of the etiologic agent, an aid in establishing appropriate antibiotic therapy. Others argue that when the signs and symptoms of early osteomyelitis are present and blood cultures are positive, prompt and aggressive antibiotic therapy without waiting for biopsy results is warranted.

The diagnostic and therapeutic approach should be individualized and depends in great measure on how advanced the process is at the time of presentation. If early intervention is the overriding necessity, positive scans in patients with compatible clinical, laboratory, and radiologic findings might dictate institution of antibiotic therapy in the absence of biopsy. This might be especially important when osteomyelitis of the spine is suspected because the spine is a site many surgeons are reluctant to biopsy. Others who believe that specific tissue findings are indispensable might use positive scans to select biopsy sites.

Scintigraphic Diagnosis

In osteomyelitis, the bone scintigram typically shows increased radiopharmaceutical uptake in the region of bone involved 24–48 h from the onset of symptoms. Inflammation, increased regional blood flow, and increased metabolic activity are the most likely explanations for the increased uptake. The specificity of these abnormal scintiscans for osteomyelitis may be increased with radionuclide angiography,[11] "blood pool,"[11] and 2–3 h delayed studies. The three-phase study is helpful in some instances to help localize better an area of involvement in a bone, and/or to depict soft tissue inflammation. In one series, three-phase scintigraphy of bone revealed that in 98 patients, the false-positive rate for osteomyelitis was decreased from 25% to 6% without altering the 92% sensitivity.[99]

Scintigraphy is also helpful when osteomyelitis arises in more than one site. Although this is rare, we have observed a small number of patients with multiple foci of osteomyelitis.

The confidence justified by a positive scintiscan in the presence of symptoms of osteomyelitis cannot be justified for a normal scan. Some patients have shown normal scintiscans or even decreased uptake in areas of subsequently proven osteomyelitis (Fig. 1-8).[2,9,77,117,146] This feature may reflect a combination of bacterial proliferation and host immune response that initially occludes local blood vessels. This explanation is reinforced by a report that high-pressure abscess will cause a cold spot or absence of radiotracer uptake on the scan.[31]

Whatever the cause, the occasional normal scintiscans in patients with osteomyelitis means that a normal bone scintiscan is no guarantee that a patient does not have osteomyelitis. When symptoms persist that the scan is normal, a repeat scan should be performed 2–3 days later (Fig. 1-14), or a gallium citrate scan may be indicated.

Ga-67 citrate is a nonspecific radiopharmaceutical that may concentrate in areas of inflammation even in the presence of a normal Tc-99m MDP scan[124] (Fig. 1-10). Gallium imaging may also provide earlier detection of osteomyelitis than is possible with Tc-99m-labelled phosphates in areas adjacent to growth plates. In some cases, Ga-67 provides better localization of the site involved with osteomyelitis than Tc-99m MDP.

Differential Diagnosis

In cellulitis overlying bone, depending on its severity, there may be reactive hyperemia of the bone resulting in a diffuse increase in the radiopharmaceutical uptake (Fig. 1-15) and suggesting concomitant osteomyelitis. If cellulitis does not produce reactive bony hyperemia, the bone scintiscan will be normal. Chronic cellulitis may show diffuse soft tissue uptake associated with faint, generalized increased uptake by adjacent bone.

In isolated septic arthritis the scan remains normal because bone-seeking radiopharmaceuticals do not enter joints to any appreciable extent. When cellulitis and hyperemia accompany the arthritis, the radiotracer concentration may be slightly or moderately increased in the bones surrounding the inflammed joint.

Followup Scintigraphy

Skeletal scintigraphy with Tc-99m MDP is not a good indicator of healing in osteomyelitis because bone repair may take place even after the infection has subsided. In this regard Ga-67 as the citrate appears to be a better indicator of cure in osteomyelitis.

Case Material

In 1976, we reported our early experience with skeletal scintigraphy in nine children (aged 2–13 years) with signs and symptoms of osteomyelitis.[154] Increased focal uptake on the scintiscans confirmed the presence of osteomyelitis in eight of these patients (including one with a subperiosteal abscess)

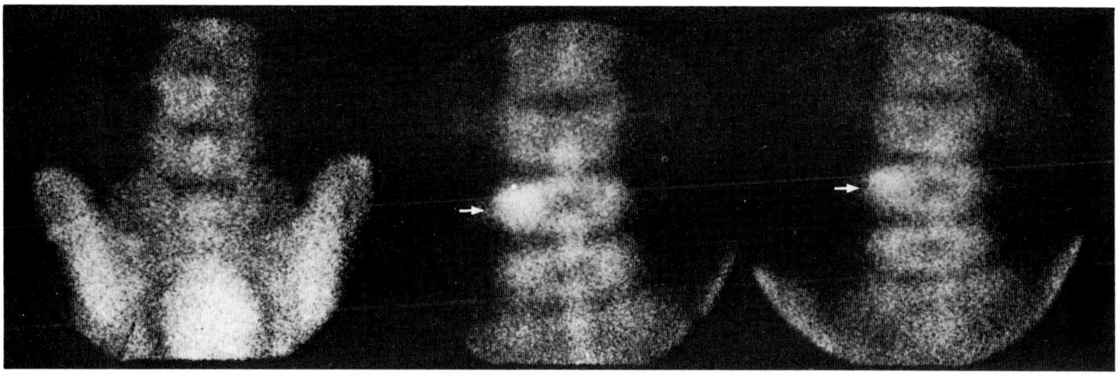

Figure 1-14. Scintigraphic evaluation of osteomyelitis. This 9-year-old boy developed left hip pain and was unable to bear weight on his left hip. The erythrocyte sedimentation rate was 9 mm/h. The initial diagnosis was toxic synovitis. The patient developed a temperature of 102°F and increased pain around his hip. His erythrocyte sedimentation rate rose to 20 mm/h with a white blood cell count of 8700/mm^3. Radiographs of his hips *(left)* and blood cultures were normal. A Tc-99m MDP bone scan is also normal. The pain, fever, nausea, and vomiting continued, and a repeat bone scan 6 days later *(center)* shows increased uptake in the body of the fourth lumbar vertebra. A blood culture at this time was positive for *S. aureus*. After treatment with intravenous antibiotics, the blood cultures became negative, and the followup bone scan (posterior view) taken 23 days later *(right)* shows reduction of the previously increased uptake of Tc-99m MDP.

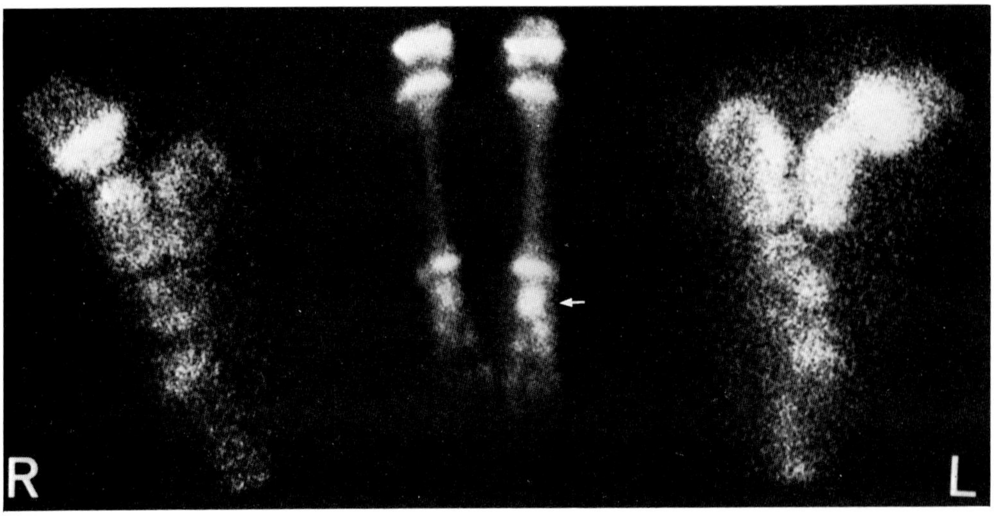

Figure 1-15. Cellulitis and osteomyelitis. This 22-month-old girl presented after 4 days of limping and pain in the left foot. Her temperature was 101.8°F with a white blood cell count of 11,000/mm^3 and erythrocyte sedimentation rate of 20 mm/h. She was treated with antibiotics and bedrest. The radiograph was normal. The bone scan shows increased uptake of Tc-99m MDP in the left ankle and tarsal bones, compatible with cellulitis. Blood culture grew *S. aureus*. After a 3-week course of antibiotics, she continued with a fever of 104°F, redness, and swelling of the left ankle. The white blood cell count was 12,000/mm^3 and the sedimentation rate had risen to 58 mm/h. After aspiration of the subcutaneous tissue yielded 1.5 ml of pus, an incision was carried down to the deeper structures until the joint of the talonavicular articulation was open and pus was again encountered. The talus was drilled but no pus was obtained. Followup radiographs 2 months later revealed regional osteoporosis, decreased soft tissue swelling, and reparative osteomyelitis. R, Right side; L, left side.

and indicated that the ninth patient had cellulitis. Only one of the eight patients with osteomyelitis showed any radiologic evidence of disease (soft tissue change); the other seven patients presumably had early disease and had not yet developed soft-tissue changes. Among these seven patients, only three showed bony changes on followup radiographs. When biopsy or drainage was performed in six patients, the scans were especially useful to the surgeon in identifying the exact sites for puncture. One of the patients had involvement of the bones adjacent to the sacroiliac joint, but initial and followup radiographs as well as repeated blood cultures were negative.[154] The sacroiliac joint is a site where an early diagnosis of infection is often difficult to determine on clinical and radiologic grounds alone.[124] Two of our patients in whom biopsy was not performed had positive blood cultures *(S. aureus)* and normal radiographs. One patient subsequently developed radiologic changes of bone destruction. The other patient, who also received high-dosage oxacillin, responded well clinically, and a repeat scintiscan and radiograph were normal.

Infarction

Theoretically, a bone infarct should show on the Tc-99m MDP scintigram as an area of decreased uptake due to vascular compromise. Although this is often the case, a healing infarct with reactive perfusion may appear as an area of increased activity on routine scintigrams (Fig. 1-16). Magnification scintigraphy may reveal that such an area actually has a core of decreased activity. Whatever its appearance, the bone infarct can confound the differential diagnosis of a number of diseases. In one series of 192 patients with sickle-cell anemia, osteomyelitis could not be differentiated from acute long bone infarction on the basis of bone or bone marrow scintigraphy.[80] Ga-67 scintigraphy is particularly useful in the identification of osteomyelitis in the patient with sickle cell disease.

Septic Arthritis

Septic arthritis usually develops after an infection of the skin or of the upper respiratory tract. Among children $<$ 2 years old, the most frequent organism

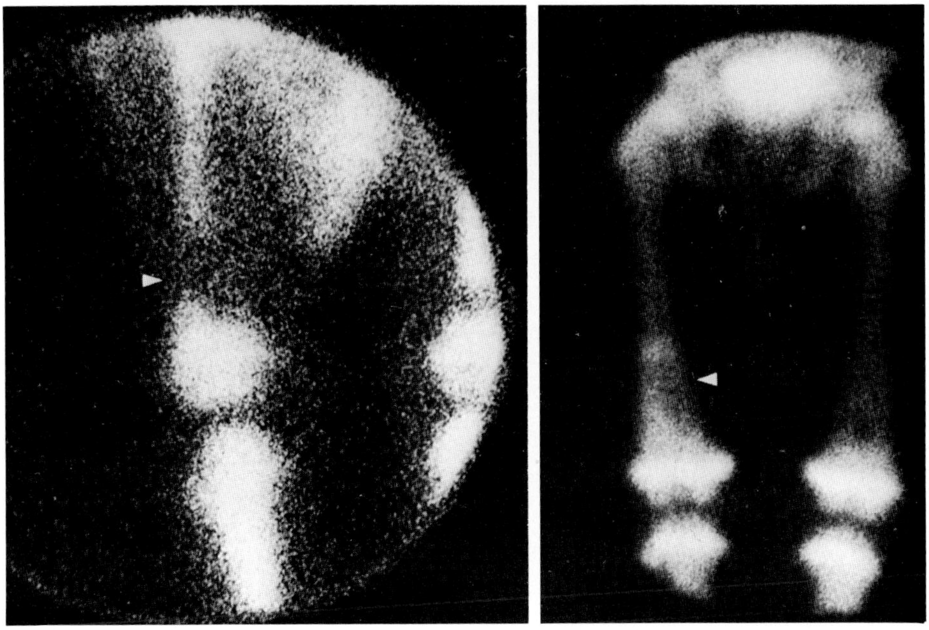

Figure 1-16. Bone infarction in sickle-cell disease. The left panel shows a Tc-99m sulfur colloid scan of the right knee of a 3-year-old patient with sickle-cell anemia. A definite focus of absent radiopharmaceutical uptake is visible in the right lower femur *(left)*. *Right:* A Tc-99m MDP scan of the same patient obtained 2 days later. An area of decreased uptake in the lower and medial aspects of the right femur is surrounded by a rim of increased uptake, which is probably reactive.

responsible for septic arthritis is *S. aureus,* but group B β-hemolytic streptococci and gram-negative enteric bacteria can also be responsible. In children 2–4 years of age, the most frequent organism encountered is *Hemophilus influenzae* type b. In this age group, staphylococci, streptococci, pneumococci, and meningococci are also involved. Septic arthritis may also result from hematogenous bacteria, from a contiguous focus of infection, or from direct inoculation of bacteria into the space in the joint.

Clinical Appearance

Local pain and swelling, systemic symptoms, and fever are common complaints. Decreased mobility of the joint involved and resistance even to passive motion may be present. Other findings include rapid erythrocyte sedimentation rate and elevated white cell count. Limp without fever may be the only symptom. After clinical or radiographic suggestion of septic arthritis, arthrocentesis will confirm the diagnosis. In young children or neonates, the clinical presentation may not be suggestive because of the relatively abundant soft tissue around the joint. Refusal to move the affected limb due to pain may be the only indication of disease.

Scintigraphic Findings

In the presence of septic arthritis of the hip, scanning may reveal decreased or even absent radiopharmaceutical uptake in the femoral head (Figs. 1-17–1-19). This is caused by ischemia due to increased pressure in the articular capsule. If pressure in the capsule is not sufficiently high, the scan may be normal or may show only faintly increased uptake in the bones surrounding the involved joint. Osteomyelitis may or may not be present with septic arthritis. Because the metaphyseal venous plexus traverses the epiphyseal plate in children under 2 years of age, osteomyelitis is more likely to be complicated by septic arthritis in these children than in older children. Radionuclide bone scanning is indicated to identify concomitant osteomyelitis before the radiographic changes take place. Con-

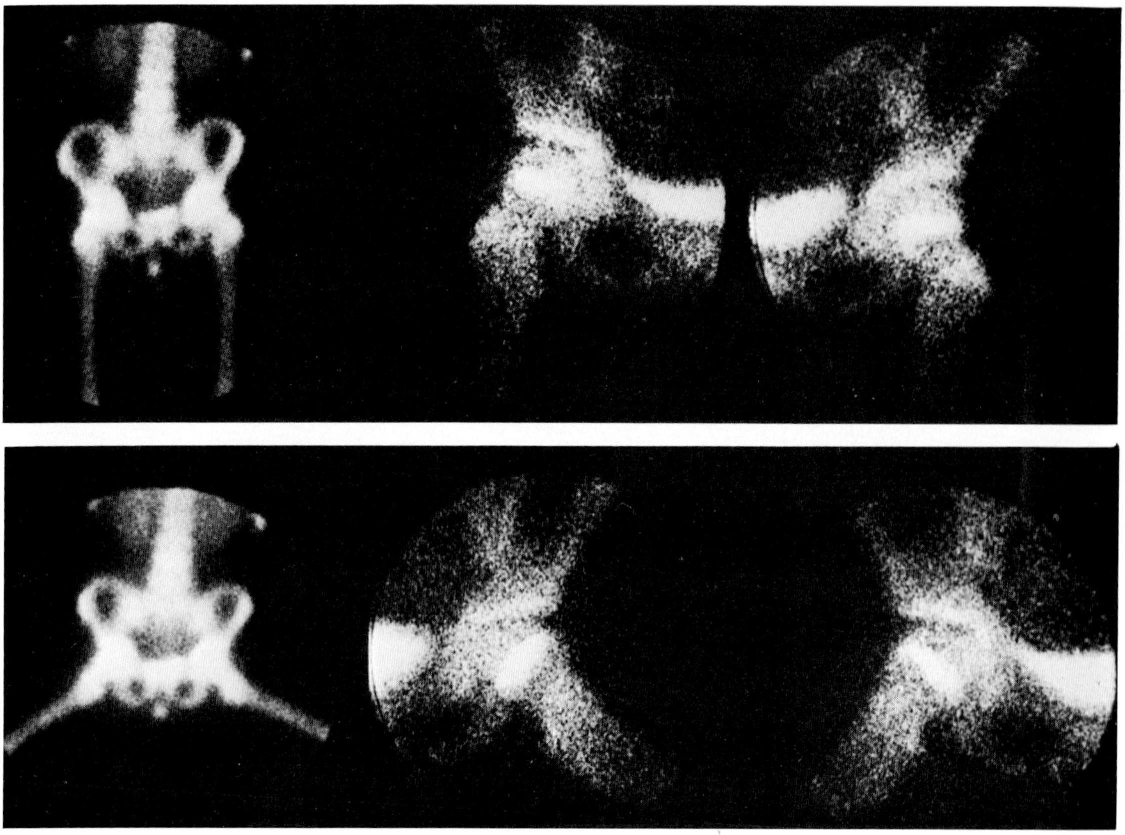

Figure 1-17. Normal Tc-99m MDP bone scan. *Top:* Normal anterior pinhole views of the hip (*left:* anterior view; *center:* right hip, anterior view; *right:* left hip, anterior view). *Bottom:* Normal frogleg views of the hip (*left:* anterior view; *center:* right hip, anterior view; *right:* left hip, anterior view).

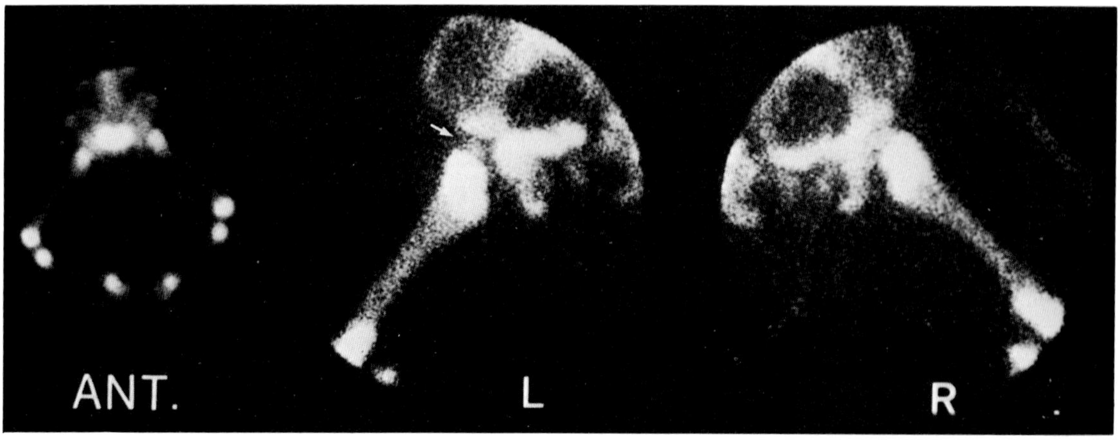

Figure 1-18. Septic arthritis of the left hip in a 9-month-old girl. *Left:* Anterior view using the high-resolution paraellel-hole collimator shows no evidence of abnormal Tc-99m MDP concentration. *Center and right:* Pinhole views obtained from the posterior projection show definite decreased uptake of Tc-99m MDP in the left femoral head. This is most likely secondary to ischemia resulting from increased pressure within the articular capsule. Increased intracapsular pressure produces a tamponade of the vessels feeding the femoral head. Ant., Anterior view; L, left side; R, right side.

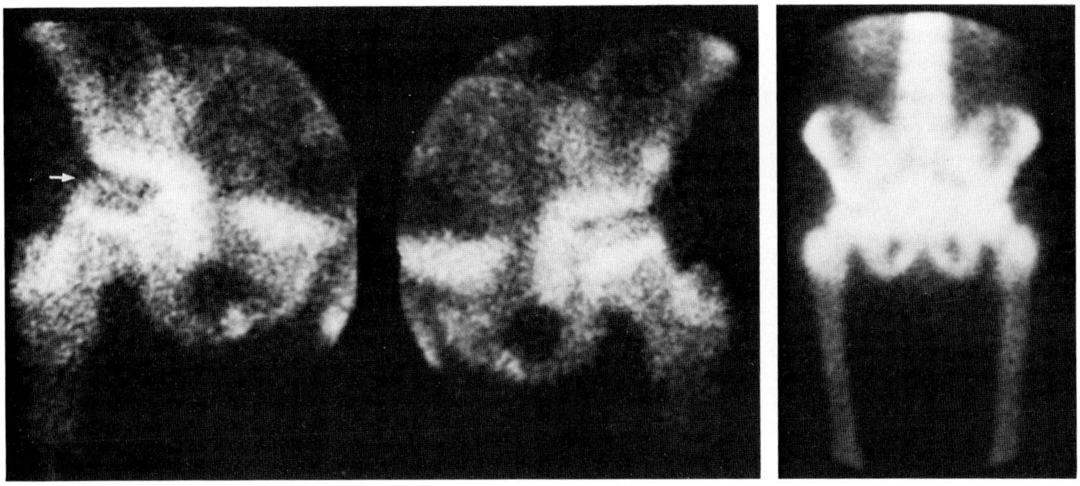

Figure 1-19. Septic arthritis of the hip in a 7-year-old boy. Anterior bone scintigram with pinhole magnification shows decreased Tc-99m MDP uptake in the right femoral head due to ischemia secondary to pressure in the intraarticular capsule.

comitant osteomyelitis will cause a focal increase of radiopharmaceutical uptake.

Aseptic Necrosis

In Legg-Calve-Perthes disease, the femoral head undergoes aseptic necrotic changes that involve the bone marrow and bony tissue but not the articular cartilage or epiphyseal plate. The cause is believed to be ischemia of the epiphysis due to vascular changes. The condition occurs most commonly between the ages of 5 and 7 years with a male: female ratio of 3:1. The disease is bilateral in about 10% of the patients. Early diagnosis of this disorder is important because early treatment may reduce the extent of subsequent damage and the time until healing. The prognosis also appears related to age (being better in younger patients) and to the degree of epiphyseal involvement.[25]

Scintigraphic and Radiographic Images

One of the most striking abnormalities visible by bone scintigraphy is that of an avascular femoral head (Figs. 1-20 and 1-21). Early in the disease there is absence of radiotracer uptake in a segment of the femoral head. Radionuclide bone scanning has a reported sensitivity and specificity > 90% in this phase of the disease,[16,18,91,147] and attempts have been made to quantitate the degree of femoral head uptake and prognosis.[39,85]

Radiologically, there may be no detectable change during the first few weeks of the disease. Later changes include a slight widening of the joint space: a linear translucency of the epiphysis appearing subchondally follows rapidly, starting anteriorly, and is accompanied by increased bone density. The scintiscan at this stage may still reveal no uptake in the femoral head and sometimes increased uptake in the acetabulum and proximal femur due to reaction.[60] After a variable period, this is followed by reossification and gradual reformation of the femoral head. Revascularization of the femoral head is accompanied by increased radiopharmaceutical uptake within it.

In the presence of fluid within the hip joint, reduced or even absent radiopharmaceutical uptake in the femoral head may be due only to ischemia secondary to increased pressure within the capsule. It would be very difficult to determine a priori if the absence of uptake in the femoral head is associated with necrosis or if it is transient. Drainage of the fluid under pressure within the hip should allow return of blood flow and uptake provided no permanent damage has occurred.

Differential Diagnosis

There are several other lesions of the hip that cause hip pain and limp. In some cases pain may also occur in the knee. These lesions include: infection, synovitis, trauma, slipped femoral epiphysis, and

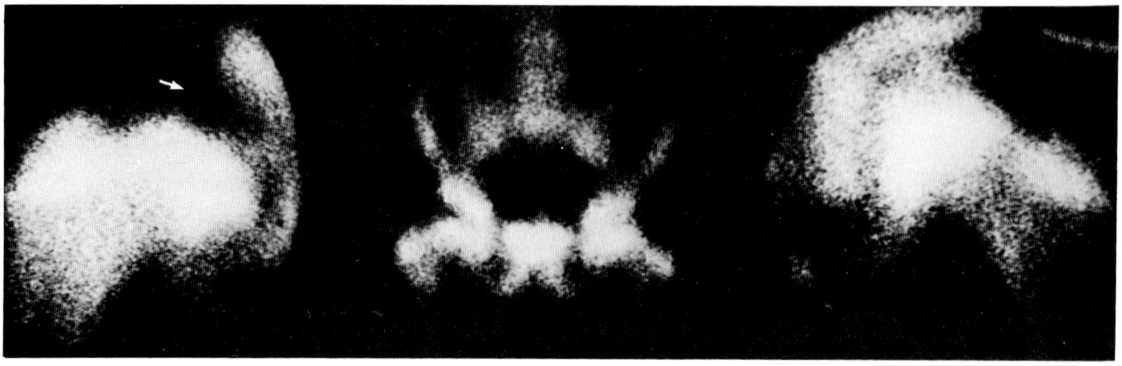

Figure 1-20. Aseptic necrosis of the femoral head. This 6-year-old boy presented with right hip pain and limited range of motion. The conventional *(center)* and magnified *(left and right)* anterior views show no uptake of Tc-99m MDP within the right femoral head. Radiographs of this patient's hips were normal.

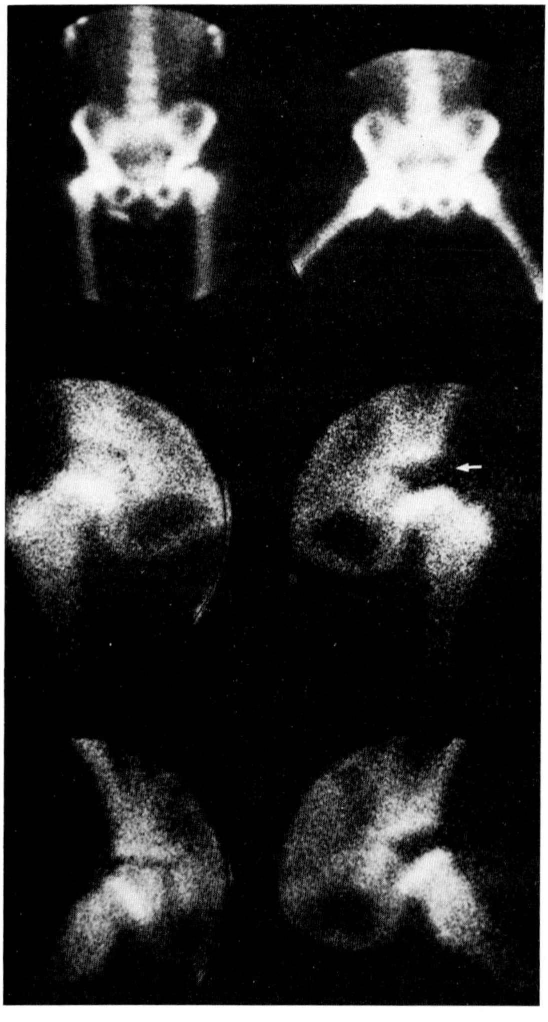

Figure 1-21. Aseptic necrosis of the left femoral head. No radiopharmaceutical uptake in the left femoral head can be seen on the conventional or magnified images. This patient had normal radiographs.

juvenile rheumatoid arthritis. Infection is usually suggested by signs of systemic involvement with fever and toxemia, local tenderness, swelling, and limitation of movement.

Toxic synovitis may produce only a faint increase in radiopharmaceutical uptake by bones around the hip joint. In the majority of cases, the scintiscan may appear entirely normal; in others there may be a faint increase in uptake in bones surrounding the joint. Synovitis associated with trauma, which is often trivial and overlooked, is a common cause of painful hips. In this disorder, there is usually joint effusion and also limitation of movement. It may be impossible to distinguish synovitis from early Legg-Calve-Perthes disease before the characteristic radiographic changes have occurred.

Decreased-to-absent uptake of radiopharmaceutical in the femoral head and other bones can also be seen in Gaucher's disease (Fig. 1-22) and in patients receiving high-dose corticosteroid therapy.[13]

Trauma

Direct trauma to bone or even the periosteum alone produces an immediate reparative response that results in increased uptake of radiotracer.[40,57] This makes bone scanning extremely sensitive for the diagnosis of trauma within 24–48 h of the injury. The pattern of abnormal uptake can be focal, well-defined, or diffuse (Fig. 1-23). When fractures are not visible radiologically or are in areas that are difficult to evaluate on routine radiographs, such as the spine and ribs (Fig. 1-24), radionuclide scanning is particularly helpful.

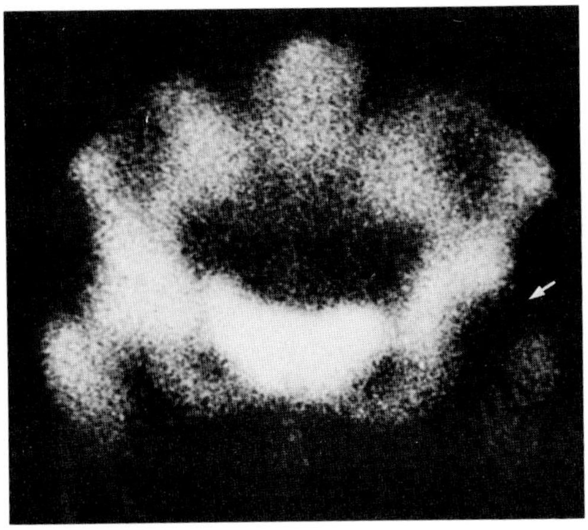

Figure 1-22. Avascularity of the femoral head in Gaucher's disease. There is no Tc-99m MDP uptake within the left femoral head and neck. Radiographs of this patient were normal.

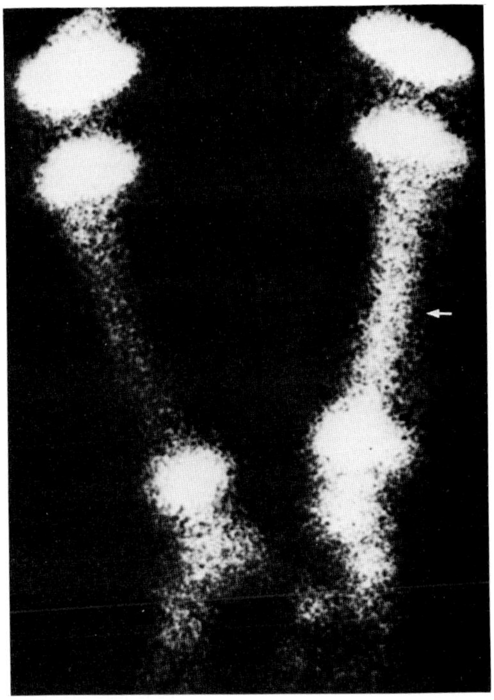

Figure 1-23. A: Hairline fracture of the left tibia in a toddler. There is a diffuse increase in uptake of Tc-99m MDP in the left tibia.

Denervation of a limb will cause changes in blood flow that can result in increased uptake of the bone-seeking pharmaceutical in the entire limb (Fig. 1-25). Soon after immobilization the increased blood flow to an extremity causes consequent increase in radiotracer uptake. If immobilization continues, there will be a diffuse reduction in uptake in the extremity involved (Fig. 1-26).

Trauma resulting in fracture of the femoral neck (uncommon in children) can result in aseptic necrosis with or without associated displacement. The bone scan in these patients will reveal no radionuclide uptake in the femoral neck accompanied by increased uptake at the fracture site.

Increased uptake in a site of fracture may be seen for several years. Battered children will demonstrate more abnormalities on the bone scan than can be demonstrated radiologically. The bone scan cannot be used reliably to predict the age of the injury, however. Similarly, the bone scan will be abnormal for many years after surgical manipulation of bone or biopsy.[161]

Stress Fractures-Stress Reaction

Stress fractures are part of a constellation of dynamic changes in the regional blood flow, metabolism, and architecture of bone. Multiple repetitive musculoskeletal stresses lead to development of an osteoclastic process that results in an inability to

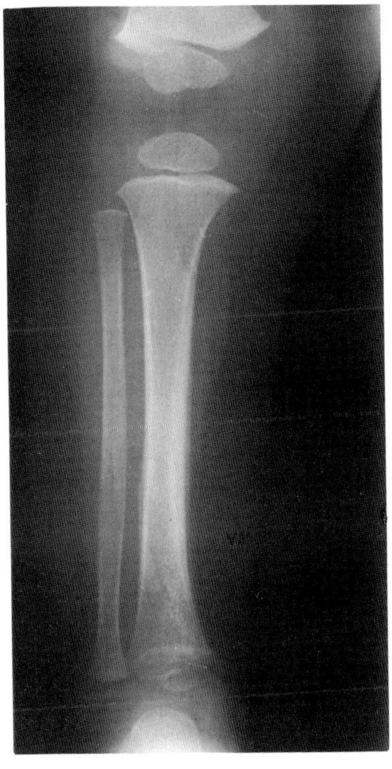

Figure 1-23. B: Radiography did not become abnormal until 7 days after the injury.

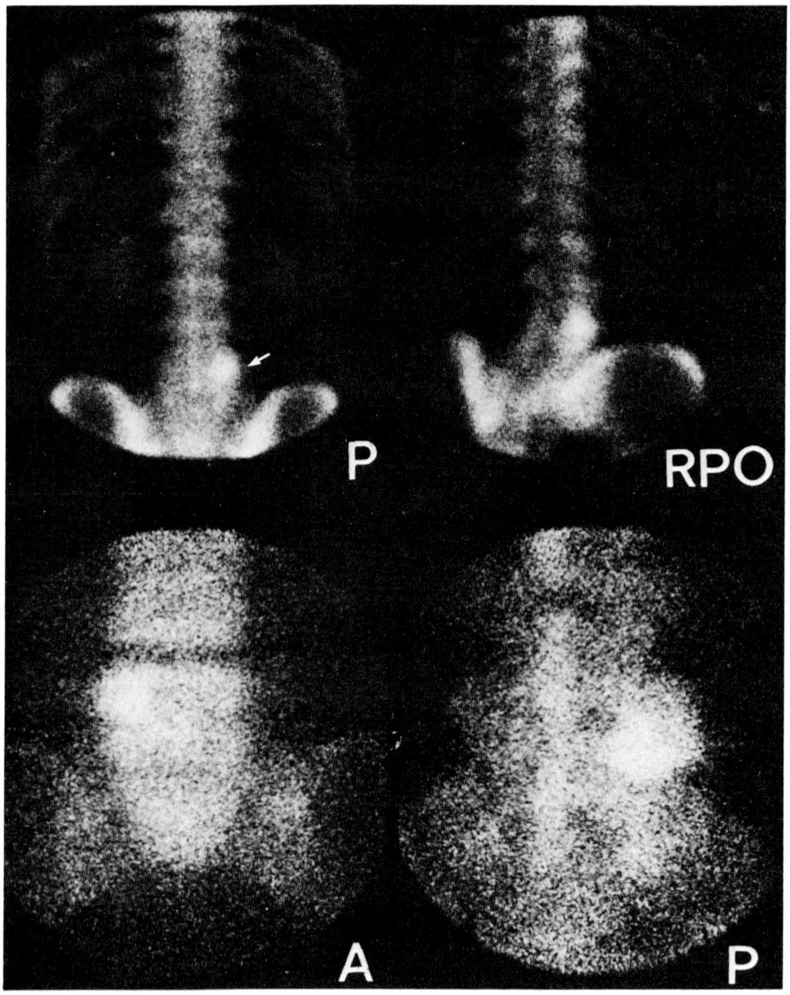

Figure 1-24

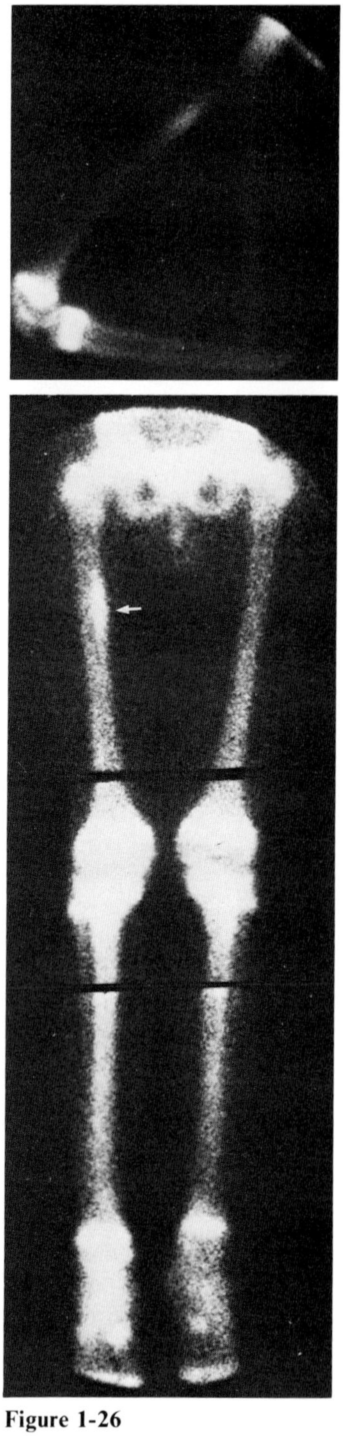

Figure 1-26

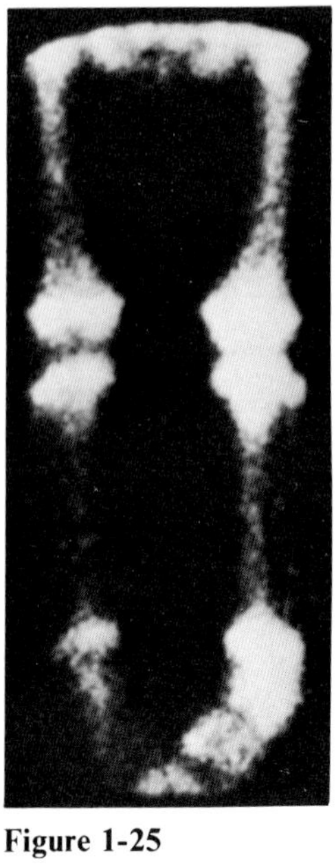

Figure 1-25

Figure 1-24. Fracture of the right pars interarticularis of the fifth lumbar vertebra. Tc-99m MDP bone scans. The *upper panel* shows conventional high-resolution images, and the *lower panel* shows images obtained with the pinhole collimator. P, Posterior view; RPO, right posterior oblique view; A, anterior view.

Figure 1-25. Left sympathectomy in an 18-month-old girl after surgery for a left Wilm's tumor. The skeletal scan shows diffusely increased uptake of Tc-99m MDP in the bones of the left lower extremity.

Figure 1-26. Disuse leading to decreased bone-seeker uptake in the left leg. This patient was walking with the aid of a crutch in order to prevent weight-bearing on the left leg, which was painful. The etiology of the pain was not known. An area of increased uptake of Tc-99m MDP in the right mid-femur is due to a stress fracture.

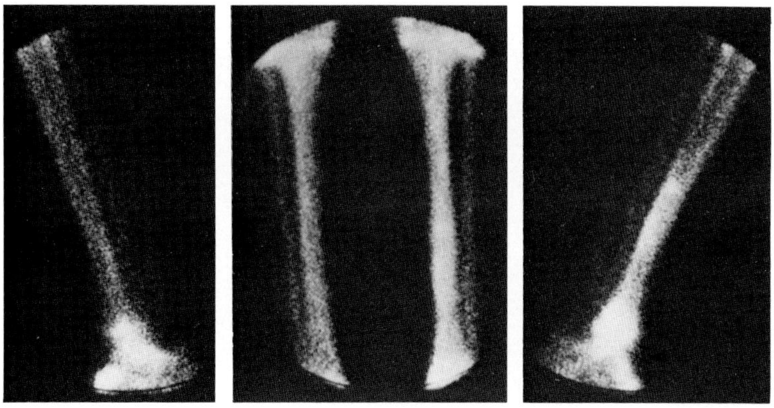

Figure 1-27. Stress fracture of the left tibia in a high jumper. There is diffusely increased uptake of Tc-99m MDP in both tibiae. The tibia of the left leg, which this athlete used for takeoff, shows a greater increase in uptake. In addition, there is an even greater increase in the uptake in the lower half of the left tibia, corresponding to a stress fracture. *Left:* right side; *center:* anterior view; *right:* left side.

maintain the architectural integrity of the bone. As the osteoclastic response surpasses the osteoblastic repair, cortical disruption occurs with the ultimate consequence of displaced fractures.

Stress fracture (reaction) develops over a period of days, weeks, or months in ballet dancers, gymnasts, swimmers, jumpers, joggers, and other individuals engaged in unaccustomed strenuous activities (Fig. 1-27). Most commonly involved are the bones of the lower extremities; the presenting symptoms are localized swelling and pain; and the onset is insidious.[43,96]

When stress fractures occur in normal bones, they usually heal without complications. These injuries, if not treated properly, may be disabling, however.[27,28,164] Stress fractures of the tibia, fibula, or metatarsals may have a protracted course if unrecognized. When the damage occurs to the femoral neck, complete fracture with displacement can be the consequence of a failure to diagnose the problem.

Skeletal scintigraphy is the only method for documenting sites of bone stress early and should be the initial examination for many patients presenting with exercise-related pain.[161] Scintigraphy should not be limited to the symptomatic site because multiple sites of stress are frequently found in these patients. For example, in runners with pain in one leg, scintigraphy of both lower extremities, the pelvis, and the lower spine should be performed (Figs. 1-28 and 1-29). In these patients, there is a characteristic diffuse increase in radiopharmaceutical uptake along the tibiae. Conventional roentgenograms should be obtained also, but the delay in radiographic appearance of stress fractures can be as long as 3 weeks.[161]

The stress reaction in bone is thought to be a normal response to an abnormal stimulus.[164] Bone responds to stress with osteonal remodeling; initial remodeling is followed by accelerated osteoblastic activity and replacement.[76] Accelerated physical activity can lead to reabsorption that exceeds the replacement capacity of the bone, resulting in cortical weakening and microfractures or even frank cortical fractures.[76] Displacement fractures can be prevented with early diagnosis and treatment.

The association of diffuse and focal abnormalities in the same site as well as asymmetric patterns may well support the theory of a continuum in scintigraphic abnormalities associated with bony stress. Early on, the resorptive changes are not radiographically detectable. Later, as reactive bone repair proceeds, radiographic changes appear (endosteal callous formation, periosteal reaction, and focal sclerosis accompanied by a fracture line.)[132,164]

In our experience, more than 60% of athletes with tibial abnormalities have exhibited bilateral changes, and associated roentgenographic abnormalities are found in almost 30% of the patients at the time of diagnosis. Thus, early diagnosis must be actively pursued to prevent the occasionally severe sequelae and associated morbidity of stress fractures.

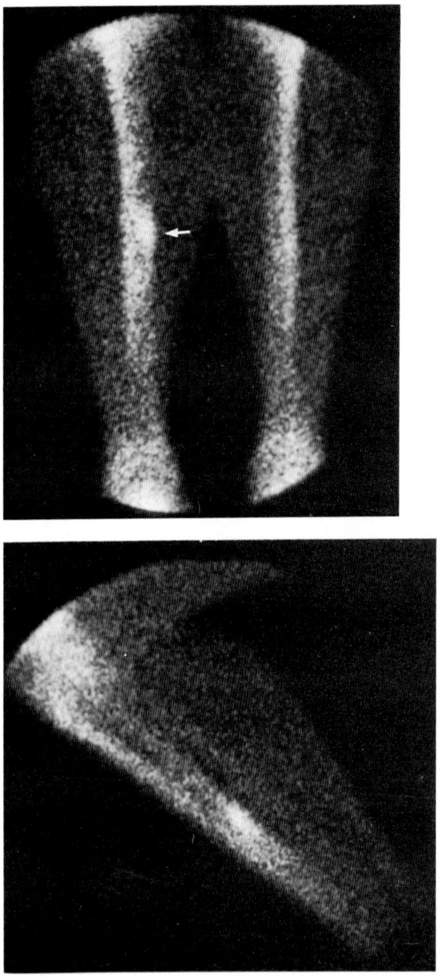

Osteochondritis Dissecans

Osteochondritis dissecans is a rather common orthopedic condition encountered most frequently in patients between 15 and 25 years of age. It is more common in males, with a ratio of 4:1 to 13:1 depending on the series. Pathologically, there is epiphyseal ischemic necrosis involving only a fragment of the peripheral osseous epiphysis under the articular cartilage. In about 85% of patients, the medial femoral condyle is affected. In about 10% of patients, two or more lesions are found and they tend to be symmetric. Other involved sites are the femoral head, the elbow, the distal humerus, and the humeral head. The cause for this lesion is not known.

Development of the condition begins when an area of bone necrosis appears in the lateral border of the medial femoral condyle and extends to the

◁ **Figure 1-28.** Stress fracture in the right tibia with stress in both tibiae in a runner. These images were obtained from a 25-year-old runner with pain referred to the right leg. The anterior scintiscan *(top)* reveals typical diffuse increase of Tc-99m MDP along the lateral aspect of both tibiae. In addition, the right lateral scintiscan *(bottom)* shows a focal area of even greater uptake in the posteromedial aspect of the right tibia. This represents a stress fracture. *Top:* anterior view; *bottom:* right lateral view.

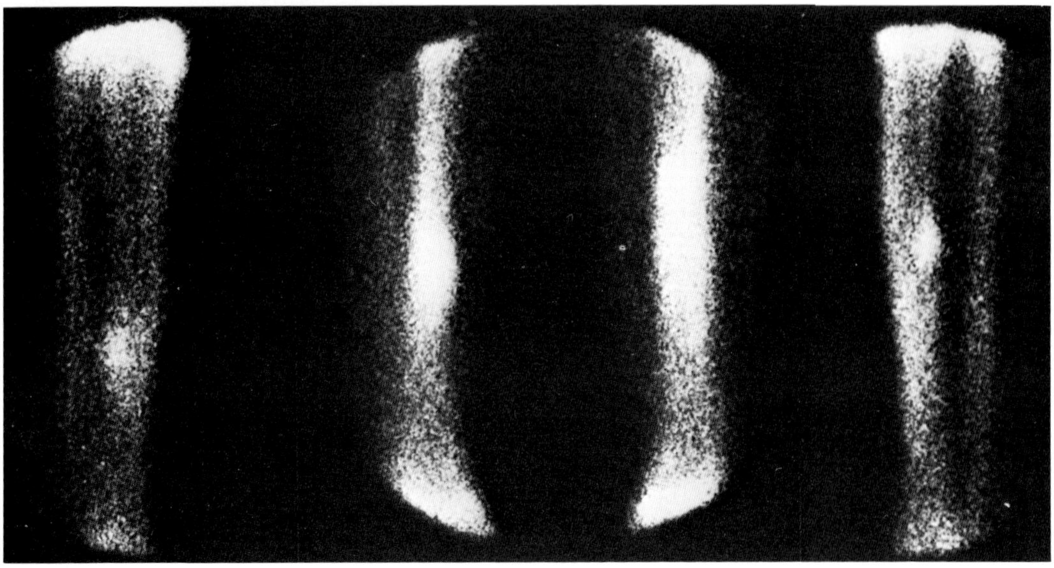

Figure 1-29. Bone scintigram of the tibiae and fibulae in an active runner. There is diffusely increased uptake of Tc-99m MDP in the tibiae. In addition, there are focal areas of increased uptake in the mid-tibiae, worse in the left. *Left:* right lateral view; *center:* right side; *right:* left lateral view.

intercondylar fossa. A fragment of bone that supports the articular cartilage then becomes necrotic and collapses. A region of hemorrhage appears around the dead bony fragment, and a capsule of granulation tissue forms with increased regional blood flow about this area. During this period, bone scintigraphy will reveal increased uptake of radiopharmaceutical in the area involved (Fig. 1-30). Using magnification scintigraphy it may be possible to observe the photon-deficient area of the infarcted bone within the area of increased uptake.

Cysts

Simple, solitary, or unicameral cysts of unknown etiology usually are found in the metaphysis of a cylindrical bone of the growing skeleton. They are ovoid and smooth and contain fluid that may be bloody, clear, or amber. These lesions may be caused by extravasation of blood into the metaphysis of growing bones.

Skeletal scintigraphy of a simple cyst may be normal, if the cyst is small and uncomplicated, or may show a focal area of decreased uptake with or without a surrounding rim of increased uptake due to stress (Fig. 1-31). If a fracture is present in the wall of the cyst, increased activity around the cyst may be the predominant scintigraphic feature. Magnification scintigraphy in some cases reveals a central core of decreased uptake.

Fibrous Dysplasia

Fibrous dysplasia is a bone disorder of unknown etiology. The involved structures lack mature bone and sometimes have islands of cartilage and cysts filled with fluid. Fibrous dysplasia may involve many or all bones and is frequently unilateral. Histologically, there is a fibrous matrix that contains trabeculae of immature bone with various degrees of calcification. The bones affected most frequently are the femur and the tibia, followed by the pelvis, fibula, humerus, radius, and ulna. Fractures and deformity are common secondary consequences of this disease. Increased growth of bones of the face and skull creates a typical facial appearance.[116] The radiologic features include sclerosis, cystlike lesions, fractures, and deformity. The long bones

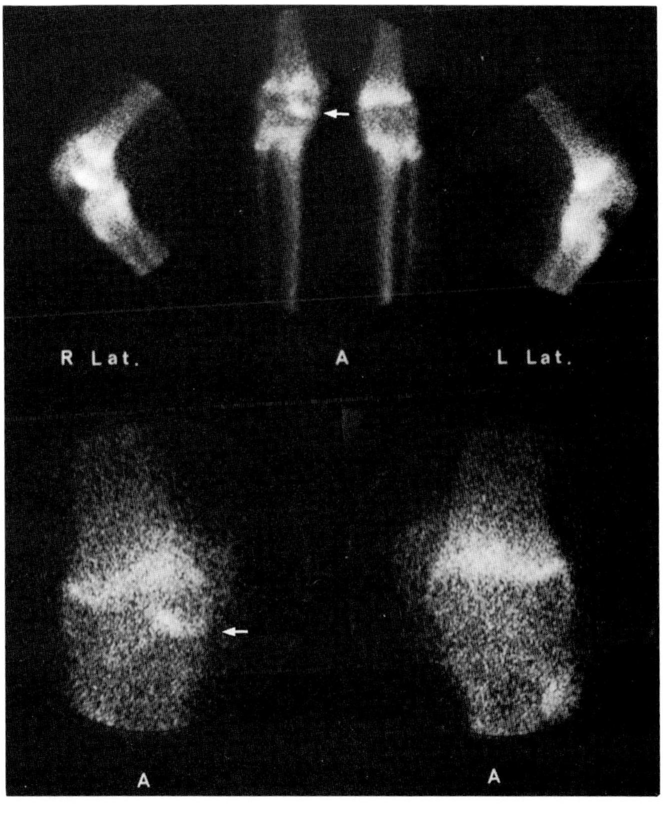

Figure 1-30. Osteochondritis dissecans of the right knee. The conventional *(top)* and magnified scintiscans of the knees reveal a well-defined area of increased uptake of Tc-99m MDP in the right medial condyle. R. Lat., Right lateral view; A, anterior view; L. Lat., left lateral view.

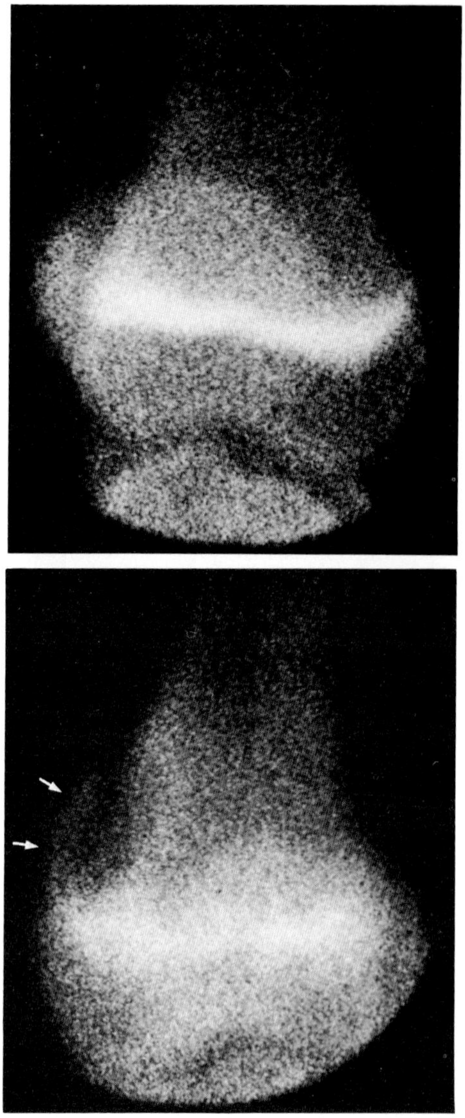

Figure 1-31. Aneurysmal bone cyst. Anterior pinhole views show a cyst in the medial aspect of the left lower femur, just above the epiphyseal growth plate. There is a rim of slightly increased uptake of Tc-99m MDP surrounding a well-defined region of decreased uptake in the cyst. *Top:* right side; *bottom:* left side.

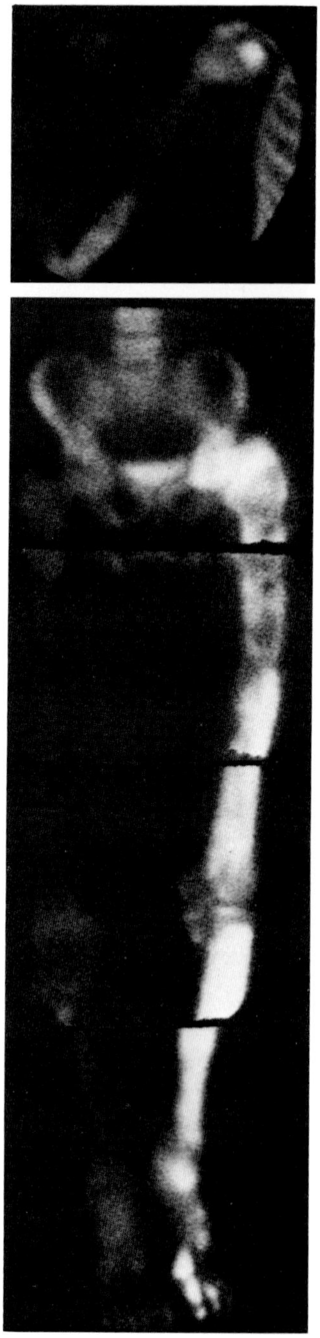

Figure 1-32. Fibrous dysplasia. In this patient several regions on the bone scan show intensely increased uptake of Tc-99m MDP and deformity of the bones. ▷

may be bowed with deformity of the femoral head. Albright's syndrome includes polyostotic fibrous dysplasia, abnormal skin pigmentation, and precocious puberty. Skeletal scintigraphy will show greatly increased radiopharmaceutical uptake in the affected bones (Fig. 1-32).

Infantile Cortical Hyperostosis

Infantile cortical hyperostosis, or Caffey's disease, is a disease of unknown etiology characterized by hyperplasia of subperiosteal bone over which there is soft tissue swelling and sometimes a brawny dis-

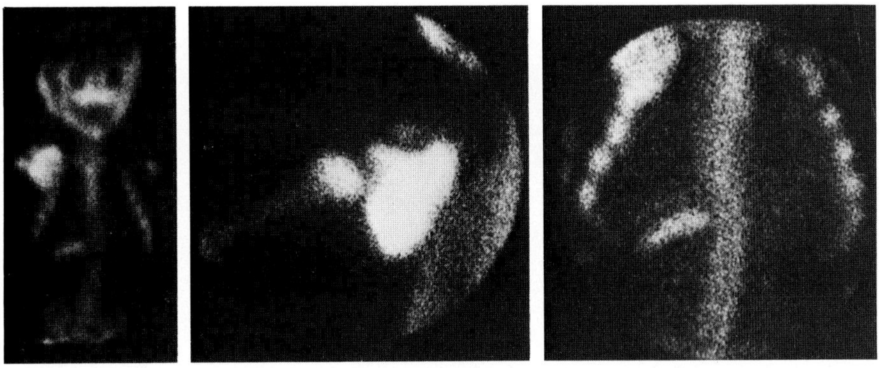

Figure 1-33. Infantile cortical hyperostosis (Caffey's disease). The skeletal scintigram in this 3-month-old boy shows markedly increased uptake of Tc-99m MDP in the right scapula and one of the ribs on the right.

coloration. Lesions of Caffey's disease have been observed in the skull, mandible, clavicles, ribs, scapulae, long bones of the extremities, and metatarsals. Recovery is the rule and usually occurs within weeks to a year. Radiologically there is periosteal new bone formation and cortical thickening of underlying bone. During healing radiographs may show laminated periosteal reaction and in the more chronic forms will show cortical thinning and shaft expansion. Scintigraphy is not indicated in this condition. During the active phase of the disease scintigraphy will reveal intense accumulation of radiopharmaceutical in the involved bones (Fig. 1-33).

Nonossifying Fibroma

Nonossifying fibroma has also been labelled nonosteogenic fibroma, metaphyseal fibrous defect, fibrous cortical defect, osteitis fibrosa, and xanthogranuloma of bone. Whatever the name, this well-defined lytic lesion is found in the metaphysis of long bones, usually in children between the ages of 4 and 8 years. Approximately 90% of the lesions appear in the distal femur and are discovered on radiographs obtained for unrelated reasons. When the nonossifying fibromas are large, they may cause pain and lead to pathologic fracture.

On the radiograph eccentric radiolucent lesions with a thin sclerotic rim characteristically appear in proximity to the epiphyseal growth plate without reaching it.[49] The lesions have been described as a "bunch of grapes" or "soap bubbles." Generally, biopsy is not indicated because the radiographic appearance is so characteristic.

Scintigraphy is not generally indicated unless the diagnosis is uncertain or complications are suspected. The scintigraphic pattern is similar to that of bone cyst: a region of decreased radiopharmaceutical uptake is surrounded by a thin rim of increased uptake (Fig. 1-34). If a fracture is present, the characteristic increase in uptake will be present.

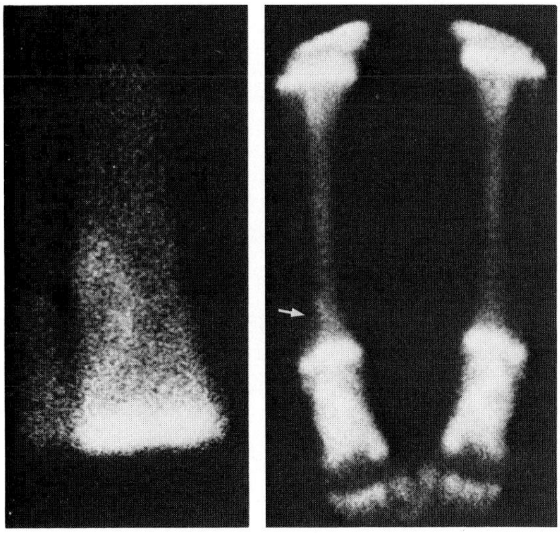

Figure 1-34. Nonossifying fibroma of the right lower tibia. An irregular area of decreased uptake of Tc-99m MDP is surrounded by a periphery of increased uptake.

Dental Disorders

Fall of deciduous teeth, recent dental extraction, dental and periodontal infections, trauma, and prostheses can cause scintigraphic abnormalities of bone. Examination of the patient and dental history are very useful to help explain the scintigraphic findings.[8,152]

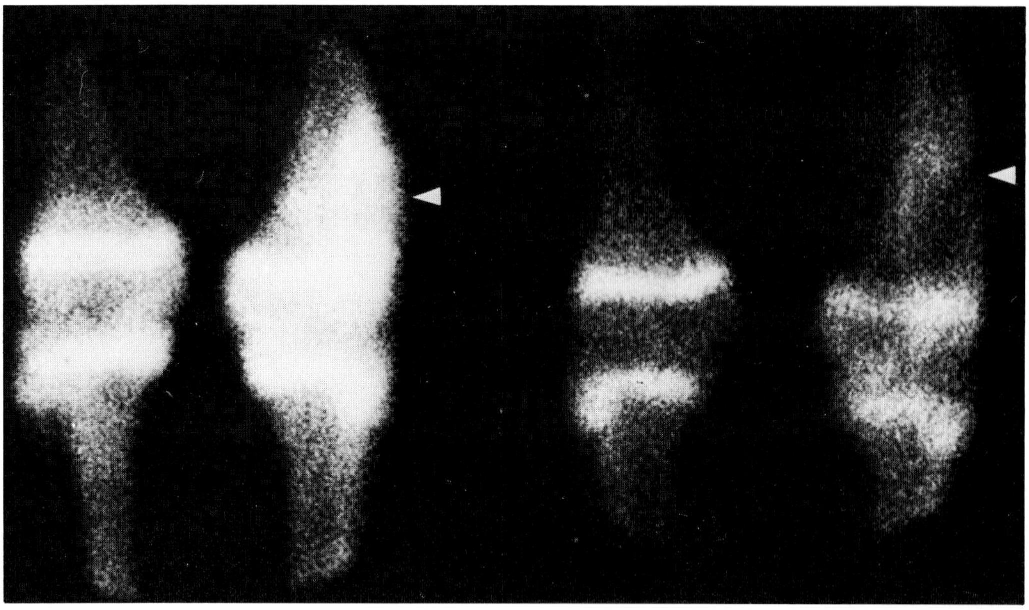

Figure 1-35. Osteosarcoma of the left distal femur. There is intense uptake of Tc-99m MDP in the region of the tumor *(left, arrowhead)*. In this unique case, the patient was treated with chemotherapy and radiotherapy. On the scan obtained months later *(right)*, there is a significant decrease in uptake of Tc-99m MDP in the region of the tumor and also the surrounding bones *(arrowhead)*.

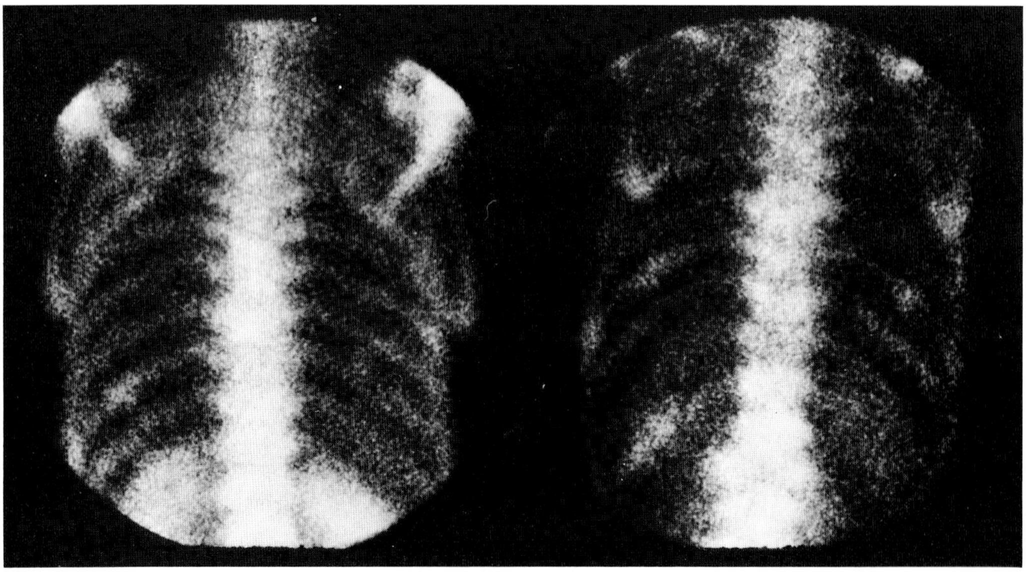

Figure 1-36. Metastatic osteosarcoma. Tc-99m MDP scintigraphy. Note the rapid extension of metastatic disease in several ribs and the spine during the 2 months between the first scan and the second scan.

Osteosarcoma

Osteosarcoma is the most commonly scanned primary neoplasm of bone in our institution. The contribution of skeletal scintigraphy to the evaluation of patients with this tumor is generally limited to delineation of the extent of the primary lesion (Fig. 1-35) and diagnosis of skeletal and soft tissue metastases (Figs. 1-36–1-39). Although this tumor is avid for Tc-99m-labelled phosphates and this char-

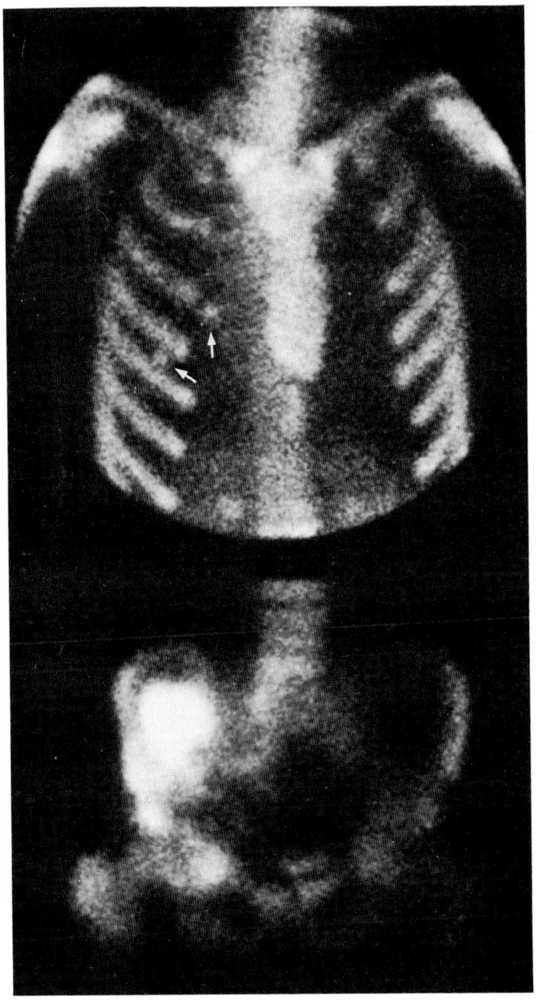

Figure 1-37. Osteosarcoma of the right iliac bone with local invasion and two soft tissue metastases in the right chest after injection of Tc-99m MDP.

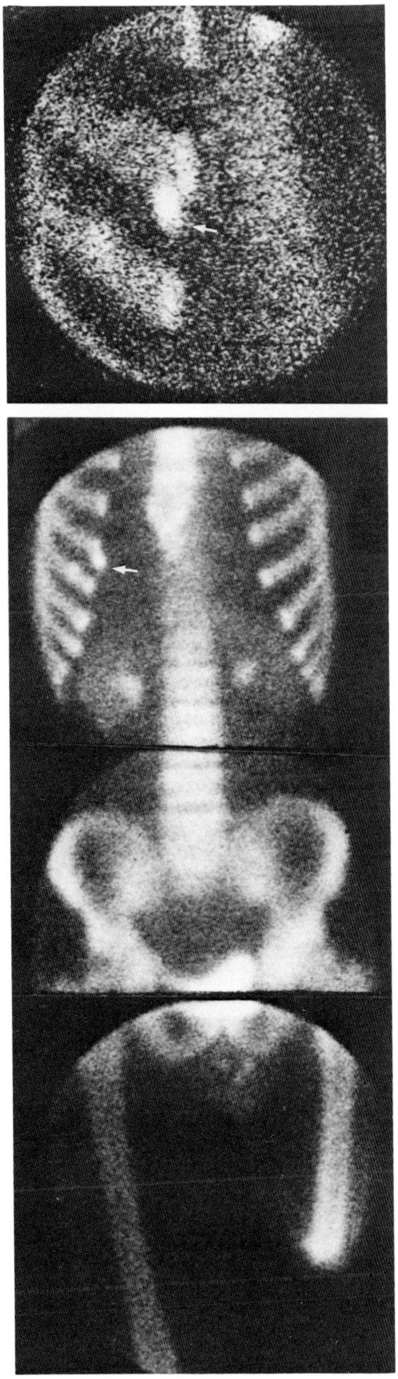

Figure 1-38. Osteosarcoma of the left distal femur. ▷ Skeletal scintigram obtained after amputation. Increased uptake of Tc-99m MDP in the remainder of the left femur is most likely due to postoperative hyperemia. There is a slight increase in uptake in the soft tissues surrounding the stump and a pulmonary metastasis that projects just below the anterior aspect of one of the right ribs.

acteristic should provide early diagnosis, the typical radiographic changes are usually obvious by the time patients become symptomatic. Thus, in practice, scintigraphy will rarely provide early detection of primary osteosarcoma in the presence of normal plain radiographs. We find scintigraphy to be less sensitive than plain chest radiographs, conventional chest tomography, and computed tomography in the diagnosis of pulmonary metastasis. For skeletal metastases, the reverse is true.

Although the yield at times may be low, bone scintigraphy is indicated at presentation and at regular intervals during followup in order to identify the existence and extent of osseous metastases

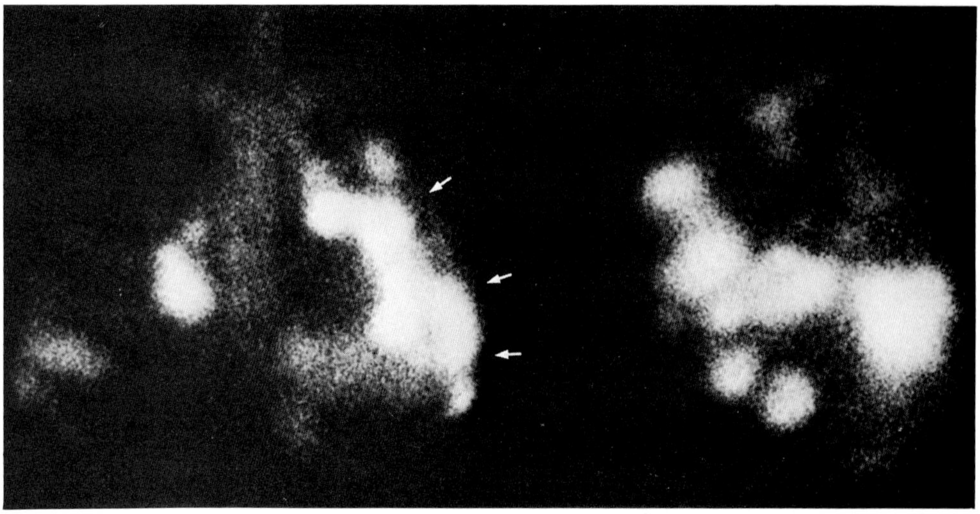

Figure 1-39. Metastatic osteosarcoma. Anterior *(left)* and left lateral *(right)* projections of the chest reveal intense uptake of Tc-99m MDP in several areas within the chest, particularly in the pericardial region.

and to provide early diagnosis in those patients who are exceptions to the typical disease course. In one study of 55 patients with osteosarcoma, radionuclide scans at presentation identified unsuspected osseous metastases in one patient and revealed proximal primary tumor extension not evident on the radiographs in another patient.[104] During followup in this same series, 11 of 20 patients with bone metastases were asymptomatic for bone involvement at the time the scans became abnormal.[104] Further, in another report of three children with the malignancy, the bone scan was helpful for confirming pulmonary metastases in two patients and for diagnosing previously unsuspected pulmonary metastases in the third patient.[83]

In the rare multicentric sclerosing osteosarcoma and in metachronous osteosarcoma, scintigraphy will reveal multiple areas of increased radiopharmaceutical uptake in the skeleton (Fig. 1-40).

In planning treatment for the disease, it is useful to know the extent of the tumor. Using skeletal scintigraphy, it is possible to outline the limits of the bony lesion on the patient's skin using the gamma camera and a small radioactive source (we use a drop of Tc-99m within the tip of a plastic needle cover). On an oscilloscope, the operator can see both the extent of abnormal uptake in the lesion and the radioactive source, which can be moved in any direction (Fig. 1-41). Since the radiopharmaceutical uptake extends slightly beyond the limit of the tumor, marking with the aid of bone scintigraphy provides an inherent margin of safety for resection.

Review of a small number of patients at Children's Hospital in Boston revealed that the bone scan and radiographic studies correlated well for 12 of 13 patients and that there was no extension of the tumor beyond the limit of surgical resection. In the single exception, radiotracer uptake throughout the shaft was slightly increased while the radiographic abnormality was confined to the distal metaphysis. Examination of the gross specimen did not reveal intramedullary spread, but there was marrow necrosis, giant cell infiltration, and granulation tissue.

Chew and Hudson [20] found extended uptake patterns in 11 of 18 preoperative scans when they compared the scintigraphic findings with the gross surgical specimens. In eight instances, the areas of extended uptake had marrow hyperemia, medullary reactive bone, or periosteal new bone.

Skeletal scintigraphy has been useful in the early detection of local recurrence and metastases in osteosarcoma. With the introduction of newer therapeutic regimens, pulmonary or skeletal metastases may occur first to be followed by metastases to soft tissues, brain, or other organs. When there has been amputation of a lower limb and a prosthesis fitted, it is usual to find increased radiopharmaceutical uptake at the end of the stump, in the region of the ipsilateral hip joint, and in the soft tissues surrounding the prosthesis. In addition, there may

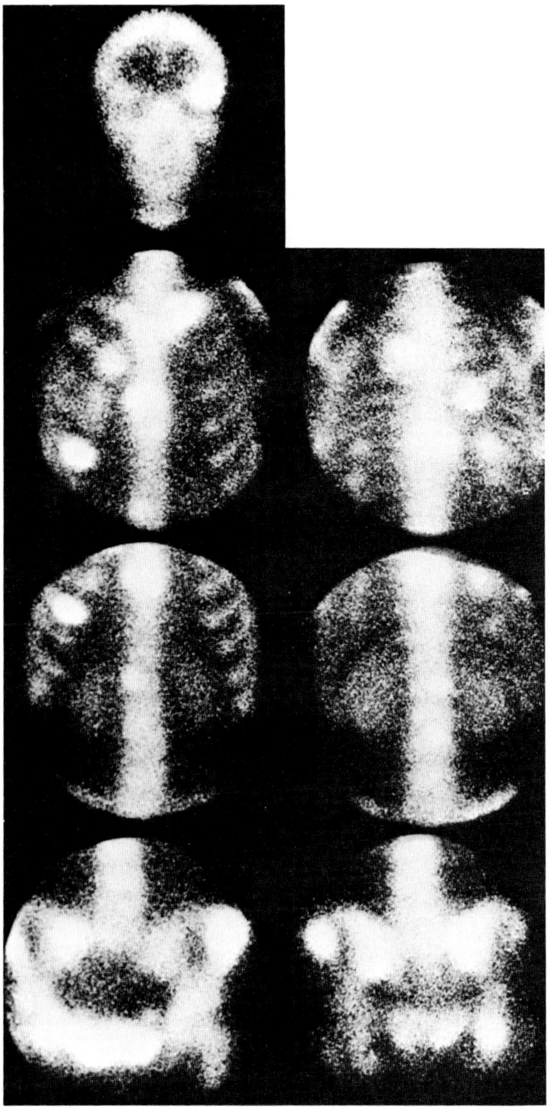

Figure 1-40. Multicentric osteosarcoma. Multiple bony and soft tissue regions of intensely increased uptake of Tc-99m MDP are seen throughout the body due to osteosarcoma.

be increased radiopharmaceutical uptake distally, all the way to the toes, due to reactive hyperemia. With disuse, the ipsilateral hip will with time reveal a decrease in radiopharmaceutical uptake.

Recent chemotherapy programs with methotrexate alone or with adriamycin and/or vincristine have increased the survival rate for patients with osteosarcoma.[69] Prior to the introduction of methotrexate, survival rates were 4–22% at 5 years after diagnosis.[14,58] More recently, a 5-year survival rate

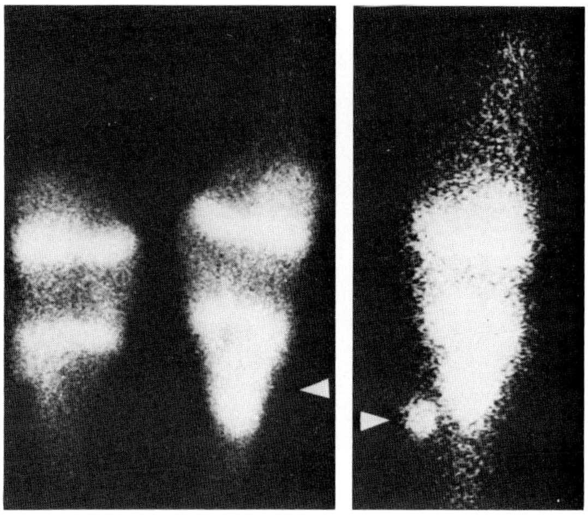

Figure 1-41. Osteosarcoma of the left proximal tibia *(left, arrowhead)* and a small radioactive source used as a marker *(right, arrowhead)*.

of 66% has been reported with no evidence of lung metastases up to 4 years.[72]

Previous work had indicated that only a small percentage of children had osseous metastases at presentation, and, in addition, no bone metastases developed before pulmonary metastases were apparent.[105] A more recent study[48] evaluated 56 patients with biopsy-proven osteosarcoma from the Children's Hospital Medical Center, Sidney Farber Cancer Institute, New England Deaconess Hospital, and Peter Bent Brigham Hospital over a period of 6 years (1972–1977). There were 38 males and 18 females (ratio 2.1:1). The average age of onset was 14.6 years with the 25th and 75th percentiles occurring at 11 and 16 years. The most common site for primary tumor was the femur (58.9%), then the tibia (21.4%), followed by the humerus, fibula, pelvis, and skull. Only two patients had metastatic disease at presentation. Thus, in this study the yield of abnormal bone scintiscans for metastatic disease was 2%. In the followup period, 57% of the patients developed osseous metastasis and/or pulmonary metastasis. In order of frequency, bone metastasis affected the ribs, pelvis, vertebrae, tibiae and fibulae, femora, skull, humeri, and other bones.

During the followup period only pulmonary metastases were found in 32% of the patients. In 39% of patients, pulmonary metastases developed sooner than osseous metastases. In 13%, pulmonary and bony metastases developed concomitantly. Of

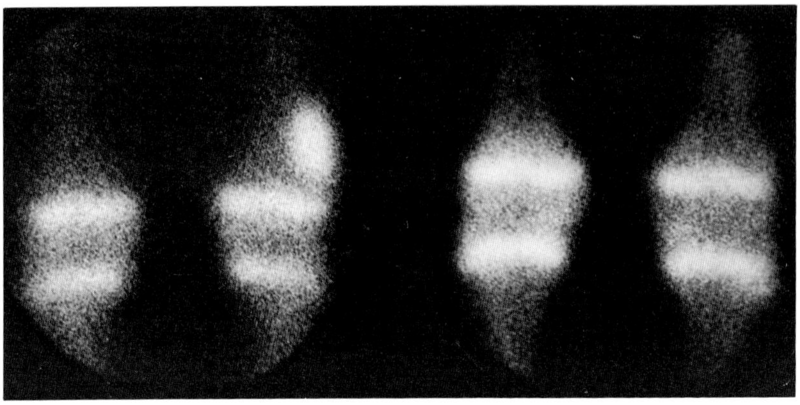

Figure 1-42. Parosteal osteosarcoma of the left distal femur. Tc-99m MDP scintiscans were taken before *(left)* and after *(right)* surgical excision of the tumor.

the 56 patients, 43 died with a median length of survival of 38 months. Once pulmonary metastases developed, the mean survival was only 8 months. Uptake of radiopharmaceutical bone seeker in lung metastases is not common—only 5% of the 29 patients in our series.

Most patients (79%) who had a leg amputated demonstrated asymmetric uptake in the pelvis and/or sacroiliac joints. Of the patients with asymmetric uptake, 35% had increased uptake on the amputated side and 65% on the other side. This asymmetry may be secondary to mechanical stress, disease, and/or the use of prostheses.

Parosteal Osteosarcoma

Parosteal or juxtacortical osteosarcoma is a malignant bone tumor that originates on the external surface of the bone in relation to the periosteum and/or the immediate parosteal connective tissue. The tumor is uncommon (3% of all osteosarcomas), has limited growth potential, and has a relatively good prognosis. The sex distribution is nearly equal between males and females. It occurs most commonly in the third decade of life, but the age range is 12–58 years. Swelling or a mass with dull aching pain or tenderness are usual presenting symptoms. The most frequent bones involved are the distal femur followed by the humerus, tibia, radius, and ulna. Other rare sites include the mandible, metacarpal bones, clavicle, and scapula.

The three histologic grades of parosteal osteosarcoma are: grade I, low grade; grade II, intermediate degree of malignancy; and grade III, high grade, malignant. Radiographically, the tumor appears irregular, lobulated, and densely radiopaque. In about 30% of patients, smooth margins can be seen. Also in about 30% of patients, the thin periosteal lucency (so-called string sign) that separates the tumor from the cortex is visible. In these patients, radiopharmaceutical accumulation appears outside the bone (Fig. 1-42).

Ewing's Sarcoma

Ewing's sarcoma is a malignant tumor of bone characterized by uniform, densely packed small cells with round cell nuclei but without distinct cytoplasmic borders or prominent nucleoli.[32,33,61,92,94] The tumor cells may derive from the connective tissue framework of bone marrow. Ewing's sarcoma makes up about 10–15% of all primary bone tumors.

Many patients with this disease have low to moderate fever, anemia, leukocytosis, and increased sedimentation rate at admission. Pain and swelling are the most common symptoms. About 70% of the patients experience intermittent pain, which may be dull to severe and becomes persistent for about a month prior to diagnosis. Visible or palpable tender swelling of rapidly increasing size is seen in most patients. Local increase in temperature with dilated blood vessels and tenderness often suggests an inflammatory lesion.

More than 80% of Ewing's sarcomas occur in the first 2 decades of life, and the tumor is quite uncommon after age 30. The youngest patient reported was 5 months old.[21] The peak incidence of Ewing's sarcoma in girls is between 5 and 9 years of age and in boys from 10 to 14 years.[45] The tumor is twice as common in males as in females. In one review the most common site of the primary tumor was the pelvis (25%) followed in order of frequency by ribs, femora, spine, tibiae, fibulae, scapulae, and other bones.[47] Another series of 167 cases showed that the long tubular bones were the most often af-

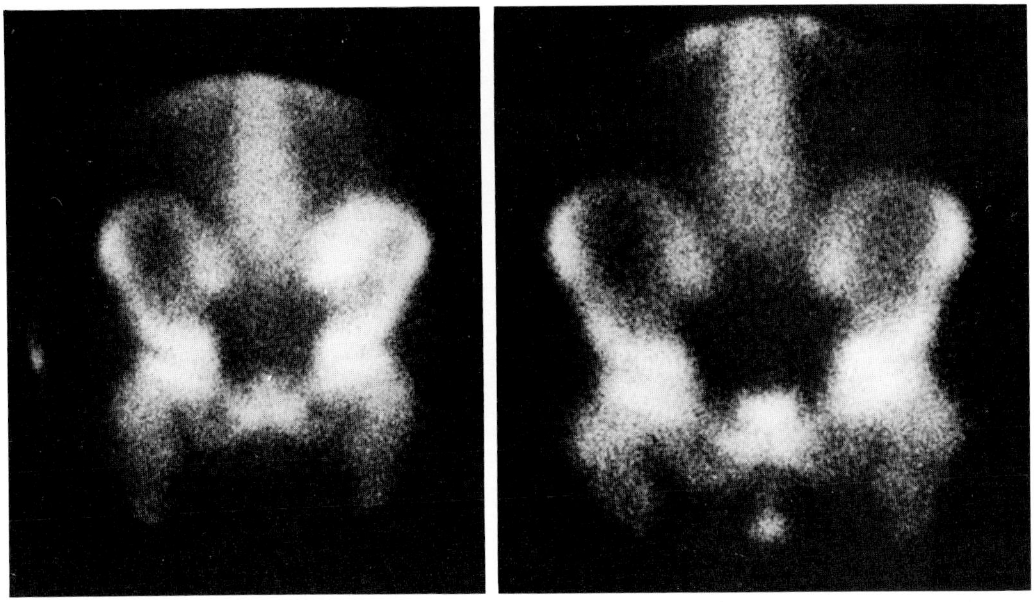

Figure 1-43. Ewing's sarcoma of the left pelvis before *(left)* and after *(right)* chemotherapy. Tc-99m MDP scintigraphy.

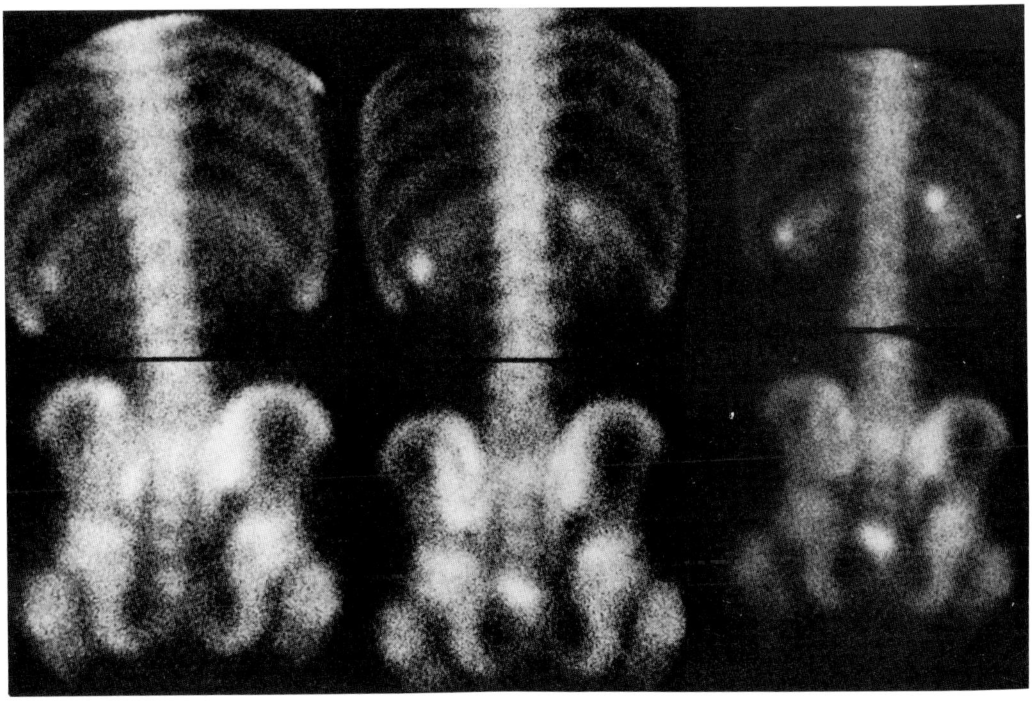

Figure 1-44. Ewing's sarcoma of the left pelvis. Shown is a series of skeletal scintiscans (Tc-99m MDP) on a 15-year-old male who presented with pain over his left iliac crest. Radiographs showed a lytic lesion in the left sacroiliac area. The initial bone scan reveals an area of diffusely increased uptake in the left iliac bone along with an apparent decrease of radiopharmaceutical uptake in the posterior aspect of the iliac bone. There is also increased uptake in the eleventh posterior left rib. Biopsy revealed Ewing's sarcoma. On the followup scintiscans, one can see the changing pattern of increased uptake in the left iliac bone after the biopsy and no new lesions.

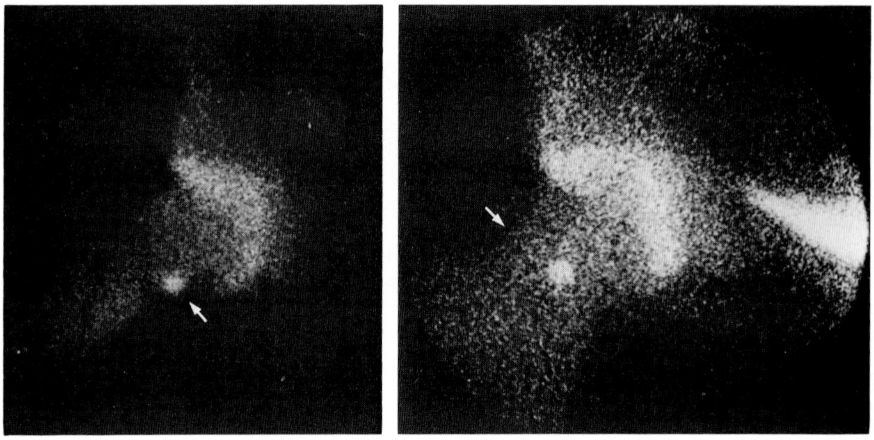

Figure 1-45. Osteoid osteoma of the posterior aspect of the right femoral neck. Images obtained with a pinhole collimator. An intense, small, well-defined area of increased uptake of Tc-99m MDP is visible on the frogleg *(left)* and anterior *(right)* scintiscans. Radiographs were normal.

fected: femora (27%); tibiae and fibulae (17%); and the humeri (9%). Among the flat bones, the pelvis was involved in 18% of the patients.[67]

The clinical and radiographic presentation of Ewing's sarcoma may mimic osteomyelitis. Both conditions may involve the metaphysis although Ewing's sarcoma is somewhat more common in the midshaft.

Currently, the 5-year survival for patients with Ewing's sarcoma treated with combinations of chemotherapy, radiation therapy, and occasionally surgery is about 75%. Unlike osteosarcoma, with which 2% of the patients have bone metastases at presentation, 11% of patients with Ewing's sarcoma present with bone metastases and another 45% develop bone metastases during the first 2 years after presentation.

Because of the importance of metastatic disease in the choice of primary and followup therapy for this tumor, bone scintigraphy should be done at presentation and at frequent intervals thereafter. The scintigraphic appearance in Ewing's sarcoma consists of intense uptake of bone seeker in the lesion[71,126] (Figs. 1-43 and 1-44).

Osteoid Osteoma

Osteoid osteoma is a benign osteoblastic lesion characterized by a well-demarcated core (nidus), usually < 1 cm in diameter, and by a distinctive surrounding zone of reactive bone formation. Pain from this lesion is accompanied by increased skin temperature in the affected region and profuse perspiration. Exquisite local tenderness can also be a striking feature. In many cases, salicylates completely relieve the symptoms. Pain is not always localized at the exact site of the lesion and it may be referred to a nearby joint. Muscle wasting, painful limping, and diminished stretch reflexes in the involved extremity may be present.

Osteoid osteoma occurs predominantly in children, adolescents, and young adults between the ages of 10 and 25 years and is rare after the age of 30 years. The youngest patient reported was 8 months old [53]; the oldest, 60 years. It is twice as common in males as in females.

Osteoid osteoma may be found in the cortex (most frequently) or the medulla of bone. Occasionally the lesion abuts the joint cartilage and, at times, may erode through it. This tumor has been known to occur in nearly every bone of the body but has a special predilection for the bones of the legs. In about half of the patients, this lesion is located in the femur or tibia. Spinal location occurs in about 10% of patients. Distal phalangeal presentation in children may result in premature closure of the epiphysis. Spinal localization has been known to cause unexplained backache and painful scoliosis in children and adults.[118] In most cases of osteoid osteoma of the spine reported in the literature, plain films usually did not demonstrate the lesion.[15,41,93] From the radiologic point of view, polytomography, computed tomography, and un-

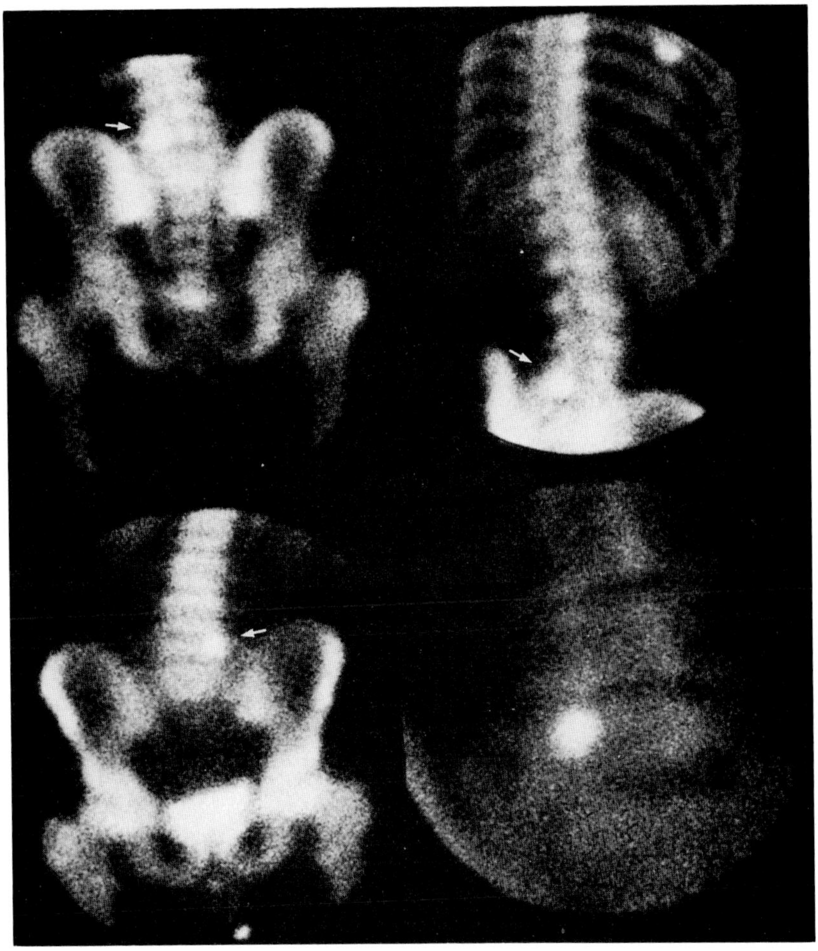

Figure 1-46. Osteoid osteoma of the spine. This 17-year-old male had had painful scoliosis for 6 months. The pain was localized to the left side of the lower back and radiated to the left knee. The pain was constant and was relieved by salicylates. Anterior lateral radiographs of the thoracolumbar spine showed mild left thoracic and right lumbar scoliosis and no soft tissue abnormality. Bone scintigraphy with Tc-99m MDP 2 days later shows a well-defined area of increased uptake on the left side of the fifth lumbar vertebra, consistent with osteoid osteoma. Tomograms showed a lytic area surrounded by a sclerotic area approximately 1.2 cm in diameter in the lamina of the vertebra.

commonly angiography may be required to pinpoint the nidus accurately.

Radiographically, osteoid osteoma frequently shows a characteristic radiolucent sphere surrounded by an exaggerated zone of sclerosis.[1] A calcified nidus may be visible in the translucent sphere. This appearance is characteristic but delays still occur in making the diagnosis.[118]

Bone scintigraphy is very useful in patients suspected of osteoid osteoma in whom the lesion is not demonstrated radiologically (Figs. 1-45 and 1-46). This is particularly important in the spine, pelvis, and femoral neck. Scintigraphy may even be performed intraoperatively in order to ensure complete removal of the lesion.[143] Imaging of the specimen using magnification scintigraphy had been used in our hospital in order to ensure that there was a margin of "normal" bone surrounding the lesion. However, intraoperative scanning using a mobile gamma camera equipped with a pinhole collimator is the recommended approach at present. The most frequent scintigraphic finding in osteoid osteoma is an intense, well-localized area of increased radiopharmaceutical uptake that may or may not be surrounded by an area of diffusely increased uptake.[44,102,139,165]

Neuroblastoma

Neuroblastoma, ganglioneuroblastoma, and ganglioneuroma arise from neural crest tissue at any site along the craniospinal axis. Their first clinical manifestations result from metastatic involvement or palpation of a large intraabdominal mass.[36,98] Most of these tumors secrete variable amounts of catecholamines or their byproducts.

The overall mortality with this tumor is high although a more favorable prognosis exists for children under 1–2 years of age. About 75% of all patients with neuroblastoma are encountered during the first 4 years of life.[4,123]

This tumor occurs in one of every 100,000 children under 15 years of age with a male:female ratio of 1.2:1.[110] Autopsies in infants under 3 months of age reveal neuroblastoma in situ in 1:200 to 1:1000 cases, suggesting that neuroblastoma may be a relatively common tumor undergoing spontaneous regression in most infants.[35] Studies of serial sections of the adrenal glands revealed in incidence of neuroblastoma in situ of 1:39.[51]

Over 55% of these tumors appear in the abdomen (over one-third in the adrenal gland) (Table 1-5). Less frequently, they appear in the chest, head and neck, and pelvis.[36] Neuroblastoma extends by local invasion and metastatic spread to the liver, bone marrow, skeleton, and intracranial dura. About 70% of children over 1 year of age and 40–50% of children under 1 year of age present with disseminated disease.

Table 1-5. Sites of Primary Neuroblastoma

Site	Frequency (%)
Abdomen	55
Adrenal	37
Nonadrenal	18
Chest	13
Neck	5
Head	2
Pelvis	4
Other	9
Unknown	12

Stages

There are five clinical stages of neuroblastoma: stage I, tumor confined to the organ of origin; stage II, tumor extending in continuity beyond organ of origin but not crossing the midline; stage III, tumor extending in continuity beyond the midline and possible regional node involvement bilaterally; stage IV, remote disease involving the skeleton, organs, soft tissue, or distant nodes; stage IVS, patients who would otherwise be stage I or II but who have remote disease confined to one or more of the following sites: liver, skin, or bone marrow (not bone).[34]

Clinical Evaluation

The clinical manifestations of neuroblastoma, especially in the very young, are abdominal swelling associated with an abdominal mass (firm, nontender, irregular). The mass is usually in one upper quadrant. Hepatomegaly may be present with liver involvement. The patient may be anemic secondary to hemorrhage into the tumor. Pain and tenderness occur in the presence of bone metastases. Tumor masses may be seen in involved superficial bones. Pancytopenia may occur with extensive involvement of the bone marrow. Skin nodules also may be present, particularly in the younger patients. Other symptoms include pain, irritability, chronic diarrhea, vomiting due to increased intracranial pressure, and possibly fever, lethargy, or anorexia. Thoracic neuroblastoma may cause dyspnea or may be found on a chest radiograph obtained for other reasons.

Evaluation of patients suspected of neuroblastoma usually requires intravenous urography, radiography of the chest, abdominal ultrasound, and hepatic and skeletal scintigraphy (Figs. 1-47–1-50). Bone marrow aspiration is done in all patients. Characteristically, these patients have high catecholamine levels in urine, particularly vanillylmandelic acid (VMA).

Scanning with Tc-99m MDP

Skeletal scintigraphy in patients with neuroblastoma is quite characteristic. Very often the bone-seeking radiopharmaceutical will concentrate in the primary tumor with varied degrees of intensity. The intensity of such uptake has not been shown to relate to the degree of malignancy or prognosis.[87,127] The uptake of Tc-99m MDP in the primary tumor appears to be more intense in the youngest patients. Even primary lesions that show no radiographic evidence of calcification may re-

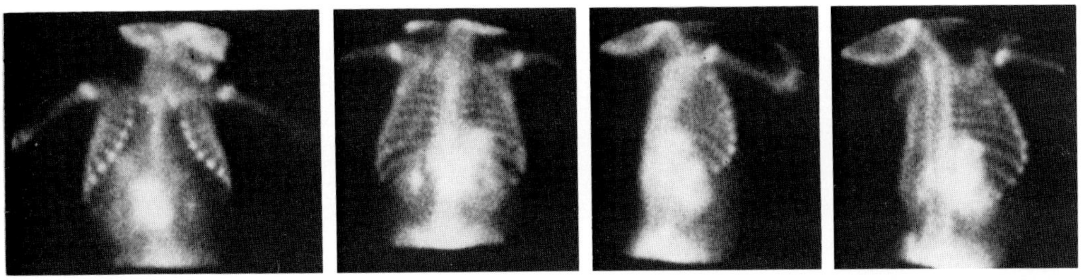

A P RLAT. RPO

Figure 1-47. Neuroblastoma, grade IV. Skeletal scintiscan of a 9-month-old girl with an abdominal mass shows intense uptake of Tc-99m MDP in the abdomen. This abnormality corresponds to the abdominal mass defined by palpation and by ultrasonography. The lesion appears to arise from the left suprarenal region, is irregular, and displaces the right kidney inferiorly and laterally. The skeleton per se appears normal, but the bone marrow aspirate was abnormal. A, Anterior view; P, posterior view; R. Lat., right lateral view; RPO, right posterior oblique view.

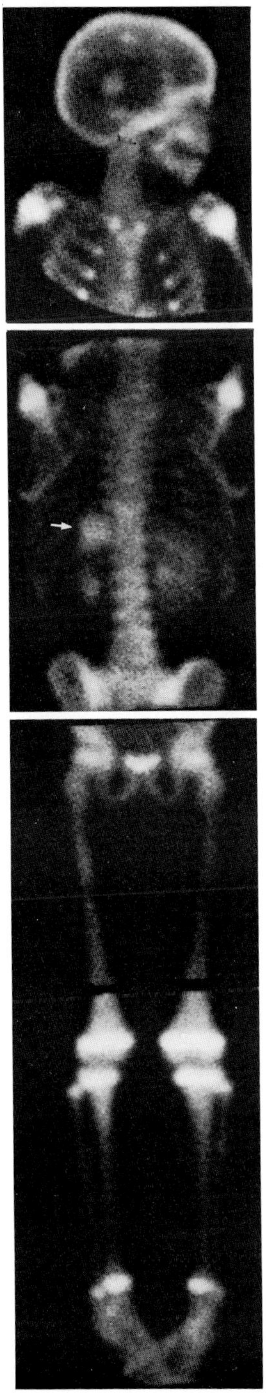

Figure 1-48. Neuroblastoma. Increased uptake of Tc-99m MDP can be seen in the primary lesion (left adrenal gland) and in bony metastases, including the skull, spine, femora, and tibiae. ▷

veal increased uptake of radiopharmaceutical. This property of Tc-99m MDP to concentrate in the primary tumor aids in defining the extent of the tumor and in detecting residual tumor (Fig. 1-47).

Skeletal scintigraphy is a sensitive detector of metastatic neuroblastoma to bone[65] and will be abnormal weeks before radiographic changes are apparent. A typical pattern of increased uptake can be seen in the proximal humeri, distal femora, and proximal tibiae. These lesions are often symmetric, and in some instances the scintiscans may be wrongly interpreted as normal, especially in the long bones. The scintiscan will also define metastatic involvement in the skull or spine (Figs. 1-48 and 1-49), and scintigraphy with Tc-99m MDP may detect associated renal abnormalities (displacement, asymmetry, obstruction).

Later in the disease, lesions of certain age that are clearly seen radiographically may not reveal increased uptake in the bone scan. Chemotherapy may reduce this abnormal uptake to such degree that the skeletal scintigram may appear normal. This normal appearance can be misleading because it does not mean that the neuroblastoma has been eradicated. We have seen recurrent increased uptake in the very same areas that had become normal a few months previously (Fig. 1-50).

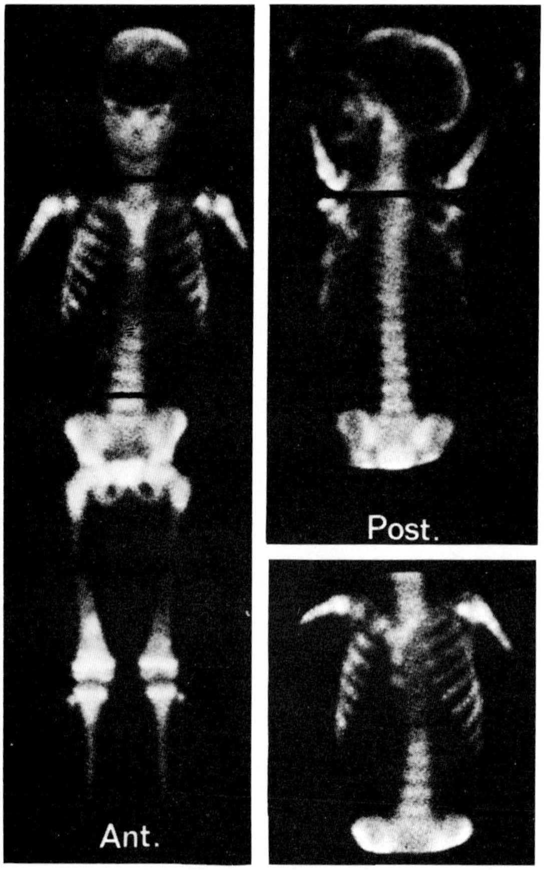

Figure 1-49. Metastatic neuroblastoma. This 5-year-old girl presented with right leg pain and intermittent fever. Workup for repeated pain revealed a lucent area in the right distal femur. Hemoglobin was 9.4 g/100 ml; hematocrit, 28%; white blood cell count, $8500/mm^3$; and platelets, 480,000. The patient at admission was febrile. A bone marrow aspirate of the left distal femur showed necrosis but not infiltrative cells. *Left:* The bone scan (Tc-99m MDP) shows multiple areas of abnormal uptake including the skull, both proximal humeri, several ribs, proximal and distal femora, and proximal tibiae. Abdominal ultrasound and intravenous pyelography were normal. A repeat bone marrow aspirate was consistent with neuroblastoma. *Below:* The bone marrow scan (Tc-99m sulfur colloid) shows multiple areas of decreased uptake suggestive of metastatic disease. Ant., Anterior view; Post., posterior view; R, right arm; L, left arm.

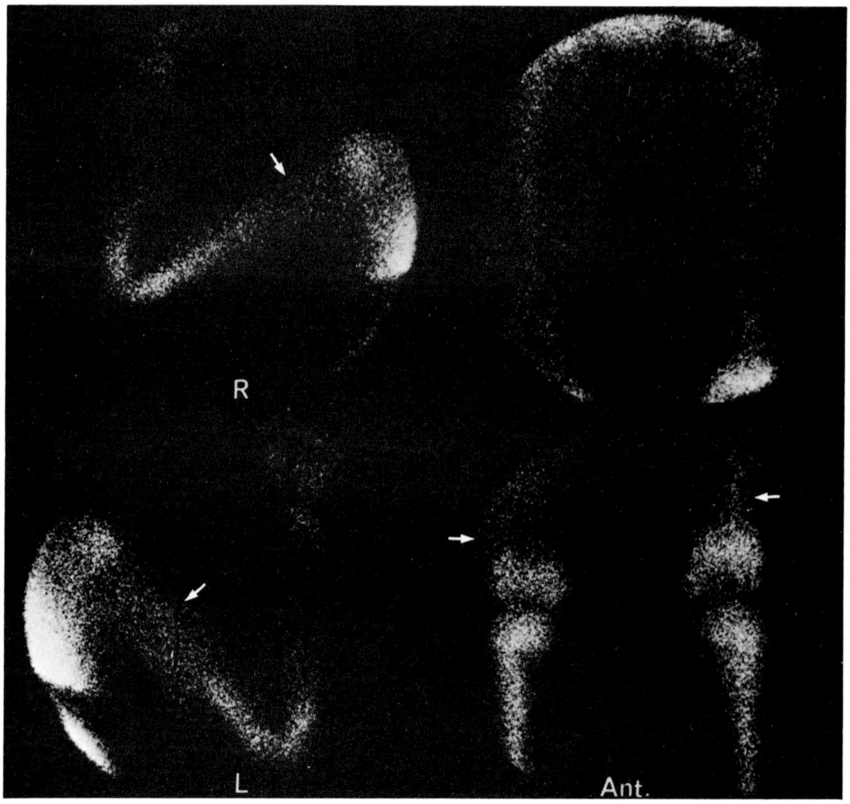

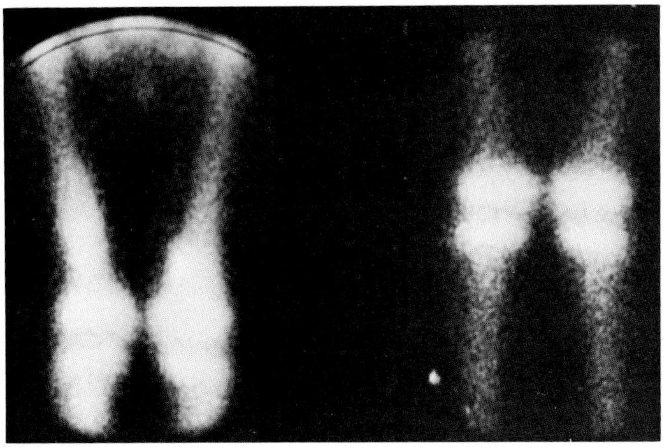

Figure 1-50. Effect of chemotherapy on metastatic neuroblastoma. Note the uptake of Tc-99m MDP by metastases in both the femora and tibiae *(left)* has become nearly normal several months after chemotherapy *(right)*. Recurrent disease appeared in the same sites a year later.

It is thus important to realize that in neuroblastoma:

1. The bone scan is useful to evaluate the extent of the primary tumor and in the early diagnosis of skeletal metastases.
2. A normal bone scan after the patient has been treated with chemotherapy is no guarantee of cure.
3. In certain lesions of advanced metastic bone disease, the bone scan may not be abnormal.

Scanning with Tc-99m Sulfur Colloid

Because metastatic involvement of the skeleton may begin in the bone marrow and then continue into the cortical bone, patients with bone marrow metastasis may have a normal bone scan early in the disease. In these patients, bone marrow scintigraphy may help to detect the bone marrow involvement. Unfortunately, only about 5% of the injected dose of Tc-99m sulfur colloid is concentrated in the bone marrow. Bone marrow imaging with this agent is thus time-consuming and results in images of relatively low information density. Because uptake of Tc-99m sulfur colloid is high in the liver and the spleen, examination of the spine and thorax is almost impossible with this agent. Bone marrow scans obtained while or after the patient has been treated with chemotherapy may be abnormal, but it may be impossible to differentiate on the scintiscan between active disease and fibrosis in the bone marrow (see Chapter 3).

Hepatic scintigraphy using Tc-99m sulfur colloid is useful in the diagnosis of hepatic involvement with neuroblastoma (see Chapter 9).

Histiocytosis

Histiocytosis is a collective term for three diseases characterized by the presence of granulomatous lesions with histiocytic proliferation: Hand-Schüller-Christian disease, Letterer-Siwe disease, and eosinophilic granuloma of bone. The wide spectrum of their clinical patterns ranges from a single lesion that grows slowly to disseminated disease that grows rapidly and is fatal (Fig. 1-51).

About 50% of the patients have lesions only in bone, most commonly the skull, legs, spine, and pelvis. Symptoms include bone pain and swelling of the involved area. Anemia and skin or mucosal eruptions may also be present. An invasive process in the hypothatamic pituitary region occasionally occurs and results in diabetes insipidus. Other patients with the disease have osseous and visceral involvement. Major visceral involvement of the liver, spleen, lungs, lymph nodes, and bone marrow is more characteristic of patients in the first year of life. Alternatively, extreme progression of the disease may be limited to one area only: lungs, lymph nodes, or liver.

Radiographic bone survey is the examination of choice to identify bone lesions in this disease.[84,120,136] A negative study may occasionally be followed by radionuclide examination in order to identify new areas of involvement. Specific diagnosis is made by biopsy.

Bone lesions in histiocytosis have a natural history of rapid growth followed by stability and eventual decrease in size. Skull lesions show this evolution most prominently.

The appearance of the bone scan is variable. When there is expansion of the marrow cavity without cortical involvement, the bone scan may be normal. Marked increase in uptake of the radiopharmaceutical is seen following pressure necrosis, in the subsequent repair phase of the disease, and in the acute phase, when the disease is in bone and periosteal stripping has occurred.[7] In one reported series, nine of ten patients with eosinophilic granuloma had abnormal scans.[44]

Review of concurrent bone scans and skeletal radiographs of 14 patients with biopsy-proven histiocytosis was carried out in our hospital to see if lesion evolution could explain reports of false-negative bone scans (i.e., normal radionuclide uptake in areas with radiographically demonstrable lesions). Our review confirmed the high false-negative rate observed by other authors: 36% of our cases had lesions radiographically but normal bone scans. We noted, however, that in patients with skull lesions, lesions with irregular edges (newer, more active lesions) were always abnormal scintigraphically while lesions with smooth edges were seldom abnormal. One patients with multiple lesions, who had serial scans and skeletal surveys, exhibited radiographic lesions without increased uptake as well as increased uptake without radiographic changes. Two of this patient's radiographic abnormalities were preceded by focally increased radionuclide uptake. Another patient had a pelvic lesion detected by bone scan after several negative radiographs. We conclude that the bone scans are more effective in detecting new lesions than old in this disease.

Leukemia

In leukemia, bone scans are obtained to establish whether bone pain is due to an infiltrative process or to osteomyelitis. Both of these conditions give rise to increased uptake of radiopharmaceuticals in the involved area. Because the cortical abnormality in leukemia is secondary to marrow involvement, bone marrow scanning may have greater value than skeletal scintigraphy. An abnormal focus of decreased activity in the bone marrow scan, when observed in association with a normal bone scan, suggests leukemic infiltration rather than infection. If the bone scan is also abnormal, however, no specific conclusion can be drawn.

Lymphoma

A malignant lymphoma of bone may occur at any age, but it is rare in the very young. In a small number of cases, there is no evidence of disease elsewhere, and the osseous lesion can be presumed to be primary. Bone scanning has been found to be a more sensitive indicator of disease than roentgenography, and marrow scanning may be more sensitive than bone scintigraphy.[44] The neoplastic process is somewhat similar to leukemia in that the bony lesion is secondary to marrow involvement (Fig. 1-52). The skeletal abnormalities may be either multicentric or solitary.

Rhabdomyosarcoma

Rhabdomyosarcoma presents as a mass, most commonly in the head and neck although it has been reported in almost every area of the body. Both sexes are affected, and the tumor occurs in all age groups. Metastases are common not only in lymph nodes, lungs, and liver but also in bone and bone marrow. Radiography usually describes the site of involvement, but radionuclide scanning may aid in defining the extent of the lesion and detecting metastatic involvement.[160] The bone scan shows nonspecific increased activity once spread has occurred (Fig. 1-53).

Fibrosarcoma

This malignant tumor does not produce osteoid material, but may show periosteal new-bone formation. The neoplastic tissue often extends beyond the lytic zone seen in the radiograph. Associated with the reactive bone formation is a marked increased in uptake of the bone agent. As mentioned previously, secondary fibrosarcoma may follow radiotherapy for another lesion; this too shows increased activity.

Wilms' Tumor

Skeletal metastases with Wilms' tumor are uncommon, but they do occur. More characteristically, skeletal metastases are seen from sarcomatous tumors in the kidney. Scintigraphically they present as foci of increased activity that are indistinguishable from the many other possible causes of a positive scan. With the longer length of survival now resulting from improved therapeutic regimens, secondary spread to bone may be seen more frequently.

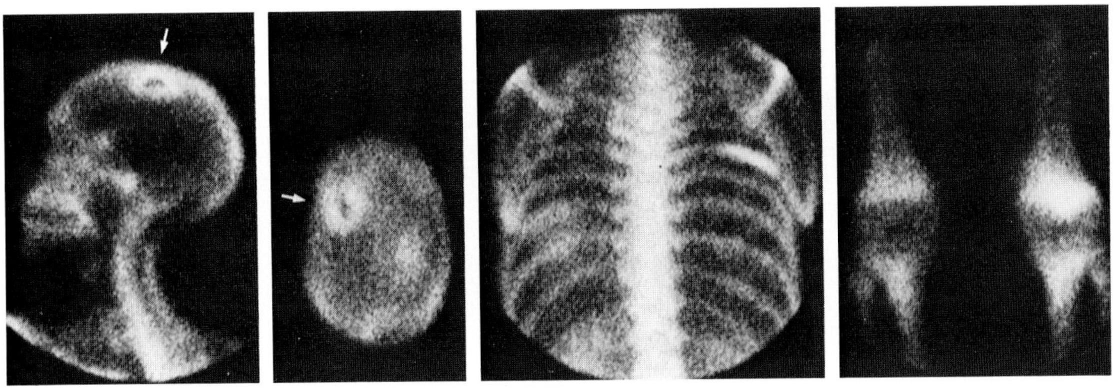

Figure 1-51. Histiocytosis. Multiple lesions of the skull, right scapula, ribs, left femur, and left tibia show increased uptake of Tc-99m MDP.

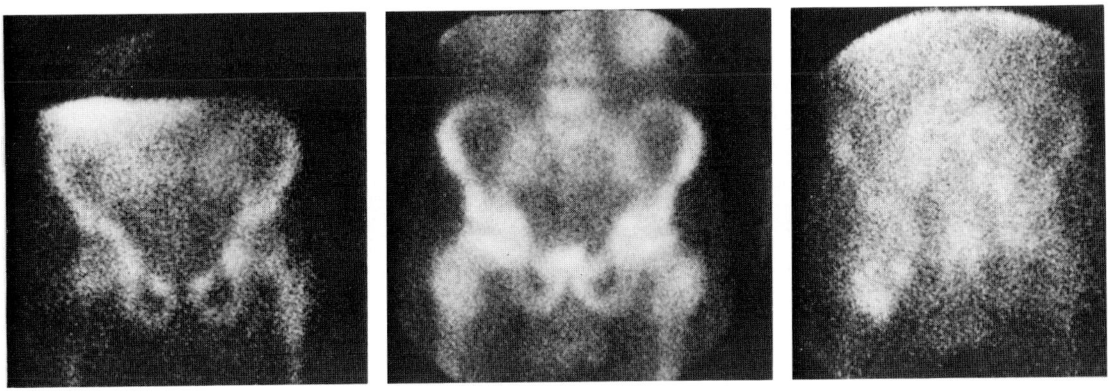

Figure 1-52. Hodgkin's lymphoma. Images obtained on a 14-year-old male with Hodgkin's disease in apparent relapse. The patient complained of leg pain. The Tc-99m sulfur-colloid bone marrow image *(left)* reveals a photon-deficient area in the right proximal femur. The Tc-99m MDP bone scan *(center)* reveals very minimal increase in uptake of radiopharmaceutical in the same region. The gallium scan *(right)* shows a marked area of radiotracer uptake in the same region plus increased uptake in the lymph nodes.

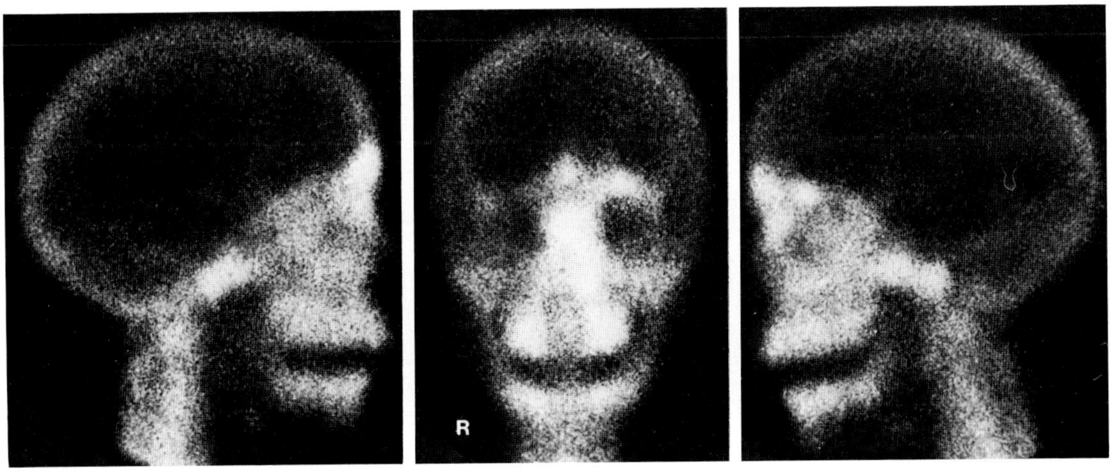

Figure 1-53. Metastatic rhabdomyosarcoma spreading to the bones around the left orbit. Scintigraphy with Tc-99m MDP. *Left:* right lateral view; *center:* anterior view; *right:* left lateral view.

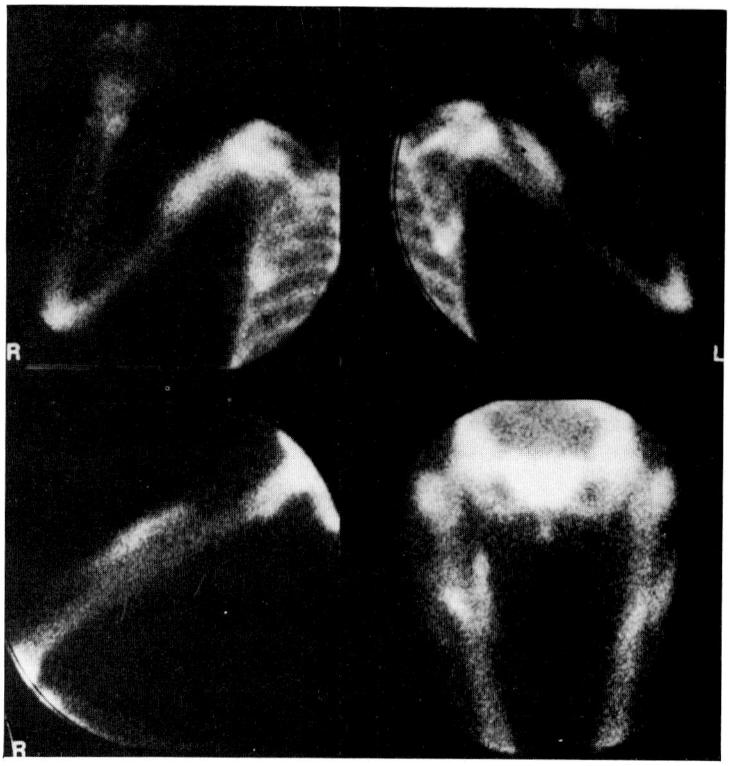

Figure 1-54. Multiple sites of extraosseous uptake of Tc-99m MDP in a patient who received multiple intramuscular injections. R, Right side; L, left side.

Extraosseous Uptake of Bone-Seeking Radiopharmaceuticals

A number of conditions may result in extraosseous concentration of bone-seeking radiopharmaceuticals (Table 1-6). Primary neuroblastoma and soft tissue metastases will frequently reveal increased radiopharmaceutical uptake on a bone scan (see section on neuroblastoma). Recent intramuscular injections of drugs such as sedatives will cause a characteristic pattern of increased uptake in the muscle(s) involved (Fig. 1-54).

Table 1-6. Extraosseous Concentration of Tc-99m Bone-Seeking Radiopharmaceuticals

1.	Neuroblastoma
2.	Recent intramuscular injection
3.	Splenic infarction in sickle-cell anemia
4.	Myocardial infarction
5.	Cerebral infarction
6.	Certain chemotherapeutic regimens. Increased renal uptake
7.	Iron overload after transfusion. Increased renal uptake
8.	Pulmonary and other soft tissue metastases in osteosarcoma and Ewing's sarcoma
9.	Ectopic calcification. Paraosteoarthropathy
10.	Necrotizing enterocolitis
11.	Renal obstruction, displacement, or toxicity

In children with sickle-cell anemia who have an infarcted spleen, the splenic silhouette may be visible on a bone scintigram performed to diagnose osteomyelitis or bone infarct (Fig. 1-55). The spleen in these children may be small, and a Tc-99m sulfur colloid scintigram will fail to highlight the organ.[38]

There is abundant literature to describe the concentration of bone-seeking technetium radiopharmaceuticals after acute myocardial infarction in adult patients. Cerebral infarction is another lesion known to concentrate Tc-99m skeletal radiopharmaceuticals avidly[37] (Fig. 1-56).

Some pulmonary metastases of osteosarcoma also concentrate these radiopharmaceuticals. In our experience only 5–15% of metastases seen on the chest radiograph are detected with conventional gamma camera scintigraphy. Detection of pulmonary metastases in osteosarcoma is carried out best at present using conventional chest roentgenograms, conventional tomography, and computed tomography. We have also observed intense

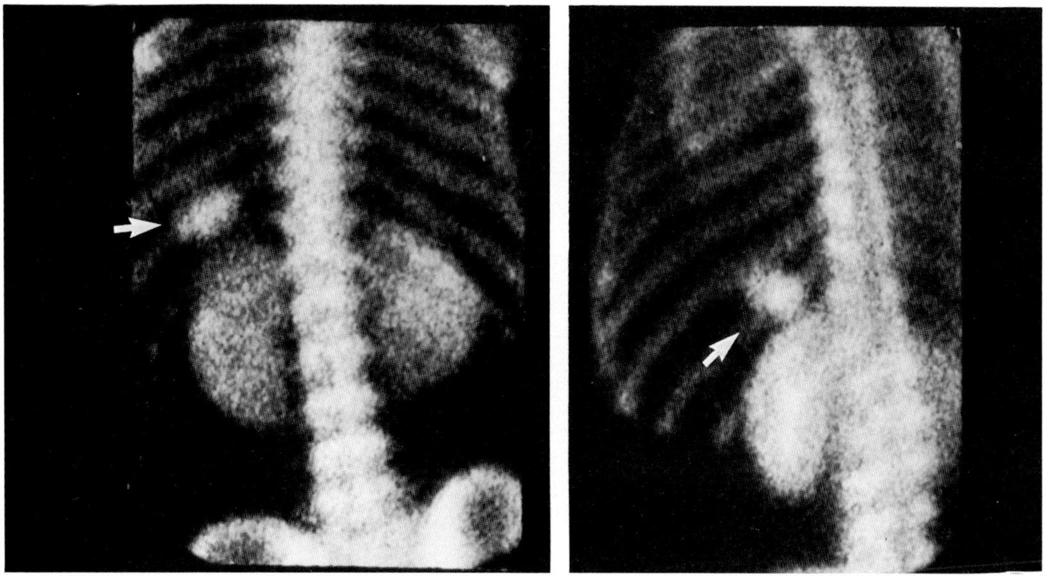

Figure 1-55. Splenic uptake of Tc-99m MDP in a patient with sickle-cell disease. *Left:* posterior view; *right:* left posterior oblique view.

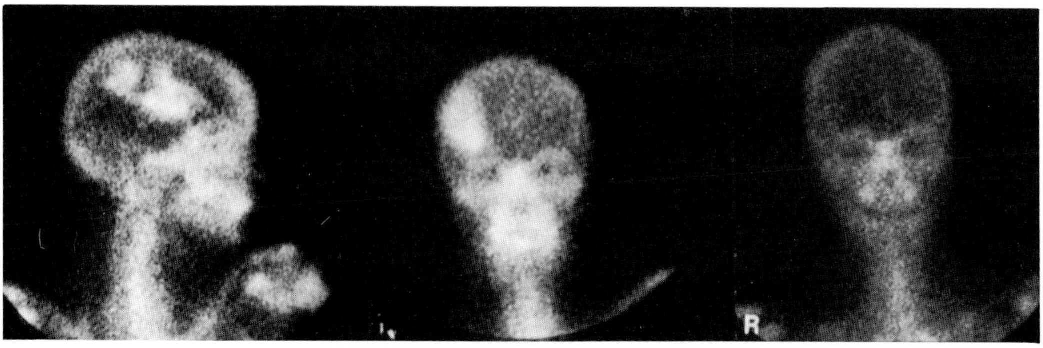

Figure 1-56. Stroke in a 15-year-old female. The right lateral and anterior view of Tc-99m MDP uptake reveal an area of intense accumulation of radiopharmaceutical in the territory of the right middle cerebral artery *(left and center)*. A followup study 4 months later *(right)* indicates normal uptake.

uptakc of radiopharmaceuticals in a patient with advanced metastatic osteosarcoma involving the pericardium. Some pulmonary and soft tissue metastases of Ewing's sarcoma may be evident on the skeletal scintigrams, but this has very little diagnostic value.

Patients who receive many blood transfusions may exhibit increased renal uptake of the bone radiotracer, probably due to the iron overload. Increased renal uptake on skeletal scintigraphy is also seen in patients under certain chemotherapeutic regimens[134] (Fig. 1-57). Occasionally skeletal scintigraphy will uncover renal disease. For example, a skeletal scintigram performed in a search for the cause of bone pain may reveal renal obstruction and nothing wrong with the skeleton. Renal displacement and ureteral obstruction due to tumors or to lack of function or agenesis of a kidney may be discovered during routine scintigraphy.

Ectopic calcification, as it occurs around the hip joints of paraplegic patients, may show intense concentration of the bone seeker during the process of calcification when the new bone is immature. As maturity is reached, the heterotopic bone forma-

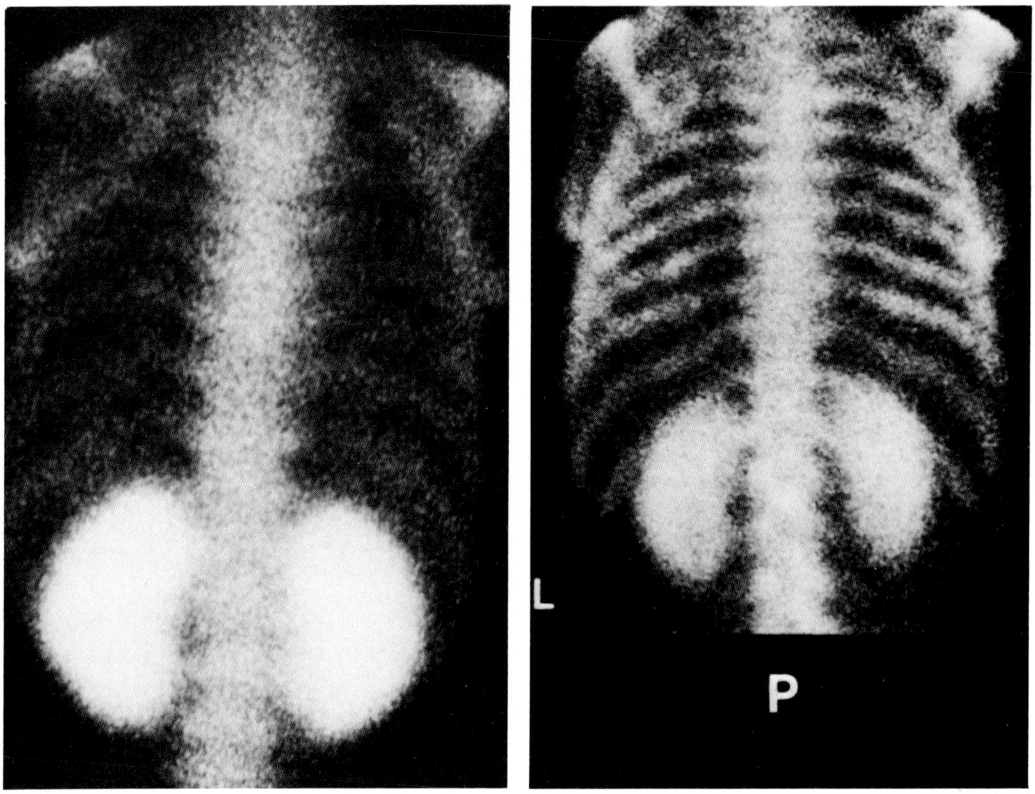

Figure 1-57. Two patients with increased renal uptake of Tc-99m MDP. *Left:* Patient during amphotericin therapy. *Right:* The second patient has leukemia. L, Left side.

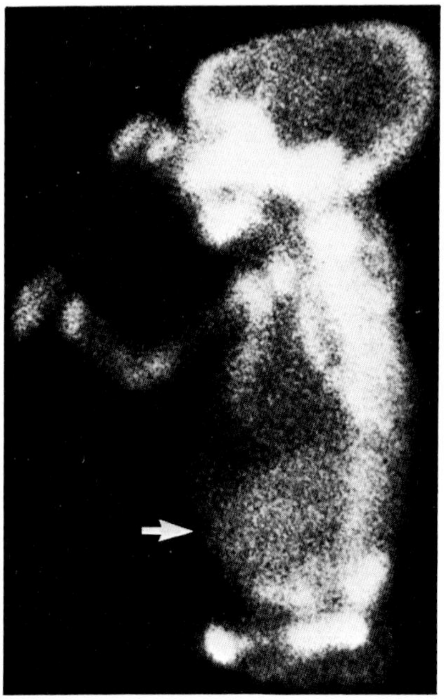

Figure 1-58. Necrotizing enterocolitis in a newborn, Tc-99m MDP. Left lateral scintiscan reveals abnormal concentration of the radiotracer in the intestine. The diagnosis was confirmed at surgery.

tion will concentrate less and less radiopharmaceutical. Serial skeletal scintigraphy has been used in paraplegic patients in order to determine the most appropriate time for surgical removal of the heterotopic calcification.[151] There appears to be a lower recurrence rate of new heterotopic bone formation if surgery is carried out when the abnormal calcification has reached maturity.

The ischemic intestine of neonates with necrotizing enterocolitis has been shown to concentrate bone-seeking radiopharmaceuticals.[133] In these neonates there is necrosis of the intestine, usually the ileum and the proximal colon but lesions may be found anywhere in the intestine. Necrotizing enterocolitis occurs in 1–2% of all premature infants and has also been found in older infants with congenital heart disease. Other predisposing factors include respiratory distress, sepsis, hypotension, and perinatal asphyxia. Vomiting, abdominal distension, gastrointestinal bleeding, and temperature instability are common. These patients have an increased white blood cell count with a deviation to the left and a decrease in platelet counts. Radiographic findings include dilated bowel loops with or without air/fluid levels, isolated unchanged bowel loop on serial examinations, pneumatosis intestinalis, and air in the portal vein or biliary tree. Abdominal scintigraphy using Tc-99m MDP or another bone seeker has been carried out in infants in whom the clinical and radiographic features of necrotizing enterocolitis are not clear (Fig. 1-58).

References

1. Aegerter E, Kirkpatrick JA. Orthopedic diseases. Physiology, pathology, radiology, 4th ed. Philadelphia: WB Saunders, 1975.
2. Ash JM, Gilday DL. The futility of bone scanning neonatal osteomyelitis: concise communication. J Nucl Med 1980; 21:417–20.
3. Atkins HL, Hauser W, Richards P. Factors affecting distribution of technetium-99m sulfur colloid. J Reticuloendothelial Soc 1970; 8:176–84.
4. Bachmann KD. Das neuroblastoma sympathicum. Klinik ude Prognose von 1030 Fallen. Kinderheilk 1962; 86:710–24.
5. Bauer GCH, Wendeberg B. External counting of ^{47}Ca and ^{85}Sr in studies of localized skeletal lesions in man. J Bone Joint Surg (Br) 1959; 41B:558–80.
6. Beamisch MR, Brown EB. A comparison of the behavior of ^{111}In and ^{59}Fe labelled transferrin on incubation with human and rat reticulocytes. Blood 1974; 43:703–11.
7. Bell EG, McAfee JG, Mahon DF. Bone scanning. In: Schneider PB, Treves S, eds. Nuclear medicine in clinical practice. Amsterdam: Elsevier, 1978.
8. Bergstedt HF. Bone scintigraphy of facial skeleton with Tc-99m disphosphonate. Acta Radiol (Diagn) 1975; 16:337–41.
9. Berkowitz ID, Wenzel W. "Normal" technetium bone scans in patients with acute osteomyelitis. Am J Dis Child 1980; 134:828–30.
10. Blair WF, Hanley SR. Stress fracture of the proximal fibula. Am J Sports Med 1980; 8:212–3.
11. Bonte FJ, Parkey RW, Graham KD, Moore J, Stokely EM. A new method for radionuclide imaging of acute myocardial infarcts. Radiology 1974; 110:473–4.
12. Bunn HF, McNeil BJ, Rosenthal DS, Krantz SB. Bone marrow imaging in pure red blood cell aplasia. Arch Intern Med 1976; 136:1169–72.
13. Burt RW, Matthews TJ. Aseptic necrosis of the knee: bone scintigraphy. AJR 1982; 138:571–3.
14. Cade S. Osteogenic sarcoma. A study based on 133 patients. J R Coll Surg Edinb 1955; 1:79–111.
15. Caldicott WJH. Diagnosis of spinal osteoid osteoma. Radiology 1969; 92:1192–5.
16. Calver R, Venugopal V, Dorgan J, Bentley G, Gimlette T. Radionuclide scanning in early diagnosis of Perthes' disease. J Bone Joint Surg (Br) 1981; 63B:379–82.
17. Capitanio MA, Kirkpatrick JA. Early roentgen observations in acute osteomyelitis. AJR 1970; 108:488–96.
18. Cavailloles F, Bok B, Bensahel H. Bone scintigraphy in the diagnosis and followup of Perthes' disease. Eur J Nucl Med 1982; 7:327–30.
19. Cheng TH, Holman BL. Radionuclide assessment of Gaucher's disease. J Nucl Med 1978; 19:1333–6.
20. Chew FS, Hudson TM. Radionuclide bone scanning of osteosarcoma: falsely extended uptake patterns. AJR 1982; 139:49–54.
21. Coley BL, Higinbotham NL, Bowden L. Endothelioma of bone (Ewing's sarcoma). Ann Surg 1948; 128:533–60.
22. Conway JJ. Radionuclide bone imaging in pediatrics. Pediatr Clin North Am 1977; 24:701–12.
23. Cortes EP, Holland JF, Wang JJ, Sinks LF. Doxorubicin in disseminated osteosarcoma. JAMA 1972; 221:1132–8.
24. Dahlin DC, Coventry MB. Osteogenic sarcoma. A study of six hundred cases. J Bone Joint Surg (Am) 1967; 49A:101–10.
25. Danigelis JA. Pinhole imaging in Legg-Calve-Perthes disease: further observations. Semin Nucl Med 1976; 6:69–82.
26. Danigelis JA, Fisher RL, Ozonoff MD, Sziklas JJ. Tc-99m polyphosphate bone imaging in Legg-Perthes disease. Radiology 1975; 115:407–13.
27. Devas MB. Stress fractures of the tibia in athletes or "shin soreness." J Bone Joint Surg (Br) 1958; 40B:227–39.
28. Devas MB. Stress fractures. London: Churchill Livingstone, 1975.
29. Dobson EL, Jones HB. Behavior of intravenously injected particulate material: its rate of disappearance from the blood stream as a measurement of liver blood flow. Acta Medica Scand (Suppl 273) 1953; 144:1–71.
30. Dobson EL, Gofman JW, Jones HB, Kelly LS, Walker LA. Studies with colloids containing radioisotopes of yttrium, zirconium, columbium and lanthanum in bone marrow, liver and spleen. J Lab Clin Med 1949; 34:305–12.
31. Erasmie U, Hirsch G. Acute haematogenous osteomyelitis in children. The reliability of skeletal scintigraphy. Z Kinderchir 1981; 32:360–6.
32. Ewing J. Diffuse endothelioma of bone. Proc NY Pathol Soc 1921; 21:17–24.
33. Ewing J. Further report on endothelial myeloma of bone. Proc NY Pathol Soc 1924; 24:93–100.
34. Evans AE, D'Angio GJ, Randolph J. A proposed

staging for children with neuroblastoma. Cancer 1971; 27:374–8.
35. Everson TC, Cole WH. Spontaneous regression of cancer: study and abstracts of reports in the world medical literature and of personal communication concerning spontaneous regression of malignant disease. Philadelphia: WB Saunders, 1966.
36. Fernbach DJ, Williams TE, Donaldson MH. Neuroblastoma. In: Sutow WW, Vietti TJ, Fernbach DJ, eds. Clinical pediatric oncology. St. Louis: CV Mosby, 1977.
37. Fischer KC, McKusick KA, Pendergrass HP, Potsaid MS. Improved brain scan specificity utilizing Tc-99m pertechnetate and Tc-99m (Sn) diphosphonate. J Nucl Med 1975; 16:705–8.
38. Fischer KC, Shapiro S, Treves S. Visualization of the spleen with a bone-seeking radionuclide in a child with sickle-cell anemia. Radiology 1977; 122:398.
39. Fisher RL, Roderique JW, Brown DC, Danigelis JA, Ozonoff MB, Sziklas JJ. The relationship of isotopic bone imaging findings to prognosis in Legg-Perthes disease. Clin Orthop 1980; 150:23–29.
40. Fordham EW, Ramachandran PC. Radionuclide imaging of osseous trauma. Semin Nucl Med 1974; 4:411–29.
41. Freiberger RH. Osteoid osteoma of the spine. A cause of backache and scoliosis in children and young adults. Radiology 1960; 75:232–6.
42. Gelfand JJ, Silberstein EB. Radionuclide imaging: use in diagnosis of osteomyelitis in children. JAMA 1977; 237:245–7.
43. Geslien GE, Thrall JH, Espinosa JE, Older RA. Early detection of stress fractures using Tc-99m polyphosphate. Radiology 1976; 121:638–7.
44. Gilday DL, Ash JM, Benign bone tumors. Semin Nucl Med 1976; 6:33–46.
45. Glass AG, Fraumeni JF. Epidemiology of bone cancer in children. J Natl Cancer Inst 1970; 44:187–99.
46. Goldstein H, Treves S. Bone scintigraphy of osteoid osteoma: a clinical review. Clin Nucl Med 1978; 3:359–63.
47. Goldstein H, McNeil BJ, Zufall E, Treves S. Is there still a place for bone scanning in Ewing's sarcoma? J Nucl Med 1980; 21:10–12.
48. Goldstein H, McNeil BJ, Zufall E, Jaffe N, Treves S. Changing indications for bone scintigraphy in patients with osteosarcoma. Radiology 1980; 135:177–80.
49. Greyson ND, Pang S. The variable bone scan appearances of nonosteogenic fibroma of bone. Clin Nucl Med 1981; 6:242–5.
50. Greenberg ML, Atkins HL, Schifer LM. Erythropoietic and reticuloendothelial function in bone marrow in dogs. Science 1966; 152:526–8.
51. Guin GH, Gilbert EF, Jones B. Incidental neuroblastoma in infants. Am J Clin Pathol 1969; 51:126–36.
52. Haase JM, Sfakianakis GN, Lobe TE, Boles ET. Prospective evaluation of radionuclide scanning in detection of intestinal necrosis in neonatal necrotizing enterocolitis. J Pediatr Surg 1981; 16:241–5.
53. Habermann ET, Stern RE. Osteoid osteoma of the tibia in an eight month old boy. A case report. J Bone Joint Surg (Am) 1974; 56A:633–6.
54. Handmaker H. Acute hematogenous osteomyelitis: has the bone scan betrayed us? Radiology 1980; 135:787–9.
55. Handmaker H, Giammona ST. The "hot joint"—increased diagnostic accuracy using combined ^{99m}Tc-phosphate and ^{67}Ga-citrate imaging in pediatrics. J Nucl Med 1976; 17:554.
56. Handmaker H, Leonards R. The bone scan in inflammatory osseous disease. Semin Nucl Med 1976; 6:95–105.
57. Harcke HT. Bone imaging in infants and children: a review. J Nucl Med 1978; 19:324–9.
58. Hayles AB, Dahlin DC, Coventry MB. Osteogenic sarcoma in children. JAMA 1960; 174:1174–7.
59. Heyman S, Davis MA, Shulkin PA, Treves S. Biologic evaluation of radiocolloids for bone marrow scintigraphy. In: Radiopharmaceuticals II. Proceedings of the 2nd International Symposium on Radiopharmaceuticals. New York: Society of Nuclear Medicine, 1979.
60. Heyman S, Goldstein HA, Crowley W, Treves S. The scintigraphic evaluation of hip pain in children. Clin Nucl Med 1980; 5:109–15.
61. Hildebrand ZC. Über das rubulare Angiosarkom oder Endotheliom des Knochens. Dtsch Z Chir 1890; 31:262–81.
62. Hoffer P. Gallium and infection. J Nucl Med 1980; 21:484–8.
63. Horn NL, Bennett LR, Marciano D. Evaluation of aplastic anemia with indium chloride In-111 scanning. Arch Intern Med 1980; 140:1299–1303.
64. Hosain, FH, McIntyre PA, Poulouse K, Sterk HS, Wagner HN. Binding of trace amounts of ionic indium-113 to plasma transferrin. Clin Chim Acta 1969; 24:69–75.
65. Howman-Giles RB, Gilday DL, Ash JM. Radionuclide skeletal survey in neuroblastoma. Radiology 1979; 131:497–502.
66. Humphry A, Gilday DL, Brown RG. Bone scintigraphy in chondroblastoma. Radiology 1980; 137:497–9.
67. Huvos A. Bone tumors. Diagnosis, treatment and prognosis. Philadelphia: WB Saunders, 1979.
68. Jaffe N. Osteogenic sarcoma. State of the art with

high-dose methotrexate treatment. Clin Orthop 1976; 120:95–102.
69. Jaffe N, Frei E. Osteogenic sarcoma: advances in treatment. CA 1976; 26:351–9.
70. Jaffe N, Frei E, Traggis D, Bishop Y. Adjuvant methotrexate and citrovorum-factor treatment of osteogenic sarcoma. N Engl J Med 1974; 291:994–7.
71. Jaffe N, Traggis D, Sallan S, Cassady R. Improved outlook for Ewing's sarcoma with combination chemotherapy (vincristine, actinomycin D and cyclophosphamide) and radiation therapy. Cancer 1976; 38:1925–30.
72. Jaffe N, Murray J, Traggis D, Cassady JR, Filler RM, Watts H, Weichselbaum R, Weinstein H. Multidisciplinary treatment for childhood sarcoma. Am J Surg 1977; 133:405–13.
73. Jaffe N, Traggis D, Cassady JR, Filler RM, Watts H, Frei E. The role of high-dose methotrexate with citrovorum factor "rescue" in the treatment of osteogenic sarcoma. Int J Radiat Oncol Biol Phys 1977; 2:261–6.
74. Javadpour N, Woltering EA, Brennan MF. Adrenal neoplasms. Curr Probl Surg 1980; 17:1–52.
75. Jeffcoat MK, McNeil BJ, Davis MA. Indium and iron as tracers for erythroid precursors. J Nucl Med 1978; 19:496–500.
76. Johnson LC, Stradford HT, Geis RW, Dineen JR, Kerley E. Histogenesis of stress fractures. J Bone Joint Surg (Am) 1963; 45A:1542.
77. Jones DC, Cady RB. "Cold" bone scans in acute osteomyelitis. J Bone Joint Surg (Br) 1981; 63B:376–8.
78. Jonsater S. Coxa plana. A histo-pathologic and arthrografic study. Acta Orthop Scand 1953; (Suppl XII):1–98.
79. Kallfelz FA, Subramanian G, Blair RJ, McAfee JG. Long term retention of ^{95m}Tc after administration of labeled polyphosphate, diphosphonate, and pertechnetate (TcO_4^-) in dogs. J Nucl Med 1973; 14:414–5.
80. Keeley K, Buchanan GR. Acute infarction of long bones in children with sickle cell anemia. J Pediatr 1982; 101:170–5.
81. Kemshead JT, Black J. Developments in the biology of neuroblastoma: implications for diagnosis and treatment. Dev Med Chil Neurol 1980; 22:816–29.
82. Khuri FJ, Alton DJ, Hardy BE, Cook GT, Churchill BM. Adrenal hemorrhage in neonates: report of 5 cases and review of the literature. J Urol 1980; 124:684–7.
83. Kirks DR, McCook TA, Merten DF, Sullivan DC. The value of radionuclide bone imaging in selected patients with osteogenic sarcoma metastatic to lung. Pediatr Radiol 1980; 9:139–43.
84. Kumar R, Balachandran S. Relative roles of radionuclide scanning and radiographic imaging in eosinophilic granuloma. Clin Nucl Med 1980; 5:538–42.
85. LaMont RL, Muz J, Heilbronner D, Bouwhuis JA. Quantitative assessment of femoral head involvement in Legg-Calve-Perthes disease. J Bone Joint Surg (Am) 1981; 63A:746–52.
86. Lavender JP, Loew J, Barker JR, Burn JI, Chaudhri MA. Gallium-67 citrate scanning in neoplastic inflammatory lesions. Br J Radiol 1971; 44:361–6.
87. Levinson ED, Spencer RP. Radionuclide and ultrasound images as potential prognostic indicators in neuroblastoma. Invest Radiol 1981; 16:373.
88. Lilien DL, Berger HG, Anderson DP, Bennett LR. ^{111}In chloride: a new agent for bone marrow imaging. J Nucl Med 1973; 14:184–6.
89. Lisbona R, Rosenthall L. Observations on the sequential use of Tc-99m-phosphate complex and Ga-67 imaging in osteomyelitis, cellulitis and septic arthritis. Radiology 1977; 123:123–9.
90. Littenberg RL, Taketa RM, Alazraki NP. Gallium-67 for localization of septic lesions. Ann Intern Med 1973; 79:403–6.
91. Lucie RS, Fuller S, Burdick DC, Johnston RM. Early prediction of avascular necrosis of the femoral head following femoral neck fractures. Clin Orthop 1981; (161):207–14.
92. Lucke A. Beitrage zur Geschwulstlehre. Virchows Arch (Pathol Anat) 1866; 35:524–39.
93. MacLellan DI, Wilson FC. Osteoid osteoma of the spine. J Bone Joint Surg (Am) 1967; 49A:111–21.
94. Markwald VA. Ein fall von multiplem intravascularem Endotheliom in den gesammten Knochen des Skelets (Myelom, Angiosarcom). Virchows Arch (Pathol Anat) 1895; 141:128–52.
95. Martindale AW, Papadimitriou JM, Turner JH. Technetium-99m antimony colloid for bone marrow imaging. J Nucl Med 1980; 21:1035–41.
96. Marty R, Denney J, McKamey MR, Rowley MJ. Bone trauma and related benign disease: assessment by bone scanning. Semin Nucl Med 1976; 6:107–20.
97. Matin P. The appearance of bone scans following fractures, including immediate and long-term studies. J Nucl Med 1979; 20:1227–31.
98. Mauer AM. Neuroblastoma. In: Vaughan VC, McKay RJ, Behrman RE, eds. Nelson's textbook of pediatrics. Philadelphia: WB Saunders, 1979.
99. Maurer AH, Chen DCP, Camargo EE, Wong DF, Wagner HN Jr, Alderson PO. Utility of three-phase skeletal scintigraphy in suspected osteomyelitis: concise communication. J Nucl Med 1981; 22:941–9.
100. McAffee JG, Subramanian G. Radioactive colloids. In: Freeman LM, Johnson PM, eds. Clinical

scintillation imaging, 2nd ed. New York: Grune & Stratton, 1975.

101. McAffee JG, Subramanian G, Aburano T, Thomas FD, Fernandez P, Gagne G, Lyons B, Zapf-Long C. A new formulation of Tc-99m minimicroaggregated albumin for marrow imaging: comparison with other colloids, In-111 and Fe-59. J Nucl Med 1982; 23:21–28.
102. McCombs RK, Olson WH. Positive ^{18}F bone scan in a case of osteoid osteoma: case report. J Nucl Med 1975; 16:465–6.
103. McIntyre PA, Larson M, Eikman EA, Colman M, Scheffel U, Hodkinson BA. Comparison of metabolism of iron-labeled transferrin (Fe-TF) and indium-labeled transferrin (In-TF) by erythropoietic marrow. J Nucl Med 1974; 15:856–62.
104. McKillop JH, Etcubanas E, Goris ML. The indications for and limitations of bone scintigraphy in osteogenic sarcoma: a review of 55 patients. Cancer 1981; 48:1133–8.
105. McNeil BJ, Cassady JR, Geiser CF, Jaffe N, Traggis D, Treves S. Fluorine-18 bone scintigraphy in children with osteosarcoma or Ewing's sarcoma. Radiology 1973; 109:627–31.
106. McNeil BJ, Holman BL, Button LN, Rosenthal DS. Use of indium chloride scintigraphy in patients with myelofibrosis. J Nucl Med 1974; 15:647–51.
107. McNeil BJ, Rappeport JM, Nathan DG. Indium chloride scintigraphy—an index of severity in patients with aplastic anemia. Br J Haematol 1976; 34:599–604.
108. Merrick MV, Gordon-Smith EC, Lavender JP, Szur L. A comparison of ^{111}In and ^{52}Fe and ^{99m}Tc sulfur colloid for bone marrow scanning. J Nucl Med 1975; 16:66–68.
109. Meurman KOA, Elfving S. Stress fracture in soldiers: multifocal bone disorder; comparative radiologic and scintigraphic study. Radiology 1980; 134:483–7.
110. Miller RW, Fraumeni JF, Hill JA. Neuroblastoma: epidemiologic approach to its origin. Am J Dis Child 1968; 115:253–61.
111. Mills GQ, Marymont JH, Murphy DA. Bone scan utilization in the differential diagnosis of exercise-induced lower extremity pain. Clin Orthop 1980; (149):207–10.
112. Murray IP. Bone scanning in the child and young adult. Part I. Skeletal Radiol 1980; 5:1–14.
113. Murray IP. Bone scanning in the child and young adult. Part II. Skeletal Radiol 1980; 5:65–76.
114. Murray IP. Photopenia in skeletal scintigraphy of suspected bone and joint infection. Clin Nucl Med 1982; 7:13–20.
115. Najean Y, Le Danvic M, Le Mercier N, Pecking A, Colonna P, Rain JD. Significance of bone marrow scintigraphy in aplastic anemia. J Nucl Med 1980; 21:213–8.
116. Nance FL, Fonseca RJ, Burkes EJ Jr. Technetium bone imaging as an adjunct in the management of fibrous dysplasia. Oral Surg 1980; 50:199–206.
117. Nelson HT, Taylor A. Bone scanning in the diagnosis of acute osteomyelitis. Eur J Nucl Med 1980; 5:267–9.
118. Omojola MF, Cockshott WP, Beatty EG. Osteoid osteoma: an evaluation of diagnostic modalities. Clin Radiol 1981; 32:199–204.
119. Oseas RS, Siddiqui AR, Wellman HN, Baehner RL. Usefulness of bone marrow imaging in childhood malignancies. J Pediatr 1982; 101:206–9.
120. Parker BR, Pinckney L, Etcubanas E. Relative efficacy of radiographic and radionuclide bone surveys in the detection of the skeletal lesions of histiocytosis X. Radiology 1980; 134:377–80.
121. Parkey RW, Bonte FJ, Meyer SL, Atkins JM, Curry GL, Stokely EM, Willerson JT. A new method for radionuclide imaging of acute myocardial infarction in humans. Circulation 1974; 50:540–6.
122. Pauwels EKJ, TeVelde J, Hermans J, Haak HL, Jurgens PJ. ^{111}Indium chloride bone marrow scintigraphy in aplastic anemia. Scand J Haematol 1981; 26:81–90.
123. Peterson DR, Bill AH Jr, Kirkland IS. Neuroblastoma trends in time. J Pediatr Surg 1969; 4:244–9.
124. Pope TL, Teague WG, Kossack R, Bray ST, Flannery DB. Pseudomonas sacroiliac osteomyelitis: diagnosis by gallium citrate Ga-67 scan. Am J Dis Child 1982; 136:649–50.
125. Rain JD, Castro-Malaspina H, Dresch C, Najean Y. Scintigraphie medullair dans les anemies per default de production. Nouv Presse Med 1975; 4:1471–6.
126. Rosen C, Caparros B, Mosende C, McCormic B, Huvos AG, Marcove RC. Curability of Ewing's sarcoma and considerations for future therapeutic trials. Cancer 1978; 41:888–9.
127. Rosenfield N, Treves S. Osseous and extraosseous uptake of flourine-18 and technetium-99m polyphosphate in children with neuroblastoma. Radiology 1974; 111:127–133.
128. Roub LW, Gumerman LW, Hanley EN, Williams CM, Goodman M, Herbert DL. Bone stress: radionuclide imaging perspective. Radiology 1979; 132:431–8.
129. Saba TM, Blumenstock FA, Weber P, Kaplan JE. Physiologic role of cold insoluble globulin in host defense: implications of its characterization as an opsonic 2-surface-binding glycoprotein. Ann New York Acad Sci 1978; 312:43–55.

130. Sanchis M, Zahir A, Freeman MAR. The experimental simulation of Perthes disease by consecutive interruptions of the blood supply to the capital femoral epiphysis in the puppy. J Bone Joint Surg (Am) 1973; 55A:335–42.
131. Saunders AJ, El Sayed TF, Hilson AJW, Maisely MN, Grahame R. Stress lesions of the lower leg and foot. Clin Radiol 1979; 30:649–51.
132. Savoca C. Stress fractures, a classification of the earliest radiographic signs. Radiology 1971; 100:519–24.
133. Sfakianakis GN, Ortiz VN, Haase GM, Boles ET. Tc-99m diphosphonate abdominal imaging in necrotizing enterocolitis: a prospective study (abstract). J Nucl Med 1978; 19:691.
134. Siddiqui AR. Increased uptake of technetium-99m-labeled bone imaging agents in the kidneys. Semin Nucl Med 1982; 12:101–2.
135. Siddiqui AR, Oseas RS, Wellman HN, Doerr DR, Baehner RL. Evaluation of bone marrow scanning with technetium-99m sulfur colloid in pediatric oncology. J Nucl Med 1979; 20:379–86.
136. Siddiqui AR, Tashjian JH, Lazarus K, Wellman HN, Baehner RL. Nuclear medicine studies in evaluation of skeletal lesions in children with histiocytosis X. Radiology 1981; 140:787–9.
137. Siddiqui AR, Cohen M, Moran DP. Usefulness of dynamic renal and static bone imaging after single foot injection of Tc-99m methylene diphosphonate (MDP) in children with abdominal masses. Twenty-fifth Annual Meeting of the Society for Pediatric Radiology, May 7–9, 1982, New Orleans, LA.
138. Sinks LF, Mindell ER. Chemotherapy of osteosarcoma. Clin Orthop 1975; (111):101–4.
139. Smith FW, Gilday DL. Scintigraphic appearances of osteoid osteoma. Radiology 1980; 137:191–5.
140. Snapper I. Bone disease in medical practice. New York: Grune & Stratton, 1957.
141. Spencer RP, Levinson ED, Baldwin RD, Sziklas JJ, Witek JT, Rosenberg R. Diverse bone scan abnormalities in shin splints. J Nucl Med 1979; 20:1271–2.
142. Staub RT, Gaston E. ^{111}In chloride distribution and kinetics in hematologic disease. J Nucl Med 1973; 14:456–7.
143. Sty J, Simons G. Intraoperative 99m technetium bone imaging in the treatment of benign osteoblastic tumors. Clin Orthop 1982; (165):223–7.
144. Subramanian G, McAfee JG, Bell EG, Blair RJ, O'Mara RE, Ralston PH. ^{99m}Tc-labeled polyphosphate as a skeletal imaging agent. Radiology 1972; 102:701–4.
145. Suit HD. Radiotherapy in osteosarcoma. Clin Orthop 1975; (111):71–75.
146. Sullivan DC, Rosenfield NS, Ogden J, Gottschalk A. Problems in the scintigraphic detection of osteomyelitis in children. Radiology 1980; 135:731–6.
147. Sutherland AD, Savage JP, Paterson DC, Foster BK. The nuclide bone scan in the diagnosis and management of Perthes' disease. J Bone Joint Surg (Br) 1980; 62B:300–6.
148. Sutow WW, Sullivan MP, Fernbach DJ, Cangir A, George SL. Adjuvant chemotherapy in primary treatment of osteogenic sarcoma. A Southwest Oncology Group study. Cancer 1975; 36:1598–1602.
149. Sutow WW, Gehan EA, Vietti TJ, Frias AE, Dyment PG. Multidrug chemotherapy in primary treatement of osteosarcoma. J Bone Joint Surg (Am) 1976; 58A:629–33.
150. Sweetnam R. The surgical management of primary osteosarcoma. Clin Orthop 1975; (111):57–64.
151. Tanaka T, Rossier AB, Hussey RW, Ahnberg DS, Treves S. Quantitative assessment of para-osteoarthropathy and its maturation on serial radionuclide bone images. Radiology 1977; 123:217–221.
152. Tow DE, Garcia DA, Jansons D, Sullivan TM, Niederman R. Bone scan in dental diseases. J Nucl Med 1978; 19:845–7.
153. Treves S. Skeletal scintigraphy in the diagnosis of acute osteomyelitis. Hosp Pract 1979; 14:66–73.
154. Treves S, Khettry J, Broker FH, Wilkinson RH, Watts H. Osteomyelitis: early scintigraphic detection in children. Pediatrics 1976; 57:173–86.
155. Truenta J. The normal vascular anatomy of the human femoral head during growth. J Bone Joint Surg (Br) 1957; 39B:358–94.
156. Valimaki M, Vuopio P, Liewendahl K. Bone lesions in chronic myelogenous leukaemia. Acta Med Scand 1981; 210:403–8.
157. Waldvogel FA, Medoff G, Swartz MN. Osteomyelitis: a review of clinical features, therapeutic considerations and unusual aspects. Part I. N Engl J Med 1970; 287:198–206.
158. Waldvogel FA, Medoff G, Swartz MN. Osteomyelitis: a review of clinical features, therapeutic considerations and unusual aspects. Part II. N Engl J Med 1970; 282:260–6.
159. Waldvogel FA, Medoff G, Swartz MN. Osteomyelitis: a review of clinical features, therapeutic considerations and unusual aspects. Part III. N Engl J Med 1970; 282:316–22.
160. Weinblatt ME, Miller JH. Radionuclide scanning in children with rhabdomyosarcoma. Med Pediatr Oncol 1981; 9:293–301.

161. Wilcox JR, Moniot AL, Green JP. Bone scanning in the evaluation of exercise related stress injuries. Radiology 1977; 123:699–703.
162. Willerson JT, Parkey RW, Bonte FJ, Meyer SL, Atkins JM, Stokely EM. Technetium stannous pyrophosphate myocardial scintigrams in patients with chest pain of varying etiology. Circulation 1975; 51:1046–52.
163. Willerson JT, Parkey RW, Bonte FJ, Meyer SL, Stokely EM. Acute subendocardial myocardial infarction in patients: its detection by technetium-99m stannous pyrophosphate myocardial scintigrams. Circulation 1975; 51:436–41.
164. Wilson E. Stress fractures. Radiology 1969; 92:481–6.
165. Winter PF, Johnson PM, Hilal SK, Feldman F. Scintigraphic detection of osteoid osteoma. Radiology 1977; 122:177–8.

Chapter 2 Skeletal Scintigraphy for Assessment of Mandibular Growth and Asymmetry

Leonard B. Kaban
S. T. Treves

General Considerations

Treatment of the adult patient with a facial deformity consists of three-dimensional analysis of the anomaly and planning of the operative correction. Treatment of the pediatric patient, on the other hand, requires consideration of a fourth dimension: growth. Assessment of skeletal growth is crucial, because the purpose of treatment is not only to correct the presenting defect, but also to unlock growth potential and to minimize secondary distortion of adjacent structures.[8,11]

Currently, facial growth is evaluated by the following methods:

1. Serial observation, correlating the patient's chronologic age with growth history (e.g., height, weight, head circumference, changes in occlusion).
2. Radiographs of the hand and wrist bones to compare their skeletal maturation with known age-adjusted standards.
3. Superimposition of serial cephalograms, the most direct method of assessing facial growth.

These techniques, however, measure only the results of past growth; they provide little information about dynamics of growth. Serial cephalograms have been used to document rate of growth, but during the observation period, deformity may worsen and longitudinal data may not be available for all patients. Prediction of facial skeletal maturity on the basis of a hand and wrist radiograph is often inaccurate; the mandible may continue to grow after the hand has matured. A physiologic or dynamic method of facial growth analysis would therefore be a major advance in the diagnosis and treatment of cranio-maxillofacial deformities.

Skeletal scintigraphy is an ideal method to measure growth dynamics because uptake of radiopharmaceutical depends on blood flow[7] and may also be related to bone formation and remodeling.[6] In the past, scintigraphy was used as a qualitative, morphologic method to document differences in uptake between two sides of the mandible in asymmetric patients.[5] However, normal age-adjusted uptake values were not established for the mandible and there was no objective method of differentiating normal versus abnormal side. We have begun to establish normal age-adjusted uptake values for technetium-99m methylene diphosphonate (Tc-99m MDP) in the human mandible.[2,9] In addition, studies using Sprague-Dawley rats[2] have demonstrated that radiopharmaceutical uptake is a sensitive indicator of growth changes in the rat mandible. This work documented that uptake changes varied not only with size of the mandibular region but also with change in length and weight per unit time, i.e., growth rate.

Computerized skeletal scintigraphy is potentially applicable for analysis of other bones in the craniofacial skeleton, such as the maxilla, nose, zygoma, and calvaria. It may be useful for assessment of craniosynostosis and the effects of prematurely fused sutures on cranial and facial growth. Normal uptake patterns, however, must be established before these other bones can be studied. Skeletal scintigraphy may also be useful for eval-

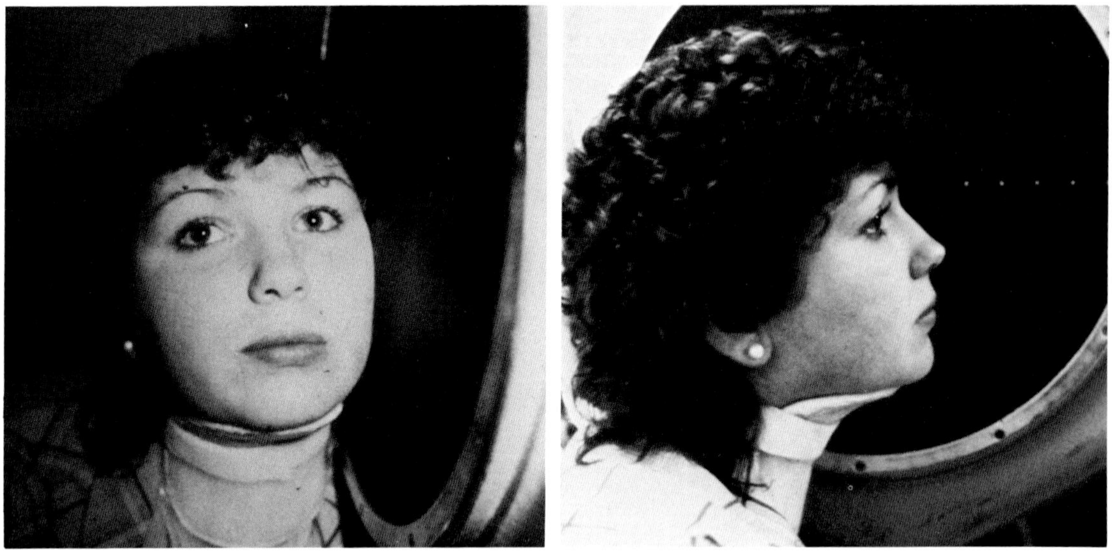

Figure 2-1. Plastic head holder hyperextends neck so that mandibular rami and condyles are not superimposed on cervical spine.

uation of long bone growth, if normal uptake patterns are established.

The most important advantage of skeletal scintigraphy is its ability to obtain physiologic information on growth dynamics with one observation. The technique is reproducible by the same examiner and by two different examiners.[2] Head position is not as critical as it is in cephalometrics, because scintigraphy is a quantitative measure of radioactivity in a given bone mass and not a morphologic representation of the facial skeleton.

Radiopharmaceuticals, Method of Examination, and Analysis

A dose of 200 μCi/kg of Tc-99m MDP is administered and imaging of the mandible is performed 2–4 h later. The gamma camera is equipped with a high-resolution collimator. The patient's head is positioned in front of the gamma camera with the neck hyperextended to separate the mandibular ramus and the cervical spine. The mandibular body is in contact with the camera; a positioner is useful to obtain reproducible alignment of the head (Fig. 2-1). Right and left mandibular views and an image of the posterior lumbar spine are obtained. All images are recorded on the computer, for a minimum of 200,000 counts each, on a 128×128 matrix format. Arbitrarily, we use the activity from a region of interest (ROI) over the fourth vertebral body as a standard.

ROIs are outined over the images of the condyles, ramus, body, and fourth lumbar vertebra (Fig. 2-2). Another region, lateral to that of the fourth vertebra, is marked for correction of background activity. The average number of counts per pixel in each ROI is determined and a ratio of uptake *(RU)* of each mandibular region (condyle, body, ramus) to the fourth lumbar vertebra is calculated:

$$RU = \frac{\text{Counts in ROI of mandible} - \text{background counts}}{\text{Counts in fourth lumbar vertebra} - \text{background counts}}$$

All radiopharmaceutical uptake results are reported as an *RU* of the ROI to the fourth lumbar vertebra.[9] Use of the ratio is necessary to normalize changes in uptake, decay, and clearance between patients.

Clinical Applications

Normal Studies

Over a 3-year period we evaluated 90 patients who were undergoing skeletal scintigraphic study for localized bone pathology distant from the craniofa-

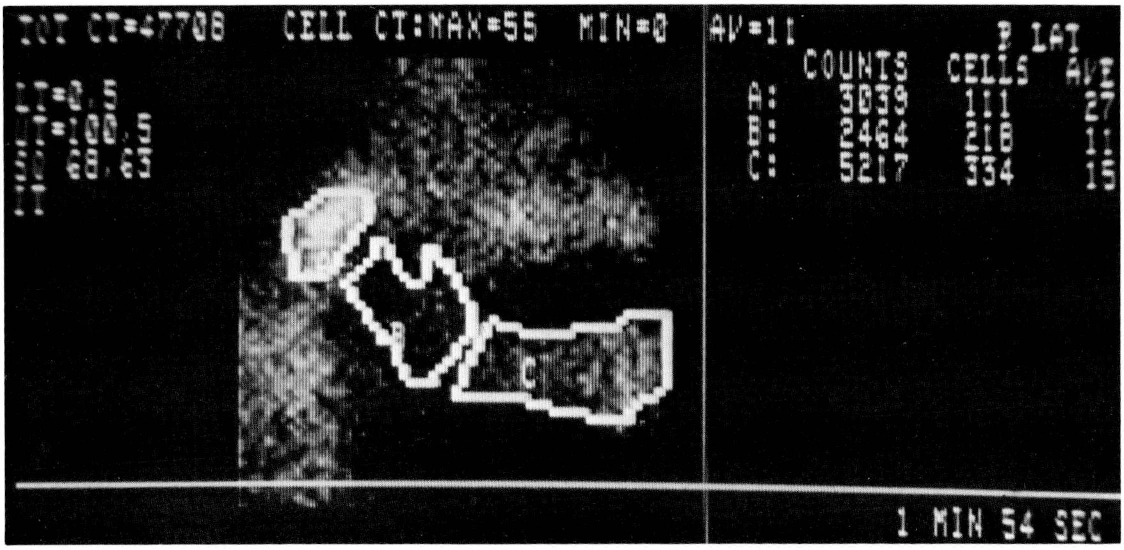

Figure 2-2. A: Right lateral mandibular image with condylar, ramus, and body regions outlined.

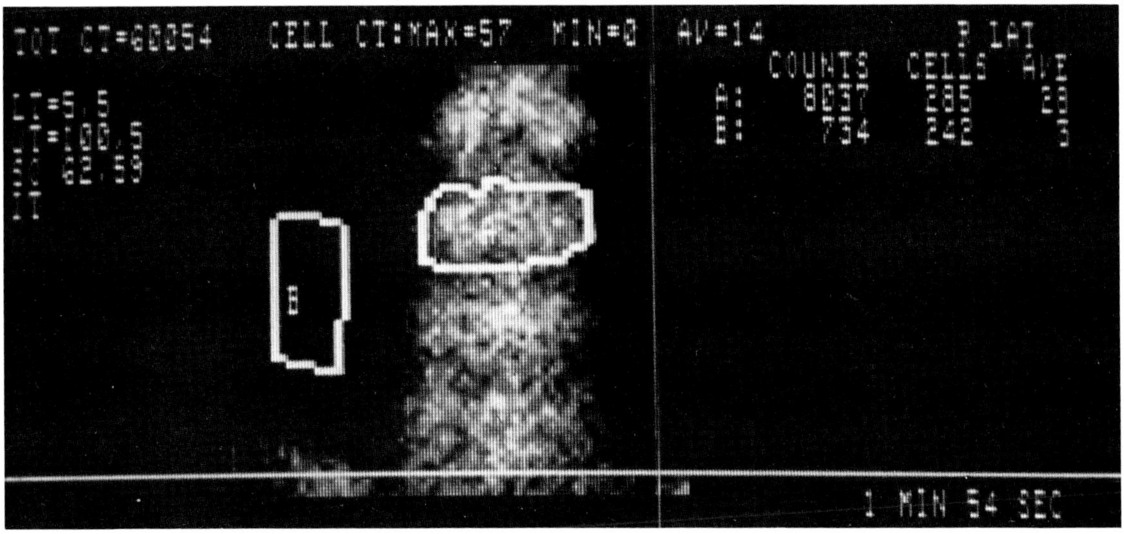

Figure 2-2. B: Posterior lumbar spine image with background counts.

cial region.[2,9] The patients chosen for study were from 2 months to 30 years of age; they had no systemic disease, and were not taking medications. In all cases, clinical examination revealed no craniomaxillofacial deformities and a normal occlusion.

The linear regression analysis in Fig. 2-3 represents mandibular skeletal age as determined by the scintigraphic ratio.[3,4] Right-to-left-sided differences were not statistically significant and data were combined to give a data base of 180 condyles in 90 patients. The technique was reproducible by the same examiner and by two different examiners.[2,3]

Assessment of Mandibular Growth and Skeletal Maturation

Establishment of age-adjusted *RU* for the normal population has made possible objective assessment of mandibular growth. With one measurement of *RU*, compared with the normal population, the level of mandibular maturation can be determined.

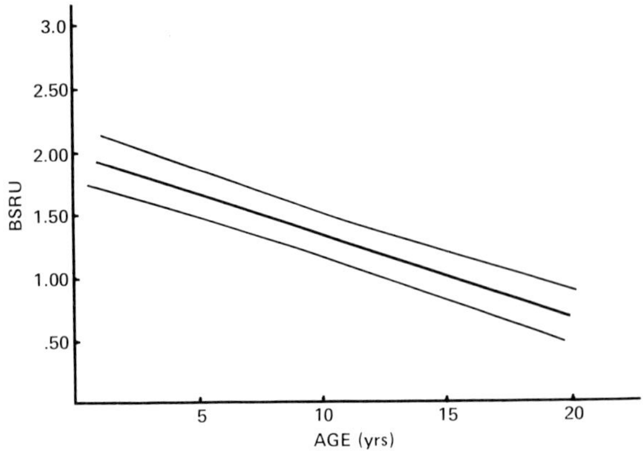

Figure 2-3. A: Linear regression analysis of age versus *RU* for normal patients. BSRU, uptake ratio to 4th lumbar vertebra.

Age	Ratio
0–2	2.0–1.85
2–5	1.85–1.65
5–10	1.65–1.30
10–15	1.30–1.10
15–20	1.10–0.70
20	<0.70

Figure 2-3. B: Approximate *RU* by age taken from linear regression analysis.

The question of whether growth has ceased in a symmetric deformity, such as mandibular prognathism, can be answered; surgical correction can then be performed without further delay. In patients with asymmetric deformities, ongoing asymmetric growth can be documented by unequal *RU*. On the other hand, equal *RU* shows that asymmetric growth has ceased. In difficult diagnostic cases, normal versus abnormal side can be determined by comparing *RU* with the normal standards. End-stage deformity can be predicted when uptake ratios approach 0.70 (adult norm). Finally, by comparing uptake ratios before and after treatment, skeletal scintigraphy can be used to assess the effects of surgical and orthodontic therapy on mandibular growth.

M.S. was a 15-year-old male who presented with a facial asymmetry. The left side of the face was flatter, and the left mandible was shorter than the right (Figs. 2-4A and B). The mandibular skeletal and dental midlines were deviated toward the left (small) side and there was a crossbite on the left.

The differential diagnosis was unilateral right condylar hyperplasia, left condylar hypoplasia, or generalized mandibular asymmetry. The first bone scan (at age 15) showed that the right condylar, ramus, and body regions had *RUs* 20–100% greater than the left, which was in the normal range for the patient's age. This was consistent with a generalized asymmetric mandibular growth pattern, normal left side, and right side hyperplasia. The patient would have to wait until asymmetric growth stopped before treatment could be started. Two years later a repeat scan showed marked decrease in the *RU* asymmetry, with the right-to-left-sided differences between condyles, ramus, and body within 1 standard deviation (right condyle 1.61; left 1.59, difference 0.02, SD 0.05). He was now exhibiting a normal, symmetric growth pattern but had not reached skeletal maturity (*RU* 0.70); surgery was deferred. One year later, at age 18, surgery was performed and the patient has had a stable anatomic result (Fig. 2-4C).

P.F., a 17-year-old white male, presented with maxillary hypoplasia and relative mandibular prognathism (Fig. 2-5A). Radiographs of the hand and wrist showed that the radius and ulnar epiphyses were not fused. Skeletal scintigraphy however, showed a condylar *RU* of 0.68 bilaterally (Fig. 2-5B). The patient had reached skeletal maturity and surgery could be planned.

G.M. was a 15-year-old patient with left hemifacial microsomia. The left side of the face was flat, the left mandible was short, and the left temporomandibular joint (TMJ) was displaced anteriorly and medially. The chin point was deviated to the left and there was considerable shortening of the midface on the affected side as evidenced by the upward cant of the occlusal plane (Figs. 2-6A and B). The only previous surgery was ear construction. The patient wanted surgical correction as soon as possible.

Skeletal scintigraphy revealed *RU* of 0.57 on the left and 0.75 on the right (Fig. 2-6C). These ratios indicated that the right side was normal and had reached skeletal maturity and that the left side was hypoplastic (*RU* beyond 2 SD from the norm). This was a stable, end-stage growth pattern. Surgery was carried out and the patient has had a stable result, as predicted by the scan, 3 years postoperatively (Fig. 2-6D).

Assessment of Mandibular Asymmetry

We have applied the standard data to study 21 patients with mandibular asymmetry.[4] Uptake on the

A

B

C

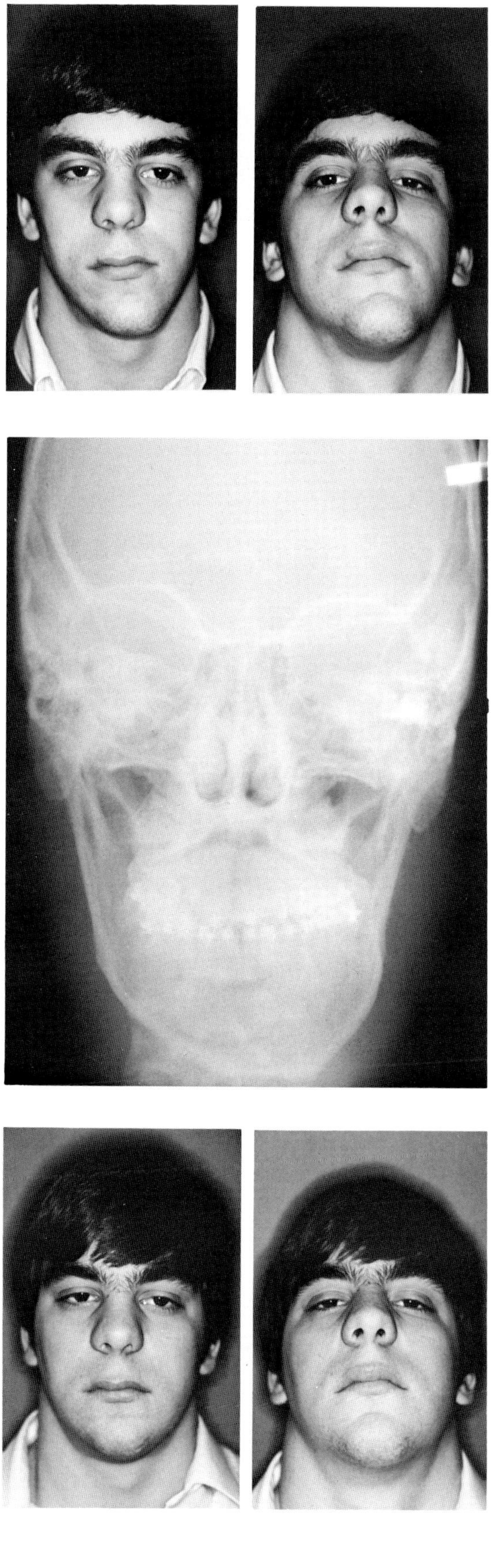

Figure 2-4. A: Frontal and submental views of patient with generalized asymmetric mandibular growth. The chin point is deviated to the left and left mandible is flatter than the right. **B:** AP cephalometric radiograph demonstrates asymmetry. **C:** Frontal and submental views 2 years postoperatively demonstrate stable result.

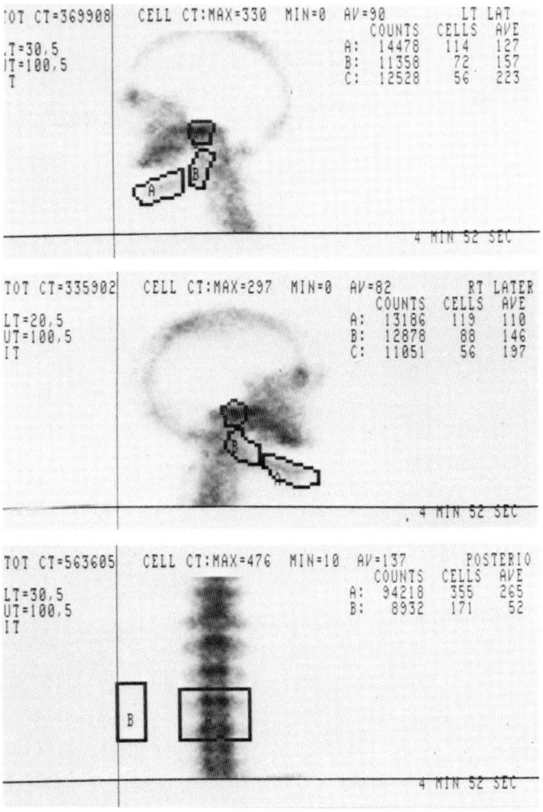

Figure 2-5. Scintigram of patient revealed right and left *RU* of 0.68. Morphologically the midface is retruded in relation to mandible.

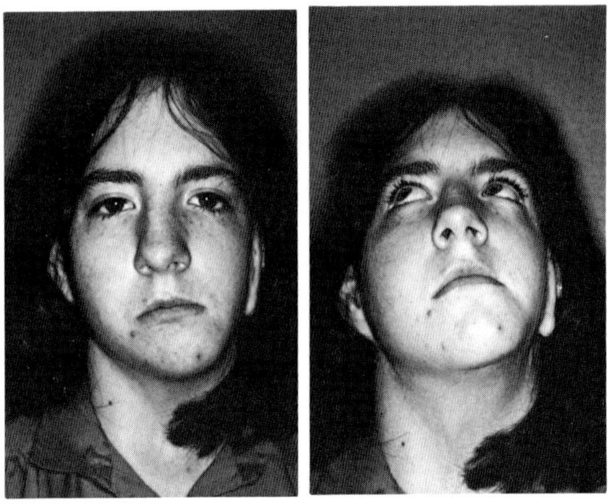

A

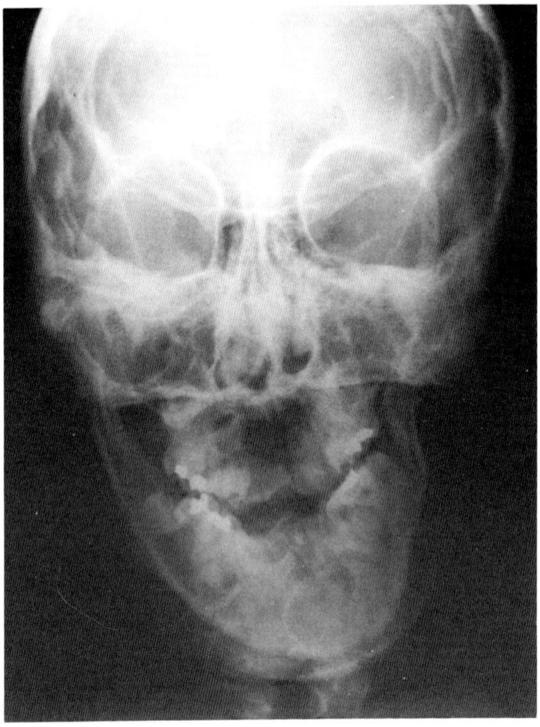

B

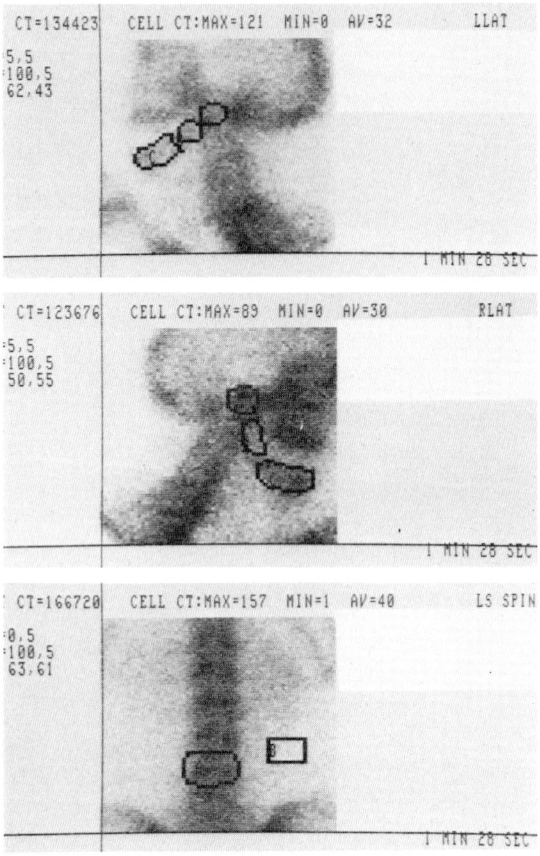

C

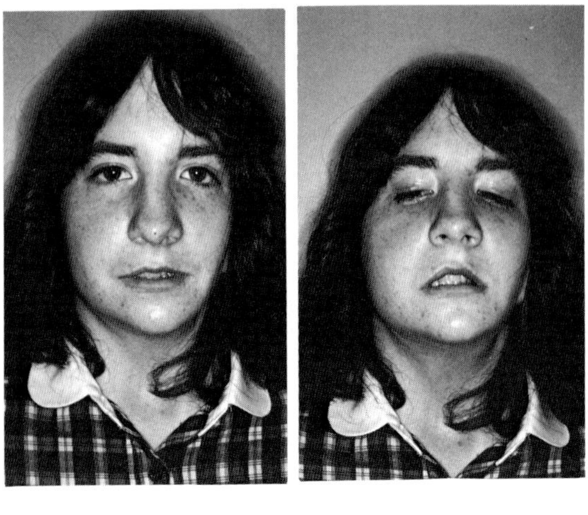

D

Figure 2-6. A: Frontal and submental views demonstrate the asymmetry. **B:** AP cephalogram demonstrates short, flat left mandibular ramus, deviated chin point, oblique cant of occlusal plane, and pyriform apertures upward toward the left. **C:** Skeletal scintigram. **D:** Frontal and submental views 3 years postoperatively demonstrate stable skeletal result.

normal side was generally at the lower end of the normal range (Fig. 2-7). Patients who had asymmetric uptake > 2 SD beyond the norm showed progression of deformity and required treatment. When right and left sides were equal in uptake there was no further progression of the asymmetry. Finally, we were able to demonstrate equalization of uptake patterns after surgical excision of condylar hyperplasia.

L.T. began to demonstrate progressive left mandibular asymmetry as a teenager. By age 20, she began to complain of pain when opening the jaw and noise in the left TMJ. Physical examination revealed an obvious mandibular asymmetry, with the left ramus longer than the right and the left body longer and more convex than the right (Fig. 2-8A). The occlusion was normal. Lateral (Fig. 2-8B), anterior-posterior cephalograms and panoramic radiographs documented the asymmetry. Clinically the patient had unilateral left condylar hyperplasia. Skeletal scintigraphy revealed a right condylar *RU* of 1.09 and a left of 1.30 (right-to-left difference 0.21, normal 0.05), confirming the diagnosis of left unilateral condylar hyperplasia.

The patient underwent left high condylectomy and contouring of the left body of the mandible. She has had a stable result with no further evidence of asymmetric growth, 4 years postoperatively (Fig. 2-8C).

K.S. was a 14-year-old boy undergoing orthodontic treatment for a malocclusion secondary to mandibular retrognathism (hypoplasia). His mother and the orthodontist were concerned about

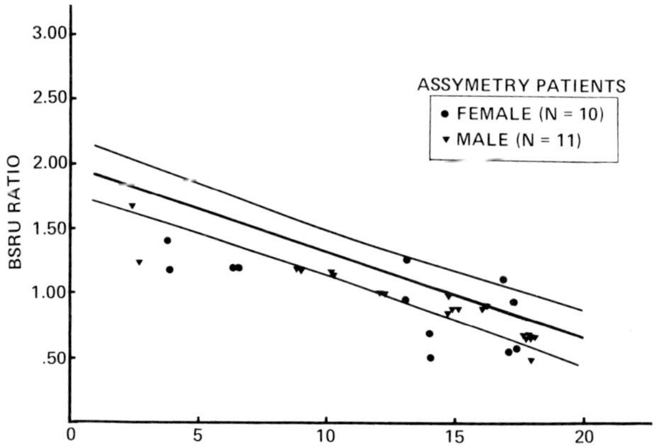

Figure 2-7. Linear regression analysis of normal patients with values of 21 asymmetry patients plotted. Circles, females; triangles, males.

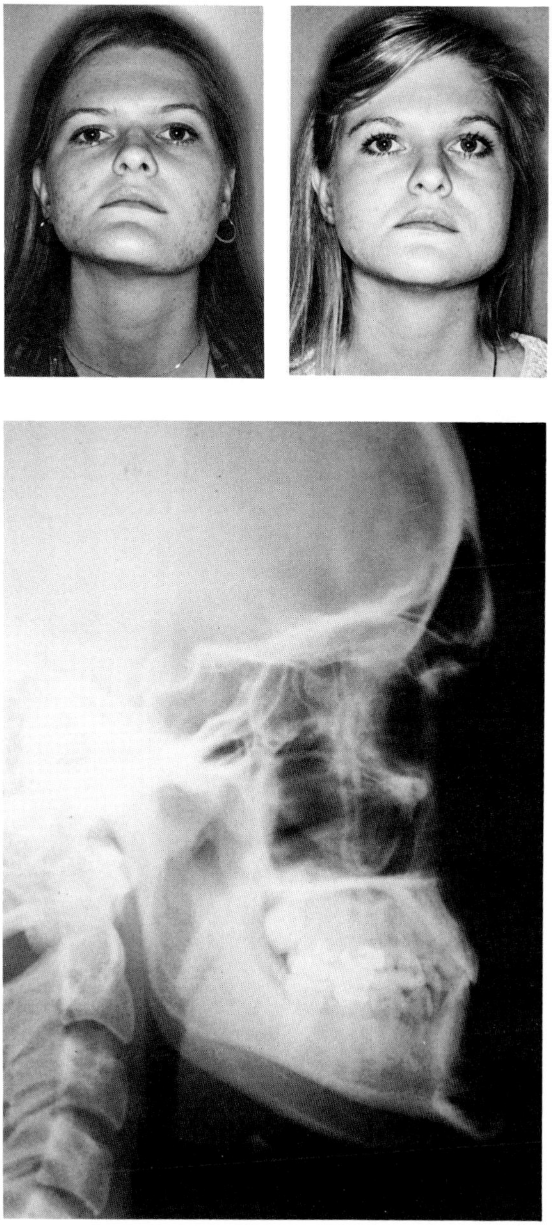

A,C

B

Figure 2-8. A: Frontal photograph demonstrates enlarged left mandible. **B:** Lateral cephalogram demonstrates length discrepancy between right and left mandible as a double contour shadow. **C:** Four years postoperatively the patient has had a stable result.

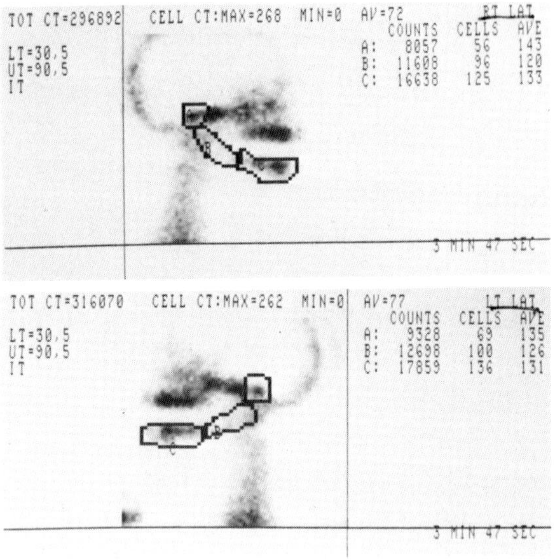

Figure 2-9. Skeletal scintigram revealed equal right and left *RU*.

a mandibular asymmetry; the right side of the jaw recently seemed to be smaller than the left. Was this a developing or ongoing asymmetric growth pattern? Skeletal scintigraphy revealed equal right and left *RU* values for the condyle, ramus, and body regions (Fig. 2-9). The deformity was the result of past asymmetric growth. The child now had a symmetric growth pattern. His orthodontic therapy was continued and did not have to be modified. This type of diagnostic information could not be provided by any other diagnostic modality.

Results of Surgical Therapy

Skeletal scintigraphy has been useful to assess the results of surgical therapy for mandibular asymmetry. When the scan confirms a diagnosis of condylar hyperplasia, a high condylectomy is performed. The purpose of surgery is to excise the abnormal condylar growth center in order to eliminate the asymmetric growth process. Patients who have demonstrated equalization of *RU* postoperatively have had a stable clinical result. Skeletal scintigraphy established the effectiveness of surgical excision of the abnormal condylar segment.

Results of Activator Therapy

The concept of stimulating facial growth with orthodontic appliances is an exciting one. McNamara[10] demonstrated that distraction forces on the mandible of growing monkeys led to apposition of bone and forward growth of the jaw. Documenting the effect of activators in humans has been difficult because of the lack of a method to assess growth dynamics. We have demonstrated equalization of *RU* between the normal and affected sides in response to activator treatment for mandibular asymmetry.[2,4] This was a demonstration of the physiologic effect of activator therapy.

A 4-year-old patient with hemifacial microsomia was begun on activator treatment to stimulate growth on the affected side (Fig. 2-10). The pretreatment *RU* was 1.2 on the affected side and 1.4 on the normal side. The difference of 0.20 was greater than 2 SD beyond the norm. After 6 months of treatment the occlusion improved and there was clinical evidence of forward growth of the mandible. Repeat scintigraphy showed equalization of uptake, but this was a result of decrease on the normal side rather than increase on the affected side. This somewhat surprising result raises the question of how activator devices work. The answer to this question remains unknown despite widespread use of these devices. Skeletal scintigraphy may be helpful in determining the mechanism of response to activators.

Summary

Skeletal scintigraphy is a useful physiologic method of measuring facial growth dynamics. It is especially helpful for evaluation of difficult growth diagnostic problems, for aiding decisions on timing of treatment in the growing child, and for assessment of the effects of surgical and orthodontic therapy. Scintigraphy is a useful research tool for assessment of facial growth.

We have begun to use skeletal scintigraphy for evaluation of abnormalities in facial growth secondary to vascular malformations.[1] As part of a large study of vascular lesions, Tc-99m MDP scintigraphy was performed on five patients with head and neck and five with extremity vascular malformations. In patients with lymphatic malformations, blood flow was not increased in the soft tissue or bone. Venous malformations showed increased blood pooling without increased osseous blood flow in the underlying bone. In contrast, the arterial lesions demonstrated early and persistently elevated blood flow and increased blood pooling. Scintigrams at 2 h showed generalized, increased uptake

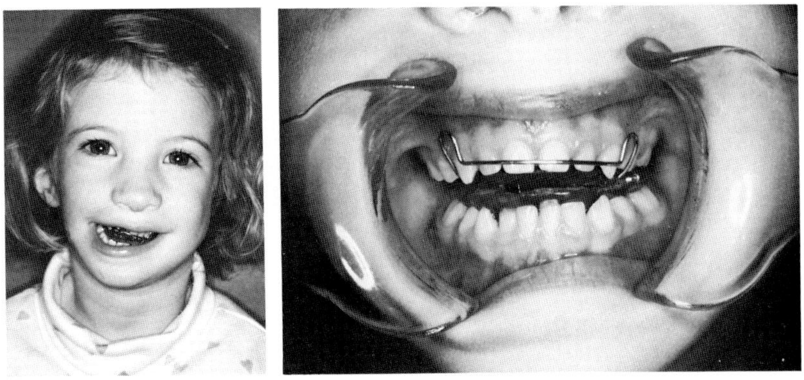

Figure 2-10. *Left:* Frontal view of patient with right hemifacial microsomia demonstrating facial asymmetry and weakness of the marginal mandibular branch of the facial nerve. Patient is wearing an activator appliance. *Right:* Intraoral view demonstrates how the appliance distracts the mandible inferiorly and toward the normal left side, placing stretch on the soft tissue of the affected side.

in the bones of the involved areas. Documenting the patterns of blood flow may help us understand the mechanisms of skeletal changes associated with vascular malformations.

In a recent study of 21 patients with mandibular asymmetry[4] we compared computerized scintigraphy with standard subjective assessment by the radiologist. In 13/21 cases diagnoses by the two methods were in agreement. In 5/8 remaining cases, subjective assessment revealed no asymmetry, but computerized scan revealed differences > 2 SD between right and left condylar regions, indicating asymmetric growth. In the remaining 3/8 patients, computerized scan showed symmetric growth whereas subjective reading showed asymmetry. The computerized scan was more accurate in all cases.

The normal, age-adjusted, standards of uptake are based on 90 patients (180 condyles, rami, and bodies). We are continuing our efforts to obtain scintgrams on patients with normal facial morphology, to accumulate 100 patients in the 0–5, 6–12, 13–16, 17–20, and > 20 years age groups. Other centers will have to corroborate these standards independently.

Acknowledgments We would like to acknowledge George J. Cisneros, D.M.D.,M.M.Sc. who spent 3 years as a Fellow in Orthodontics and Pediatric Dentistry at the Children's Hospital Medical Center and Harvard School of Dental Medicine, Boston. Dr. Cisneros worked with us to accumulate most of the data presented in this chapter. The work formed the basis for his Master of Science thesis awarded by Harvard University in June, 1982.

References

1. Boyd B, Mulliken JB, Kaban LB, Upton J, Murray JE. Skeletal changes associated with vascular malformations, Plast Reconstr Surg 1984 (in press).
2. Cisneros GJ. The use of bone seeking radiopharmaceutical uptake in the assessment of facial growth and development. Master of Science in Oral Biology, Thesis, Harvard University, June 1982.
3. Cisneros GJ, Kaban LB. Use of skeletal scintigraphy for assessment of mandibular and facial growth. In: Bell WH, Proffitt WR, and White RP, eds. Surgical correction of dentofacial deformities, Vol. III. Philadelphia; W.B. Saunders, 1984 (in press).
4. Cisneros GJ, Kaban LB: Computerized skeletal scintigraphy for assessment of mandibular asymmetry. J. Oral Maxillofac Surg 1984 (in press).
5. Donoff RB, Jeffcoat MK, Kaplan ML. Use of a miniaturized detector in facial bone scanning. Int J Oral Surg 1973; 7:482–7.
6. Fleisch H, Russell RG, Francis MD. Diphosphonates inhibit hydroxyapatite dissolution in vitro and bone resorption in tissue culture and in vivo. Science 1969; 165:1262–4.
7. Genant HK et al. Bone seeking radionuclides: an in vivo study of factors affecting skeletal uptake. Radiology 1974; 113:373–82.
8. Kaban LB, Mulliken JB, Murray JE. Three dimensional approach to analysis and treatment of hem-

ifacial microsomia, Cleft Palate J 1981; 18:90–9.
9. Kaban LB, Cisneros GJ, Heyman S, Treves S. Assessment of mandibular growth by skeletal scintigraphy. J Oral Maxillofac Surg 1982; 40:18–22.
10. McNamara JA. Neuromuscular and skeletal adaptation to altered function in the orofacial region. Am J Orthod 1973; 64:578–606.
11. Murray JE, Mulliken JB, Kaban LB, Belfer M. Twenty year experience with maxillo-craniofacial surgery. Ann Surg 1979; 190:320–31.

Chapter 3 Bone Marrow

S. T. Treves

Whole-body bone marrow scintigraphy is a convenient and sensitive method for viewing the distribution of active bone marrow and monitoring its changing patterns with age, stress, and disease.[17] Bone marrow scan abnormalities may precede conventional bone scan and radiographic findings.

Scintigraphy of the bone marrow in children has been performed with technetium-99m (Tc-99m) sulfur colloid and with indium-111 (In-111) as chloride. Some examples of Tc-99m sulfur colloid images are shown in the previous chapters.

Clinical Applications

Sickle-Cell Disease

Scanning with Tc-99m sulfur colloid provides a method for diagnosing bone marrow infarction in patients with sickle-cell anemia (Fig. 3-1). Most patients with sickle-cell anemia show increased marrow activity with expansion to the long bones and skull.

In a study by Alavi et al.[1] 8 of 17 asymptomatic patients with sickle-cell anemia who had no crisis during this study had regions of decreased bone marrow uptake thought to be due to previous infarction and subsequent fibrosis. Two patients who were scanned both while asymptomatic and thereafter during a crisis showed no new infarcts.

In the same study, another group of patients was studied first during crisis and then at subsequent intervals. Six of 10 patients in this group had areas of decreased activity in the bone marrow corresponding to focal pain in the same area, clinically thought to correspond to infarction. Four of these patients repopulated their marrow within 12 months.

Radiographic studies are not helpful in the early diagnosis of bone infarction in patients with sickle-cell disease. Further, infarcts often resolve without ever producing radiographic changes. In sickle-cell anemia, red marrow extends to the ankles, wrists, skull, and much of the long bone shafts. In a study by Lutzker and Alavi[10] half of the bone marrow scans in over 30 patients with sickle-cell disorders showed focally reduced activity probably representing fibrosis from previous infarctions. In the same study, 9 of 12 patients evaluated during an acute crisis showed focal areas of reduced radiocolloidal uptake corresponding to sites of pain.

Hematologic Disorders

In-111 chloride has been used to locate erythropoietic marrow, and several reports have shown its efficacy in such varied hematologic disorders as aplastic anemia, leukemia, and lymphoma.[2,4–9,11–15,18] In-111 imaging is useful in evaluating bone marrow erythroid activity and following the response to therapy in patients with aplastic anemia and myelofibrosis[16] (Figs. 3-2–3-4).

Chu et al.[3] reported irregular distribution of Tc-99m sulfur colloid in four patients with Fanconi's anemia. Normal-to-increased activity was seen in the humeri, tibiae, femora, radii, and ulnae. Skip areas of normal distribution were seen in the proximal diaphyses of the humeri and femora. These

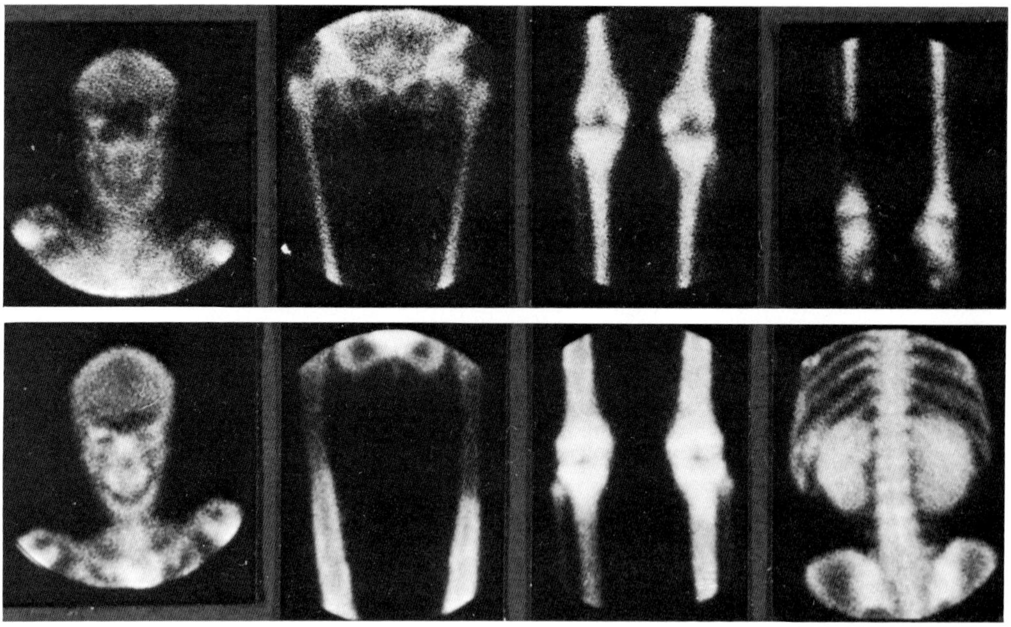

Figure 3-1. Tc-99m sulfur colloid (Tc-99m SC) scan in a patient with sickle-cell disease *(top)*. There is an increase in peripheral bone marrow activity and an area of absent marrow uptake in the right distal tibia. The Tc-99m methylene diphosphonate (MDP) scan *(bottom)* in the same patient shows abnormal distribution of the tracer. Intense and irregular radionuclide uptake is evident in both distal femora, in the left tibia, and in the proximal right tibia, presumably due to bony reaction after infarction. The spleen is small and concentrates the radiotracer, suggesting splenic infarction. The kidneys are large and show abnormal concentration of Tc-99m MDP as in cases of iron overload.

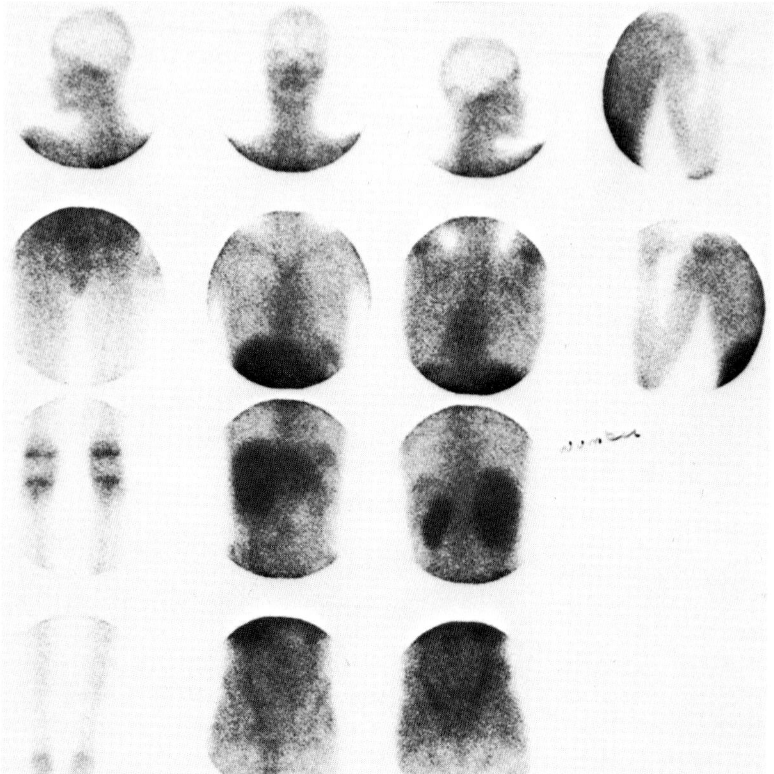

Figure 3-2. In-111 chloride whole-body bone marrow scan (48 h) in a patient with aplastic anemia. There is minimal uptake of radiotracer in the bone marrow.

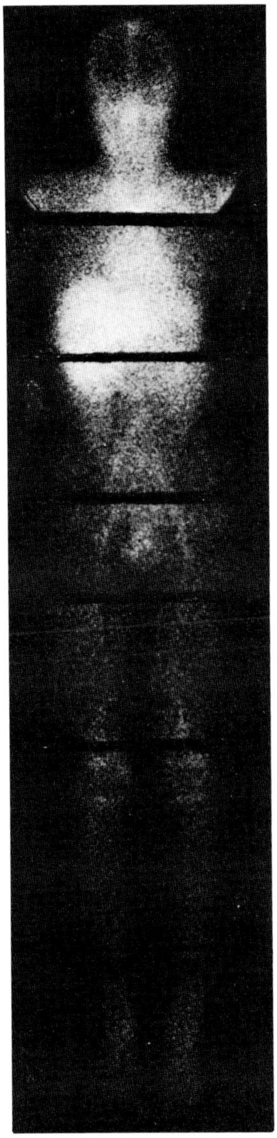

Figure 3-3. Aplastic anemia. In-111 chloride scan.

authors suggest that bone marrow scintigraphy may have some value in the differential diagnosis of pancytopenia.

Childhood Malignancies

Marrow involvement of malignancies usually is reflected by decreased uptake of radiotracers in the areas involved. This finding may be accompanied by normal bone scanning and radiographs. Persistent bone marrow defects in patients with neuroblastoma in remission may represent local myelofibrosis rather than active disease.

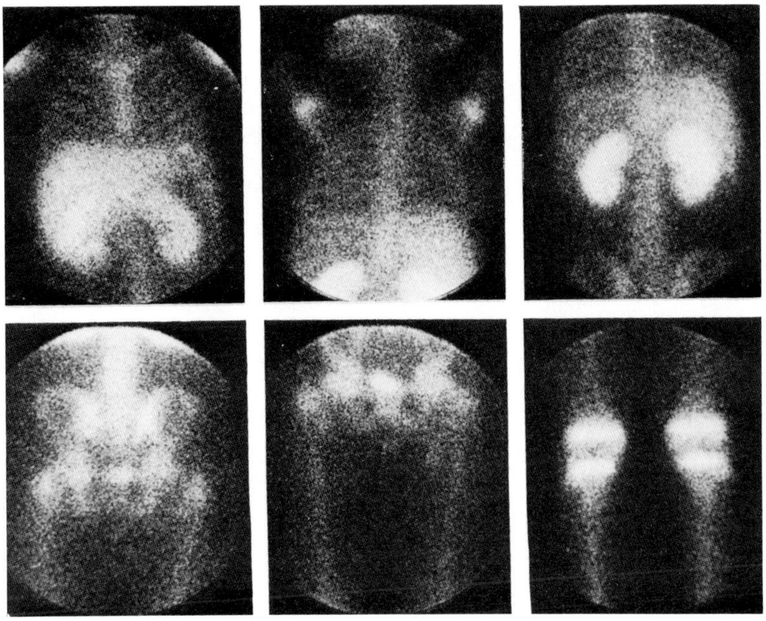

Figure 3-4. In-111 chloride scan in a patient with aplastic anemia several weeks after successful bone marrow transplantation. There is uptake of the radiotracer throughout the bone marrow spaces.

References

1. Alavi A, Bond JP, Kuhl DE, Creech RH. Scan detection of bone marrow infarcts in sickle cell disorders. J Nucl Med 1974; 15:1003–10.
2. Bunn HF, McNeil BJ, Rosenthal DS, Krantz SB. Bone marrow imaging in pure red blood cell aplasia. Arch Intern Med 1976; 136:1169–72.
3. Chu JY, Ho JE, Monteleone PL, O'Connor DM. Technetium colloid bone marrow imaging in Fanconi's anemia. Pediatrics 1979; 64:635–9.
4. Gilbert EH, Earle JD, Glatstein E, Goris ML, Kaplan HS, Kriss JP. ^{111}Indium bone marrow scintigraphy as an aid in selecting marrow biopsy sites for the evaluation of marrow elements in patients with lymphoma. Cancer 1976; 38:1560–7.
5. Gilbert EH, Earle JD, Goris ML, Kaplan HS, Kriss JP. The accuracy of $^{111}InCl_3$ as a bone marrow scanning agent. Radiology 1976; 119:167–8.
6. Gilbert EH, Glastein E, Goris ML, et al. Value of ^{111}indium chloride bone marrow scanning in the differential diagnosis of blood count depression in lymphoma. Cancer 1978; 41:143–52.
7. Helmer RE III, Sayle BA, Alperin JB, Gardner FH. ^{111}In chloride bone marrow scintigraphy and ferrokinetic studies in a case of sickle cell anemia with transient erythroid aplasia. Acta Haematol 1979; 61:330–3.

8. Horn NL, Bennett LR, Marciano D. Evaluation of aplastic anemia with indium chloride In-111 scanning. Arch Intern Med 1980; 140:1299–1303.
9. Lilien DL, Berger HG, Anderson DP, Bennett LR. ^{111}In chloride: a new agent for bone marrow imaging. J Nucl Med 1973; 14:184–6.
10. Lutzker LG, Alavi A. Bone and marrow imaging in sickle cell disease: diagnosis of infarction. Semin Nucl Med 1976; 6:83–93.
11. McNeil BJ, Holman BL, Button LN, Rosenthal DS. Use of indium chloride scintigraphy in patients with myelofibrosis. J Nucl Med 1974; 15:647–51.
12. McNeil BJ, Rappeport JM, Nathan DG. Indium chloride scintigraphy—an index of severity in patients with aplastic anemia. Br J Haematol 1976; 34:599–604.
13. Merrick MV, Gordon-Smith EC, Lavender JP, Szur L. A comparison of ^{111}In and ^{52}Fe and ^{99m}Tc sulfur colloid for bone marrow scanning. J Nucl Med 1975; 16:66–8.
14. Najean Y, Le Danvic M, Le Mercier N, Pecking A, Colonna P, Rain JD. Significance of bone marrow scintigraphy in aplastic anemia. J Nucl Med 1980; 21:213–18.
15. Pauwels EKJ, TeVelde J, Hermans J, Haak HL, Jurgens PJ. ^{111}Indium chloride bone marrow scintigraphy in aplastic anemia. Scand J Haematol 1981; 26:81–90.
16. Sayle BA, Helmer RE, Birdsong BA, Balachandran S, Gardner FH. Bone marrow imaging with indium-111 chloride in aplastic anemia and myelofibrosis: concise communication. J Nucl Med 1982; 23:121–5.
17. Siddiqui AR, Oseas RS, Wellman HN, Doerr DR, Baehner RL. Evaluation of bone marrow scanning with technetium-99m sulfur colloid in pediatric oncology. J Nucl Med 1979; 20:379–86.
18. Staub RT, Gaston E. ^{111}In chloride distribution and kinetics in hematologic disease. J Nucl Med 1973; 14:456–7.

Chapter 4 Kidneys

S. T. Treves
Robert L. Lebowitz
Alvin Kuruc
Sydney Heyman
Paul Rosen

Early diagnosis and treatment can lead to far less morbidity and mortality associated with abnormalities of the urinary tract in children. The precise incidence of congenital malformations of the urinary tract has not yet been established because systematic screening in early childhood has not been done. With the increased utilization of ultrasonography in obstetrics a clearer idea of the incidence of renal disease in the prenatal and neonatal periods is being developed. While about 10% of all people are affected, many abnormalities are minor and have no clinical significance. Excluding polycystic kidneys, the incidence of major malformations has been estimated to be 4–7/1000.[13] Collectively, congenital abnormalities account for about 45% of cases of chronic renal failure.[26] The incidence of preexisting lesions has been reported to be 15–23% in children showing serious renal injury following relatively minor trauma.[62] Associated anomalies of other organs are not uncommon, especially when the kidney is involved. Infections of the urinary tract affect 3–5% of all children. In the neonatal period males are more commonly affected, but after the age of 3 months, the female:male ratio becomes about 3:1.[16]

Assessment of patients with urinary problems usually includes history, physical examination, and a urine specimen for microscopy and culture. Tests reflecting global renal function commonly used include urinalysis, blood urea nitrogen, serum creatinine, electrolytes, and acid-base status. Other more complex tests include clearance studies to measure glomerular filtration rate (*GFR*) and effective renal plasma flow (ERPF). Intravenous urography, voiding cystouretherography, and ultrasonography provide information about anatomy of the genitourinary tract, and to a lesser extent, function. Of particular interest is the observation that a normal urinalysis and intravenous urogram or ultrasonogram does not necessarily exclude urologic problems, such as significant reflux. More invasive diagnostic procedures include endoscopy, antegrade pyelography, renal angiography, and biopsy. Individual renal function may be assessed by split renal function studies.

With recent advances in nuclear medicine, there has been a renewed interest in the radionuclide evaluation of the urinary tract. Radionuclide techniques can be used safely in severely ill patients, in patients with renal insufficiency, and in premature and newborn infants. These techniques allow evaluation of morphology and quantitation of function simultaneously and thus provide information that cannot be obtained easily by other diagnostic modalities. The tracers used in these studies do not cause any toxic or even pharmacologic effect, nor do they produce an osmotic and/or hemodynamic load. Unlike radiographic contrast agents, radiopharmaceutical administration does not provoke allergic reaction.

Radionuclide studies should be considered a unique and important adjunct to the diagnosis of renal disorders and the evaluation of renal function in children.

Method

Radiopharmaceuticals

Tc-99m DTPA

Tc-99m DTPA (technetium-99m stannous diethylenetriamine pentacetic acid complex) is handled largely by glomerular filtration at a slightly lower rate than iodine-125 (I-125) iothalamate and thus, inulin.[4,18,30,31,41,49,51,61,65,76,84,112] About 10% of the Tc-99m activity appears to be bound to plasma proteins. Dynamic imaging of the kidneys, the collecting system, ureters, and the bladder can be performed with Tc-99m DTPA but this agent is not adequate for static renal scintigraphy because it does not label the renal parenchyma.

Estimates of radiation absorbed doses with Tc-99m DTPA are shown in Table 4-1. These estimates are for children with normal renal function so that the doses to patients with decreased renal function will generally be higher and have a different distribution.

Tc-99m DMSA

After intravenous administration, Tc-99m DMSA (dimercaptosuccinic acid) is distributed in the plasma bound to plasma proteins (90%). Only a very small fraction of the injected activity is eliminated in the urine. The cumulative urinary excretion of Tc-99m DMSA is about 6% at 1 h, 12% at 2 h, and 28% at 14 h.

The blood disappearance of Tc-99m DMSA follows a single-exponential decrease in most normal individuals. At 14 h after injection, 6–9% of the dose is present in the blood. The mean half-time of this tracer in blood is about 50 min. Red cell binding of Tc-99m DMSA is 0–5%. At 1 h 50% of the injected dose is in the kidneys and at 24 h it reaches about 70%.[32] This activity is found principally in the proximal convoluted tubules, with only minimal activity elsewhere in the kidney (Fig. 4-1).[137] The fractional distribution of Tc-99m DMSA between the right and left kidneys correlates well with renal blood flow as determined by strontium-85 (Sr-85) microsphere distribution ($r = 0.95$). Changes in renal mass correlate well with changes in Tc-99m DMSA distribution in dogs (percent uptake of left versus right kidney).[19] Activity of Tc-99m DMSA complex has been shown in subcellular studies to be with cytosol proteins, to the mitochondria, and to a lesser extent, to nuclei and microsomes.[131] We found a good correlation in the regional and relative renal distributions of Tc-99m DMSA and cobalt-57 (Co-57) microspheres in normal and obstructed kidneys (Table 4-2) (DiPietro M, Caldicott W, Treves S, unpublished data). In patients, Taylor et al. found a good correlation between the relative renal accumulation of Tc-99m DMSA at 24 h and relative effective renal plasma flow to each kidney measured with I-131 orthoiodohippurate (I-131-OIH).[123] Tc-99m DMSA is well suited for static scintigraphy. Excellent images of renal cortex can be obtained 4–24 h after injection. Estimates of radiation exposure for Tc-99m DMSA are shown in Table 4-3.

Table 4-1. Tc-99m DTPA Usual Administered Activity and Absorbed Radiation Dose

Age (yr)	Newborn	1	5	10	15
Weight (kg)	3.5	10	20	30	50
Administered dose (mCi)	0.5	1.0	2.0	4.0	6.0
Absorbed dose (rad)					
Bladder[a]	1.05	1.30	1.28	2.0	1.36
Kidneys	0.11	0.042	0.11	0.14	0.10
Ovaries	0.08	0.086	0.11	0.14	0.13
Testes	0.07	0.087	0.09	0.12	0.11
Whole body	0.042	0.041	0.05	0.06	0.07

From the Radiopharmaceutical Internal Dose Information Center, Oak Ridge Associated Universities, Oak Ridge, TN.

[a]Bladder wall dose calculated on assumption that bladder was emptied at intervals of 4.8 h.

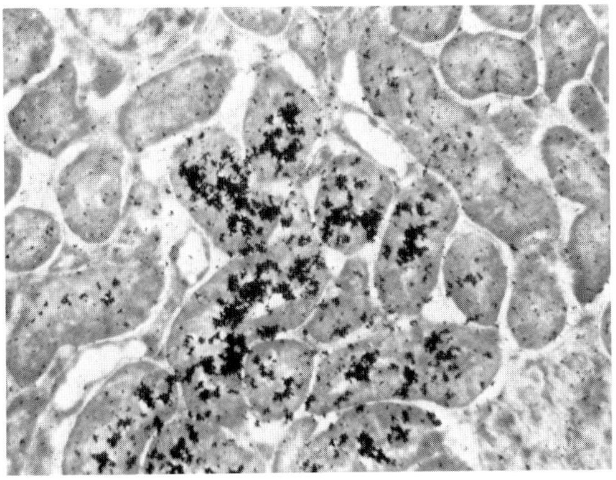

Figure 4-1. Tc-99m DMSA. Frozen section autoradiography from a rat kidney 1 h following intravenous administration of Tc-99m DMSA. The activity concentrates principally in the proximal convoluted tubules. Minimal or no activity is seen elsewhere. Hematoxylin and eosin stain.

Tc-99m Glucoheptonate

Tc-99m glucoheptonate is rapidly taken up by the kidneys and eliminated in the urine. Within 1 h after intravenous injection, about 2% of the initial activity is present in the blood, and about 25% of the administered activity appears in the urine. Tc-99m glucoheptonate permits excellent dynamic imaging with rapid visualization of renal parenchyma collecting system and ureters. The mechanism of uptake of Tc-99m glucoheptonate is not well known but it appears to be partly filtered by the glomeruli and also transported actively by the renal tubular cells. There is initial rapid secretion of the agent in the urine; however, about 20% of the injected activity remains in the kidney, labelling the cells of the proximal convoluted tubules.[137] This permits static renal scintigraphy at 2–4 or more hours after the injection of the agent. In patients with severe renal failure, delayed static images (4–6 h) will show activity within the bowel, limiting evaluation of the renal parenchyma.

I-131, I-123 Orthoiodohippurate (OIH)

This agent is handled by the kidneys similarly to para-aminohippuric acid (PAH).[129] PAH is the standard compound for measuring the effective renal plasma flow. About 20% of PAH is eliminated by glomerular filtration and 80% by tubular secretion. About 90% of this substance is extracted by the kidney in a single pass.[17] Because of its selectivity for renal tissue, sodium I-131 OIH is a useful agent for dynamic renal imaging. Series of gamma camera images obtained after injection of this tracer permit visualization of the renal outlines, the collecting system, the ureters, and the bladder. Drawbacks of I-131 OIH are the low photon yield, the high energy of I-131 (364 keV) which precludes efficient detection with gamma cameras, and the presence of undesirable beta radiation, which contributes significantly to radiation dose to patients. The clearance values of I-131 OIH are apparently lower than those of PAH (OIH/PAH = 0.85).[77] The blood clearance of a substance cleared by the tubules gives a measure of the plasma flow if the secretion of such substance is complete. The rate of blood flow to the kidneys is directly proportional to the arteriovenous difference of the concentration of the agent. The calculated blood clearance would give the total renal

Table 4-2. Percent of the Total Renal Uptake in a Single Obstructed Kidney in Rabbits

Tc-99m DMSA	Co-57 Microspheres
46	46
48	47
49	48
46	51
49	49
25	31
48	47

Table 4-3. Tc-99m DMSA Administered Doses and Radiation Absorbed Doses

Age (yr)	Newborn	1	5	10	15
Weight (kg)	3.5	10	20	30	50
Administered dose (mCi)	0.5	0.7	1.0	1.5	2.0
Absorbed dose (rad)					
Whole body	0.08	0.05	0.04	0.04	0.03
Kidneys	3.65	2.03	1.6	1.5	1.66
Ovaries	0.07	0.06	0.05	0.05	0.04
Testes	0.04	0.04	0.03	0.03	0.02

plasma flow if the compound was totally extracted in a single pass. In reality, the calculated clearance will be slightly lower than the total renal plasma flow.

I-123 OIH is a superior radiopharmaceutical and should be used if available. I-123 provides a higher photon flux than I-131 and does not produce beta radiation. Unfortunately, the availability of I-123 OIH is limited at the present time.

Effects of Radiographic Contrast Agents on Radionuclide Imaging of the Kidneys

Contrast agents used on intravenous urography and angiography result in a reduction of renal uptake of tracers accompanied by a prolongation of their intrarenal transit time. This effect usually lasts 24–48 h. Therefore, it is suggested that radionuclide studies of the kidneys be performed either before or 48 h after the administration of contrast agents.

Examination Technique

Tc-99m DTPA Studies

Patients are examined in their normal state of hydration. If possible, before beginning the examination the patient is asked to empty his or her bladder. Children are examined in the supine position with the gamma camera placed underneath the examining table and viewing the area of the kidneys and bladder. Recipients of renal transplants are also examined in the supine position and the gamma camera views the kidney from an anterior projection. An intravenous drip infusion of saline is started before administration of the radiotracer and maintained during the entire examination. This is advantageous as it maintains a level of hydration, prevents accidental extravasation of tracer, and makes the administration of furosemide, when needed, convenient.

Patients suspected of having urinary tract obstruction and/or vesicoureteric reflux who cannot or will not void may require a resical catheter, which should be allowed to drain throughout the study.

The Tc-99m DTPA study may consist of a radionuclide angiogram followed immediately by serial imaging for 30–40 min (one frame/0.5–1 min). Radionuclide angiography, however, may be omitted. Radionuclide angiography is recorded on the computer at a rate of one frame/sec for 1 min. This is followed immediately by a recording rate of one frame/0.5–1.0 min for 40 min. For renal radionuclide angiography a dose of Tc-99m DTPA of 200 μCi/kg of body weight is usual, with a minimal dose of 1–2 mCi. Radionuclide angiography in most clinical instances rarely provides information not available on series of images obtained over a period of 30–40 min. If radionuclide angiography is not desired, the administered dose of Tc-99m DTPA may be reduced (30–50 μCi/kg of body weight) and the entire study may be recorded at a rate of one frame/0.5–1.0 min for 30–40 min. The study is monitored on a persistence oscilloscope in order to assess renal uptake and drainage of the tracer. If there is no retention of tracer within the pelvicalyceal system or the ureter(s), urinary obstruction is ruled out and the study is terminated at 15–20 min. If urinary obstruction is present or suspected, furosemide is administered approximately 15 min after injection of the tracer and recording is continued either until the end of 40 min or earlier in the absence of retention. Additional delayed images should be obtained in patients who show tracer retention during the initial part of the study. These patients should be encouraged to walk and/or change position in order to promote drainage before obtaining additional images.

A normal Tc-99m DTPA study reveals relatively rapid and intense concentration of the tracer in the renal parenchyma at 1–3 min after injection. Passage of the tracer into the renal calyces and the renal pelves occurs at 2–6 min and the ureters are rarely visualized. By 10–20 min the bolus of Tc-99m DTPA activity has usually cleared the kidneys. Small areas of persistent activity in the pelvicalyceal system are usually not significant and they disappear rapidly with change of the position of the patient or after voiding. Activity within the bladder appears at 2–6 min after the injection of tracer and its level increases with time as more Tc-99m DTPA is filtered by the kidneys. Background activity, which is a reflection of blood clearance of the tracer, decreases as the study progresses (Fig. 4-2). Monitoring the blood level of Tc-99m DTPA with the gamma camera or with an external probe and a blood sample at the end of the study can be used to calculate *GFR* simultaneously with imaging.

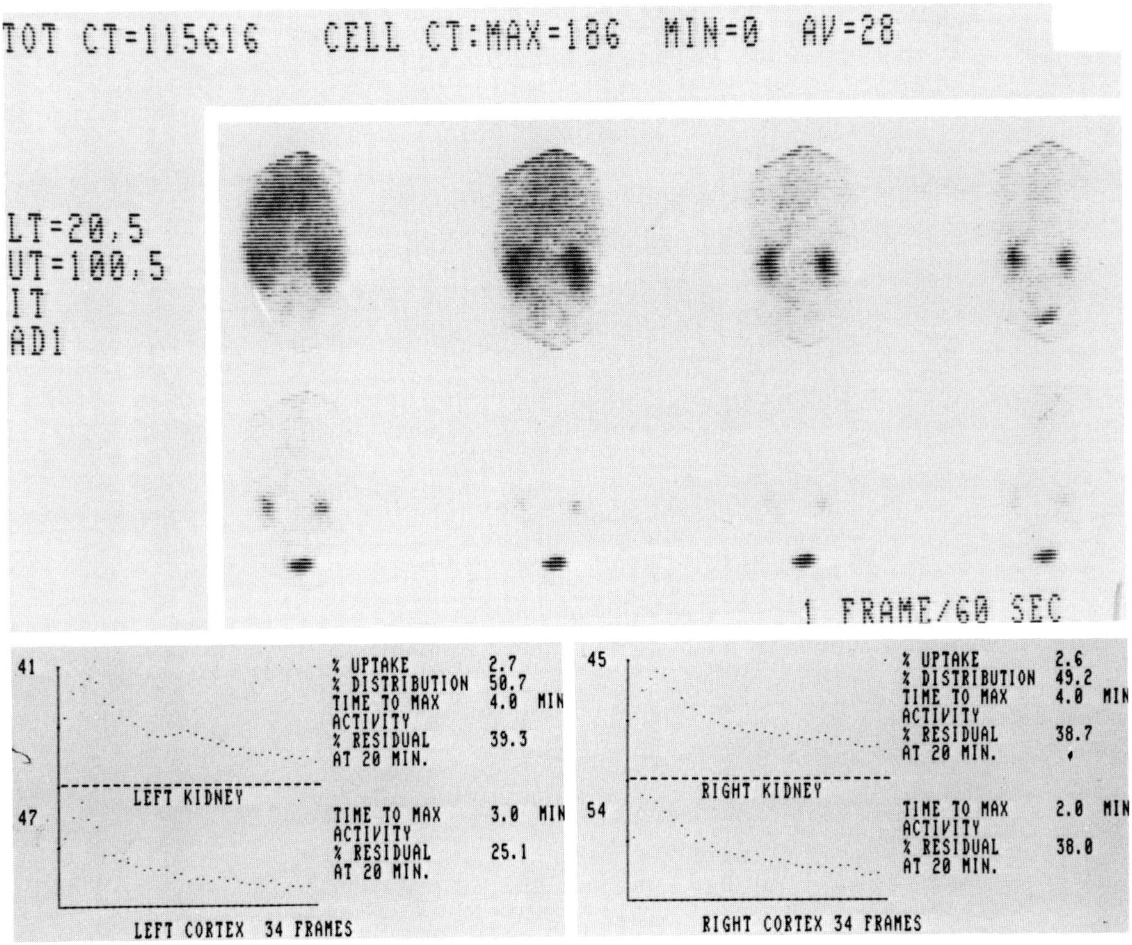

Figure 4-2. Normal Tc-99m DTPA study. One-month-old infant suspected of having renal vein thrombosis. *Top:* Each frame represents 2 min. *Bottom:* Normal time-activity curves from areas of the kidneys and cortices.

Tc-99m DMSA Study

Tc-99m DMSA is administered intravenously in a usual dose of 0.5–3.0 mCi (Table 4-1). Imaging should begin at about 4 h after injection in the absence of urinary obstruction.

The patient is examined in the supine or prone position and a posterior image with 300,000–500,000 counts using a high-resolution collimator is recorded. Another image of the kidneys together with a radioactive ruler calibrated in centimeters is obtained. This image is used to measure the size of the kidneys (Fig. 4-3). Regions of interest (ROI) of each renal silhouette and an area of background are outlined. The distribution of regional activity after background subtraction is calculated. A special case is that of renal duplication in which it may also be necessary to outline the upper and lower poles of the kidney(s) in order to estimate the distribution of functioning renal parenchyma (Fig. 4-4).

Magnified images using a pinhole collimator are very useful to examine the kidneys not only in infants in whom magnification is mandatory but also in older children (Fig. 4-5). Small infarcts, scars, duplication, and fetal lobation can be outlined with pinhole magnification and not with high-resolution collimator. Posterior and posterior oblique projections are used to outline the renal silhouettes better.

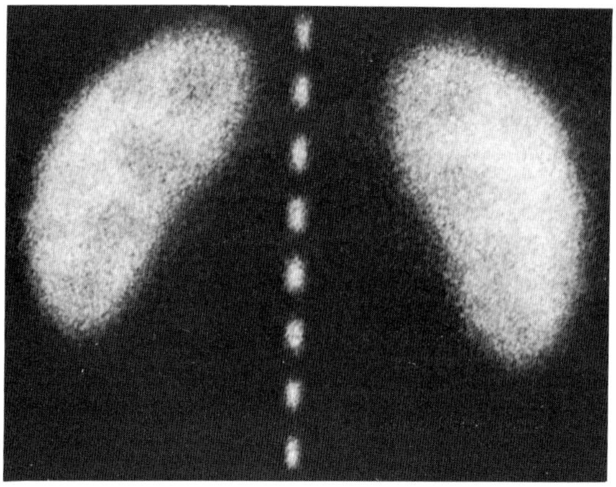

Figure 4-3. Normal Tc-99m DMSA scintiscan from a renal donor. Posterior view. Areas of low uptake correspond to the pelvicalyceal system. A radioactive ruler used for measuring the kidneys, with marks at 1 cm is seen between the renal outlines.

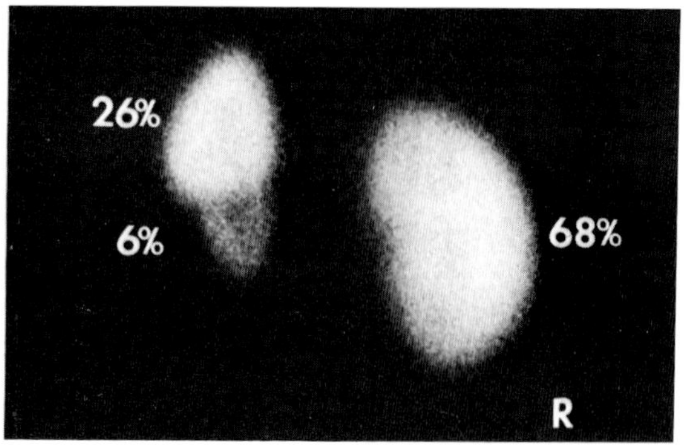

Figure 4-4. Duplication of the left kidney in a 7-year-old female with recurrent urinary tract infections. Posterior view of a Tc-99m DMSA renal scan. The right kidney is enlarged with adequate distribution of activity. The left kidney shows a clear demarcation between the upper pole, which functions well, and the lower pole, which is small and shows reduced concentration of the tracer.

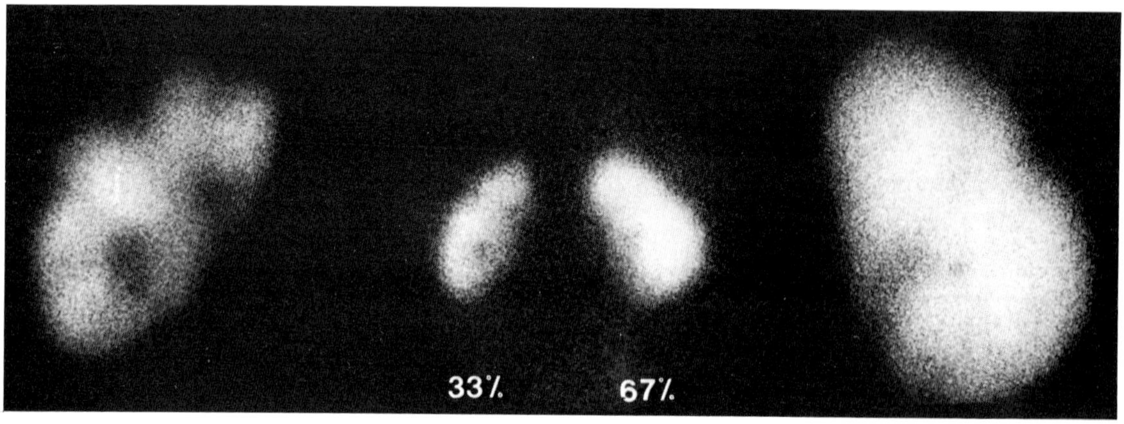

Figure 4-5. Renal scarring. Tc-99m DMSA renal scan from a 6-year-old male with a history of fever and vomiting. He was found to have bilateral reflux with scarring of the left kidney which was reduced in size on intravenous urography. The scintiscan reveals large bilateral intrarenal focal defects more pronounced on the left. These defects are appreciated better on the images obtained with the pinhole collimator shown on either side of the panel.

Each magnified image is obtained for about 150,000 counts.

In cases of severe obstruction, some amount of the Tc-99m DMSA activity may be present in the collecting system which tends to overestimate renal uptake. Delayed images up to 24 h after the injection are useful as they allow most of the tracer in the renal calyces and pelves to drain, permitting a better quantitation of the distribution of functional renal parenchyma. Normally, the distribution of functioning parenchyma in the two renal units as assessed by Tc-99m DMSA is from 50–50% to 45–55%.

Correction for Tissue Attenuation and Detection of Extrarenal Activity

For quantitative analysis of dynamic renal scintigraphy, one would like to know the amount of activity in each kidney as a function of time. In practice, the amount of renal activity is approximated by time-activity curves obtained from ROIs over the kidneys (Fig. 4-2). Tissue attenuation and detection of extrarenal activity can introduce error into this approximation. It is therefore desirable to attempt to correct for these factors. Correction for extrarenal activity (that is background correction) is usually based on the time-activity curve obtained from an ROI adjacent to the kidneys. This ROI is termed the background region. Various background regions have been proposed. An area between the kidneys,[59] an area around the kidneys,[110] an area superior to the kidneys,[50,83] and an area inferolateral to the kidneys[43] have all been used.

Allowing $R(t)$ and $B(t)$ to be the renal and background time-activity curves, respectively, the background-corrected renal time-activity curve, $R_c(t)$, is computed using the formula:

$$R_c(t) = R(t) - S\,B(t)\,(A_R/A_B) \qquad [1]$$

in which A_R, A_B, and S are the area in pixels of the renal ROI, the area in pixels of the background ROI, and a scaling factor (usually equal to 1), respectively.[59] In order to correct for the effect of tissue attenuation, it is necessary to know the distance, x, of the kidney from the surface of the body. This distance may be measured by the gamma camera, using a lateral view, or by ultrasonography. Alternatively, this distance may be estimated from the patient's height and weight by using a nomogram.[106] Attenuation correction is implemented by multiplying the background-corrected renal time-activity curve by e^{ux} where u is the linear attenuation coefficient of the radiotracer in soft tissues.[43,83]

Deconvolution Analysis

After correction for background activity and tissue attenuation, the renal time-activity curve obtained during radionuclide renography approximates the amount of tracer in the kidney as a function of time. This time-activity curve may be considered to be a composite of two separate functions, the amount of radiotracer entering the kidney as a function of time (that is the input function) and the fraction of radiotracer remaining in the kidney after it enters as a function of time (that is the retention function). The input function, and hence the observed renal time-activity curve, is affected by factors that have no bearing on the function of a particular kidney such as the function of the other kidney, loss of radiotracer from the intravascular space, and occasionally, continued input of radiotracer from a partially extravasated injection.[23]

Clearly, it would be desirable to separate the retention function, which depends solely on the function of the kidney of interest, from the input function. The input function is commonly assumed to be proportional to the plasma tracer concentration in the blood entering the kidney. This is difficult to measure directly. In practice, the input function may be approximated as being proportional to a time-activity curve obtained from the abdominal aorta,[22] heart,[95] liver,[95] or brain. There are two possible sources of error in this approximation: temporal differences in tracer concentration between the plasma in the pool being monitored and the renal artery, and possible contamination of the observed blood pool curve by detection of extravascular activity. However, approximation of the input function by externally detected time-activity curves has been found to work well in practice.[33]

Theoretically, the retention function of the kidney can be measured directly by injecting an instantaneous pulse of tracer into the renal artery and preventing its recirculation. The resulting renal time-activity curve is termed the unit impulse response *(UIR)* of the kidney. Such an invasive approach is clearly not practical. It is possible, however, to estimate indirectly the UIR of a kidney from any observed renal time-activity curve, if the input function is known. This is done by modeling the kidney as a linear, time-invariant system and using a mathematical technique known as deconvolution. Several investigators have reported using deconvolution to estimate the renal *UIR*.[22,37,59,132] One problem with the method is that small random data errors may lead to physiologically unrealistic negative values and high-frequency oscillations in the computed *UIR*.[42] In order to circumvent this problem, we have found it useful to introduce constraints, derived from physiologic considerations of the renal system, into the deconvolution process. Specifically, the computed *UIR* is constrained to be nonnegative and nonincreasing. *UIRs* computed using this technique have been shown to be relatively insensitive to random data errors.[67]

Interpretation of the Renal UIR

The physical meaning of the computed *UIR* is analogous to the result of a renal time-activity curve obtained after an instantaneous intraarterial injection of a radiotracer without recirculation, as described in the previous section. Consider such a curve obtained with a substance that is handled like PAH (for example I-131 OIH). All tracer arriving in the kidney subsequently enters the tubular space, either by glomerular filtration or tubular secretion, and leaves via the ureter. The corresponding *UIR,* shown schematically in Fig. 4-6A, consists of a tubular plateau phase (from time 0 to the minimal tubular transit time) followed by a tubular washout phase. Now consider such a curve obtained with a material that is handled like inulin (for example Tc-99m DTPA). A fraction of the tracer equal to the filtration fraction will enter the tubular space by glomerular filtration and leave via the ureter. The remainder of tracer will remain in the vascular space and leave the kidney via the renal vein. The corresponding *UIR,* shown schematically in Fig. 4-6B, consists of a vascular plateau phase (from time 0 until the minimal vascular transit time), a vascular washout phase (until the maximal vascular transit time), a tubular plateau phase (until the minimal tubular transit time), and a tubular washout phase. The amplitude of the tubular plateau divided by the amplitude of the vascular plateau is equal to the filtration fraction. The vascular phase occurs quite rapidly, however, and may be difficult to delineate at the frame rates commonly used for dynamic renal imaging. It is sometimes useful in interpretation to eliminate the vascular phase of the *UIR* by setting the *UIR* values prior to a set time (chosen to be greater than the maximal vascular transit times and less than the minimal tubular transit time) equal to the *UIR* value at that time. The resulting curve is termed the tubular *UIR.*

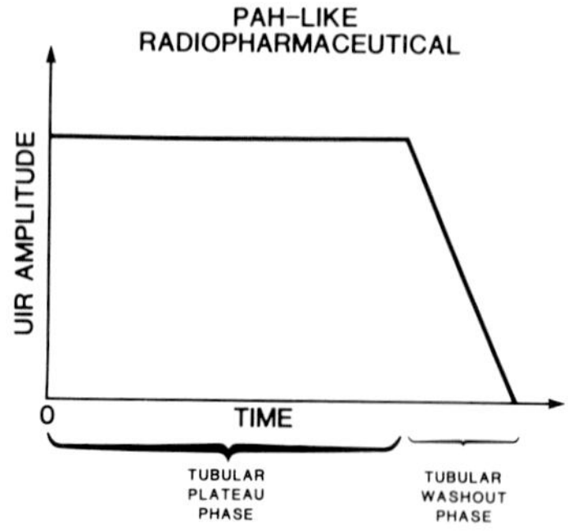

Figure 4-6. A: Deconvoluted renal time-activity histogram from a substance behaving like PAH.

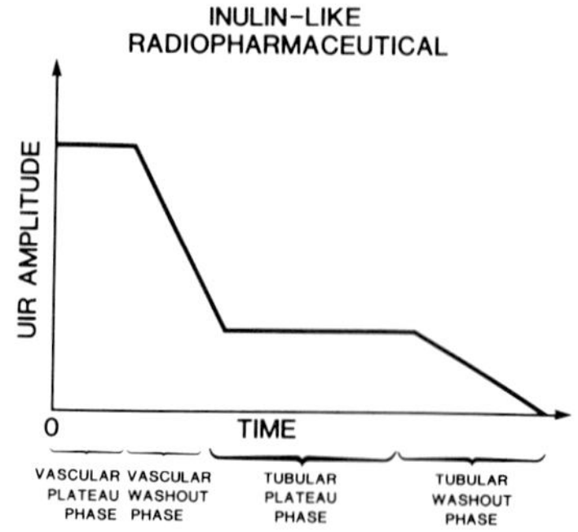

Figure 4-6. B: Deconvoluted renal time-activity curve from a substance behaving like inulin.

Computed *UIR*s may be used to calculate indices of relative renal function (that is, left vs. right). Relative effective renal plasma flow *(ERPF)* may be estimated from the relative initial amplitudes of the *UIRs* obtained using a tracer that is handled like PAH.[37,59] Relative *GFR* may be estimated from the relative initial amplitudes of the tubular *UIRs* obtained using a tracer that is handled like inulin.[22] Relative *GFR* calculated by this method has been shown to correlate well with individual kidney creatinine clearance.[56] Computed *UIRs* are also useful for quantitating transit times of radiotracer through the kidney. The mean tubular transit time *(MTTT)* (that is the mean time that filtered or secreted radiotracer remains in the kidney) has been shown to be of value in distinguishing obstructive and nonobstructive renal disease.[95] *MTTT* may be computed using the formula:

$$MTTT = \sum_{i=1}^{N-1} i(UIR[i+1] - UIR[i])/UIR[1] \qquad [2]$$

in which $UIR[i]$ $(i = 1, N)$ is the N point tubular *UIR* curve.

Glomerular Filtration Rate (GFR)

GFR may be estimated following intravenous injection of a radiotracer that is handled like inulin. The substance most commonly used for this purpose is stannous Tc-99m DTPA. There are two basic approaches for the estimation of *GFR.* The first approach is based on clearance of the radiotracer from the plasma. The second approach is based on the rate of tracer uptake by the kidney.

Both approaches are feasible, and the choice between them is a matter of convenience. In the method using plasma clearance, it is assumed that the radiotracer leaves the body solely through the urine. Single-injection techniques have largely replaced the classic, but tedious, constant-infusion techniques. The tracer is administered by rapid intravenous injection. The concentration of the tracer in the plasma as a function of time may be monitored by counting a series of blood samples. Alternatively, plasma concentration of the tracer may be recorded by an external detector over the heart or head. The resulting time-activity curve must be calibrated by one or more blood samples. External detector introduces a possible source of error because activity outside of the intravascular space may be detected. In practice, however, it results in similar estimates of *GFR*[89,104] and has the advantage of reducing the number of blood samples needed.

Equations for calculating the clearance of a radiotracer after a single injection are usually derived from a single- or multiple-compartment model.[12,105] The parameters of the model are estimated by fitting a single[53,104] or multiple[96,102] exponential curve to the plasma concentration curve. More generally, it can be shown that *GFR* may be calculated from the dose injected, *D*, and the total area under the plasma concentration curve (interpolated and extrapolated to infinity), *A*, using the formula[45]:

$$GFR = D/A \qquad [3]$$

From this point of view, exponential curve fitting is merely a method for interpolating and extrapolating the plasma radiotracer concentration curve (Fig. 4-7). Single-injection clearance methods for estimating *GFR* have been shown to correlate well with inulin,[53] iothalamate, and creatinine[96] clearances obtained using the constant infusion technique.

The other approach to estimation of *GFR*, based on the uptake of the tracer by the kidney, assumes that the radiotracer remains in the kidney for at least some fixed period of time after it enters (typically 2–3 min). It also assumes that the amount of intravascular activity is negligible relative to the amount of intratubular activity during the time of measurement. Changes in radiotracer concentration in the plasma may or may not be taken into account.

Piepsz et al.[93] reported a method by which *GFR* was estimated from the cardiac and renal time-activity curves obtained during the first 3 min after injection of Tc-99m DTPA. *GFR* was calculated using the formula:

$$GFR = (dR(t)/dt)/P(t) \qquad [4]$$

in which $R(t)$ and $P(t)$ represent total renal activity and plasma activity concentration as functions of time. The method was found to correlate with 24-h creatinine clearances in a series of 45 children.[94] Gates[43] reported a method by which *GFR* was estimated from the percentage of the Tc-99m DTPA dose taken up by the kidney in the 2–3-min interval following injection. The percentage of uptake was found to correlate well with 24-h creatinine clearance values in a series of 31 adults. It is not clear, however, that the method will work quantitatively in children because of their greatly varying volumes of distribution.

For the past eight years, our laboratory has been using a method similar to that reported by Gates to quantify the percent uptake of Tc-99m DTPA on images at 60–120 sec after injection. The percentage of Tc-99m DTPA renal uptake has been helpful in estimating global and individual renal function. With this method it is possible to monitor changes in renal function in patients on surgical and/or medical treatment for a variety of renal diseases. It is also possible to estimate differential *GFR* from the relative percentage of uptake by the two kidneys after correction for background activity and tissue attenuation. This method for esti-

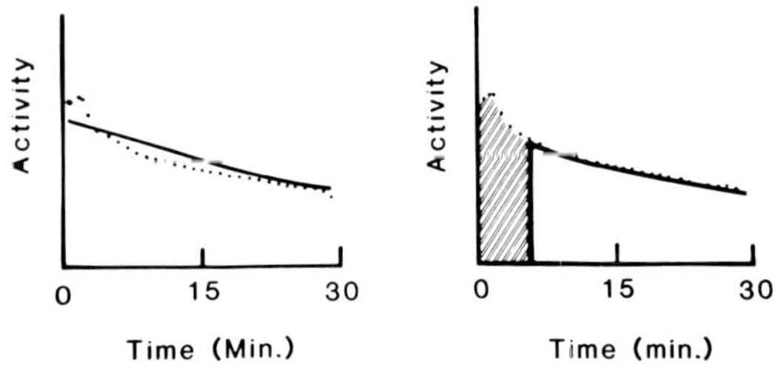

Figure 4-7. Calculation of *GFR* using Eq. [3] required an estimate of the area under the tracer disappearance curve. The area may be estimated as the area under an exponential fit to the data curve *(left:)*. Greater accuracy may be obtained by numerically integrating the first 5 min of the data curve and adding the area under an exponential fit to the remainder *(right)*.

mating differential *GFR* has been shown to correlate well with separate kidney iothalamate[96] and Cr-51 ethylenediaminetetraacetic acid (EDTA)[9] clearance values obtained by ureteric catheterization.

ERPF

ERPF may be estimated in the same manner as *GFR* if a radiotracer that is handled like PAH rather than like inulin is used. The most commonly used radiotracers for this purpose are I-131 and I-123 OIH. Both the plasma clearance and renal uptake approaches have been used. The technique using plasma clearance is essentially the same one used for estimating *GFR* from inulin-like radiopharmaceuticals. *ERPF* is calculated using a formula analogous to Eq. [3].

As in the estimation of *GFR*, the concentration of the tracer in plasma may be followed by either multiple blood samples or external detection. Both methods have been found to give similar results. Blaufox et al.[12] found a good correlation in the measurement of *ERPF* using I-131 OIH with serial blood sampling and external detection using a scintillation probe over the patient's head. Similarly, Ram et al.[98] and Razzak et al.[100] found good agreement in the values of *ERPF* calculated by serial blood sampling and by external detection over the precordium. Ram et al.[98] reported a strong correlation between *ERPF* estimates obtained by single-exponential extrapolation of I-125 OIH time-activity curves obtained from over the precordium and PAH clearance. Mackay et al.[74] reported the estimation of *ERPF* from a I-123 OIH time-activity curve obtained over the abdomen and a single blood sample using single-exponential extrapolation. *ERPF* estimates were found to correlate closely with PAH clearances but tended to be slightly lower. They averaged 89% of the PAH clearance values. Heidenreich et al.[50] reported their clinical experience in the estimation of *ERPF* from the clearance of I-123 OIH in 153 children. The renal uptake approach to *ERPF* estimation has also been used.[106] Thompson et al.[125] reported the 1–2 min renal uptake of I-131 OIH correlated well with PAH clearances.

Relative *ERPF* may also be estimated from the relative percentage of uptake of the two kidneys.[50,83,121] Relative uptake of I-123 OIH in the 0.5–2.5 min after injection has been shown to correlate well with separate kidney PAH clearance values obtained by ureteric catheterization.[74]

Clinical Applications

Neonatal Period

Radionuclide studies have proven to be useful adjuncts to both excretory urography and ultrasonography in the evaluation of renal abnormalities in the newborn. Because of the poor concentration of contrast agents by the kidneys and the relatively high doses of hypertonic agents that must be used for intravenous pyelography, radionuclide scintigraphy is particularly useful in the first week of life.[78,115] In the newborn the intravenous urogram is unsatisfactory in a significant percentage of cases for technical and physiologic reasons.[27] This is not surprising, as the *GFR* per unit of surface area is about 30% lower in the newborn than in the adult. In the first few days of life, there is a dramatic rise in the corrected *GFR* followed by a more gradual increase, so that adult levels are reached at about 1 year of age. Absolute values for the tubular maximum of PAH in newborns and infants are low even when corrected for body weight or surface area, kidney weight, and *GFR*.

In newborns, renal uptake of tracers is lower than in older children and adults. In addition, intrarenal transit time and excretion of these tracers are normally longer at this age than later in life.

A normal Tc-99m DTPA renal study in newborn infants during the first week of life generally demonstrates faint and delayed renal uptake of the tracer with or without delayed appearance of activity within the bladder. If activity is seen in the bladder within 2–5 min, the amount present will be lower than in older children. Background levels of activity will be high throughout the study reflecting low blood clearance of the tracer. This is due to normally slow *GFR* in patients in this age group. Some normal newborns, however, will demonstrate normal uptake and excretion of the tracer (Figs. 4-8 and 4-9).

Low tracer uptake and delayed transit time may also be observed in studies with OIH.

Immaturity of renal function may also be evident in studies with Tc-99m DMSA. Images obtained with this agent may show relatively low kidney-to-background ratio.

This immaturity in renal function does not affect

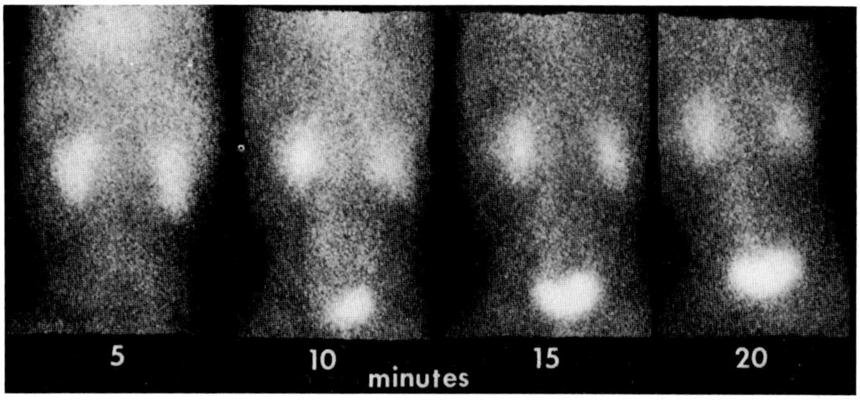

Figure 4-8. Normal Tc-99m DTPA study on a premature infant. This patient was dehydrated and mildly acidotic. There was some concern that the kidneys could not be palpated. This study was performed to evaluate function, size, and location of the kidneys. There is good uptake and excretion of tracer bilaterally (some delay in transit time is normal in this age group).

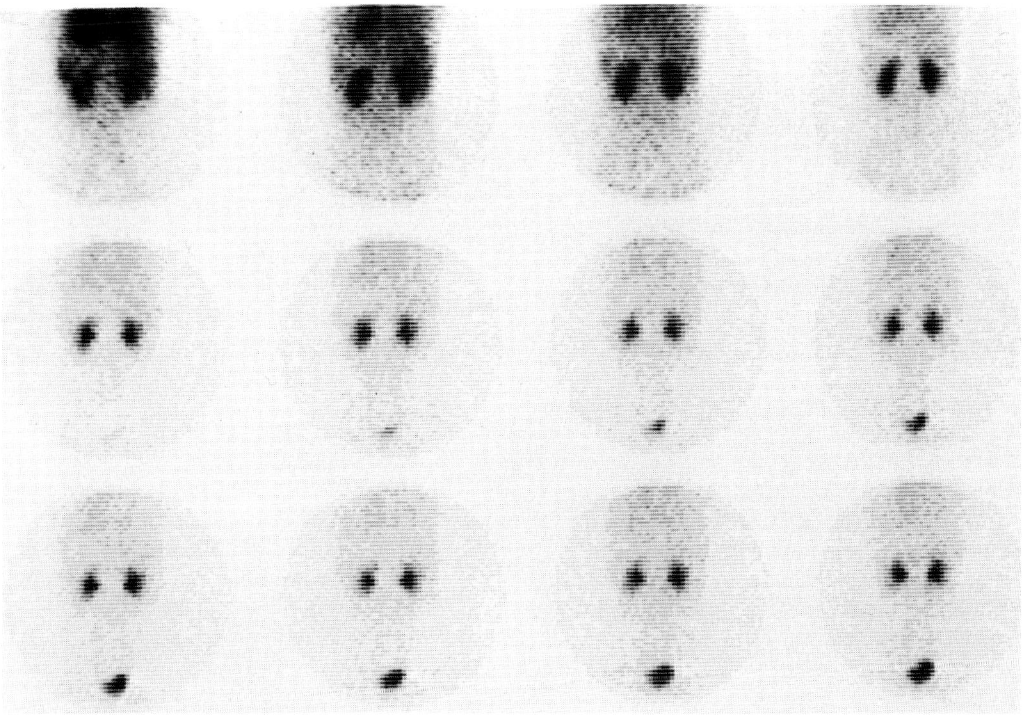

Figure 4-9. Normal Tc-99m DTPA study in an infant. One frame represents 1 min. Tracer is taken up rapidly by the kidneys and appears in the renal pelves as early as 4 min after injection. The bladder is seen at 5 min.

the ability of radionuclide studies to provide information on relative renal function. As renal function matures with age, renal uptake, intrarenal transit time, and excretion of tracers approach normal values.

A frequent indication for radionuclide renal studies in the neonatal period is unilateral or bilateral *flank masses*. A large mass may be due to severe hydronephrosis, multicystic dysplastic kidneys, polycystic kidneys, renal vein thrombosis, or

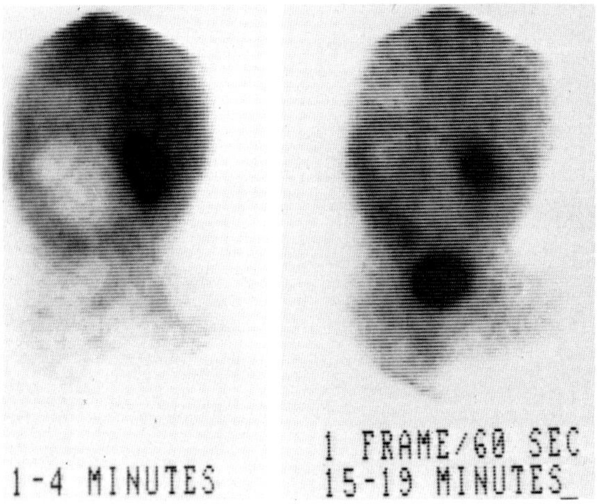

Figure 4-10. Hydronephrosis of the left kidney in a neonate. Tc-99m DTPA study, posterior view. The image on the *left* (1–4 min) reveals a dilated left collecting system surrounded by a thin rim of functional renal parenchyma. The right kidney appears normal. At 15–19 min later *(right)*, tracer is seen in the left renal parenchyma and also within the dilated left collecting system. The right kidney has drained much of the radiotracer into the bladder.

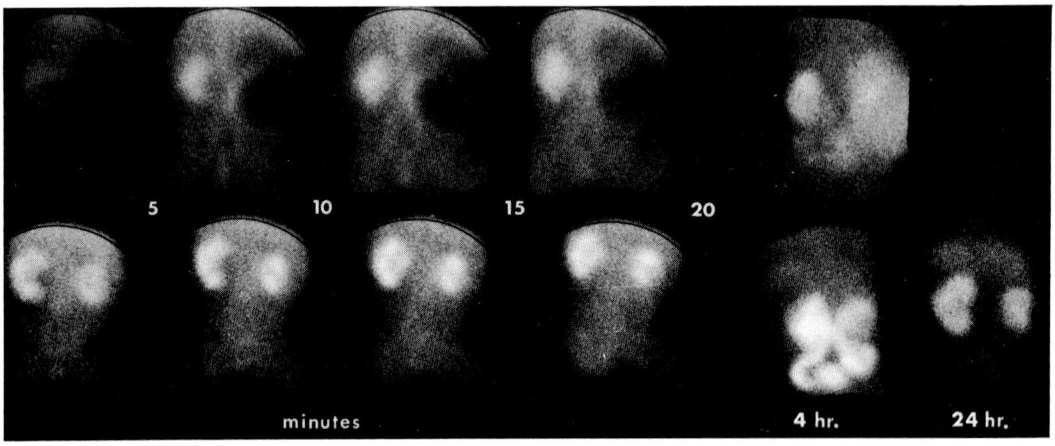

Figure 4-11. Hydronephrosis. Effect of decompression. Male infant with a right flank mass detected soon after birth. Intravenous urography and voiding cystography revealed bilateral hydronephrosis, more severe on the right, and posterior urethral valves. Tc-99m DMSA scan *(upper row)* shows decreased uptake and excretion of the tracer by the left kidney with a dilated pelvis. The right kidney reveals minimal or no uptake of the tracer with a large "photon-deficient" area corresponding to a grossly dilated renal pelvis. An image 4 h after the injection shows tracer within the large right renal pelvis. A week following surgical drainage of the right kidney another Tc-99m DTPA renal scan was obtained *(lower row)*. The right kidney is smaller and exhibits improved renal function. At 4 h postinjection, both ureters which are dilated and redundant are visualized. A Tc-99m DMSA scan performed 24 h later *(below, right)* shows a small right kidney.

nephroblastoma (Wilm's tumor). In cases of hydronephrosis due to *obstruction* at the ureteropelvic junction, scintigraphy will demonstrate abnormalities in structure and function on the involved side (Fig. 4-10). With obstruction distal to the ureterovesical junction, such as in posterior uretheral valves, there is bilateral renal involvement. Those patients presenting in early infancy have severe obstruction with impaired renal function. It should be emphasized that the evaluation of function in the presence of obstruction does not give a reliable indication of the potential for recovery. Renal function may improve once the obstruction has been relieved (Fig. 4-11).

The appearance of the scan in *polycystic renal disease* will depend on the degree of renal involvement. When function is moderately compromised, prolonged transit of the tracer will be evident. In more severe cases, there may be no evidence of functioning renal tissue (Figs. 4-12 and 4-13).

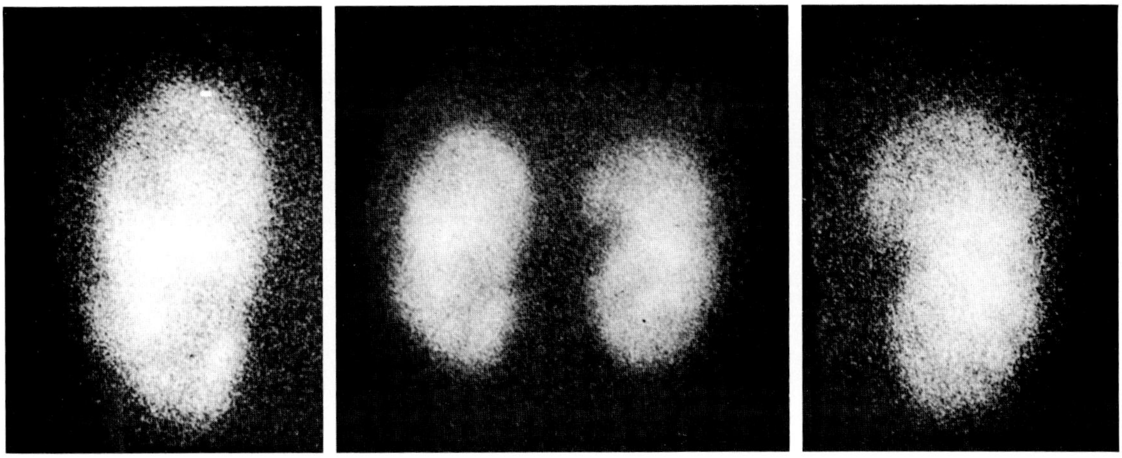

Figure 4-12. Polycystic renal disease. Tc-99m DMSA renal scintigraphs. In the center of the panel an image of 500,000 counts obtained with a high-resolution collimator is seen. On each side of the panel magnified images with a pinhole collimator are shown. Multiple intrarenal areas of decreased-to-absent uptake are visualized and they most likely represent cysts. This scan is from a 2.5-year-old female with polycystic renal disease who developed hypertension.

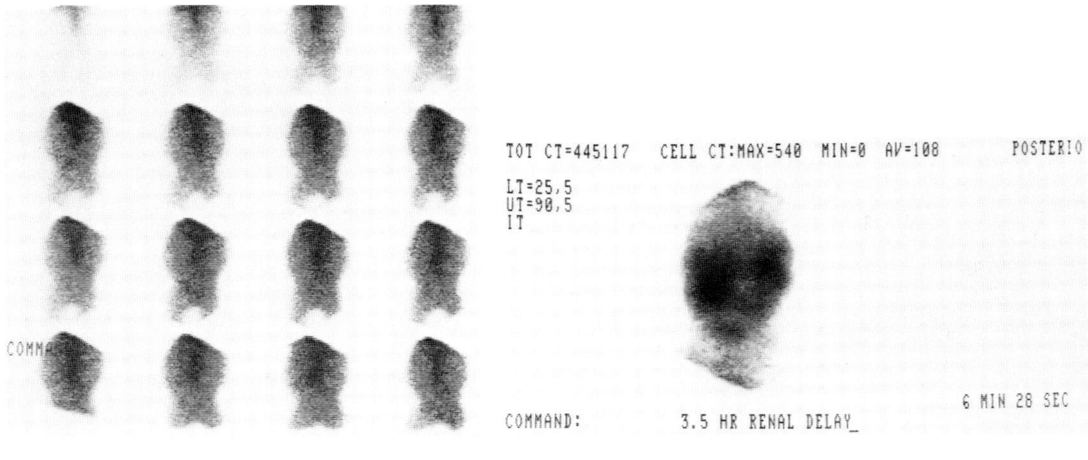

Figure 4-13. Polycystic renal disease. *Left:* Tc-99m DTPA study. One frame represents 1 min. There is no evidence of selective renal uptake of the tracer. *Right:* Tc-99m DMSA image reveals poor tracer uptake in large, dilated kidneys.

While *ascites* in the newborn is frequently due to an obstructive uropathy, anarsarca is not always renal in origin and the kidneys may be normal in size and function.

Enlarged kidneys may also be found in *multicystic dysplastic kidneys.* The scintigraphic appearance reveals minimal or no renal uptake of the tracer (Fig. 4-14). Renal dysplasia may occur without cysts. The kidneys are usually small (Fig. 4-15).

Adrenal hemorrhage may give rise to unilateral or bilateral flank masses, usually within the first few days of life. Scintigraphically, adrenal hemorrhage presents as a suprarenal photon-deficient area seen best immediately after injection of the tracer during the phase of whole-body distribution (Fig. 4-16). If the hemorrhage is large, there is usually renal displacement or compression. Renal function is preserved unless there is an associated lesion, such as renal vein thrombosis. A possible

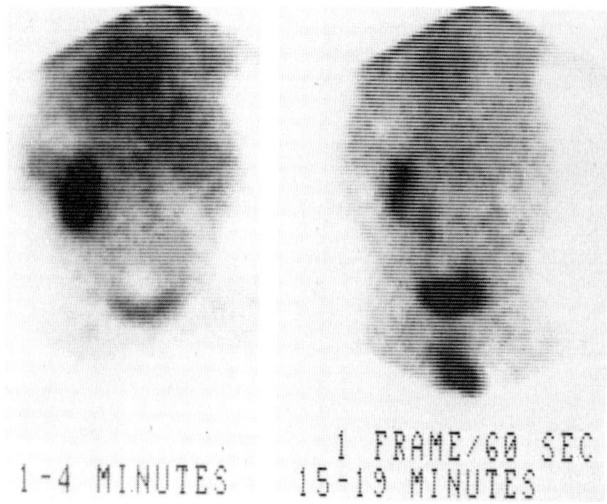

◁**Figure 4-14. A:** Multicystic dysplastic kidney in an infant. Tc-99m DTPA study, posterior view. Each image represents 5 min. The left kidney is normal but there is no evidence of selective tracer uptake in the right one. Radioactivity is already visualized in the bladder *(left)*. Fifteen to twenty minutes later there is still no uptake of tracer on the right kidney *(right)*. The left kidney has drained more tracer into the bladder.

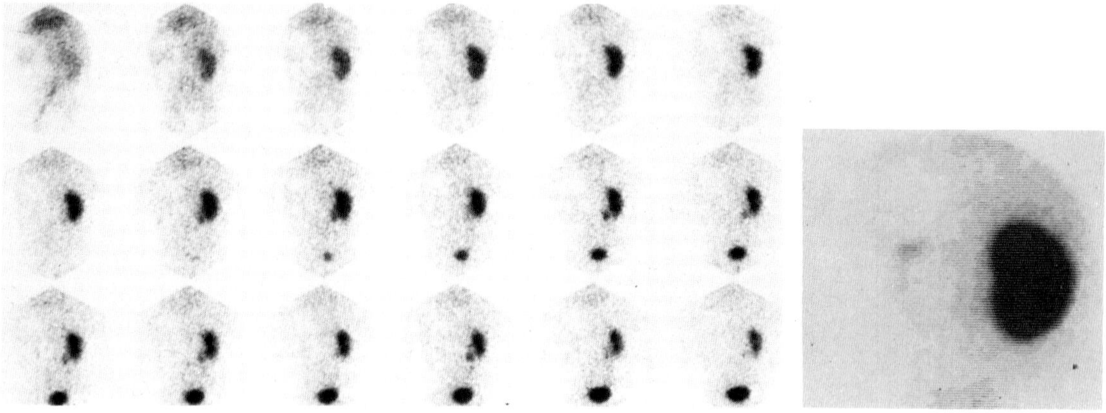

△ **Figure 4-14. B:** Left multicystic, dysplastic kidney in another infant. Series of 1-min Tc-99m DTPA images *(left)* showing no function of the left kidney. The right kidney assumes most of the renal function. Tc-99m DMSA with computer enhancement reveals a minimal amount of functioning left renal parenchyma *(right)*.

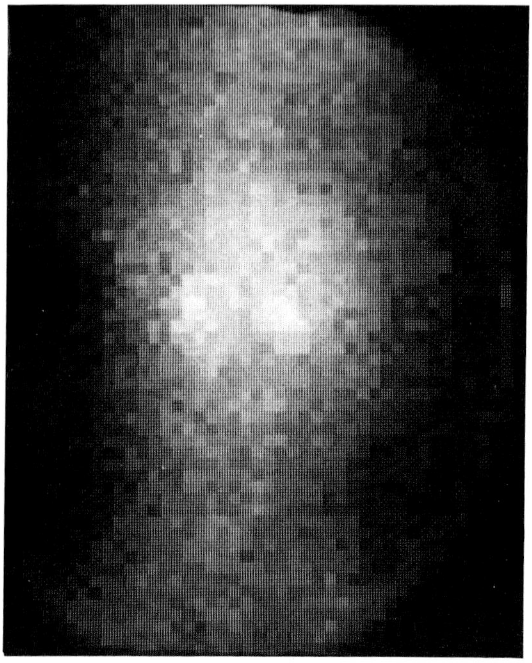

◁ **Figure 4-15.** Dysplastic renal disease. Tc-99m DMSA scintigram done 24 h after the injection of the tracer. This was done on a 7-year-old male with findings consistent with congenital renal dysplasia with an associated salt-losing tendency and tubular defect for glucose and HCO_3^- which led to metabolic acidosis, hyponatremia, and dehydration. Serum creatinine was elevated. Ultrasonography suggested only a small left kidney. The radionuclide scan reveals two small and poorly functioning kidneys.

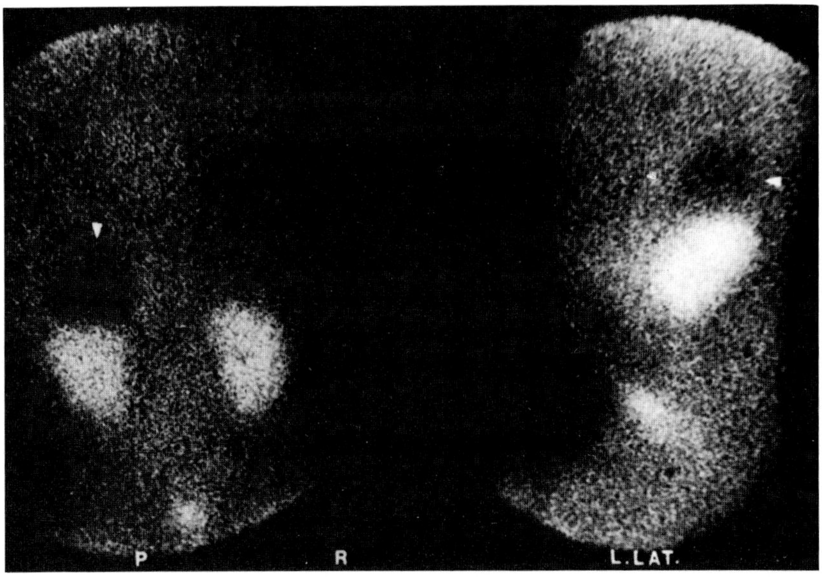

Figure 4-16. Adrenal hemorrhage. Tc-99m DTPA images from a 48-h-old post-mature male, obtained 10 min after injection. This patient was born after a difficult delivery with an Apgar score of 1. Examination of his urine revealed heavy sediment with proteinuria, raising the question of acute tubular necrosis secondary to hypoxia. A left abdominal mass was palpable. The scintiscans reveal whole-body distribution of the tracer and clear visualization of both renal units and activity in the urinary bladder. The left kidney is deformed by an avascular mass representing an adrenal hemorrhage.

source of confusion in the scintigraphic detection of adrenal hemorrhage is a distended gastric fundus, which may simulate a left suprarenal mass.

Most types of acquired renal disease in newborns are due to circulatory disturbances, such as renal arterial or venous *thrombosis*. Renal vein thrombosis in infants is probably related to venous stasis secondary to shock, septicemia, or dehydration. This disorder is also seen in infants of diabetic mothers. Consumptive coagulopathy or intravascular coagulation may be a feature in some of these patients. The infant presents with a flank mass, oliguria, and hematuria. Hypertension, which is not frequent in this condition, has been a feature in several patients we have studied. In severe cases, there is no perfusion or function in the involved side (Fig. 4-17). A followup study is useful in demonstrating the residual renal function after recovery. Occasionally the diagnosis of renal vein thrombosis is presumed on the basis of mild hematuria, proteinuria, and poor renal opacification by intravenous pyelography. Radionuclide studies may reveal information of prognostic significance, a normal study predicting a rapid and complete recovery.

Most newborns pass urine within 24 h. If micturition is delayed beyond 36 h, there may be cause for concern. Serious causes for *delayed onset of micturition* are rare in the absence of either enlarged kidneys or a palpable hypertrophied bladder. Radionuclide studies are useful for demonstrating normal renal function and morphology (Fig. 4-18). On the other hand, patients who have been anuric for 48 h with no demonstrable renal function may have renal agenesis or severe dysplasia.

The Postnatal Period

Hydronephrosis

Hydronephrosis is one of the most common indications for radionuclide evaluation of the kidneys in pediatric patients. The findings on radionuclide evaluation vary depending on the severity of the disease, site of obstruction, whether it is uni- or bilateral, presence or absence of reflux, and recent surgery. On studies performed with Tc-99m DTPA or similar substances, the hydronephrotic kidney

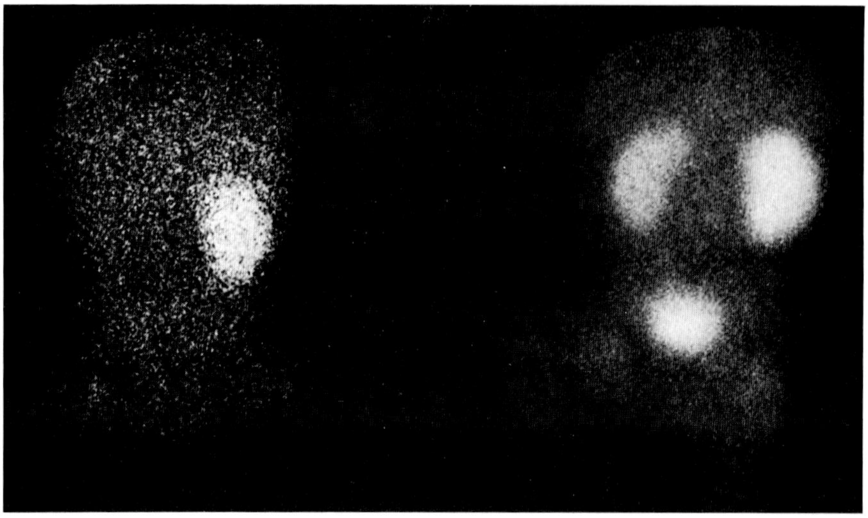

Figure 4-17. Renal vein thrombosis. Tc-99m DMSA scans. Premature, 1400 g female patient who developed hypertension after withdrawal of an umbilical artery line. Ultrasonography revealed two kidneys of normal size. The initial Tc-99m DMSA scan *(left)* reveals non-visualization of the left kidney. The patient was treated with hydralazine for 3 weeks and became normotensive. A second Tc-99m DMSA reveals return of function to the left kidney.

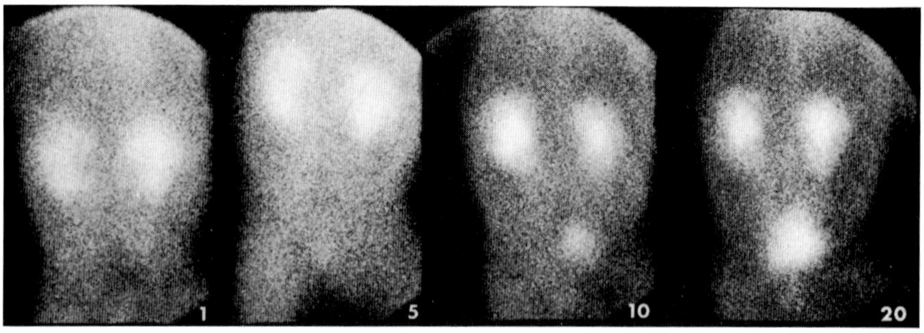

Figure 4-18. Anuria. This study was performed on a 36-h-old male infant because of anuria. The Tc-99m DTPA study reveals prompt and symmetric uptake of the tracer with no evidence of obstruction. The intra-renal transit time is slightly prolonged but this may be normal in a small infant. The bladder is visualized between 5 and 10 min after injection of the tracer. The patient produced urine within the next 12 h.

will generally appear on the early images (0–5 or even 10 min) as having an area devoid of tracer in the region corresponding to the renal pelvis and collecting system. The size of this photon-deficient area will depend on the degree of dilatation of the pyelocalyceal system. This area will be surrounded by a rim of activity corresponding to tracer within the renal parenchyma (Figs. 4-19 and 4-20).

As the study progresses in time, the pelvicalyceal system will begin to fill with radiotracer leaving the renal parenchyma. The rate of appearance of the tracer in the pelvicalyceal system will depend on the function of the hydronephrotic kidney. In some cases, tracer will begin to accumulate within 3–6 min in the pelvicalyceal system in spite of severe dilatation; in others, however, this time will be prolonged from several minutes to several hours after the injection of the tracer. The apparent function of the hydronephrotic kidney will depend on the degree of urinary obstruction increasing the pressure in the pelvicalyceal system and on the presence and degree of renal damage. The amount of radiotracer

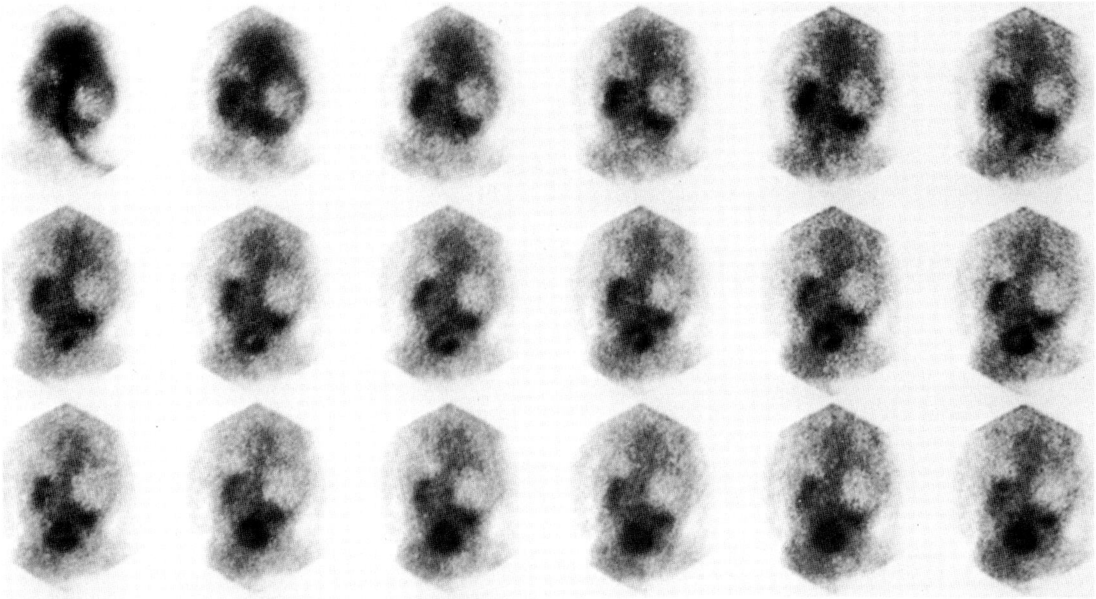
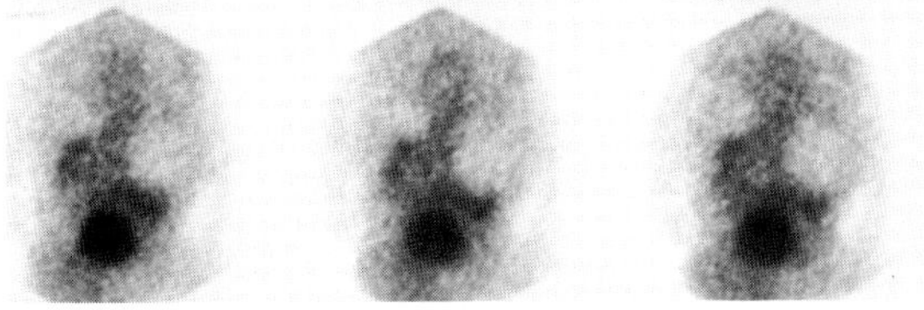

Figure 4-19. Hydronephrosis of the right kidney. Tc-99m DTPA study (one frame/60 sec) reveals a large photon-deficient area in the region of the right kidney corresponding to right hydronephrosis. The left kidney appears normal and drains well into the bladder.

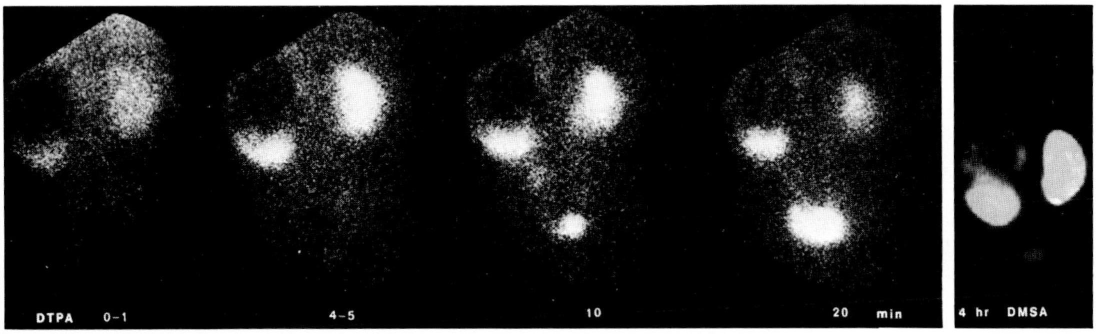

Figure 4-20. Obstruction of the upper pole of a duplicated left kidney. Series of Tc-99m DTPA images show a photon deficient area in the upper pole of the left kidney that is surrounded by a rim of parenchymal uptake of the tracer. No activity is seen within the upper collecting system of the left kidney up to 20 min. The lower pole is also obstructed but shows good function. A Tc-99m DMSA renal scan done 4 h after injection shows a hydronephrotic left upper pole with patches of functioning renal parenchyma. The left lower pole and the right kidney contain functioning parenchyma.

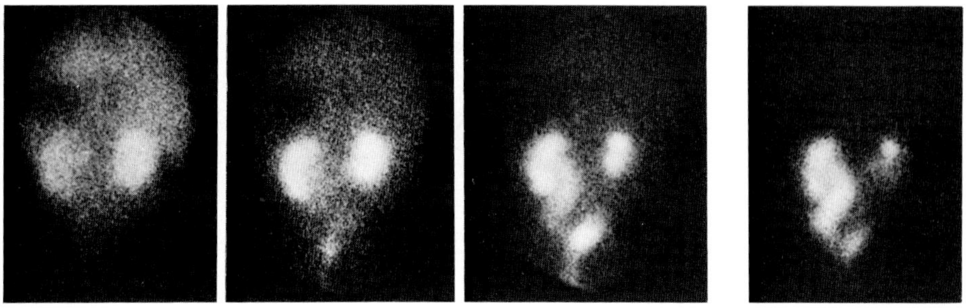

Figure 4-21. Ureterovesical junction obstruction. The right kidney is almost normal except for mild delay radionuclide transit time within the right collecting system. The left kidney exhibits less function than the right and shows prolonged retention of the tracer within the collecting system and the ureter all the way to the ureterovesical junction. Even after the administration of furosemide and voiding the left pelvis and ureter fail to drain.

uptake in the renal parenchyma is directly related to the functioning capacity of the kidney in question. Renal function as assessed in an obstructed kidney may not represent the true functional potential of such a kidney. It does indicate, however, the minimal function that may be expected. High pressure in the pelvicalyceal system results in a reduction of renal blood flow and function that may be reversed after relief of the obstruction (see above). An accurate assessment of renal functional capacity can be attained after the obstruction is relieved.[24,79]

In patients in whom the kidney(s) are not visualized by radionuclide imaging, it is not possible to determine with these studies whether there is recoverable renal function. Even extremely poor renal function due to chronic obstruction is potentially reversible.[108] In these patients, ultrasonography and/or antegrade pyelography should be done to search for surgically correctable lesions. Serial renal scanning is then useful to assess recovery.

Kalika et al. suggest that when cortical time-activity curves appear more nearly normal than the total kidney curve in preoperative patients, there is a strong likelihood of improvement after the obstruction is relieved. Abnormal cortical curves have been associated with a poor prognosis for functional improvement in their patients.[57] In some instances it is possible to identify the site of obstruction at the ureterovesical or the pelvicalyceal junction (Figs. 4-21 and 4-22). In other cases, particularly when there is obstruction at both the pelvicalyceal and ureterovesical junctions, it may be difficult to detect the ureterovesical obstruction. Detection of the level of obstruction also depends on adequate renal function and the presence or absence of dilatation of the pelvicalyceal system and ureter.

Furosemide Stimulation Test. Radionuclide studies using hydration and intravenous furosemide (Lasix) may be helpful in some instances, to differentiate urinary obstuction from a dilated nonobstructed kidney. Thrall et al. and Koff et al. modified conventional renography to include the administration of furosemide. They reported that in dilated nonobstructed kidneys increased diuresis causes a washout of tracer from the kidney. In significantly obstructed kidneys, activity in the renal area fails to decrease in response to diuresis. They reported that the major limitation with this approach was the presence of poor renal function limiting the diuretic response.[64,127] Meller et al.[80] studying children with dilated upper urinary tracts found that furosemide studies had an overall sensitivity of 87% for the detection of obstruction. They also reported a sensitivity for the diagnosis of pelviureteric junction obstruction of 93%. Shore et al.[109] evaluated diuretic renography in a group of 20 children. These authors found good correlation with other indicators of obstruction. They found a sensitivity of 83% and a specificity of 94% in their studies. We agree with their comment that severe hydroureteronephrosis may partly or totally mask the effect of diuresis on the emptying of the tracer from the renal pelvis. These authors suggest that kidneys that drain only with a change in patient position should not be considered obstructed.[109]

We employ furosemide routinely in the evaluation of children suspected of having urinary ob-

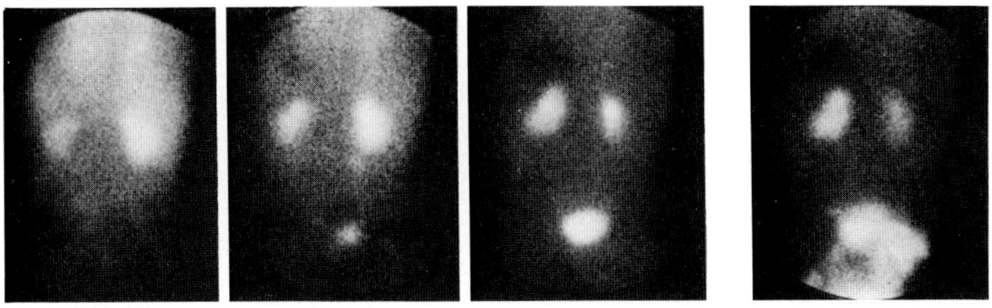

Figure 4-21. Ureterovesical junction obstruction. The right kidney is almost normal except for mild delay radionuclide transit time within the right collecting system. The left kidney exhibits less function than the right and shows prolonged retention of the tracer within the collecting system and the ureter all the way to the ureterovesical junction. Even after the administration of furosemide and voiding the left pelvis and ureter fail to drain.

struction. Before giving Tc-99m DTPA, an intranvenous saline infusion is begun and is maintained for the duration of the study. Series of 1-min images are evaluated for 12–15 min after injection of the tracer. At this time, and depending on the apparent drainage of radiotracer from the pelvicalyceal system(s), a decision is made as to whether to administer furosemide. If retention of tracer is apparent, furosemide (0.3–1.0 mg/kg) is administered into the intranveous line and imaging is continued for an additional 10–20 min or even later in order to assess the effect of diuresis on drainage. If there is no retention of tracer, furosemide is not administered and the study is terminated as usual.

Diuretic renal scintigraphy is useful when it can clearly establish the absence of presence of obstruction (Fig. 4-23). In certain instances, however, it is not possible with diuretic scintigraphy to determine whether obstruction is present: severely depressed renal function, dilatation of the pelvicalyceal system, bladder overdistention, overlapping kidney or ureter, reflux, prune belly syndrome, ectopic kidney (Fig. 4-24). As mentioned before, catheterization of the bladder is often helpful to rule out obstruction.

When there is retention of the tracer in the renal collecting system, it is helpful to have the patient empty the bladder and then obtain an image to determine if such retention was due to bladder distention and not to fixed obstruction. In infants it is useful to maintain a catheter in the bladder in order to avoid confusing results due to bladder distension. Bladder catheterization is also helpful in the interpretation of radionuclide studies in ectopic kidneys. In trying to localize the obstruction, it is important to evaluate carefully the series of images and the time-activity curves from the renal cortex, the kidneys, and the ureters.

In some patients the forced diuresis caused by furosemide will cause or reproduce flank pain, especially in those with intermittent hydronephrosis. These are usually patients who complain of intermittent pain. In these patients, perhaps there is a balance of urine inflow and outflow in the renal pelvis that usually causes no discomfort. Transient overdistension in these systems may cause pain. In other patients a relatively stable balance of urinary flow and drainage may exist in dilated systems and may cause no pain or discomfort.

Patients in whom radionuclide diagnosis of obstruction is difficult include those with urinary diversions. The dynamics of urinary flow in urinary diversions are usually different than in normal kidneys even in the absence of obstruction. Sometimes, overlap of kidney and the ileal or colonic diversion causes confusing images. Removal and replacement of external plastic bags containing radioactive urine, images in various projections, and attempts at postural drainage of the diversion are helpful maneuvers.

Studies using Tc-99m DMSA are very helpful in assessing the presence, distribution, and quantity of functioning renal cortex in obstructed kidneys. In instances of severe obstruction, delayed DMSA imaging at about 24 h after injection is helpful. With time the activity from Tc-99m DMSA continues to increase within the renal cortex while the small amounts of tracer eliminated in the urine drain, allowing for a better assessment of distribution of functioning renal parenchyma (Fig. 4-25).

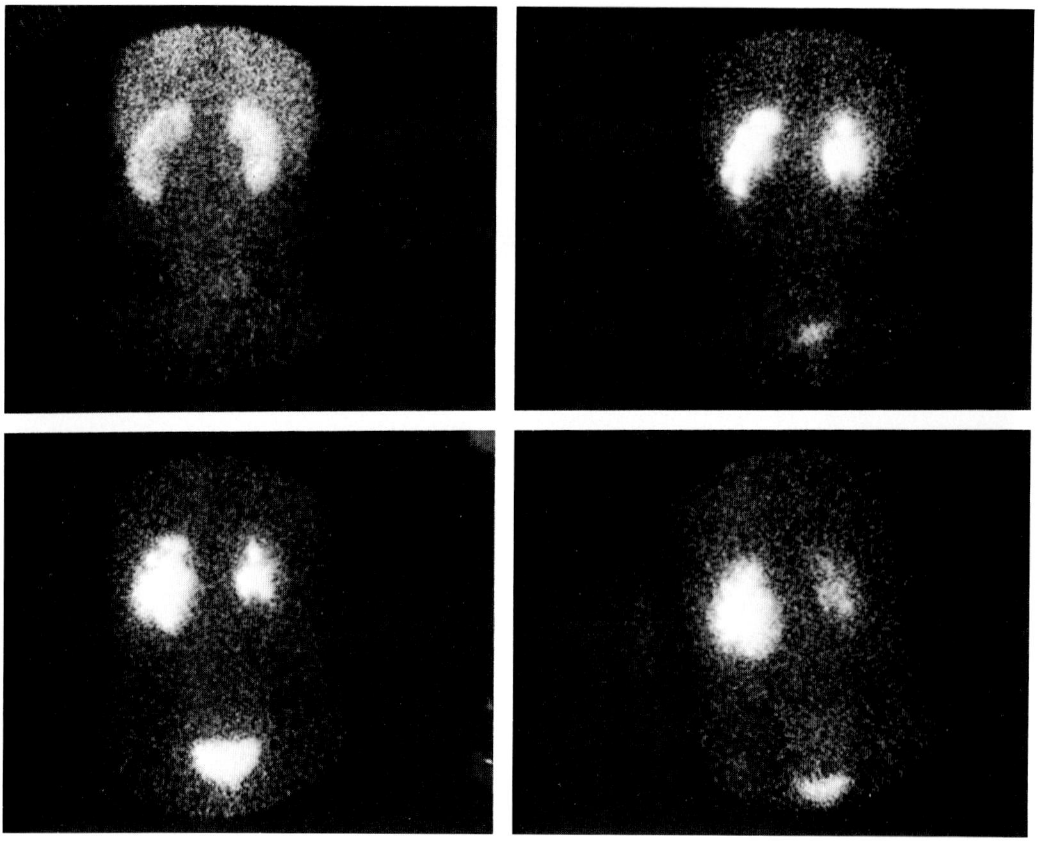

Figure 4-23. Left ureteropelvic junction obstruction. Selected frames from a Tc-99m DTPA study. *Upper left:* Two minutes after the injection of the tracer the right kidney appears normal; the left kidney takes up less amount of the tracer and shows a photon-deficient area corresponding to dilatation of the renal pelvis. *Upper right:* Ten minutes after injection. There is some retention of the tracer in the right collecting system and delayed parenchymal transit time in the left kidney. *Lower left:* Thirty minutes after injection. Some drainage has occurred from the right kidney; however, significant retention is present in a dilated left renal pelvis. *Lower right:* Fifteen minutes following administration of furosemide and after voiding. The right kidney has cleared almost completely. However, there has been no significant drainage from the left renal pelvis. In addition, the patient complained of left flank pain a few minutes following the administration of the diuretic.

Pyelonephritis

The presenting signs and symptoms of children with renal infection are varied and sometimes confusing. Clinically it is frequently difficult or impossible to differentiate infection of the bladder and ureters from actual renal parenchymal infection. Patients may present with fever, malaise, irritability, leukocytosis, and bacteriuria but no indication that there is renal parenchymal infection. Other patients with pyelonephritis may present as one of those often puzzling cases of fever of unknown origin.

The lack of sensitivity of intravenous urography and ultrasonography in the demonstration of early renal infection is well known. A relatively small number of patients with severe renal infection will demonstrate abnormalities on intravenous urography. In an excellent paper, Handmaker points out that nuclear medicine procedures are rarely mentioned in review articles dealing with imaging strategies in patients with sudden onset of fever, flank pain, and pyuria or bacteriuria.[47] This is true in spite of the fact that several nuclear medicine studies reveal renal involvement in these patients. Intravenous urograms have been found to be abnormal in only 24–26% of patients with acute pyelonephritis.[29,114] Possible abnormal urographic findings include a renal pelvis of small volume, dilated and distorted pelvicalyceal structures, renal

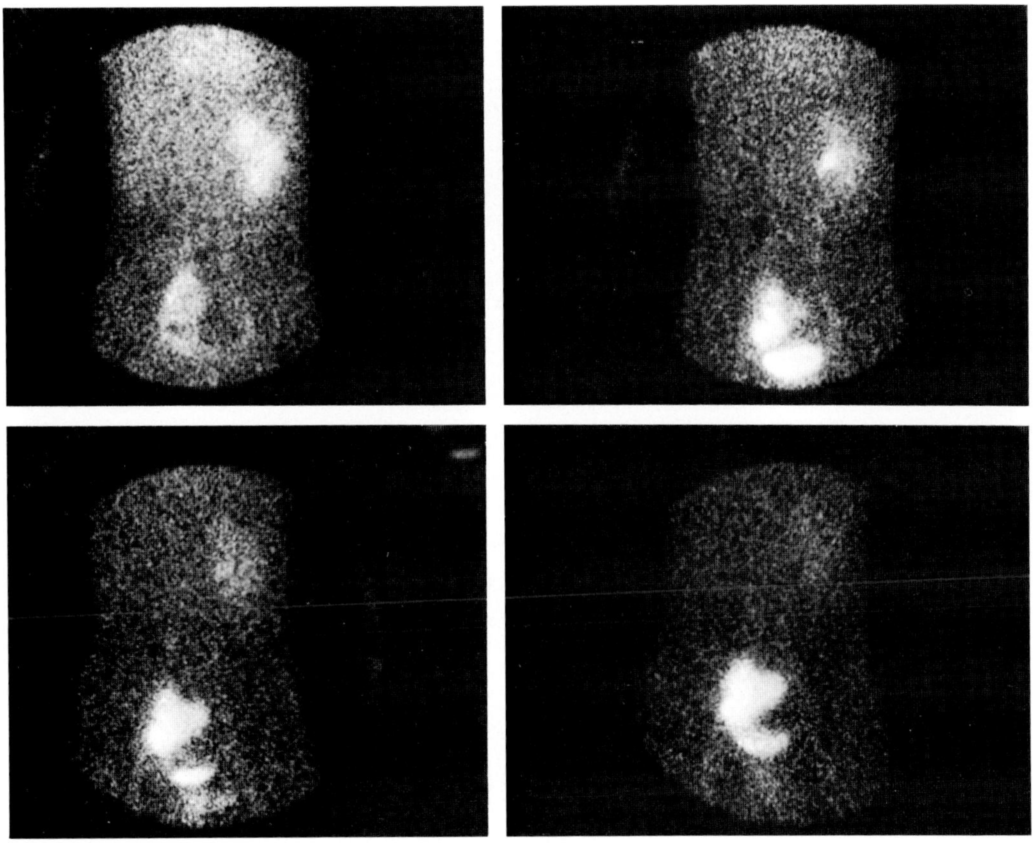

Figure 4-24. Obstructed, ectopic (pelvic), left kidney. Selected frames from a Tc-99m DTPA study. *Upper left:* Two minutes following injection. The right kidney is normal in size, shape, location, and function. The ectopic left kidney is small and shows less uptake. *Upper right:* Frame taken 15 min after the injection of the tracer shows retention in the collecting system of the ectopic kidney. *Lower left:* Frame taken immediately after voiding still shows retention of the tracer in the collecting system of the pelvic kidney. *Lower right:* Frame obtained 15 min after the administration of furosemide and after voiding also confirms the presence of significant obstruction.

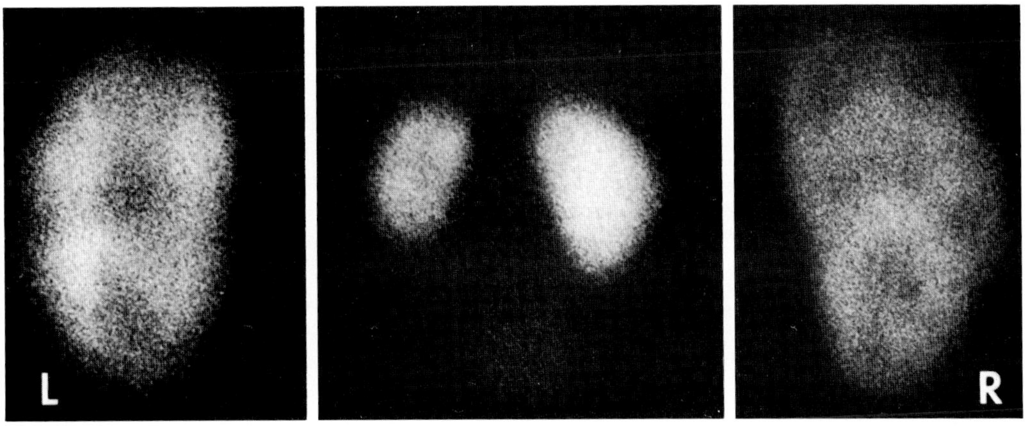

Figure 4-25. Bilateral obstruction in a 2½-month-old male. The patient had urinary tract infection with reflux diagnosed at birth. Tc-99m DMSA scintigraphy reveals reduced function of the left kidney. Pinhole magnified images seen on either side of the image reveal multiple areas of decreased-to-absent uptake due to renal damage.

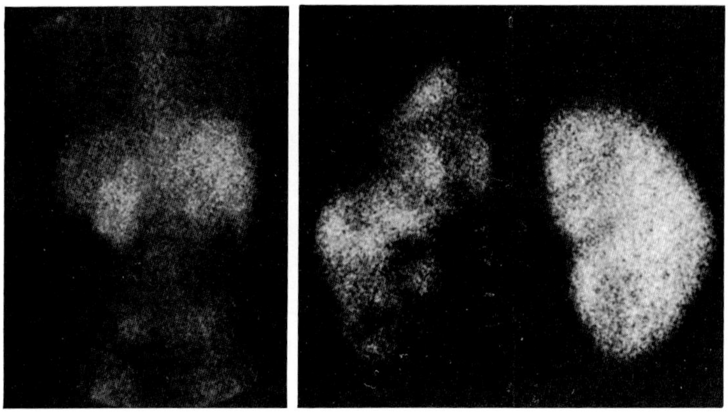

Figure 4-26. Bilateral pyelonephritis. The figure depicts a Ga-67 scan *(left)* showing intense concentration of the tracer in both kidneys with greater concentration in the left one. A Tc-99m DMSA scan *(right)* obtained on the same patient reveals multiple areas of loss of parenchymal function, worse in the left kidney.

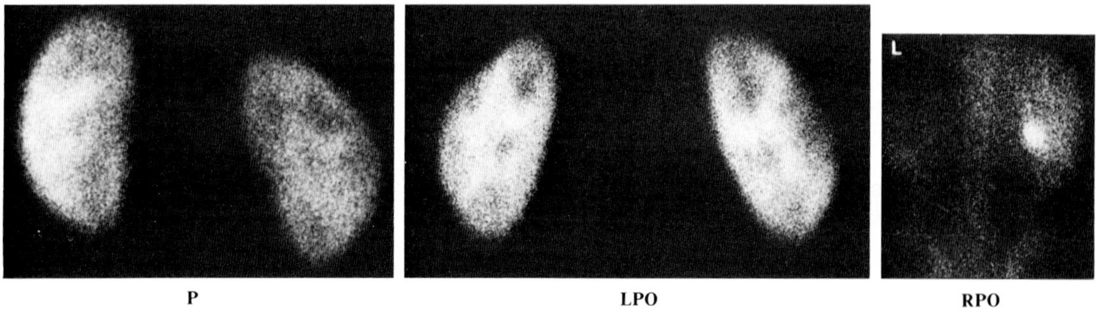

Figure 4-27. Right renal abscess. *Left and center:* Tc-99m DMSA renal scans revealing a defect in the lateral aspect of the right kidney. P, Posterior view; LPO, RPO, left and right posterior oblique projections, respectively. *Right:* Ga-67 scan obtained 48 h following intravenous injection of the tracer reveals a focus of intense radiotracer uptake in the area of the right kidney. This corresponds to the defect seen on the Tc-99m DMSA scan.

enlargement, delayed pyelogram, reduced concentration of urographic material, and dilatation of the ureter without obstruction. Ultrasonography is very useful in diagnosing renal or perirenal abscesses. In acute pyelonephritis, however, ultrasonography is less valuable, in some cases showing renal enlargement as the only abnormal finding.[107]

In the presence of reflux and recurrent urinary tract infections, radionuclide studies are sensitive methods of detecting renal damage. Functional loss can be detected with radionuclide techniques before morphologic changes are evident radiographically.

Kessler et al.[60] reported that Ga-67 citrate could be used in the diagnosis of acute pyelonephritis,[60] and since then other investigators have confirmed these findings[14,46,47,52,81,92] (Figs. 4-26 and 4-27). Ga-67 citrate concentrates in infected renal tissue early in the development of pyelonephritis even before the formation of abscess (Figs. 4-26 and 4-27). Ga-67 imaging can be also used to assess the effectiveness of antibiotic therapy (Fig. 4-28). Ga-67 may not differentiate renal from perirenal infection. A serious problem with Ga-67 is its intense accumulation within the intestine sometimes overshadowing abnormal renal concentration. In some patients it is difficult to differentiate normal from abnormal Ga-67 in the kidney.[38,47] Ga-67 accumulation in the kidneys is not specific for infection. Acute tubular necrosis, vasculitis, leukemic infiltrates, and other disorders have also been reported to accumulate Ga-67 in the kidneys.[66] Renal uptake of Ga-67 has been shown to increase in kidneys of rats with antibiotic-induced nephritis, and at least three nephrotoxic antibiotics are known to produce this effect (gentamicin, amphotericin B, and neomycin).[124]

Scintigraphy using In-111-labelled leukocytes has been reported for the detection of inflammatory renal disease, specifically renal abcess, acute pyelonephritis, and acute focal bacterial nephritis (acute lobar nephronia).[35]

Tc-99m DMSA is valuable in identification of renal damage due to early pyelonephritis. Even in the absence of urographic or ultrasonographic abnormalities, regional parenchymal uptake of DMSA may be altered in acute pyelonephritis. Handmaker reports that in his experience all patients with proven pyelonephritis had an abnormal DMSA cortical scan.[47] One or more areas of decreased tracer uptake within the renal cortex can be seen in these patients. In renal abscess, DMSA imaging will show one or more cortical defects corresponding to that lesion (Figs. 4-27 and 4-28). Tc-99m DMSA is useful to quantify the degree of renal damage, to follow the progress of antibiotic therapy, and to assess recovery and/or residual renal damage. Images with Tc-99m DMSA should also be made with the pinhole collimator in the posterior and posterior oblique projections in order to attain high resolution.

Imaging with Tc-99m DMSA facilitates detection of cortical scarring in pyelonephritis. Unlike urography, cortical scanning can detect cortical defects that do not deform the renal outline or the collecting system. Therefore, it is possible to detect renal scarring on Tc-99m DMSA scintigraphy and not on urography.[48,55]

Merrick et al. found that Tc-99m DMSA imaging had a greater sensitivity than urography for the detection of renal scars in children with pyelonephritis. After studying 79 children with bacteriologically proven urinary tract infection these authors found that both techniques agreed as to the presence or absence of abnormality in 93.5% of the kidneys studied. They found that intravenous urography had a sensitivity of 86% and a specificity of 92%. Scintigraphy showed a sensitivity of 96% and a specificity of 98%.[82] Davies et al. found renal cortical defects with mercury-197 (Hg-197) chlormerodryn scanning in 10 of 50 patients with the clinical diagnosis of chronic pyelonephritis and normal urography. This was accomplished despite the use of a tracer with low photon flux and equipment yielding poor image resolution.[21]

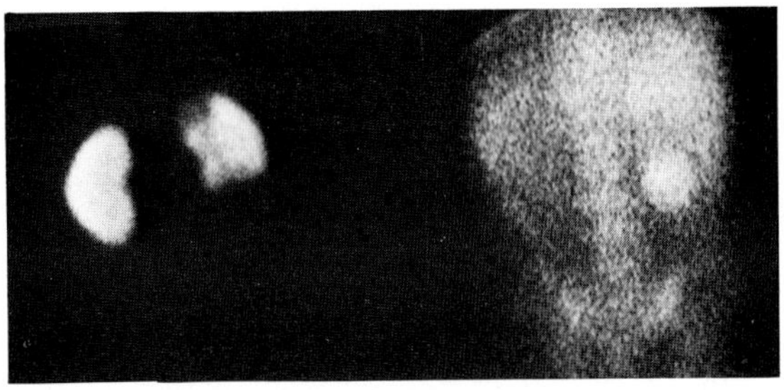

Figure 4-28. A: Abscess in the right lower pole. *Right:* Tc-99m DMSA scan shows a normal left kidney. The right renal silhouette reveals two defects, a large one in the lower pole and a smaller one in the upper pole. A Ga-67 scan reveals an intense focus of increased uptake corresponding to the defect seen on the lower pole of the right kidney. There is no increased uptake of Ga-67 in the upper pole of the right kidney, probably indicating no active infection.

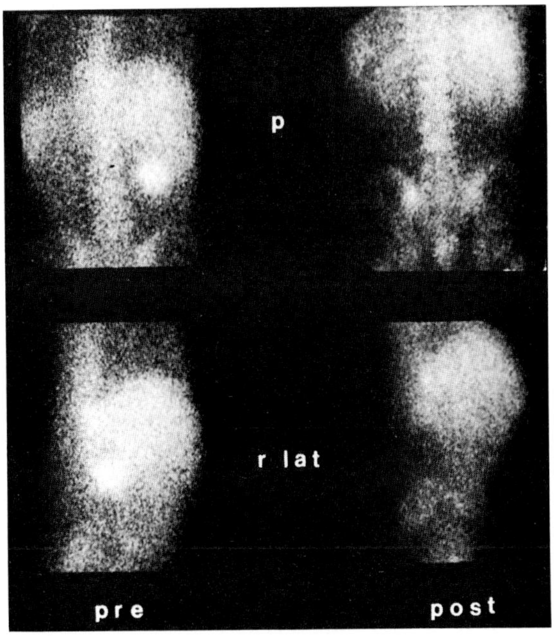

Figure 4-28. B: Ga-67 images in the same patient before *(left)* and after *(right)* 3 months of antibiotics.

Renal Vein Thrombosis

Renal vein thrombosis should be suspected in a patient, particularly a neonate, in whom hematuria and an enlarged kidney develop shortly after a period of asphyxia, shock, dehydration, or sepsis.[34,58,99,119,133] About two-thirds of all cases occur in the pediatric age group, with a majority seen in the neonatal period. In older children renal vein thrombosis may develop in patients with severe illness, toxemia, and sepsis. Renal vein thrombosis has been described as a bilateral disease but with asymmetric involvement. In this way a minor lesion in the apparently noninvolved kidney may be missed.[1] Most frequently the thrombous originates in the interlobar or arcuate veins and less commonly in the main renal vein. The thrombus may extend into the main renal vein and the inferior vena cava and/or in a retrograde fashion involve the renal cortex. Venous obstruction results in infarction and hemorrhage. Blood leaking into the interstitium and renal tubules may ultimately result in fibrosis. Increased susceptibility for the development of renal vein thrombosis has been reported in infants of diabetic mothers and in children with congenital heart disease.[1,5,120]

The variability with which renal vein thrombosis can be identified on urographic studies is considerable. Quigley et al. suggest that renal scintigraphy is a more sensitive method than intravenous urography in the screening of patients having renal vein thrombosis.[97] Findings on serial renal scintigraphy that show the evolution of renal function correlate well with the ultimate outcome. In most patients with renal vein thrombosis the kidney involved is not visualized by intravenous urography. Duncan et al. have stated that affected renal units that are not visible on initial urographic examination virtually ensures an atrophic, functionless kidney later.[28] Inferior vena cavagraphy may be normal or it may show a radiolucent image within the lumen of the vein.

With the advent of more sensitive methods of detecting renal function and an increasing knowledge of the natural history of the disease, a more accurate view of the final outcome of an affected kidney is possible. Ultrasonography may demonstrate an enlarged or a normal kidney. Most patients with renal vein thrombosis are treated medically with maintenance of normal fluid and electrolyte balance.[119] Recovery of renal function can be documented with serial Tc-99m DMSA scintigraphy (Fig. 4-17).

Renal Trauma

In patients who have had abdominal trauma, radionuclide evaluation is a sensitive technique for detecting functional and structural damage to the kidney (Fig. 4-29). Radionuclide studies should be obtained routinely in those patients having liver-spleen scans for suspected splenic trauma because there is often coexisting renal damage in these cases. One approach is to obtain both intravenous pyelography and renal scintigraphy initially, and then to follow the patient with the radionuclide study in order to assess recovery or residual damage. When the defect is not severe and the patient remains stable, the results of nonoperative treatment can be assessed easily by sequential renal studies.

Freeman et al.[40] evaluated the use of static renal scintigraphy in renal trauma. Trauma appeared, depending on its severity as a focal area of mildly or moderately decreased tracer accumulation, or as a generalized decrease or even absent uptake of tracer in the kidney. In 5 of 28 cases renal scintigraphy revealed an abnormality in the presence of normal urography. Percutaneous aortography and selective renal angiography failed to show any abnormality in 7 of 20 patients with hematuria, but radionuclide renal scans were abnormal in two of these. The angiogram was never abnormal on the face of a normal scan. Minor renal injuries usually recovered without surgery as assessed by renal scanning.[40]

Renal Infarction

Renal infarction can occur in patients with cyanotic congenital heart disease, polycythemia, atrial fibrillation, dehydration, umbilical artery catheter, and trauma. Figure 4-30 shows a renal scan on a patient with cyanotic heart disease who developed a renal infarct and its recovery with time.

Hypertension

The incidence of hypertension in children is 1.4–2.3%.[11] The reported incidence of secondary hypertension varies with the source of patients.[54,72,87] Selected referral populations report an incidence of 65–85% secondary hypertension, whereas a primary clinic incidence of 7% is cited.[72] In 563 patients with secondary hypertension were reported in the pediatric literature: 78% had a renal abnormality, and 12% were diagnosed as having renal artery disease.[72] Although thorough medical histories and physical examinations fail to give spe-

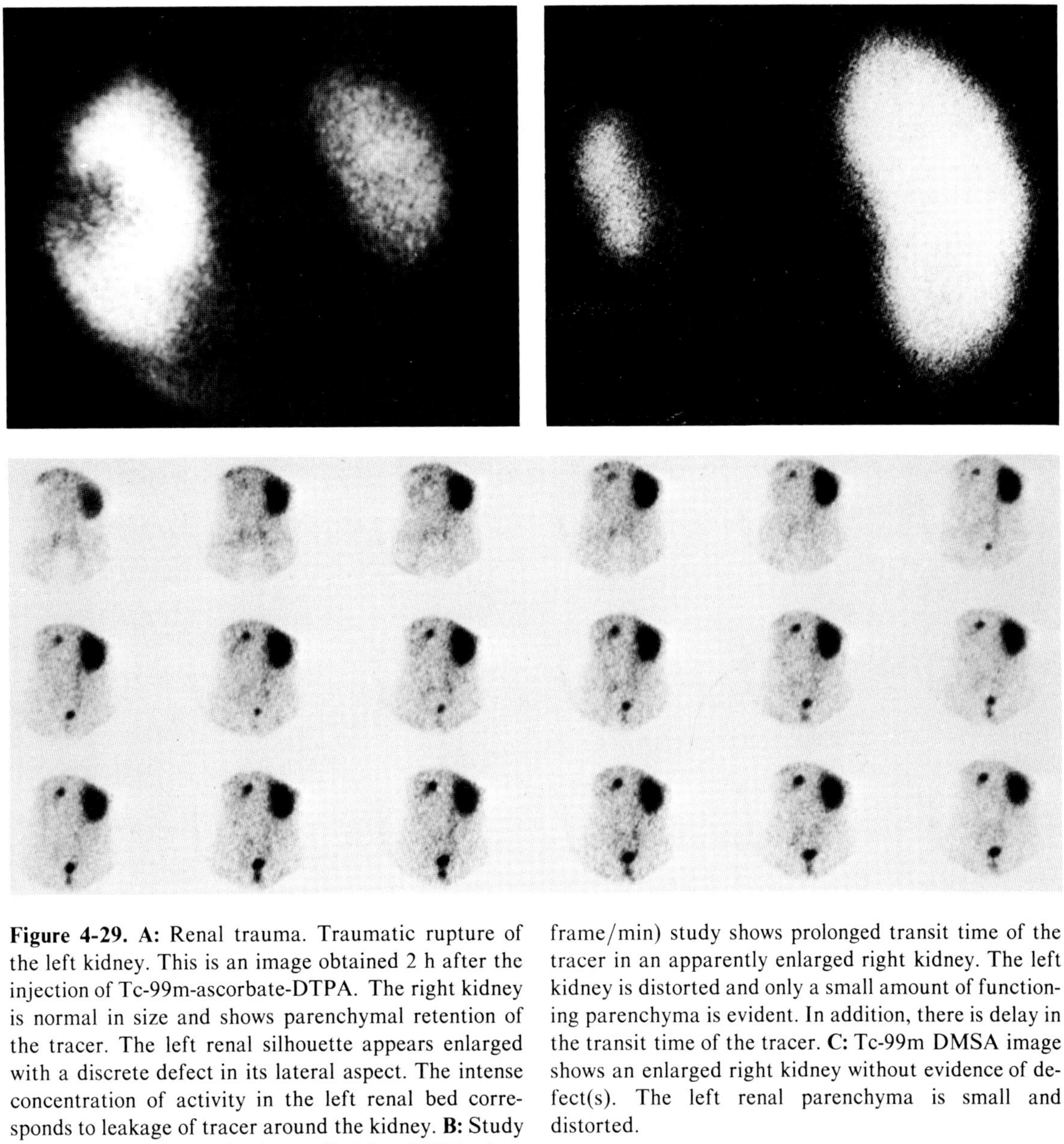

A C B

Figure 4-29. A: Renal trauma. Traumatic rupture of the left kidney. This is an image obtained 2 h after the injection of Tc-99m-ascorbate-DTPA. The right kidney is normal in size and shows parenchymal retention of the tracer. The left renal silhouette appears enlarged with a discrete defect in its lateral aspect. The intense concentration of activity in the left renal bed corresponds to leakage of tracer around the kidney. **B:** Study obtained several months later. Tc-99m DTPA (one frame/min) study shows prolonged transit time of the tracer in an apparently enlarged right kidney. The left kidney is distorted and only a small amount of functioning parenchyma is evident. In addition, there is delay in the transit time of the tracer. **C:** Tc-99m DMSA image shows an enlarged right kidney without evidence of defect(s). The left renal parenchyma is small and distorted.

cific guidance to establishing an etiology for hypertension, efforts are focused upon the kidneys, for which a guide for sequential evaluation has been advocated.[54,71,72,101] A proposed initial evaluation includes urinalysis, urine culture, intravenous urography (IVP), and clinical estimates of renal function.[54,101] Additional phases of evaluation are progressively more specific with subsequent inclusion of invasive procedures that require hospitalization. These progressive phases of assessment are implemented when abnormalities are revealed in the initial evaluation or clinical factors indicate a need for expeditious, definite evaluation.

IVP has been the initial imaging procedure in hypertension because of its excellent capability for imaging renal structure despite its limitations in detecting renal vascular disease.[8,63,117,118,126] Urography may suggest the presence of renal abnormalities such as renal cortical scarring from pyelonephritis, obstructive uropathy, renal masses

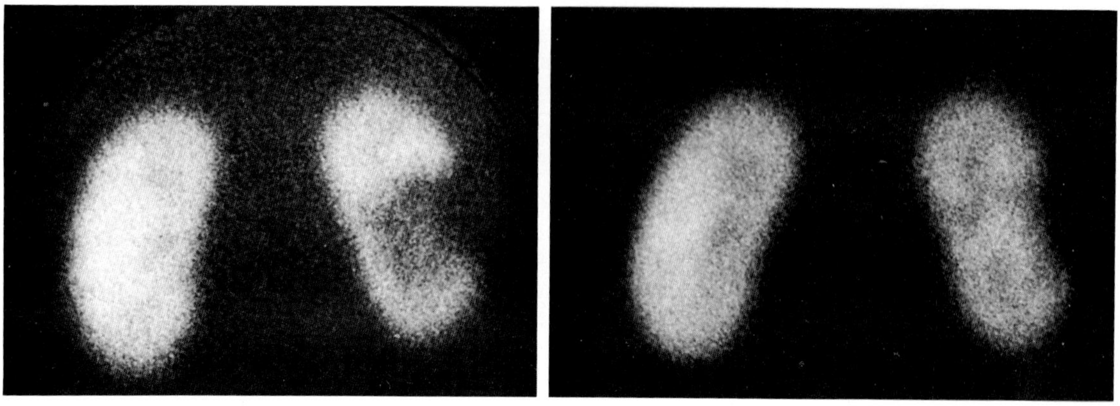

Figure 4-30. Renal infarction in a 16-year-old male who had several operations for cyanotic congenital heart disease. He presented with severe right flank pain. The initial Tc-99m DMSA scan *(left)* shows a well-defined defect in the right kidney interpreted as being a renal infarct. A repeat study about 1.5 months later shows a considerable reduction in the size of the lesion.

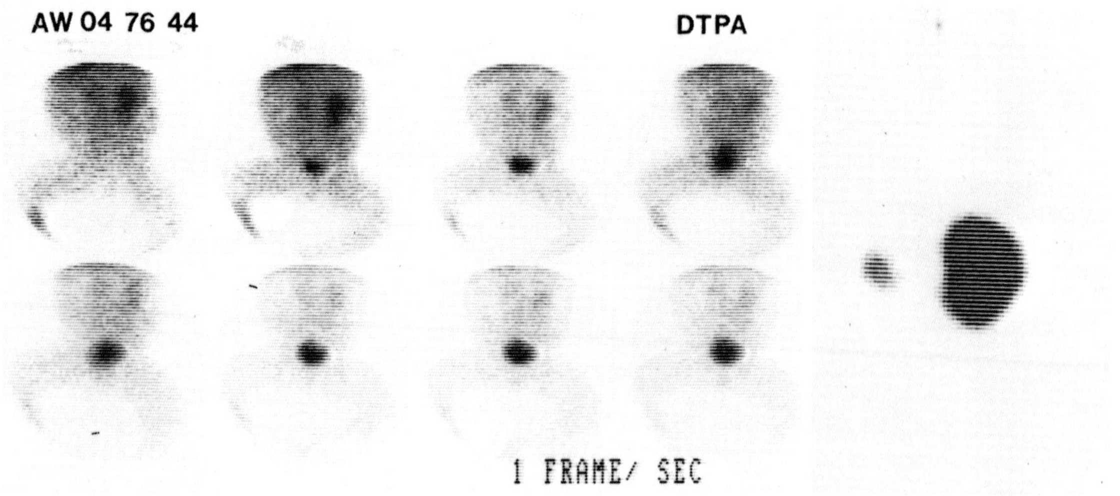

Figure 4-31. Hypertension in a premature baby following withdrawal of an umbilical artery catheter. *Left:* Tc-99m DTPA study (one frame/min). The right kidney is normal. The left kidney is small. *Right:* Tc-99m DMSA image confirms that the functioning mass of the left kidney is very low, presumably due to a complication of the umbilical artery catheter.

from cysts, tumors, or trauma, or chronic, diffuse parenchymal disease as evidenced by renal atrophy. With respect to renal vascular disease, rapid-sequence urography has been advocated. Delay in contrast appearance, discrepancy in renal length, hyperconcentration in late films, ureteric notching, and local decrease in the renal parenchyma are considered signs of renal vascular disease. However, positive studies occur in only 27–65% of patients with renal vascular disease demonstrated by arteriography.[63,126,135]

Recent advances in nuclear medicine have increased the role of renal scintigraphy in the evaluation of renal structure and function. Initial efforts using radionuclides in evaluating renal function focused on the use of I-131 OIH probe renography with the capacity to determine effective renal plasma flow and relative renal function. Interpretation was dependent upon the analysis of time-activity curves for each kidney without visual correlation of structure and function. A high number of true-positive studies were reported, but accuracy

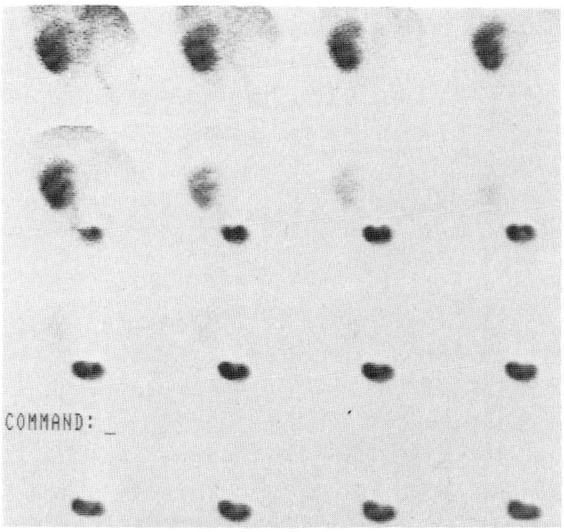

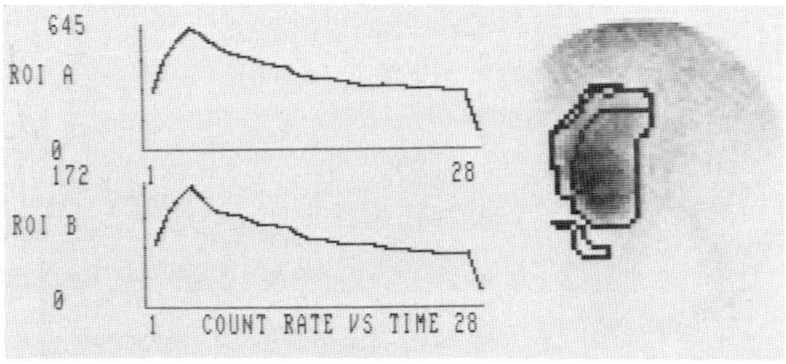

Figure 4-32. Renal transplant (living donor). Tc-99m DTPA (one frame/min). Transplant in the right iliac fossa showing excellent renal function.

and specificity were low with a high incidence of false-positive studies.[101] The introduction of gamma cameras and Tc-99m compounds have resulted in improved imaging and decreased radiation exposure[122] (Fig. 4-31).

In an evaluation of Tc-99m DTPA for the diagnosis of unilateral renovascular hypertension, Arlart et al.[2] were able to achieve a sensitivity of 82% in 105 patients with known unilateral vascular lesions. In a group of 45 patients with essential hypertension, 26% had false-positive Tc-99m DTPA studies.

Tc-99m DMSA provides improved images of the renal cortex in conjunction with quantitative data reflecting regional and differential renal function.[123] The lack of significant interference from pelvicalyceal activity enhances the capacity to detect small focal lesions of the renal parenchyma such as infarcts and pyelonephritic scars[47,134] and allows detection of focal and segmental anomalies of renal perfusion. Vivian et al.[134] reported the results of Tc-99m DMSA studies in 13 children with documented renal vascular lesions. Intravenous urography detected one of three patients with extrarenal lesions and three of eight with intrarenal arterial stenosis. Tc-99m DTPA detected none of those with extrarenal lesions and three of eight with intrarenal lesions. Tc-99m DMSA detected two of four cases with extrarenal lesions, and seven of nine with intrarenal lesions. This represents a significant improvement in the accuracy of diagnosis of renal arterial stenosis prior to angiography.

Rosen and Treves[103] report the results of renal scintigraphy using Tc-99m DTPA and Tc-99m DMSA in the evaluation of hypertensive pediatric and adolescent patients. A sensitivity of 54% was achieved with Tc-99m DTPA, as compared with 92% for Tc-99m DMSA. The specificity of both agents exceeded 95%. Tc-99m DTPA appears unable to reveal renal cortical detail in patients with chronic pyelonephritis and regional vascular lesions. The clear superiority of Tc-99m DMSA is undoubtedly a reflection of this agent's capacity to generate both anatomic and functional data.

Renal Transplantation

When a living donor is available, renal scintigraphy is usually performed to exclude unsuspected abnormality (Fig. 4-32). Several reports in the literature recommend the use of radionuclide studies to assess and follow function of a transplanted kidney and to detect early and late complications.[6,7,36,73,75,139] This technique can predict rejection and recovery of function 24–48 h before chemical changes occur in the blood or before clinical evidence of trouble. It also can detect recovery 1 or 2 days prior to return to normal blood chemistries. It is possible with this technique to assess perfusion of the transplant in the early and late postoperative periods. The radiotracer solutions produce no osmotic load and no pharmacologic effects whatsoever and can be used safely even in the presence of severe renal transplant dysfunction. When patients are on a regimen of dialysis, radionuclide studies are especially useful because biochemical findings are not helpful in assessing functional changes in this setting.

Sequential renal scintigraphy is valuable in the early diagnosis of rejection and in the avoidance of unnecessary therapy when rejection is ruled out. In patients with rejection reaction radionuclide angiography shows a reduction in the perfusion of the transplant.[15]

In the immediate postoperative period a baseline evaluation of the transplant is obtained (Fig. 4-31). Subsequent studies are performed depending on the patient's progress. Renal transplants from *living* relatives usually function immediately after transplantation. The initial perfusion and uptake of the tracers is normal and even more intense than in the normal. The intrarenal transit time is normal or even faster than normal. After a few days, provided that no complications are present, the handling of tracers by the transplant becomes identical to that of normal kidneys (Fig. 4-33). When rejection develops, the scintigraphic findings are very similar to those generated by rejecting cadaveric allografts.

Cadaveric allografts are frequently affected with acute tubular necrosis which occurs within the first few hours of transplantation and persists usually for 1–3 weeks (Fig. 4-34). The duration appears to be related to the duration of the ischemic period to which the kidney has been subjected prior to transplantation. Recovery usually follows unless rejection or other complications appear. Rejection of a transplant may develop at any time; however, in cadaveric transplants it does not generally occur until the end of the first postoperative week.[25,39]

Differentiation of acute tubular necrosis from rejection by radionuclide studies is difficult, but some nonspecific scintigraphic features may suggest the appropriate diagnosis. In acute tubular necrosis, radionuclide angiography with one of the Tc-99m renal agents will generally demonstrate relatively well-preserved perfusion. Studies with I-131 OIH or Tc-99m DTPA in acute tubular necrosis will show a relatively slow uptake and drainage of the tracer by the transplant. Usually serial Tc-99m DTPA images in acute tubular necrosis first demonstrate preserved perfusion, followed by weak uptake of the tracer. Images from 10–20 min after injection will show washout of the tracer from the kidney.

In acute tubular necrosis delayed images obtained with OIH several hours after the administration of the tracer will reveal retention of the radionuclide within the renal parenchyma with little, if any, accumulation or passage of activity into the renal pelvis, ureter, or bladder. These changes reflect decreased renal clearance. Preserved perfusion as assessed by a Tc-99m renal agent and accumulation of tracer in the kidney means that the transplant is viable and that chances of recovery of function are good, provided there is no ureteric obstruction, ureteric necrosis, or urinary leakage. The size of the renal silhouette will not change significantly in acute tubular necrosis while it may enlarge in rejection. In rejection reaction, perfusion of the transplant is reduced more than in acute tubular necrosis. The uptake and transit times of renal tracers by the transplant in rejection will vary and depend on the severity of the rejection episode. Delayed uptake and slow transit of the tracers is frequently combined with quantitative reduction of tracer uptake into the collecting system and the bladder.

Urinary obstruction, a rare complication of renal transplantation, may not be detected in the presence of severe renal dysfunction, as in cases of acute tubular necrosis or rejection. When function improves, delayed ureteral transit time or retention of the tracer in the pelvis and/or ureter are scintigraphic signs that suggest urinary obstruction. Retention of tracer within the pelviureteric system soon after surgery may be due to edema and/or inflammation in the region of the ureterovesical junction, however, and not necessarily to obstruction. Close observation with followup renal scintigraphy will help to determine whether there is true obstruction. In renal failure, the transit time, parenchymal uptake, and urinary concentration of Tc-99m DTPA are so depressed that the diagnosis of obstruction may not be made. Agents with greater parenchymal avidity (such as OIH) sometimes may demonstrate urinary obstruction even in severe renal failure.

The presence of urinary leak is easily detected with serial scintigraphy and with greater sensitivity than with other methods, because of the high contrast of the radiotracer technique (Fig. 4-35).[116] However, urine extravasation occurring over the renal or vesical areas may be seen better on urograms. Multiple delayed images at several minutes to several hours after the injection of tracer may be necessary in order to detect urinary leakage. Urinary leakage appears on the series of scintigrams as a diffuse area of increasing tracer accumulation outside the confines of the transplant, the ureter, or the bladder (Fig. 4-35).

Urinoma usually appears as a photon-deficient

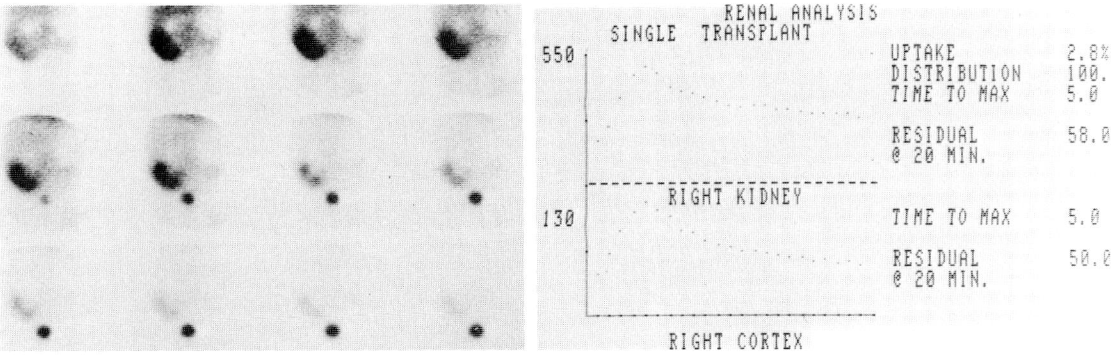

Figure 4-33. Normal function of a renal transplant in a 2-year-old male 1 week following transplantation. Tc-99m DTPA study (one frame/min).

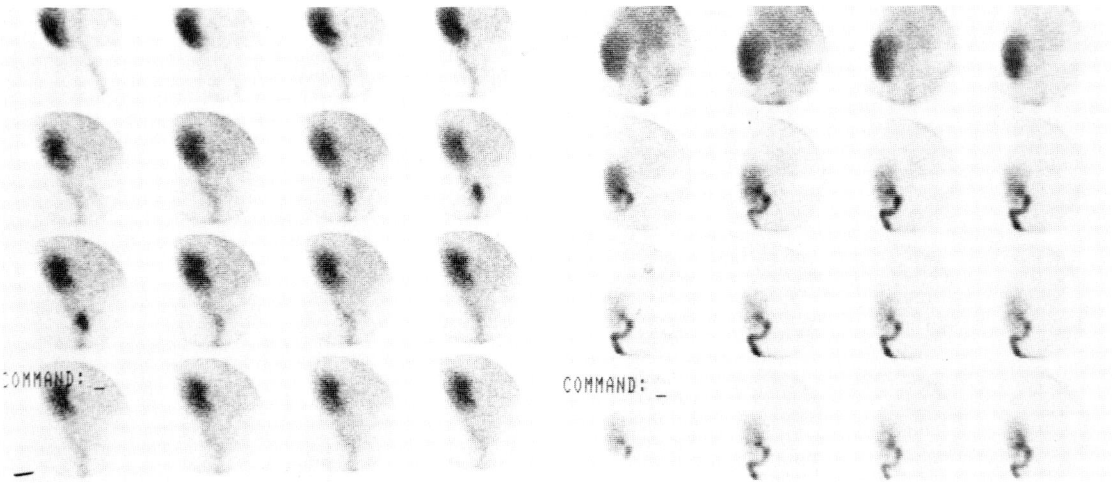

Figure 4-34. *Left:* Cadaveric renal transplant 1 day after transplantation showing low uptake and prolonged transit time consistent with acute tubular necrosis. *Right:* Same patient 3 days later showing significant improvement in renal function. Tc-99m DTPA study (one frame/min).

area on early images (5–10 min). On later images tracer accumulates within this region. If the photon-deficient area seen on early images does not concentrate radiotracer on later images, this region may represent a hematoma or a lymphocele.

A normal radionuclide angiogram on a transplant will show peak renal activity at 3–6 sec after peak aortic activity. The maximal concentration of activity within the transplant will be similar or greater than the apparent aortic concentration at the time of peak renal activity (Fig. 4-36). Normal time-activity curves from the renal area exhibit a relatively sharp peak of activity, which will be similar in shape to that obtained over the aorta. It is very important that the method of radionuclide angiography be standardized (injection, recording technique, analysis) and reproducible in order to avoid artifacts.

Complete renal artery occlusion or total renal vein obstruction with subsequent infarction cannot be distinguished by radionuclide imaging. Similarly, these two complications cannot be differentiated from hyperacute rejection (rejection within a few hours of transplantation). All of these conditions reveal lack of renal blood flow to the transplant on the radionuclide angiogram and failure to visualize the kidney on subsequent serial images. In necrotic or avascular renal transplants radionuclide

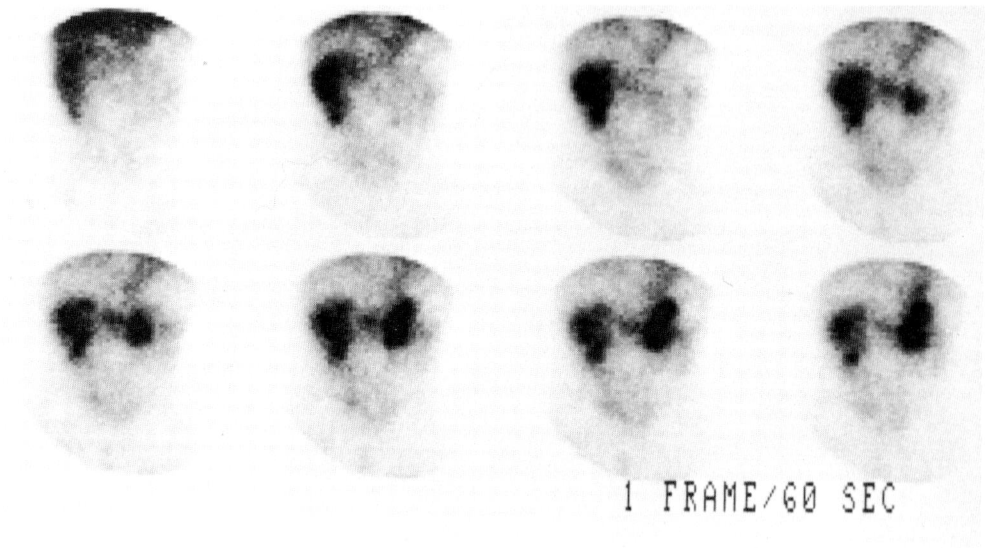

Figure 4-35. A: Urinary leak in a renal transplant. Tc-99m DTPA renal scan, anterior projection; each frame represents 2 min. The tracer concentrates rapidly in the renal transplant located in the right lower quadrant. The series of images reveals diffuse distribution of the tracer into the peritoneal cavity. A pool of radiotracer is seen in the left lower quadrant.

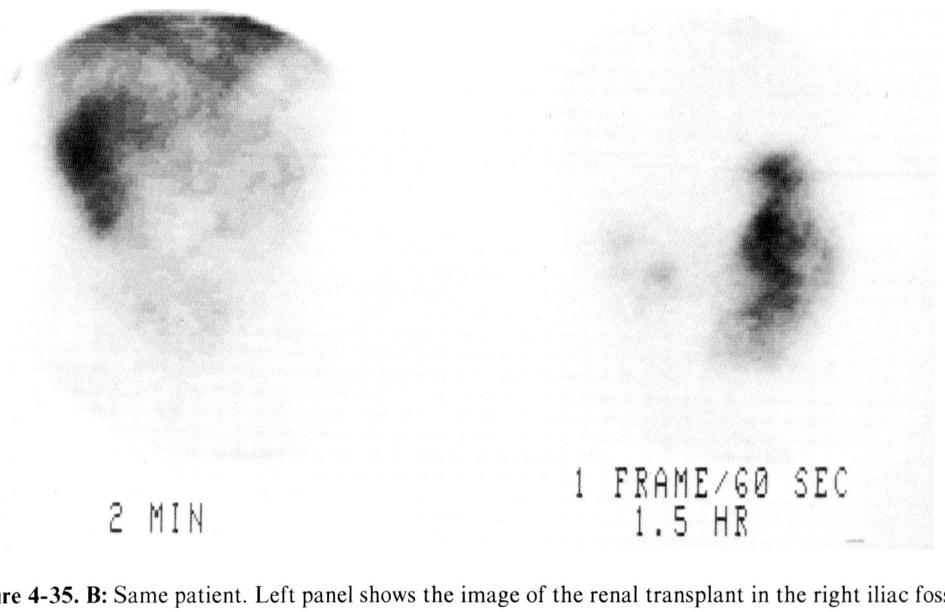

Figure 4-35. B: Same patient. Left panel shows the image of the renal transplant in the right iliac fossa. An image obtained 1.5 h later reveals distribution of the tracer with the peritoneal cavity, principally in the left hemiabdomen.

angiography will show a photon-deficient area (less activity than background) in the region of the kidneys. Chances of recovery of renal function in these patients are remote and surgical removal is generally indicated. Apparent lack of perfusion of a renal transplant on radionuclide angiography does not necessarily signify occlusion of the main renal artery leading to the transplant, but reflects actual lack of blood flow to the kidney (Fig. 4-36).

If tracer activity within the transplant is similar

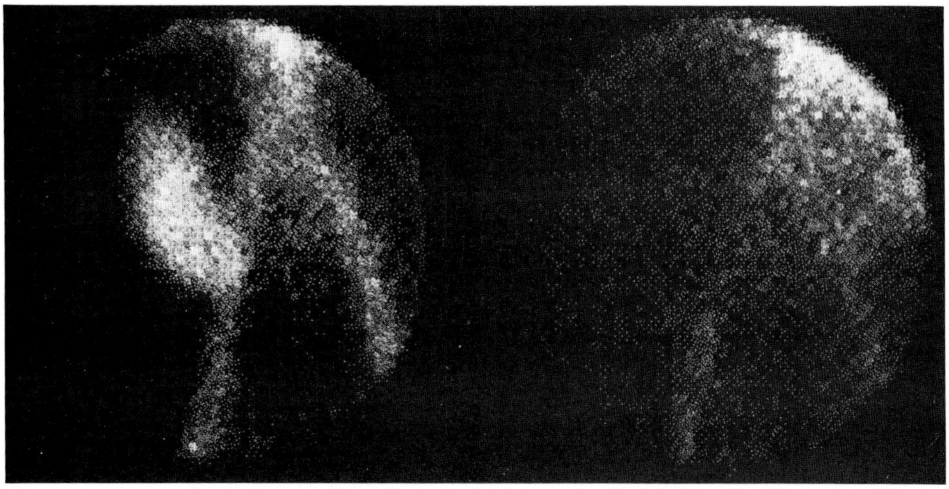

Figure 4-36. *Left:* Normal radionuclide angiogram in a renal transplant. *Right:* Absent blood flow with massive rejection. The renal artery is patent but there is no cortical capillary network to produce an image of the kidney.

to background on radionuclide angiography and on later images, it means severe depression of renal function; however, the kidney should not be assumed dead. This pattern of radionuclide uptake can be seen in severe acute tubular necrosis or severe rejection and any degree of functional recovery is possible in either case. Infarction of renal transplants can be detected rather well on Tc-99m DMSA images obtained at 4 or more hours after injection. Infarction may be due to operative ligation or thrombosis of an accessory renal artery. Segmental renal parenchymal defects may be due to infarction in an otherwise normal transplant, or to chronic rejection (Fig. 4-37).

Polycystic Renal Disease

Many less severe hereditary or developmental renal abnormalities may be present after the neonatal period. These include less severe forms of polycystic disease (Fig. 4-38).

Ectopic Kidneys-Solitary Kidney

One or both kidneys may be displaced in association with or independent of other renal malformations. Ectopic kidneys situated in the pelvis may be difficult to visualize on intravenous urography partly because of interfering surrounding bony structures (Fig. 4-24). Radionuclide studies along with ultrasonography may also be helpful in the diagnosis of a solitary kidney. Another example of renal ectopia is crossed-fused renal ectopia. In the image shown in Fig. 4-39, both kidneys are located on the right side, the left kidney being smaller and inferior to the normally placed right kidney.

Horseshoe-Shaped Kidney

In horseshoe-shaped kidneys, there is usually fusion between the lower poles. Radionuclide studies are useful in assessing functional abnormalities when there are symptoms referable to the kidney, such as infection, hypertension, and hematuria. Static images (including anterior views) will show whether the kidneys are joined by functioning renal tissue or a fibrous band (Fig. 4-40).

Duplication

Duplication of the ureter and renal pelvis is one of the most common abnormalities of the urinary tract. It occurs bilaterally in 25–30% of patients. The upper pole ureter tends to insert more caudally and medially than the normally placed lower pole ureter. The ureter from the lower pole is more often affected by reflux while the upper ureter is more often obstructed. When surgery is contemplated, the radionuclide study is useful to evaluate the relative function of the upper and lower renal segments. This is done very well with Tc-99m DMSA (Fig. 4-41).

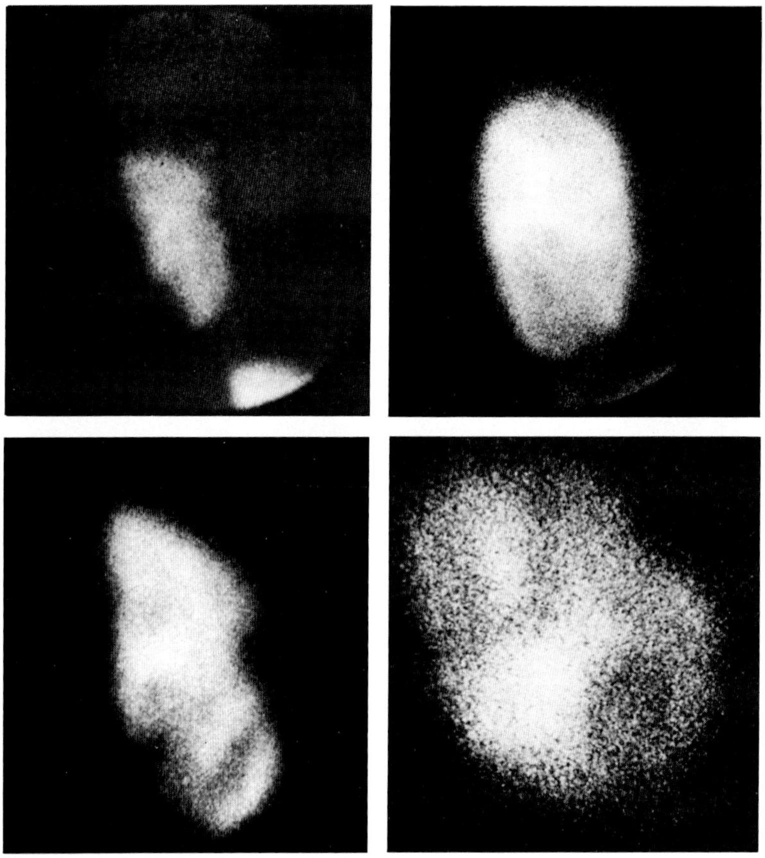

Figure 4-37. Four Tc-99m DMSA images of renal transplants showing segmental defects due to infarction or chronic rejection.

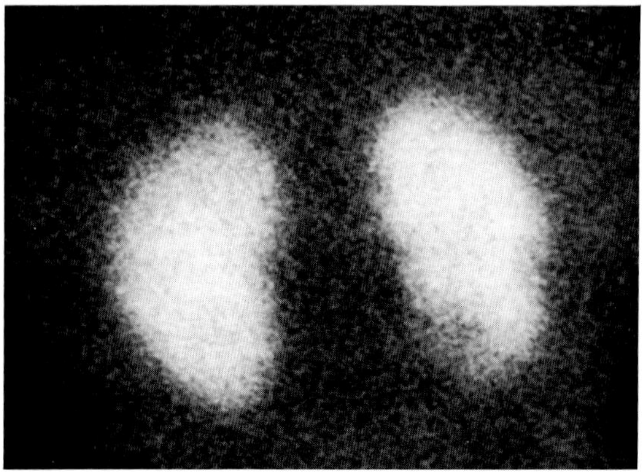

Figure 4-38. Cystic disease. Tc-99m DMSA image from an 18-month-old male who presented with hepatosplenomegaly. A liver biopsy revealed microcystic disease of the liver. The left renal silhouette appears normal. The right kidney reveals two well-defined areas of decreased uptake, one in the lower pole medially and the other laterally.

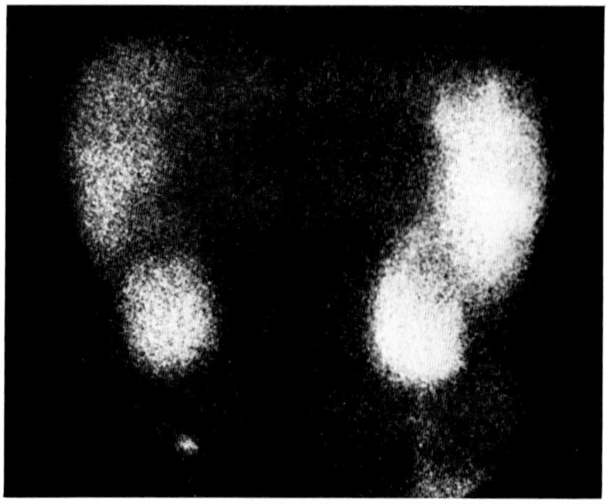

Figure 4-39. Crossed fused renal ectopia. Tc-99m DMSA scan from an 11-month-old female who was born with multiple congenital abnormalities. Both renal units are on the right side. *Left:* anterior; *right:* posterior view.

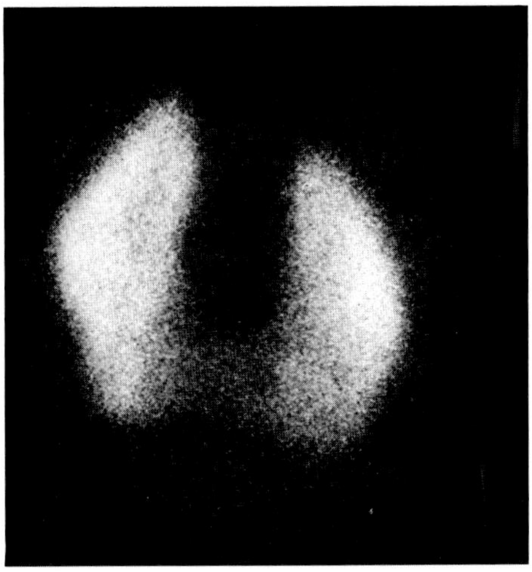

Figure 4-40. Horseshoe-shaped kidney. Tc-99m DMSA scintigraphy from a 15-year-old female with hypertension.

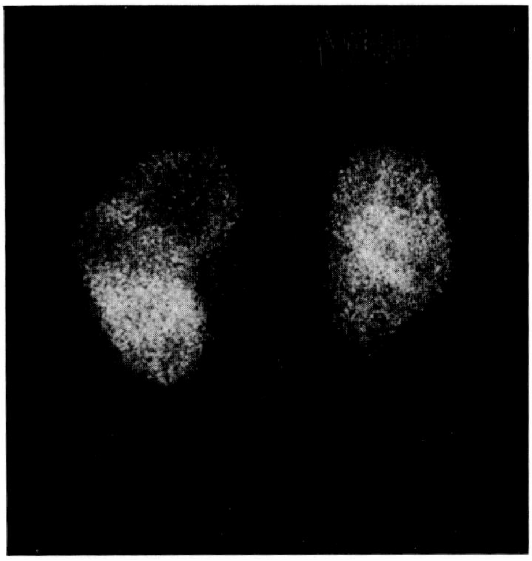

Figure 4-41. A: Duplication of the left kidney. Tc-99m DMSA scan from a 1-month-old female demonstrating dilatation and loss of function of the left upper pole. Images were obtained with a pinhole collimator. The remainder of the left kidney and the right kidney are normal.

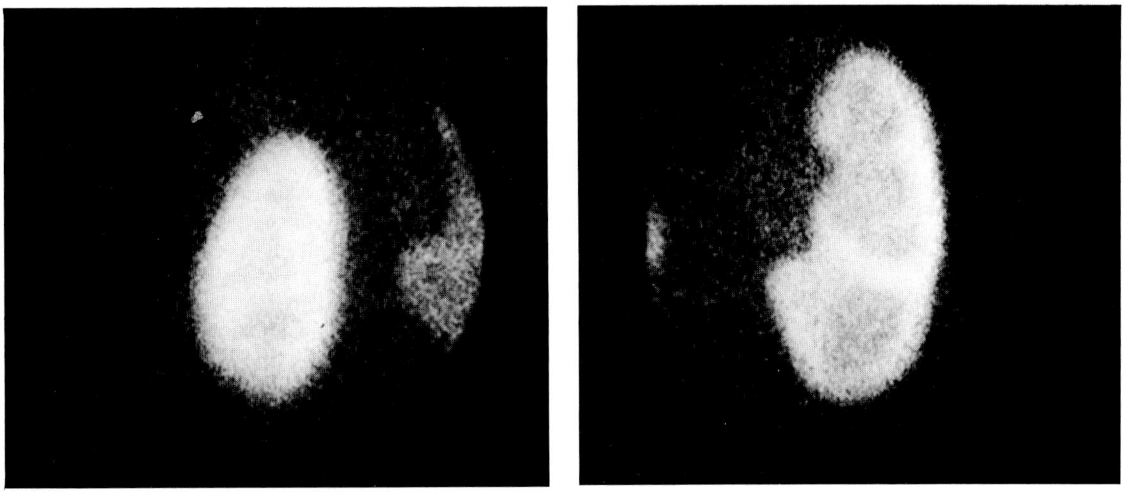

Figure 4-41. B: Magnified Tc-99m DMSA images from a 1-month-old infant with duplication of the right kidney.

Acute Renal Failure

In acute renal failure the radionuclide study has a predictive value. Improvements in function detected on such study usually precede biochemical changes by 1 or 2 days. Figure 4-42 demonstrates the improvement in renal function in a few days in a patient with acute renal failure. Similarly, radionuclide studies have been used to follow functional changes in patients with acute glomerulonephritis. In cases of acute renal failure due to severe hemolytic uremic syndrome, serial studies have been useful in assessing the response to therapy.

Nephrotic Syndrome

The nephrotic syndrome in childhood usually carries a favorable prognosis. An unusual complica-

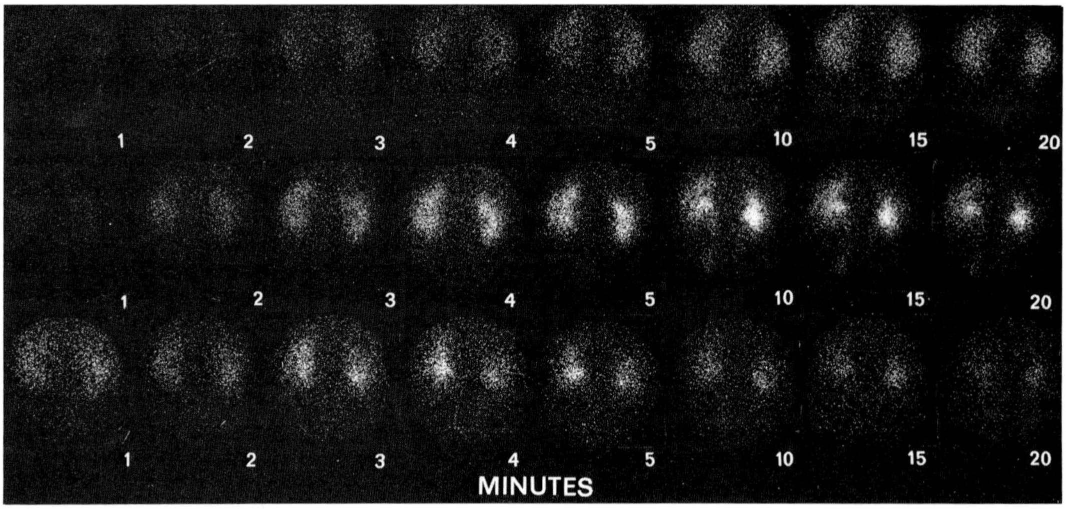

Figure 4-42. Acute renal failure and recovery. Three I-131 OIH studies from a 14-year-old male. He had a 4-month history of diarrhea and bloody stools and was admitted with severe anemia. Following transfusion of blood he became febrile and developed anuria. An intravenous urogram failed to visualize the kidneys. The first renal scan *(top row)* shows bilateral reduction of function with markedly delayed transit time. The second scan, 2 days later, reveal a dramatic improvement a day before diuresis resumed. The third scan, one week later, is normal.

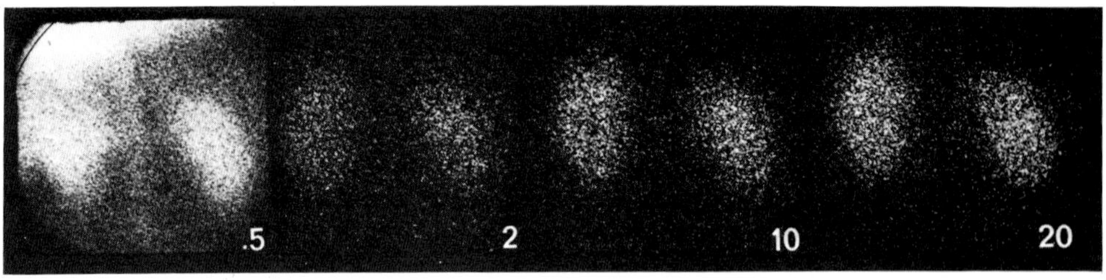

Figure 4-43. Nephrotic syndrome. A radionuclide angiogram with Tc-99m DTPA *(left)* shows good perfusion of both kidneys. Series of images obtained following injection of I-131 OIH reveal slow uptake of the tracer and prolonged intrarenal transit time. This study was from a 12-year-old male with increasing swelling of the abdomen, extremities, and face. Clinically, the patient was thought to have nephrotic syndrome (cholesterol 408 mg/dl, total protein 4.3 g/dl, protein 1.5). A renal biopsy showed lipoid nephrosis.

tion is acute renal failure, usually occurring in patients who have relapsed following an initial remission. There is often an associated febrile illness. Reversible ischemia may be differentiated from end-stage disease. In the former, there is prompt uptake of radiotracer with delayed cortical clearing (Fig. 4-43). With end-stage renal disease, there is a marked reduction in both uptake and excretion of the tracer. The reversible renal failure is probably due to a fluid deficit associated with an extravascular shift as well as fluid loss associated with a febrile illness, often with vomiting and diarrhea.

Tumors

Renal scintigraphy is not frequently utilized in the investigation of renal tumors. Wilm's tumor (nephroblastoma) is one of the most common abdominal neoplasms of early life. About two-thirds appear before the age of 3 years, but are rarely present at birth. Bilateral renal involvement is rare (Fig. 4-44). Scintigraphic findings in this condition are nonspecific and other diagnostic modalities are usually indicated. Other space-occupying lesions of the kidney seen less commonly include hematomas.

Siddiqui et al. performed Tc-99m methylene di-

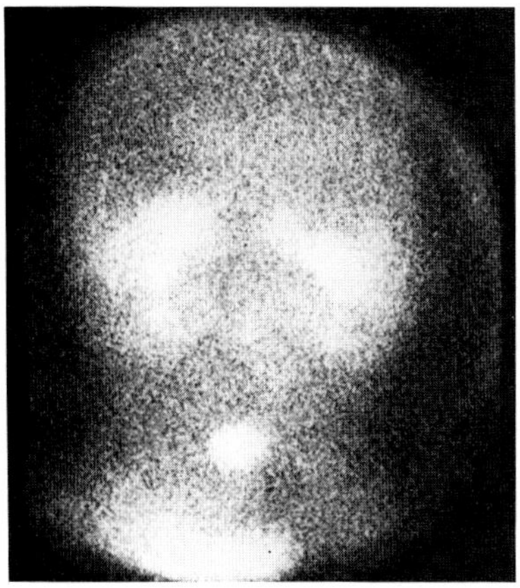

Figure 4-44. Bilateral Wilm's tumors. Six-week-old male with hypertension and bilateral flank masses. Selected Tc-99m DTPA image shows enlargement and distortion of both renal units with multiple intrarenal areas of reduced-to-absent uptake of the tracer.

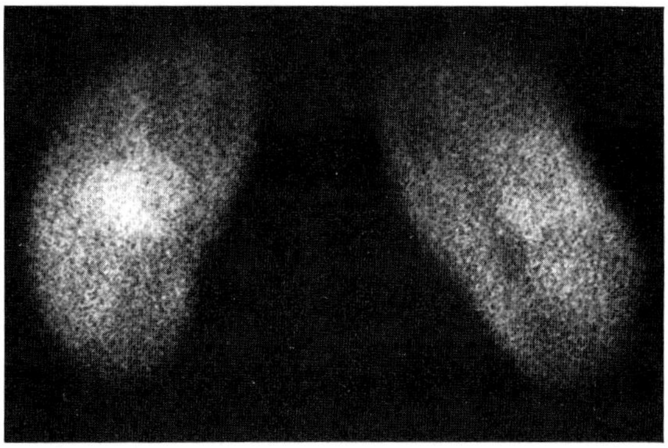

Figure 4-45. Hypertrophy of a column of Bertin. Tc-99m DMSA image obtained with a pinhole collimator reveals a round area of increased uptake in the midportion of the left kidney. This corresponded to a mass seen on an intravenous urogram and represents a hypertrophic column of Bertin.

phosphonate (MDP) imaging in children with abdominal masses. Radionuclide inferior vena cavagrams were performed with serial images for 30 min. Routine bone imaging was obtained at about 3 h. The radionuclide inferior vena cavagrams diagnosed total obstruction and displacement to the left, but partial obstruction and displacement to the right was not as easily detectable. Early renal imaging with Tc-99m MDP demonstrated displacement, distortion, obstruction, and nonvisualization of the kidney. All of the patients with Wilm's tumor demonstrated either nonvisualization or distortion of the renal parenchyma. Patients with neuroblastoma and other tumors had displacement and obstruction. There was soft tissue uptake of Tc-99m MDP in two of eight Wilm's tumors and in 12 of 17 neuroblastomas.[111]

Hypertrophy of a renal column of Bertin may appear as a mass that at times is difficult to distinguish from neoplasm or cyst at urography. Cortical radionuclide imaging can firmly establish the diagnosis of normal renal cortex and absence of tumor. Images obtained with the pinhole collimator that reveal greater structural detail than conventional collimators are very important in the diagnosis of these lesions[69,85,90] (Fig. 4-45).

Lymphomatous involvement of the kidneys can be detected with radionuclide imaging. This technique also may be used to assess response to treatment (Fig. 4-46).

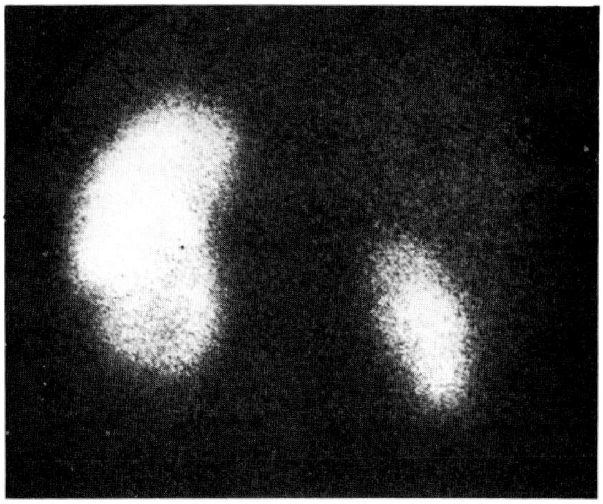

Figure 4-46. Lymphoma involving the kidneys.

Effect of Radiotherapy

Radiation therapy causes transient or permanent functional defect(s) in the kidney that correspond to the portal of irradiation. This can be appreciated on renal scintigraphy as one or more regions in the kidney showing reduced-to-absent uptake of tracer.

Prune Belly Syndrome

Prune belly syndrome includes dilatation of the urinary bladder and ureters with a bizarre, wrinkled, flabby abdominal wall in male infants.[10,44,91,136] The

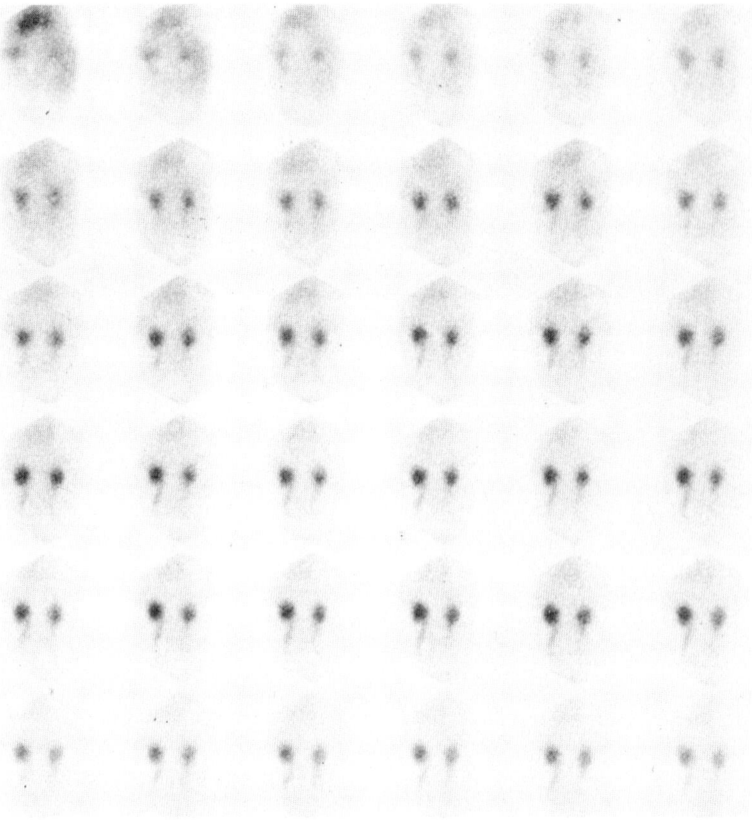

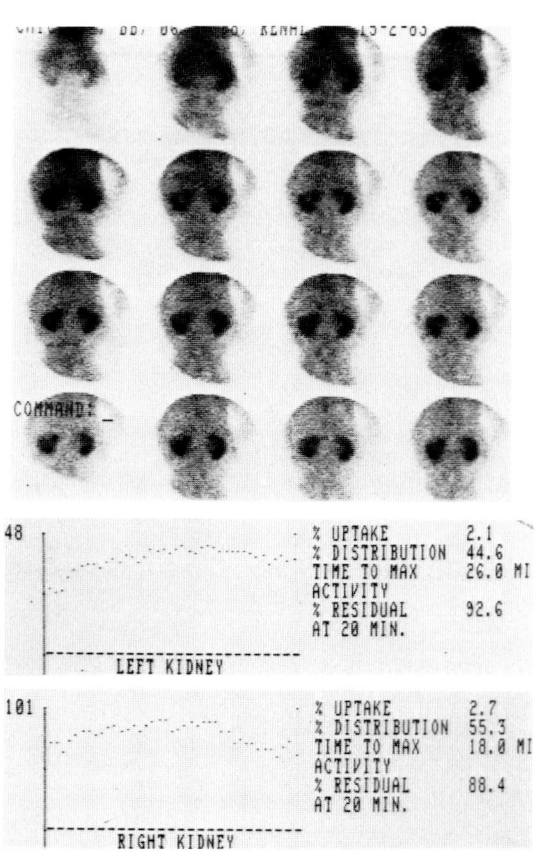

△ **Figure 4-47.** Prune belly syndrome. **A:** Tc-99m DTPA study. Each frame represents 1 min. There is delayed uptake and transit time of the tracer bilaterally.

◁ **Figure 4-47. B:** Another Tc-99m DTPA study in a 2-week-old female with prune belly sundrome. There is symmetric uptake of the tracer, dilatation of the collecting system, and delayed transit time. *Below:* Time-activity curves showing significant delay in intrarenal transit time.

cause of the abdominal muscular deficiency in this syndrome is not well known. The most severely affected patients may die soon after birth or may be stillborn. Associated abnormalities in this syndrome include pulmonary hypoplasia, renal dysplasia, urethral obstruction, weak chest wall muscles, vesicoureteric reflux, and undescended testes. Treatment of this disorder depends on the abnormalities present (obstruction, reflux, etc.).

In patients with the prune belly syndrome renal scintigraphy with Tc-99m DTPA reveals a spectrum of findings: some are normal, some show dilatation of the pelvicalyceal systems without obstruction, and others reveal dilatation with obstruction (Fig. 4-47). In addition others have vesicoureteric reflux. Tc-99m DMSA scintigraphy can help to determine regional distribution of functioning renal parenchyma, to detect renal scarring, and to evaluate the course of the renal disease. Delayed imaging is necessary to allow for drainage of the tracer from the dilated ureters.

References

1. Arneil GC, MacDonald AM, Murphy MV, Sweet EM. Renal venous thrombosis. Clin Nephrol 1973; 1:119–31.
2. Arlart I, Rosenthal J, Adam WE et al. Predictive value of radionuclide methods in the diagnosis of unilateral renovascular hypertension. Cardiovasc Radiol 1979; 2:115–25.
3. Ash JM, Antico VF, Gilday DL et al. Special considerations in the pediatric use of radionuclides in kidney studies. Semin Nucl Med 1982; 12:345–69.
4. Atkins HL, Cardinale KG, Eckelman WC, Hauser W, Klopper JF, Richards P. Evaluation of ^{99m}Tc-DTPA prepared by three different methods. Radiology 1971; 98:674–7.
5. Avery ME, Oppenheimer EH, Gordon HH. Renal vein thrombosis in newborn infants to diabetic mothers. N Engl J Med 1957; 256:1134–8.
6. Awad W, Bennet LR, Martin DC. Detection of renal homograft rejection reaction with a single dose of radiohippuran. J Urol 1968; 100:233–7.
7. Awad W, Boake RC, Bennet LR, Martin DC. Double isotope scan in kidney transplantation. Am Surg 1968; 34:768–74.
8. Bailey SM, Evans DW, Fleming HA. Intravenous urography in investigation of hypertension. Lancet 1975; ii:57–59.
9. Bailey RR, Reddy J, Boniface GR, Turner JG, McRae CU. Estimating unilateral renal function with non-invasive methods. N Z Med J 1983; 96:12–13.
10. Berdon WE, Baker DH, Wigger HJ, Blanc WA. The radiologic and pathologic spectrum of the prune belly syndrome. Radiol Clin North Am 1977; 15:83–92.
11. Blaufox MD. Systemic arterial hypertension in pediatric practice. Pediatr Clin North Am 1971; 18:577–93.
12. Blaufox MD, Potchen EJ, Merrill JP. Measurement of effective renal plasma flow in man by external counting methods. J Nucl Med 1967; 8:77–85.
13. Bois E, Feingold J, Benmaiz H, Briard ML. Congenital urinary tract malformations: epidemiologic and genetic aspects. Clin Genet 1975; 8:37–47.
14. Brugh R,Gooneratne NS, Rittenberg GM, Rous SN. Gallium-67 scanning and conservative treatment in acute inflammatory lesions of the renal cortex. J Urol 1979; 121:232–5.
15. Burke JR, Counahan R, Hilson AJ, Maisey MN, Bewick M, Ogg CS, Chantler C. Serial quantitative imaging with Tc-99m in pediatric renal transplantation. Clin Nephrol 1979; 12:174–7.
16. Burko H, Rhamy RK. Lower urinary tract problems related to infection: diagnosis and treatment. Pediatr Clin North Am 1970; 17:233–53.
17. Chervu LR, Freeman LM, Blaufox MD. Radiopharmaceuticals for renal studies. Semin Nucl Med 1974; 4:3–22.
18. Cohen ML, Smith FG Jr, Mindell RS, Vernier RL. A simple reliable method of measuring glomerular filtration rate using single, low dose sodium iothalamate I-131. Pediatrics 1969; 43:407–15.
19. Daley JJ, Jones WA, Rudd TG, Tremann JA. Differential Tc-99m dimercaptosuccinic acid (DMSA) renal localization: correlation with renal function. J Nucl Med 1977; 18:594–95.
20. Daly MJ, Henry RE. Defining renal anatomy and function with Tc-99m DMSA: clinical and renographic correlation. J Urol 1981; 126:509.
21. Davies ER, Roberts M, Roylance J, Penry JB, Stadden G. The renal scintigram in pyelonephritis. Clin Radiol 1972; 23:370–376.
22. Diffey BL, Hall FM, Corfield JR. The Tc-99m DTPA dynamic renal scan with deconvolution analysis. J Nucl Med 1976; 17:352–5.
23. Diffey BL, Hall FM, Piepsz A, Erbsmann F. Renal deconvolution and the poor injection. Eur J Nucl Med 1978; 3:145–6.
24. Djurhuus JC, Dorph S, Christiansen J et al. Predictive value of renography and I.V. urography for the outcome of reconstructive surgery in patients with hydronephrosis. Acta Chir Scand (Suppl) 1976; 472:37–41.
25. Dossetor JB, Zweig SM, Treves S, Ross WM. The I-131 orthoiodohippurate photoscan in human renal allografts. Can Med Assoc J 1970; 102:1373–8.
26. Drummond KN. The urinary system. Development abnormalities. In: Vaughan VC, McKay RJ, eds. Nelson textbook of pediatrics. Philadelphia: WB Saunders, 1975.
27. Dunbar JS, Nogrady N. Excretory urography in the first year of life. Radiol Clin North Am 1972; 10:367–91.
28. Duncan RE, Evans AT, Martin LW. Natural history and treatment of renal vein thrombosis in children. J Pediatr Surg 1977; 12:639–45.
29. Elkin M. Emergency uroradiology for the nontraumatized patient. Radiol Clin North Am 1978; 16:135–46.
30. Elwood CM, Sigman EM. The measurement of

glomerular filtration rate and effective renal plasma flow in man by iothalamate ^{125}I and iodopyracet ^{131}I. Circulation 1967; 36:441–8.
31. Elwood CM, Sigman EM, Treger C. The measurement of glomerular filtration rate with ^{125}I-sodium iothalamate (Conray). Br J Radiol 1967; 40:581–3.
32. Enlander D, Weber PM, dosRemedios LV. Renal cortical imaging in 35 patients: superior quality with ^{99m}Tc-DMSA. J Nucl Med 1974; 15:743–9.
33. Erbsmann F, Strugven J, Ham H, Piepsz A. Analysis of errors and systemic biases in the calculation of the renal retention function. In: Brill AB, Price PR, McLain WJ, Landay MW, eds. Information processing in medical imaging (Proceedings of the Vth International Conference, Nashville, 1977; ORNL/BCTIC-2), 1978:526–35.
34. Fallon ML. Renal vein thrombosis in the newborn. Arch Dis Child 1949; 24:125–8.
35. Fawcet AD, Goodwin DA, Lantieri RL. In-111 leukocyte scanning in inflammatory renal disease. Clin Nucl Med 1981; 6:231–7.
36. Figueroa JE, Maxfield WS, Batson HM, Birchall R. Radioisotope renal function studies in human renal allografts: value in differential diagnosis of oliguria in presence of obstructive disease with and without urinary extravasation. J Urol 1968; 100:104–8.
37. Fleming JS, Goddard BA. A technique for the deconvolution of the renogram. Phys Med Biol 1974; 19:540–9.
38. Frankel RS, Richman SD, Levenson SM, Johnston GS. Renal localization of gallium-67 citrate. Radiology 1975; 114:393–7.
39. Freedman GS, Schiff M, Lange RC, Brown RS, Weiss RM, Treves S, Lytton B. Functional assessment of renal homografts by means of ^{99m}Tc-DTPA and a gamma scintillation camera. Invest Urol 1972; 9:490–5.
40. Freeman LM, Kay CJ, Meng CH. Contribution of renal scanning in evaluation of renal trauma. Radiology 1966; 86:1021–9.
41. Gagnon JA, Schrier RW, Weis TP, Kokatis W, Mailloux LU. Clearance of iothalamate ^{125}I as a measure of glomerular filtration rate in the dog. J Appl Physiol 1971; 30:774–8.
42. Gamel J, Rousseau WF, Katholi CR, Mesel E. Pitfalls in digital computation of the impulse response of vascular beds from indicator-dilution curves. Circ Res 1973; 32:516–23.
43. Gates G. Glomerular filtration rate: estimation from fractional accumulation of Tc-99m DTPA (stannous). AJR 1982; 138:565–70.
44. Guthrie L. Case of congenital deficiency of the abdominal muscles with dilatation and hypertrophy of the bladder ureters. Trans Pathol Soc Lond 1896; 47:139–45.
45. Hall JE, Guyton AC, Farr BM. A single-injection method for measuring glomerular filtration rate. Am J Physiol 1977; 232:F72–76.
46. Hampel N, Class RN, Persky L. Value of gallium-67 scintigraphy in the diagnosis of localized renal and perirenal infection. J Urol 1980; 124:311–4.
47. Handmaker H. Nuclear imaging in acute pyelonephritis. Semin Nucl Med 1982; 12:246–53.
48. Handmaker H, Young BW, Lowenstein JM. Clinical experience with Tc-99m DMSA (dimercaptosuccinic acid), a new renal imaging agent. J Nucl Med 1975; 16:28–32.
49. Hauser W, Atkins HL, Nelson KG, Richards P. Technetium-99m DTPA: a new radiopharmaceutical for brain and kidney scanning. Radiology 1970; 94:679–84.
50. Heidenreich P, Lauer O, Fendel H, Oberdorfer M, Pabst HW. Determination of total and individual kidney function in children by means of I-123 hippuran whole body clearance and scintillation camera. Pediatr Radiol 1981; 11:17–27.
51. Houwen B, Donker AJM, Woldring MG. Simultaneous determination of glomerular filtration rate with ^{125}I-iothalamate and effective renal plasma flow with ^{131}I-hippuran. In: Proceedings of symposium on dynamic studies with radioisotopes in medicine, Vienna: International Atomic Energy Commission, 1971.
52. Hoving L, Meulen J, Reitsma WD. Gallium-67 scintigraphy for inflammatory masses (letter to the editor). N Engl J Med 1976; 295:1320.
53. Huttunen K, Huttunen NP, Koivula A, Ahonen A, Pauklsa R. ^{99m}Tc DTPA—a useful clinical tool for the measurement of glomerular filtration rate. Scand J Urol Invest 1982; 16:237–41.
54. Ingelfinger JR. Pediatric hypertension. Philadelphia: WB Saunders, 1982.
55. Kahn PC. Renal imaging with radionuclides, ultrasound, and computed tomography. Semin Nucl Med 1979; 9:43–57.
56. Kainer G, Milveen B, Hoschl R, Rosenberg AR. Assessment of individual renal function in children using Tc-99m DTPA. Arch Dis Child 1979; 54:931–6.
57. Kalika V, Bard RH, Iloreta A, Freeman LM, Heller S, Blaufox MD. Prediction of renal functional recovery after relief of upper urinary tract obstruction. J Urol 1981; 126:301–5.
58. Kaufmann HJ. Renal vein thrombosis. Am J Dis Child 1958; 95:377–84.
59. Kenny RW, Ackery DM, Fleming JS, Goddard BA, Grant RW. Deconvolution analysis of the scintillation camera renogram. Br J Radiol 1975; 48:481–6.
60. Kessler WO, Gittes RF, Hurwitz SR, Green JP. Gallium-67 scans in the diagnosis of pyelonephritis. West J Med Aus 1974; 121:91–3.

61. Klopper JF, Hauser W, Atkins HL, Eckelman WC, Richards P. Evaluation of ^{99}Tc-DTPA for the measurement of glomerular filtration rate. J Nucl Med 1972; 13:107–10.
62. Koenigsberg M, Blaufox MD, Freeman LM. Traumatic injuries of the renal vasculature and parenchyma. In: Freeman LM, Blaufox MD, eds. Radionuclide studies of the genitourinary system. New York: Grune & Stratton, 1975.
63. Koenigsberg M, Freeman LM, Blaufox MD. Radionuclide and ultrasound evaluation of renal morphology and function. In: Edelman CM, ed. Pediatric renal disease. Boston: Little Brown, 1978.
64. Koff SA, Thrall JH, Keyes JW. Assessment of hydroureteronephrosis in children using diuretic radionuclide renography. J Urol 1980; 123:531–4.
65. Kountz SL, Yeh SH, Wood J, Cohn R, Kriss JP. Technetium-99m (V)-citrate complex for estimation of glomerular filtration rate. Nature 1967; 215:1397–9.
66. Kumar B, Coleman RE. Significance of delayed Ga-67 localization in the kidneys. J Nucl Med 1976; 17:872–5.
67. Kuruc A, Caldicott WJH, Treves S. An improved deconvolution technique for the calculation of renal retention functions. Comp Biomed Res 1982; 15:46–56.
68. Lebowitz RL, Fellows KE, Colodny AH. Renal parenchymal infections in children. Radiol Clin North Am 1977; 15:37–47.
69. Leonard JC, Allen WA, Goin J, Smith CW. Renal cortical imaging and detection of renal mass lesions. J Nucl Med 1979; 20:1018–22.
70. Loggie JMH, Kleinman LI, Van Maanen EF. Renal function and diuretic therapy in infants and children. Part I. J Pediatr 1975; 86:485–96.
71. Loggie JMH, New MI, Robson AM. Hypertension in the pediatric patient: a reappraisal. J Pediatr 1979; 94:685–99.
72. Londe S. Causes of hypertension in the young. Pediatr Clin North Am 1978; 25:55–66.
73. Lubin E, Lewitus Z, Rosenfeld J, Levi N. Kidney scanning with hippuran, a necessary complement for correct interpretation of renography in the transplanted kidney. In: Medical radioisotope scintigraphy. Proceedings of a symposium. Vienna: International Atomic Energy Commission, 1969; 2:219–223.
74. Mackay A, Eadie AS, Cumming AMM, Graham A, Adams FG, Horton PW. Assessment of total and divided renal plasma flow by I-123 hippuran renography. Kidney Int 1981; 19:49–57.
75. Magnusson G, Collste L, Franksson C, Lundgren G. Radiorenography in clinical transplantation. Scand J Urol 1967; 1:132–51.
76. Maher FT, Nolan NG, Elveback LR. Comparison of simultaneous clearances of ^{125}I-labelled iothalamate (Glofil) and of inulin. Mayo Clin Proc 1971; 46:690–1.
77. Mailloux L, Gagnon JA. Measurement of effective renal plasma flow. In: Blaufox MD, ed. Progress in nuclear medicine. Vol. 2. Evaluation of renal function and disease with radionuclides. Baltimore: University Park Press, 1972.
78. Martin DJ, Gilday DL, Reilly BJ. Evaluation of the urinary tract in the neonatal period. Radiol Clin North Am 1975; 13:359–68.
79. McAfee JG, Singh A, O'Callaghan JP. Nuclear imaging supplementary to urography in obstructive uropathy. Radiology 1980; 137:487–96.
80. Meller ST, Eckstein HB. Renal scintigraphy: quantitative assessment of upper urinary tract dilatation in children. J Pediatr Surg 1981; 16:123–6.
81. Mendez G, Morillo G, Alonso M, Isikoff MB. Gallium-67 radionuclide imaging in acute pyelonephritis. AJR 1980; 134:17–22.
82. Merrick MV, Uttley WS, Wild SR. The detection of pyelonephritic scarring in children by radioisotope imaging. Br J Radiol 1980; 53:544–556.
83. Moser E, Jocham D, Beer M, Brill U. Effects of obstruction on single-kidney function. Clinical and experimental results with I-131 hippurate and Tc-99m DMSA. J Nucl Med 1980; 19:257–62.
84. Oester A, Wolf H, Madsen PO. Double isotope technique in renal function testing in dogs. Invest Urol 1969; 6:387–92.
85. Older RA, Korobkin M, Workman J, Cleeve DM, Sullivan D, Webster GD. Accuracy of radionuclide imaging in distinguishing renal masses with normal variants. Radiology 1980; 136:443–8.
86. Olkkonen H, Penttila IM, Uimarehuhta A. Application of the gamma function for the calculation of effective renal plasma flow by 131-I hippuran clearance. Scand J Clin Invest 1977; 37:49–51.
87. Olson DL, Lieberman E. Renal hypertension in children. Pediatr Clin North Am 1976; 23:795–806.
88. Otnes B, Rootwelt K. Mathisen W. A comparison between urography and radioisotope renography in the followup of surgery of hydronephrosis. Scand J Urol Nephrol 1975; 9:50–56.
89. Owen JE, Walker RG, Williams D, Guignard PA, D'Apice AJ. Cadmium telluride detectors in the external measurement of glomerular filtration rate using ^{99m}Tc-DTPA(Sn): comparison with ^{51}Cr-DTPA and ^{99m}Tc-DTPA(Sn) plasma sample methods. Clin Nephrol 1982; 18:200–3.
90. Parker JA, Lebowitz RL, Mascatello V, Treves S. Magnification renal scintigraphy in the differential diagnosis of septa of Bertin. Pediatr Radiol 1976; 4:157–60.
91. Parker RW. Case of an infant in whom some of

the abdominal muscles were absent. Trans Clin Soc Lond 1895; 28:201–3.
92. Patel R, Tanaka T, Mishkin F, Savage A, Das M. Gallium-67 scan: aid to diagnosis and treatment of renal and perirenal infections. Urology 1980; 16:225–8.
93. Piepsz A, Dobbeleir A, Erbsman F. Measurement of separate kidney clearance by means of Tc-99m DTPA complex and a scintillation camera. Eur J Nucl Med 1977; 2:173–7.
94. Piepsz A, Davies R, Ham HR, Dobbeleir A, Schulman C, Erbsmann F. A simple method for measuring separate glomerular filtration rate using a single injection of Tc-99m DTPA and the scintillation camera. J Pediatr 1978; 93:769–74.
95. Piepsz A, Ham HR, Erbsman F, Hall M, Diffey BL, Boggin MJ, Hall F, Miller JA, Lumbroso J, DiPaola R, Basin JP, DiPaola M, Fries D. A co-operative study on the clinical value of dynamic renal scanning with deconvolution analysis. Br J Radiol 1982; 55:419–33.
96. Powers TA, Stone WJ, Grove RB, Plunkett JM, Kadir S, Palton JA, Bowen RD. Radionuclide measurement of differential glomerular filtration rate. Invest Radiol 1981; 10:59–64.
97. Quigley JM, Druy EM, Rich JL. Acute renal vein thrombosis with a diagnostic renal scintigram. AJR 1981; 137:1066–68.
98. Ram MD, Evans K, Chisholm GD. A single injection method for measurement of effective renal plasma flow. Br J Urol 1968; 40:425–8.
99. Rasoulpour M, McLean RH. Renal venous thrombosis in neonates. Initial and followup abnormalities. Am J Dis Child 1980; 134:276–9.
100. Razzak MA, Macintyre WJ, Pritchard WH. External monitoring of hippuran I-131 disappearance as a measure of renal blood flow. Int J Appl Radiat 1967; 18:825–8.
101. Robson AM. Special diagnostic studies for the detection of renal and renovascular forms of hypertension. Pediatr Clin North Am 1978; 25:83–98.
102. Rootwelt K, Falch D, Sjokvist R. Determination of glomerular filtration rate (GFR) by analysis of capillary blood after single shot injection of ^{99m}Tc DTPA. Eur J Nucl Med 1980; 5:97–102.
103. Rosen PR, Treves S. The efficacy of Tc-99m DTPA and Tc-99m DMSA renography in the screening of pediatric patients for renal etiologies in hypertension. J Nucl Med 1983; 24:22.
104. Rossing N, Bojsen J, Frederiksen PL. The glomerular filtration rate determined with ^{99m}Tc DTPA and a portable cadmium telluride detector. Scand J Clin Lab Invest 1978; 38:23–28.
105. Sapirstein LA, Vidt DG, Mandel MJ, Hanuslk G. Volumes of distribution and clearances of intravenously injected creatinine in the dog. Am J Physiol 1955; 181:330–6.
106. Schlegal JU, Hamway SA. Individual renal plasma flow determination in 2 minutes. J Urol 1976; 116:282–5.
107. Schneider M, Becker JA, Staiano S, Campos E. Sonographic radiographic correlation of renal and perirenal infections. AJR 1976; 127:1007–14.
108. Sherman RA, Blaufox MD. Obstructive uropathy in patients with nonvisualization on renal scan. Nephrology 1980; 25:82–86.
109. Shore RM, Uehling DT, Bruskewitz R, Polycn RE. Evaluation of obstructive uropathy with diuretic renography. Am J Dis Child 1983; 137:236–40.
110. Short MD, Glass HI, Chisholm GD, Vernon P, Silvester DJ. Gamma camera renography using ^{123}I-hippuran. Br J Radiol 1973; 46:289–94.
111. Siddiqui AR, Cohen M, Moran DP. Abdominal masses in children: multiorgan imaging with Tc-99m methylene diphosphonate. AJR 1982; 139:35–38.
112. Sigman EM, Elwood CM, Reagen ME, Morris AM, Catanzaro A. The renal clearance of ^{131}I-labeled sodium iothalamate in man. Invest Urol 1965; 2:432–8.
113. Sigman EM, Elwood CM, Knox F. The measurement of glomerular filtration rate in man with sodium iothalamate-^{131}I (Conray). J Nucl Med 1966; 7:60–68.
114. Silver TM, Kass EJ, Thornbury JR, Konnak JW, Wolfman MG. The radiological spectrum of acute pyelonephritis in adults and adolescents. Radiology 1976; 118:65–71.
115. Slutsky LJ, Golimbu M, Braunstein P, Al-Askari S, Genieser N, Golumbu C. Urographic imaging in neonatal period; radionuclide scan and x-ray. Urology 1977; 10:169–72.
116. Spigos DG, Tan W, Pavel DG, Mozes M, Jonasson O, Capek V. Diagnosis of urine extravasation after renal transplantation. AJR 1977; 129:409–13.
117. Stanley JC, Fry WJ. Pediatric renal artery occlusive disease and renovascular hypertension. Arch Surg 1981; 116:669–76.
118. Stanley P, Gyepes MT, Olson DL, Gates GF. Renovascular hypertension in children and adolescents. Radiology 1978; 129:123–31.
119. Stark H. Renal vein thrombosis in infancy: recovery without nephrectomy. Am J Dis Child 1964; 108:430–5.
120. Takeuchi A, Benerschke K. Renal vein thrombosis of the newborn and its relation to maternal diabetes. Biol Neonate 1961; 3:237–56.
121. Tauxe WN, Tobin M, Dubovsky EV, Bueschen AJ, Kontzen F. A macrofunction for computer processing of comprehensive renal function studies. Eur J Nucl Med 1980; 5:103–8.
122. Taylor AT. Quantitative renal function scanning:

a historical and current status report on renal radiopharmaceuticals. In: Freeman LM, Weissman HS (eds). Nuclear Medicine Annual New York: Raven Press, 1980.

123. Taylor AT. Quantitation of renal function with static imaging agents. Semin Nucl Med 1982; 12:330–44.

124. Taylor AT, Nelson H, Vasquez M, Hollenbeck J. Renal gallium accumulation in rats with antibiotic induced nephritis: clinical implications. J Nucl Med 1980; 21:646–9.

125. Thompson IM, Boineau FG, Evans BB, Schlegel JU. The renal quantitation scintillation camera study for determination of renal function. J Urol 1983; 129:461–5.

126. Thornbury JR, Stanley JC, Fryback J. Hypertensive urogram: a nondiscriminatory test for renovascular hypertension. AJR 1982; 138:43–49.

127. Thrall JH, Koff SA, Keyes JW. Diuretic radionuclide renography and scintigraphy in the differential diagnosis of hydroureteronephrosis. Semin Nucl Med 1981; 11:89–104.

128. Treves S, Martinez DA, Davis MA and Hedley-Whyte ET. Cellular localization of Tc-99m radiopharmaceuticals by radioautography. J Nucl Med. 1976; 17:536–537.

129. Tubis M, Posnick E, Nordyke RA. Preparation and use of ^{131}I labeled sodium iodohippurate in kidney function tests. Proc Soc Exp Biol Med 1960; 103:497–8.

130. Tveter KJ, Nerdrum HJ, Mjolnerod OK. The value of radioisotope renography in the followup of patients operated upon for hydronephrosis. J Urol 1975; 114:680–3.

131. Vanlic-Razumenic N, Petrovic J. Biochemical studies of the renal radiopharmaceutical compound. Dimercaptosuccinate. I. Subcellular localization of Tc-99m DMS complex in the rat kidney in vivo. Eur J Nucl Med 1981; 6:169–72.

132. Van Stekelenburg LHM. Hippuran transit times in the kidney: a new approach. Phys Med Biol 1978; 23:291–301.

133. Verhagen AD, Hamilton JP, Genal M. Renal vein thrombosis in infants. Arch Dis Child 1965; 40:214–17.

134. Vivan G, Stringer D, deBruyn R, et al. Tc-99m DMSA in renovascular hypertension in children. In: Raynmud C, Proceedings of the third world congress of nuclear medicine and biology. Paris: Pergamon Press, 1982; IV:2663.

135. Webb JAW, Tainer LB. The role of intravenous urography in hypertension. Radiol Clin North Am 1979; 17:187–95.

136. Williams DI, Burkholder GV. The prune belly syndrome. J Urol Aust 1967; 98:244–51.

137. Willis KW, Martinez DA, Hedley-White E, Davis MA, Judy PF, Treves S. Renal localization of Tc-99m stannous glucoheptonate and Tc-99m stannous dimercaptosuccinate in the rat by frozen section autoradiography. The efficiency and resolution of technetium-99m. Radiat Res 1977; 69:475–88.

138. Winter CC, Elliott J, Grace D, Robertson A. Radioisotope renography in the assessment of renal function in the newborn. J Urol 1968; 100:99–103.

139. zum Winkel K, Harbst H, Schenck P, Franz HE, Ritz E, Ruhl L, Ziegler M, Ammann W, Maier-Borst W. Sequential scintigraphy in renal transplantation. In: Medical radioisotope scintigraphy. Proceedings of a symposium. Vienna: International Atomic Energy Commission, 1969; II:197.

Chapter 5 Radionuclide Voiding Cystography

U. V. Willi
S. T. Treves

Study of the ureters and bladder in pediatric nuclear medicine is limited to the use of radionuclide cystography for evaluation of suspected vesicoureteric reflux. This failure of the ureterovesical valve mechanism may be caused by a congenital variation, pathologic process, or immaturity that distorts the anatomy or function of the ureterovesical junction. The principal longterm consequence of vesicoureteric reflux of infected urine is the development of pyelonephritic scars that in turn may lead to hypertension and chronic renal failure.

Several passive and active factors characterize a normal valve mechanism of the ureterovesical junction. The passive factors include an oblique entry of the ureter into the bladder; an adequate length of intramural ureter, particularly of its submucosal segment; and an adequate ratio of the length of the submucosal tunnel to the diameter of the ureter. The active factors are contraction of the ureterotrigonal muscles, which close the ureteral meatus and the submucosal tunnel, and active ureteral peristalsis, as during diuresis.[33]

The incidence of vesicoureteric reflux in the general population (noninfected) is not known. In a study by Ransley,[34] only seven (1%) of 535 apparently normal neonates, infants, and children had vesicoureteric reflux. We reviewed radionuclide voiding cystograms in 37 siblings of patients with known vesicoureteric reflux and found that 12 (32%) of them exhibited reflux. The dysfunction was unilateral in eight patients and bilateral in four patients. Using radiographic cystography, Jerkins and Noe[21] found a similar incidence among siblings.

The intravesical ureter becomes longer with age, often producing sufficient length to convert a refluxing ureterovesical junction into a nonrefluxing one. Normand and Smellie in 1979 reported spontaneous cessation of reflux in 71% of children and 79% of the ureters in their patients.[30] The most important factor in the spontaneous resolution of reflux seemed to be the diameter of the ureter: resolution took place in 85% of ureters of normal caliber but only in 41% of dilated ureters. In addition, these authors reported that 63% of ureters associated with scarred kidneys also ceased to reflux spontaneously.

Followup radiographic voiding cystograms (VCUG) every 12 months or so are often obtained in patients with reflux in order to follow its evolution. Cessation of reflux usually eliminates the need for continuing antiinfectious prophylaxis. Because of the concern about gonadal radiation to children from these multiple studies, radionuclide cystography with its much lower radiation dose has become a desirable alternative.

Management of vesicoureteric reflux remains controversial. In view of its tendency to resolve spontaneously. Persistent reflux, depending on the individual patient, may call for further antibiotic treatment with continuous monitoring or surgical correction. The degree of ultimate damage to the kidneys or subsequent pathology does not appear to change with the treatment chosen.

Radionuclide cystography was introduced in the late 1950s by Winter,[56] and since then several reports on this topic have appeared.[1,3,10,16,39,51–53,57] Conway and his coworkers refined the method for application to pediatric patients.[4,7,29]

Radionuclide cystography permits continuous

monitoring of bladder filling and emptying. Reflux can be detected and its dynamics recorded at any and all times during the study. Using computerized gamma cameras, estimates of the capacity of the bladder and the volume of reflux can be made. Simultaneous recording of intravesical pressure permits assessment of reflux dynamics and analysis of the relationship between intravesical volume, pressure, and reflux.

Indications

In our institution radionuclide cystography is used in the following situations:

1. As a screening test to detect reflux in children who have had urinary infection
2. Followup a few months to a year after the initial diagnosis of vesicoureteric reflux in patients on longterm antibiotic treatment
3. Following antireflux surgery
4. In siblings of patients with known vesicoureteric reflux.

Method

Patient Preparation

A complete explanation of the procedure should be given to the patient and/or the parents. When done with patience and understanding, such a conversation will reduce anxiety caused by the examination. In addition, we find it helpful to give or mail a brochure with information and instructions for preparation to our patients.[17,24] If a patient is unusually apprehensive about the procedure, we perform the study on another day. We do not use sedation.

The patient is instructed to void in the bathroom before the examination if possible, and then to lie supine on the examination table for the entire study. The examination table is covered with absorbent paper in order to avoid contamination.

Equipment

A computerized gamma scintillation camera with a field of view sufficiently large to include both kidneys and the bladder should be used. The camera should be equipped with a high-sensitivity or diverging collimator.

Radiopharmaceuticals

The radiopharmaceutical used is technetium-99m (Tc-99m) as sodium pertechnetate: 1 mCi dissolved in a 500 ml bottle of sterile saline. This bottle is connected to the intravesical catheter by means of standard intravenous tubing.

Catheterization

Sterile urethral catheterization trays prepared for each study contain the following items: three small containers, cotton, and a sterile towel with a central opening. Other materials needed include antiseptic solution (Betadine®), sterile water, anesthetic jelly (lidocaine), a bright light source, a 10-ml syringe with a blunt, tapered adaptor, and aqueous lidocaine (0.5%). Catheters of two sizes are used: a 2.6-mm diameter catheter (French size No. 8) for most patients and a 1.5-mm diameter catheter (French size No. 5) for babies. For simultaneous pressure recordings, we use a 3-mm diameter, double-lumen catheter (French No. 9, Reusch, West Germany).

Success of the examination depends to a great extent on a careful catheterization technique. Inexperience is the most frequent cause of iatrogenic damage to the male urethra. If necessary, a parent or aide assists in restraining the patient, who lies supine and is encouraged to relax. The so-called frog position is useful in catheterizing females. The periurethral area (girls) or the glans penis (boys) is carefully cleansed with antiseptic solution and sterile water. These fluids should be warmed to body temperature before use. The catheter is lubricated with the anesthetic jelly in order to facilitate a smooth insertion. The urethral orifice in girls is identified before attempting catheterization.

In girls, the catheter should be introduced easily in one motion without hesitation. Any additional contact with the area surrounding the urethral orifice should be avoided because it causes discomfort. This cannot be emphasized enough because a child who has had a bad first experience with this procedure is not likely to cooperate in the future.

In males, the urethra is anesthetized. The penis is held with one hand, while lidocaine (5–10 ml) is slowly injected into the urethra using the blunt adaptor. Slow and deep breathing helps to relax the sphincter and allows anesthetizing of the entire urethra. Slightly squeezing the anterior portion of the penis for a minute prevents the lidocaine from draining out. The catheter is then gently and continuously introduced into the bladder. Deep breathing and/or instructing the patient to void may relax the sphincter. If the sphincter remains closed, the catheter should be kept under continuous and mild pressure against it. In the majority of cases, the catheter will eventually glide through the sphincter.

Do not try to overcome a closed or spastic sphincter by repeated back-and-forth motions of the catheter as this may result in urethral injury. In the rare instance when it is necessary to repeat the urethral anesthesia, a second attempt at catheterization is almost always successful.

Once the catheter has been advanced beyond the sphincter, the majority of children will cooperate. In girls, the catheter is fixed with adhesive surgical tape to the inner thigh; in boys, to the dorsal shaft of the penis. Leaving the catheter in place until the end of the study has the advantage of allowing a repeat examination in case of failure as well as additional filling of the bladder, if necessary, in order to initiate voiding. It is important to ensure that there is no skin contamination of the radionuclide as it may be confused with reflux during analysis.

Recording

The radionuclide cystogram is recorded on the computer in a series of 5-sec frames for the duration of the study. In addition, an analog record is made at one frame per 30 sec duration for the entire study.

Filling and Voiding

The bottle with the radionuclide is suspended 70–90 cm above the examination table and is connected to the catheter. The child is encouraged to lie quietly on the table (Fig. 5-1). Sand bags alongside the patient's body help to maintain positioning, and dim light during the procedure seems to have a quieting effect.

The entire examination is monitored on a persistence oscilloscope by the operator. The end of the filling phase is indicated by a bladder volume appropriate for the patient's age (Fig. 5-2) and a reduction of the rate of flow of the infusate.

With filling of the bladder to its capacity, voiding is usually initiated without delay. Careful and complete collection of the voided fluid is necessary for quantitation. We use a plastic urinal for both girls and boys. In girls, its lower border is gently pressed against the perineum and inner thighs.

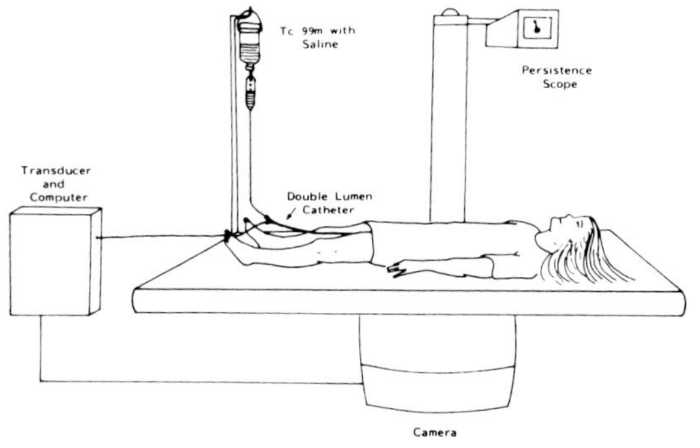

Figure 5-1. Method of radionuclide voiding cystography.

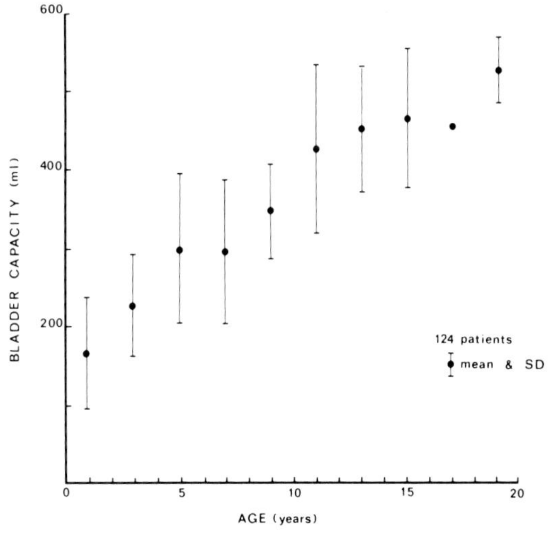

Figure 5-2. Bladder volume as a function of age.

Analysis

The sequential images of the cystogram are displayed on the computer monitor and evaluated visually. Contrast enhancement is helpful in identifying small volumes of reflux. If reflux is present, regions of interest (ROIs) are drawn over the kidneys and bladder. In addition, another region equidistant from the bladder is selected in order to correct for background scatter.

It is important to determine if there has been any patient motion during the study because it will invalidate any attempts at quantitation. If motion has not occurred, time versus activity curves are calculated for each ROI (Fig. 5-3).

In order to obtain an estimate of the volumes of reflux, bladder capacity, and residual capacity, a

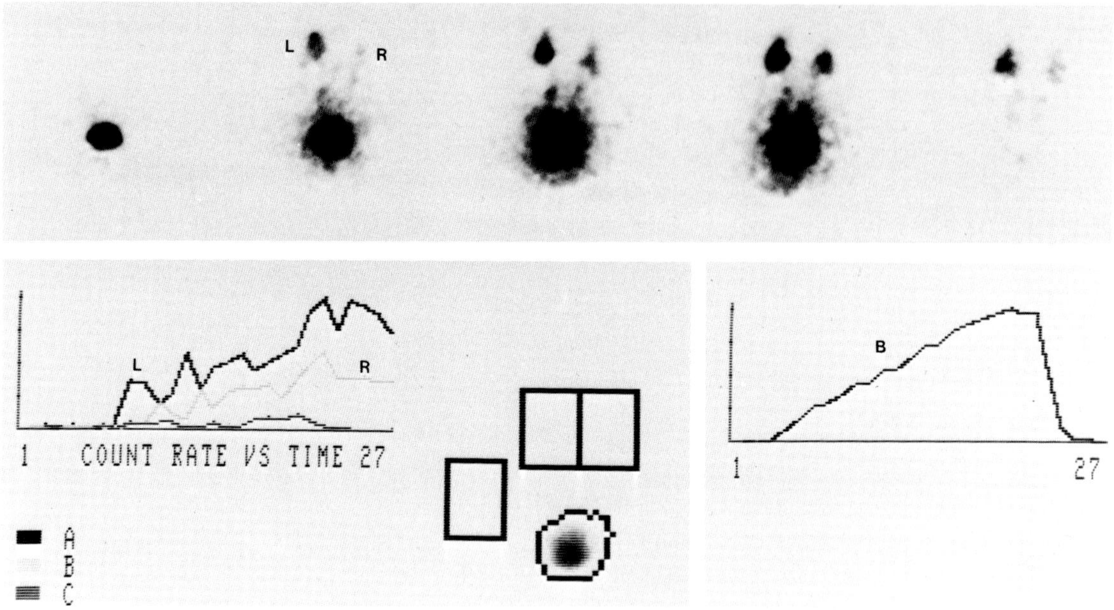

Figure 5-3. Bilateral vesicoureteric reflux in a 5-year-old female with documented reflux by conventional voiding cystography 1 year previously. L, Left ureter; R, right ureter; B, bladder.

relationship between activity and volume is obtained. Assuming that attenuation of the gamma rays is constant, that the isotope is well mixed with the solution of saline, and that a negligible amount of urine is produced by the kidneys during the study, the counts recorded will be proportional to the volume(s).

$$V = RC \qquad [1]$$

when V is volume, R is constant, and C is counts. Note that 0 counts represents zero volume.

The constant R is calculated by relating the voided volume to the drop in total vesical counts during the voiding phase of the study. At the beginning of the voiding phase, the volume is V_0 and the counts are C_0. At the end of the voiding phase, the volume will be V_e and the counts C_e. Substituting these values into Eq. [1] yields:

$$V_0 = RC_0 \qquad [2]$$

$$V_e = RC_e \qquad [3]$$

Subtracting Eq. [3] from Eq. [2] yields:

$$R = \frac{V_0 - V_e}{C_0 - C_e} = \frac{\Delta V}{\Delta C} = \frac{\text{Change in volume}}{\text{Change in counts}} \qquad [4]$$

Once the ratios are calculated, it is easy to obtain any volume of interest for any particular time of the study (e.g., maximum volume of reflux). One simply has to multiply the ratio R by the number of counts over a particular region at a given frame.

After the counts in each region are converted to volumes, it is possible to calculate rates of flow. In order to obtain the average voiding flow rate, the count loss during voiding must be divided by the time of voiding and multiplied by the constant R.

$$\text{Average flow rate} = R\frac{\Delta V}{\Delta T} \qquad [5]$$

Parameters obtained in this way include the following:

1. Volume of the bladder at the first occurrence of reflux and at the time of maximum reflux during filling and/or voiding
2. Maximum bladder volume (end of filling)
3. Volumes of reflux (initial, maximum, residual)
4. Residual bladder volume
5. Average voiding flow rate.

Interpretation

Radiologic Grading

We agree with Ransley[34] that grading of vesicoureteric reflux is convenient for communication but need not be applied too rigidly in an individual case. Recently a report by an international group studying vesicoureteric reflux adopted a classification of reflux based on its radiographic appearance[35] (Fig. 5-4). This classification represents a continuum, and some cases may not fall precisely within one of its five grades. Further, the same patient may have a grade II reflux during one examination and a grade I or III during another.

Typically, patients with reflux of low grade (I through III) are candidates for nonsurgical treatment and continuous antibiotic therapy. With higher grades of reflux (significant ureteral and pelvicalyceal dilatation), spontaneous resolution of reflux can occur but is less likely. Continuous antibiotic therapy may be given to these patients provided that their urine remains sterile, that frequent urine cultures are performed, and that serial evaluation for reflux is carried out. This routine requires careful compliance by the patient and parents.

Surgical treatment in experienced hands has a high degree of success (~95%), offers an immediate correction of the anatomic problem, and reduces the risk of pyelonephritis. Neither medical nor surgical treatment, however, offers a clear advantage as far as subsequent development of hypertension or impairment of renal growth. Whichever form of therapy is chosen, longterm followup and observation are essential to assess the patient's progress and the presence of complicating factors, such as residual vesicoureteric reflux, new scars, pyelonephritis, hypertension, or obstruction.

Reflux

An analysis of 135 consecutive radionuclide studies in our hospital revealed a 32% incidence of vesicoureteric reflux, usually grades I–III. Reflux was present in 47% of the nonsurgical patients and in 11% of the patients evaluated following surgery. It was unilateral in 60% and bilateral in 40%. Unilateral reflux occurred in the right or the left ureter with equal frequency. In the 59 refluxing renal units, reflux occurred during filling and voiding in 80% while reflux during voiding only was present in 17% of the ureters. The remaining 3% of ureters refluxed during bladder filling only. Almost 80% of those patients with reflux during filling and voiding exhibited an increase in the refluxed volume during voiding of 2–34 ml (average 7 ml).

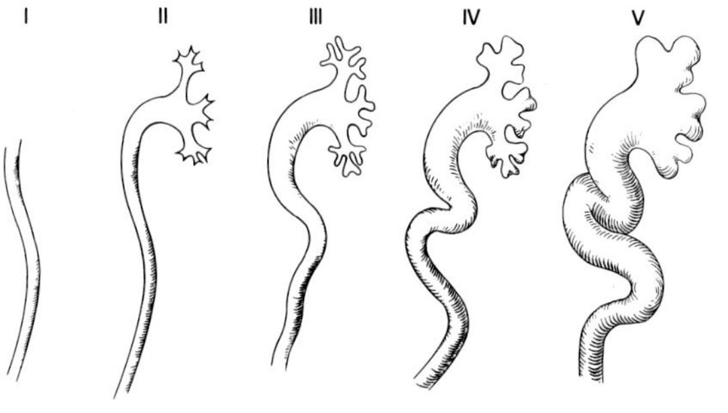

Figure 5-4. Radiographic classification of reflux. International Study Classification. I, Ureter only. II, Ureter, pelvis, and calices. No dilatation, normal caliceal fornices. III, Mild or moderate dilatation and/or tortuosity of ureter and mild or moderate dilatation of renal pelvis but no or slight blunting of fornices. IV, Moderate dilatation and/or tortuosity of ureter and moderate dilatation of renal pelvis and calices. Complete obliteration of sharp angle of fornices but maintenace of papillary impressions in majority of calices. V, Gross dilatation and tortuosity of ureter. Gross dilatation of renal pelvis and calices. Papillary impressions are no longer visible in the majority of calices.

Comparing the five radiographic grades of reflux with radionuclide cystography is not easy and may not be appropriate due to inherent technical peculiarities of these methods. In radionuclide cystography, however, it is possible to see three degrees. The less severe degree will show reflux limited to the ureter without reaching the renal pelvis (Fig. 5-5). This corresponds to grade I reflux. Another appearance is that of a small volume of vesicoureteric reflux reaching the renal pelvis with minimal or no visualization of the ureter (Figs. 5-6–5-9). This corresponds to radiographic grades II or III as it is not possible by the radionuclide technique to finely assess the diameter of the ureter and the anatomy of the pelvicalyceal system. Finally, the radionuclide cystogram could reveal a large volume of reflux reaching a dilated pelvicalyceal system with definite or marked dilatation (and even redundancy) of the ureter corresponding in appearance to radiologic grades IV and V (Figs. 5-10 and 5-11).

The radionuclide cystogram is more sensitive than conventional radiographic voiding cystography for the diagnosis of vesicoureteric reflux.[4] It also permits an estimation of the refluxed volume. Experiments with phantoms in our institution using volumetric flasks (bladders) and small containers

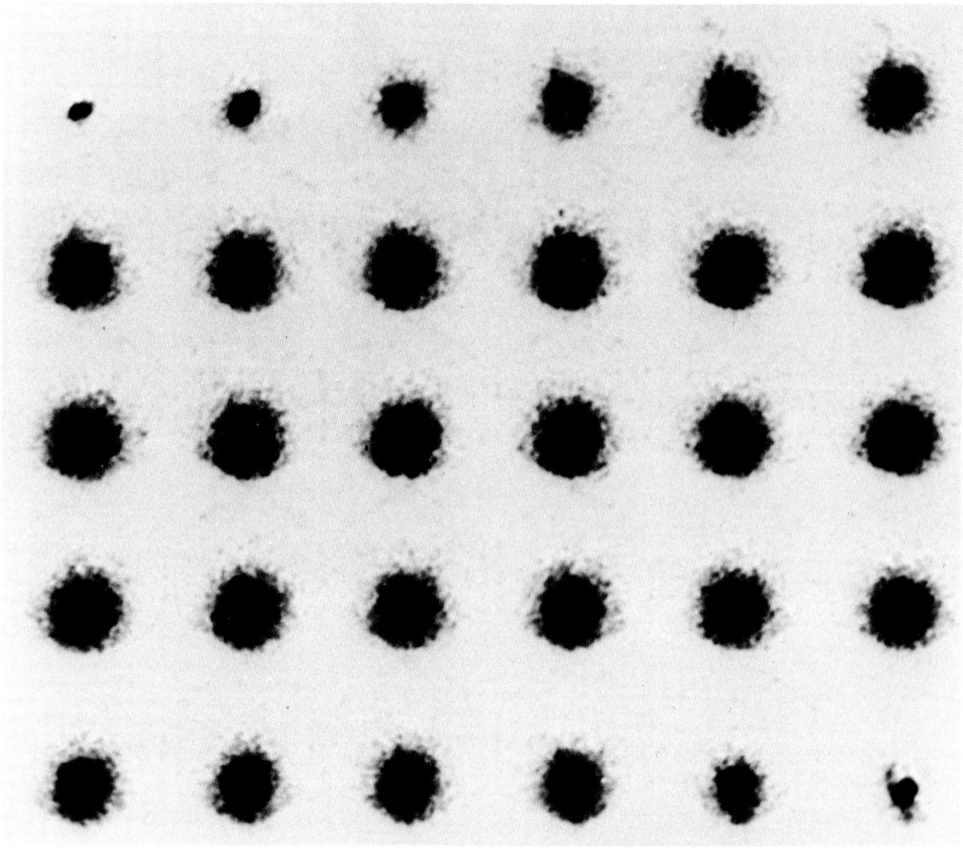

Figure 5-5. Small, intermittent left vesicoureteric reflux in an 8-year-old female with previously documented left grade I–II reflux. At the end of the top row, vesicoureteric reflux is within the ureter and appears to reach the left renal pelvis. The last frame shows reflux into the distal left ureter.

(refluxes) of various volumes and several scatter thicknesses were carried out in order to determine the sensitivity of this technique. The same radiopharmaceutical specific activity, collimator, and frame rate as used in the clinical studies were employed. Under these conditions, it was determined that: the minimum detectable volume of reflux was 0.20 ml (240 ml flask and 3.5 cm of scatter); and the minimum distance from the projected edge of the flask at which 0.20 ml of reflux was detectable was 2 cm. Actual estimate of the volume of reflux if it was < 1 ml yielded a $> 50\%$ error. Volumes in the smaller container (reflux) of 1 ml or greater yielded an error in the estimated volume of 10% when using 3.5 cm of scatter and 20% with 6 cm of scatter.

Three cadaveric kidneys containing 1.0, 5.0, and 10.0 ml of test solution in their pelvicalyceal systems were imaged along with a 240-ml flask ("bladder") using 3.5 cm of scatter. Estimations of "reflux" volume under these conditions carried an error of 10%.

Patterns of Reflux

The ability to monitor continuously during radionuclide cystography permits observation of several dynamic patterns of reflux (with no increase in radiation dose). Continuously increasing reflux characteristically occurs during the early or mid-filling phase supposedly through a patulous ureteral orifice that allows the bladder and ureter(s) to behave as a single chamber (Fig. 5-6). Occurrence of reflux in this condition appears to be independent of intravesical pressure, which is usually low during the beginning of bladder filling. This corresponds to Lattimer's group 3: reflux at low pressures and low volumes.[23]

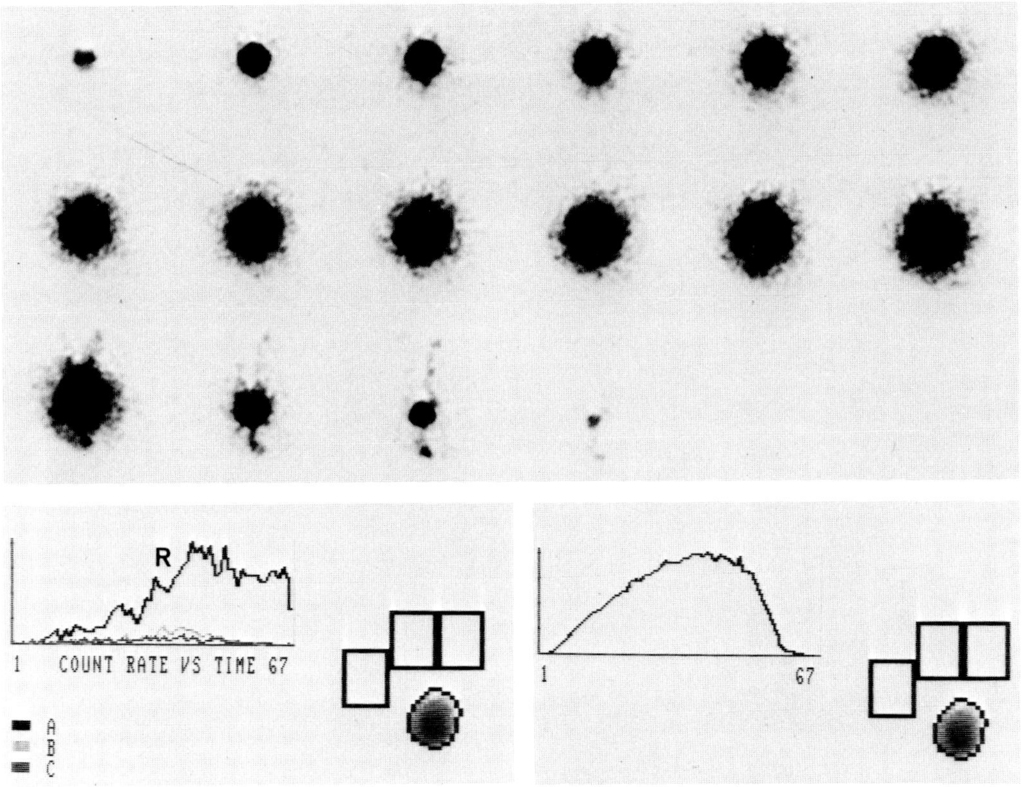

Figure 5-6. Bilateral vesicoureteric reflux in a 6-year-old female observed mainly during voiding. A year previously, this patient showed unilateral reflux. Left reflux is minimal and it does not seem to reach the renal pelvis. The reflux into the right ureter is greater than into the left, still small, and it reaches the renal pelvis.

Most commonly, vesicoureteric reflux does not start until a certain threshold of bladder volume has been reached and then either continues to increase until the end of the filling phase or shows intermittent increases and decreases in volume (Fig. 5-12). In some patients, however, there may be only transient episodes of reflux during the filling phase (Fig. 5-5). Some children who are unwilling or unable to void during the cystogram are asked to urinate in the bathroom and a postvoiding image is obtained. In some cases the postvoid image will show the only evidence of vesicoureteric reflux (Figs. 5-13 and 5-14). In certain cases of bilateral reflux, one ureter can be seen to begin refluxing at a certain bladder volume and then reflux begins into the contralateral ureter at a greater bladder volume (Figs. 5-3, 5-7, 5-12, and 5-15).

If reflux has occurred during the filling phase, it may (Fig. 5-10) or may not increase in volume during the voiding phase, and in certain instances it may decrease or disappear altogether during voiding (Figs. 5-6, 5-8, 5-12, and 5-14). In other cases reflux only occurs during or after voiding (Fig. 5-6 and 5-14). Refluxed fluid may continuously drain into the bladder immediately after completion of voiding and despite the fact that at this time the intravesical pressure frequently reaches its maximum. Reflux, therefore, may not have as much to do with intravesical pressure as with the state of bladder filling and contraction insofar as they affect the ureterovesical junction.

Bladder Capacity

Information about bladder capacity on previous studies, mean standard values, and observation of the infusion flow rate should aid the operator in filling the patient's bladder to its approximate capac-

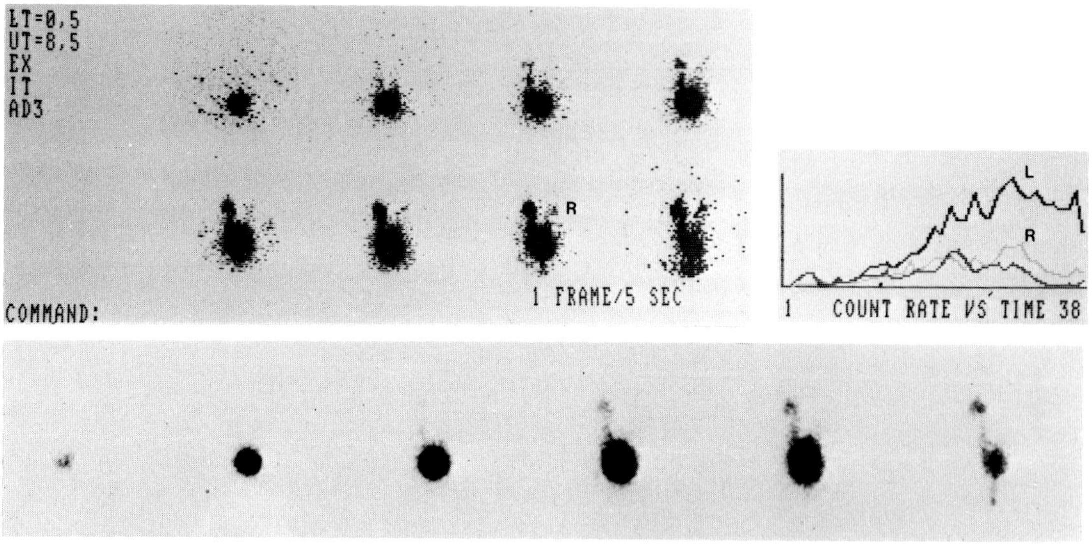

Figure 5-7. Bilateral vesicoureteric reflux 6 months following surgical repair of megaureters. Left reflux is greater than right. Enhanced computer images *(top left)* reveal the right reflux clearly while analog images *(bottom)* show only left reflux. Time-activity curves over the ureters reveal the dynamics of reflux *(top right)*.

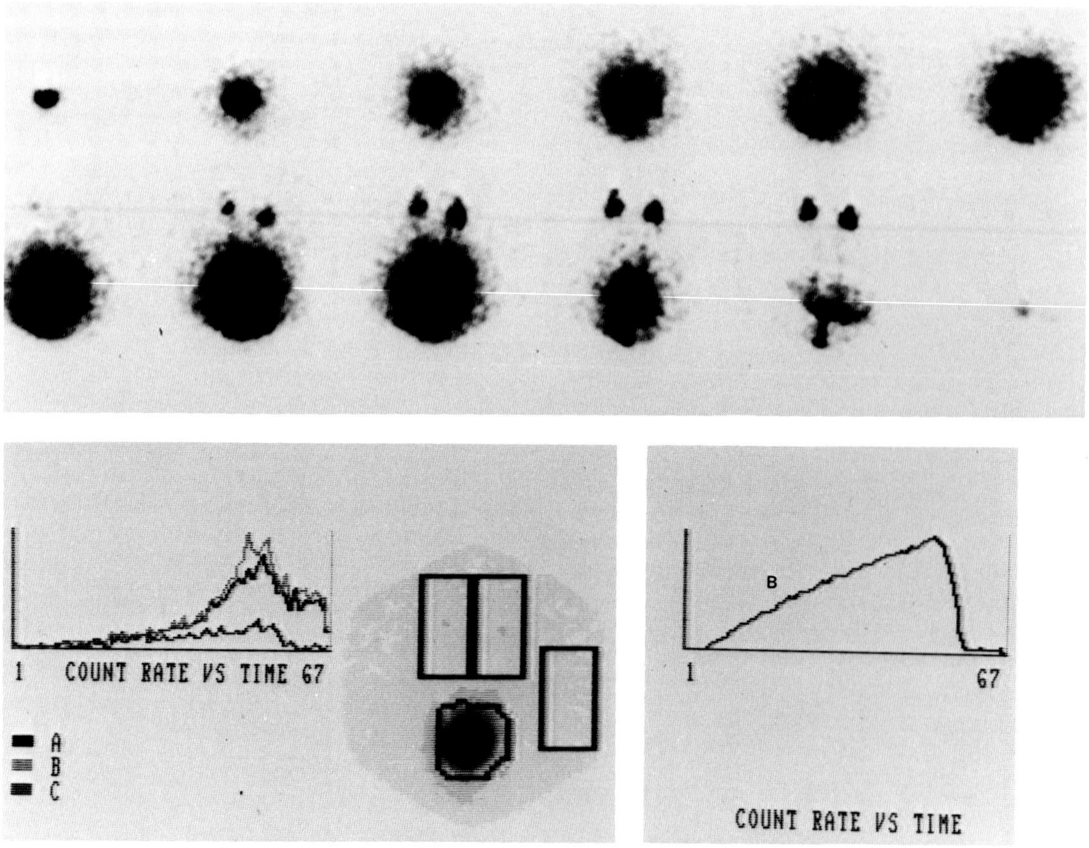

Figure 5-8. Bilateral reflux 1 year followup in an 8-year-old female with previous left grade III reflux by voiding cystography. Reflux occurs in both ureters at almost the same bladder volume (200 ml). Reflux extends into both renal pelves and it drains to completion with voiding.

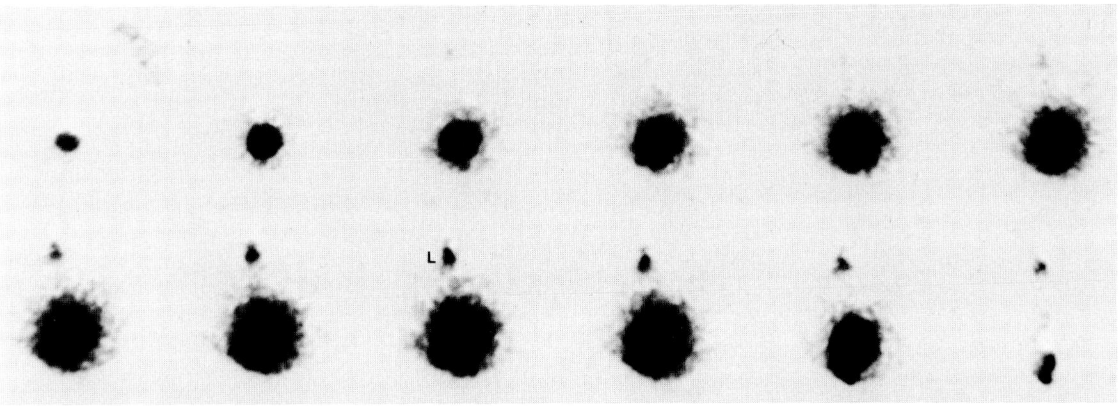

Figure 5-9. Five-year-old female with left vesicoureteric reflux 4 months after right ureteral reimplantation. There is no evidence of right vesicoureteric reflux.

ity. These and other guides are highly variable, however. For example, bladder capacity generally increases with the age of the patient (Fig. 5-2), but its variability at a given age or in a given patient may correspond to 100% or more of the mean volume. Similarly, subjective criteria of complete bladder filling produced by the patient (toes curling upward, restless legs, urgency) should be noted, but their value is questionable.

Influences operating at the time of examination may cause the functional capacity to be quite different from the actual capacity. Mechanical factors, such as rapid filling of the bladder, irritation from the catheter, or low temperature of the instilled fluid can induce high bladder tonus and thus lower bladder capacity. Apprehension may provoke the same response. Uninhibited bladder contractions due to irritability from severe inflammation characteristically cause intermittent pain and urgency and tend to keep bladder capacity low. In most children with urinary tract infection in our series, however, bladder capacity seemed not to be affected. However, Starfield[45] established values of functional bladder capacity in nonenuretic and enuretic children and showed that the bladder capacities were significantly lower in the latter group.

Intravesical Pressure

Our method of examination permits, if desired, simultaneous recording of the radionuclide cystogram and intravesical pressures in the computer. Using a double-lumen catheter (see Method), one channel is used for infusion while the other is connected to a pressure transducer. The pressure transducer output is connected through an analog-to-digital converter to the computer. Time-activity and time-pressure waves can then be displayed on the same computer monitor.

In a study in our institution aimed at establishing normal and abnormal ranges of intravesical pressure, measurements during radionuclide cystography were obtained in 40 patients. There were 16 normal children, 15 children with reflux, and 9 children who had surgery previously. In the normal children, maximum intravesical pressures during filling were 15–80 cm H_2O (average 42 cm H_2O) and during voiding or postvoiding 24–136 cm H_2O (average 78 cm H_2O). There was no significant difference between these, the patients with reflux, and those who had prior reimplants. The initial voiding pressure was always slightly higher than the maximum filling pressure. Intravesical pressures decreased with increasing bladder capacity. During filling of the bladder, the intravesical pressure showed a continuous increase until full bladder capacity was reached. Toward the end of voiding, a pressure peak that occurred after contraction characterized the pressure curve. In most instances, the highest recorded intravesical pressure was reached during this moment after contraction.

There is no satisfactory proof of the concept that intravesical pressure causes vesicoureteric reflux.[41] A relationship between intravesical pressure and cortical renal damage in the absence of infection remains widely debated[2] although in patients with vesicoureteric reflux there are alterations in renal blood flow during voiding.[31] Renal damage from

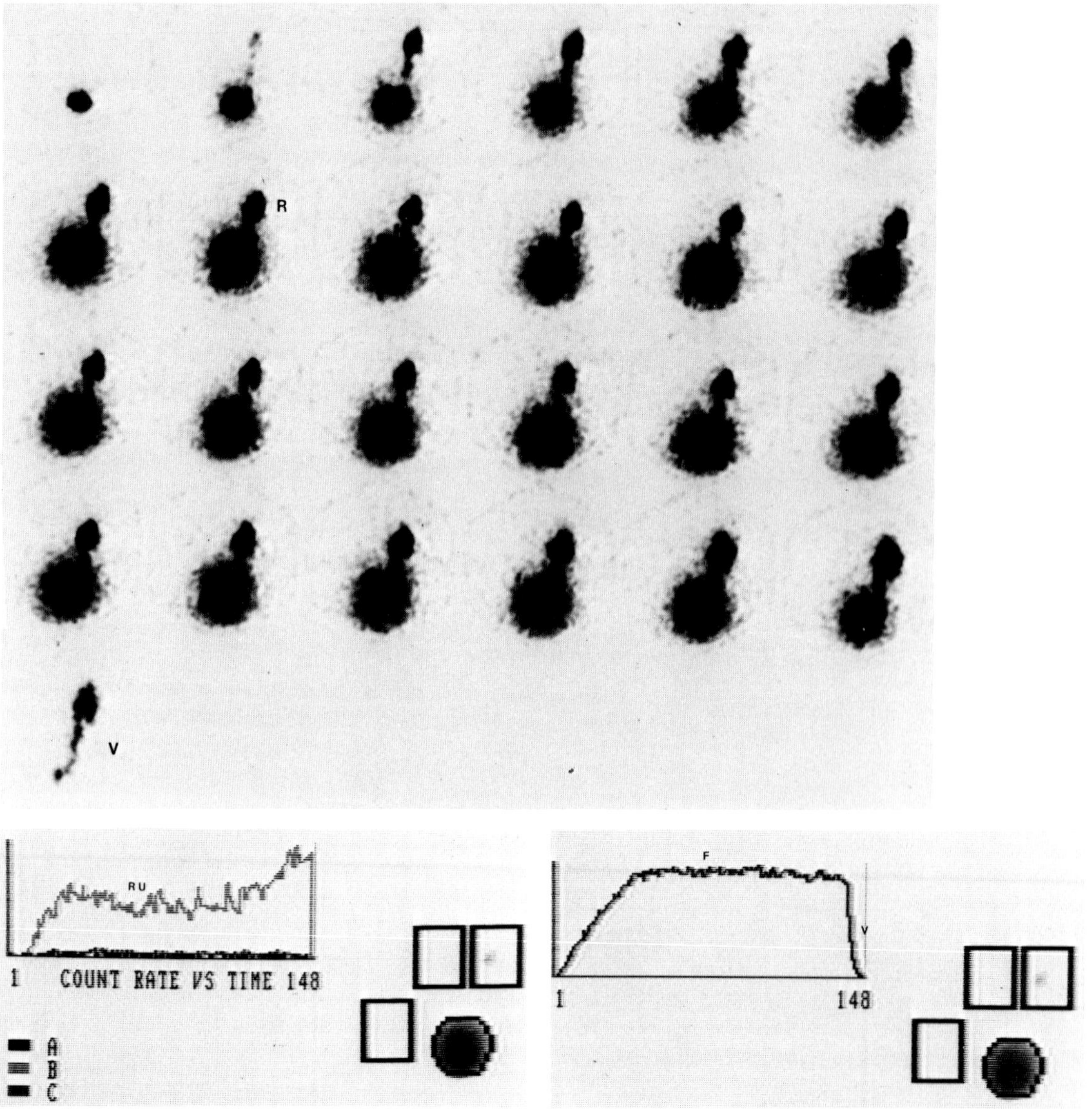

Figure 5-10. Five-year-old female with previous pyelonephritis and bilateral vesicoureteric reflux. Previous left ureteral reimplantation. There is right vesicoureteric reflux only (R) which occurs at a small bladder volume (150 ml) and increases at the end of bladder filling (F) and during voiding (V).

pyelotubular backflow of contrast material has also been considered.[22] It has been clearly demonstrated that in children under 6 years of age, but mainly in infants, massive reflux in the presence of urinary tract infection leads to renal damage.[8,18,36,38,40,41]

Intrarenal reflux seems to play an important role in the etiology of renal damage.[37] Since intravesical pressure is higher in younger children than in older ones, it follows that intravesical pressure decreases with increasing bladder capacity. With renal damage mainly occurring in younger children, perhaps there is some relationship between intravesical pressure and reflux nephropathy. In the absence of a barrier at the ureterovesical junction, the upper urinary system and the bladder act as a single chamber. Studies in our laboratory seem to indicate that intravesical pressure is probably least important in terms of etiology, management, and

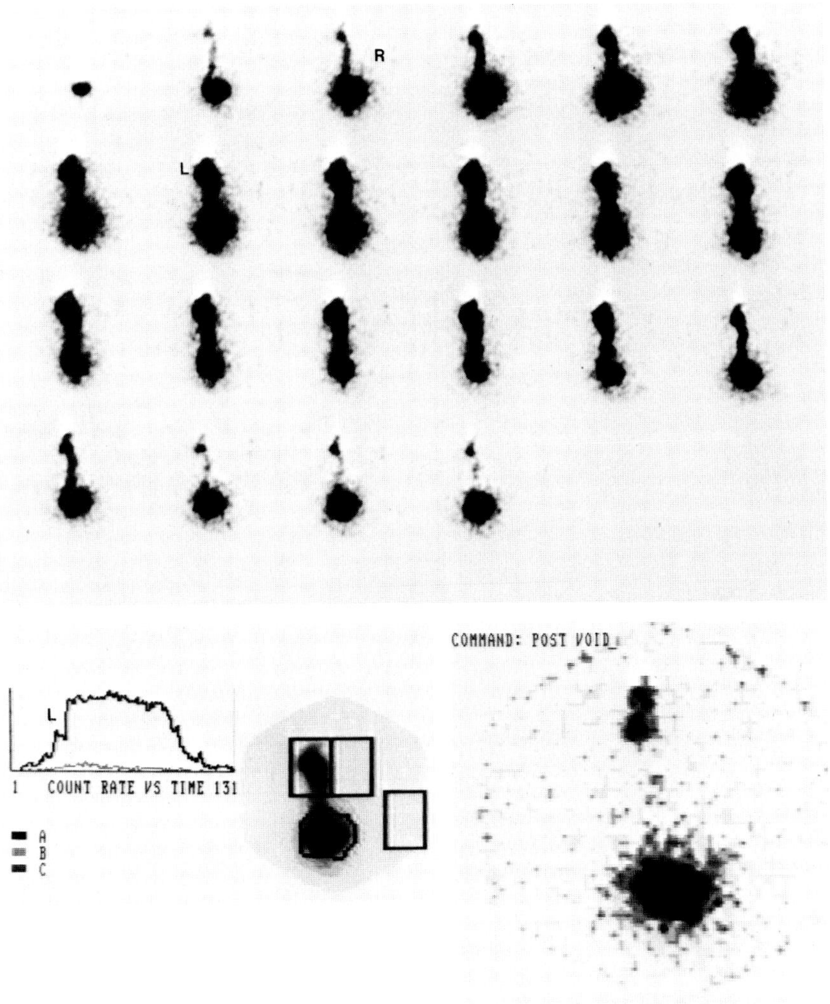

Figure 5-11. Four-year-old male with severe left vesicoureteric reflux. Reflux occurs at a relatively small bladder volume (150 ml). A postvoid image *(below right)* reveals retention of radiotracer within the left renal pelvis. On the third image *(above)* there is evidence of right vesicoureteric reflux to the distal ureter only.

prognosis of reflux provided that no distal obstruction or neurogenic dysfunction coexists. The majority of our patients exhibited reflux during filling at a relatively large bladder volume. The increasing bladder volume during the cystogram probably influences the anatomy and competence of the ureterovesical junction more than the increase in pressure.

In the growing child, maturation of the ureterovesical junction probably implies not only lengthening of the intravesical ureter, but also strengthening of the specific musculature related to the ureterovesical junction. Therefore, decreasing occurrence of reflux with age is to be expected.[4,19,49,50] Controversy still exists about maturation of the ureterovesical junction.[28,47] Reflux only during voiding may be related to the changing anatomic condition of the ureterovesical junction during

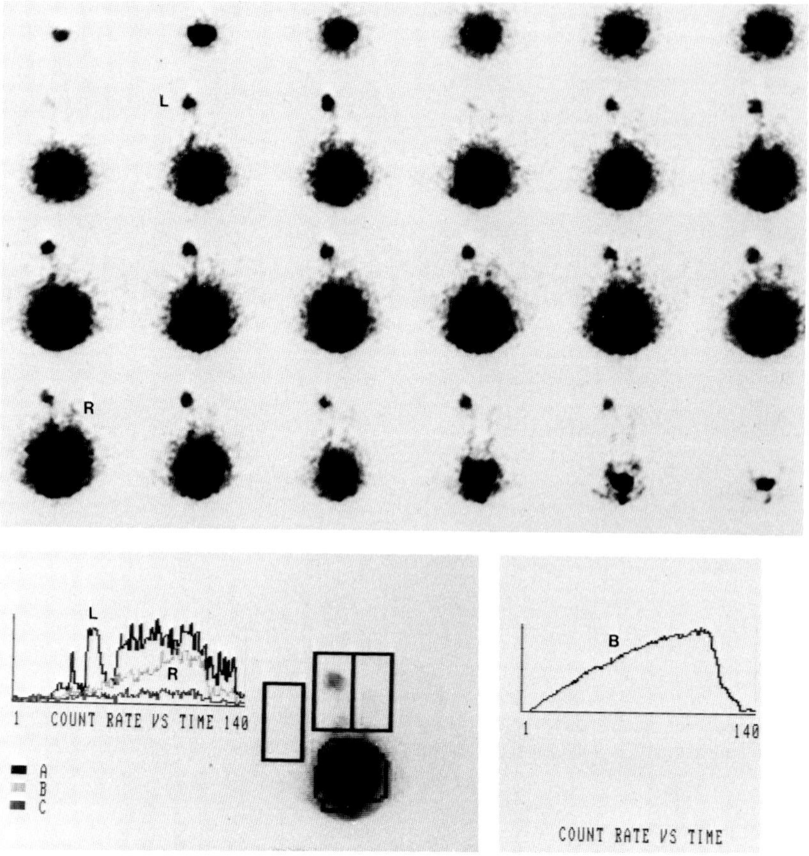

Figure 5-12. Bilateral vesicoureteric reflux in a 9-year-old female, 1 year followup. Reflux in the left ureter (L) occurs at a bladder volume of 230 ml while right reflux (R) occurs at nearly 400 ml of bladder capacity. Note the dynamic nature of the reflux and the complete emptying of activity from the renal pelvis after voiding. B, Bladder time-activity curve.

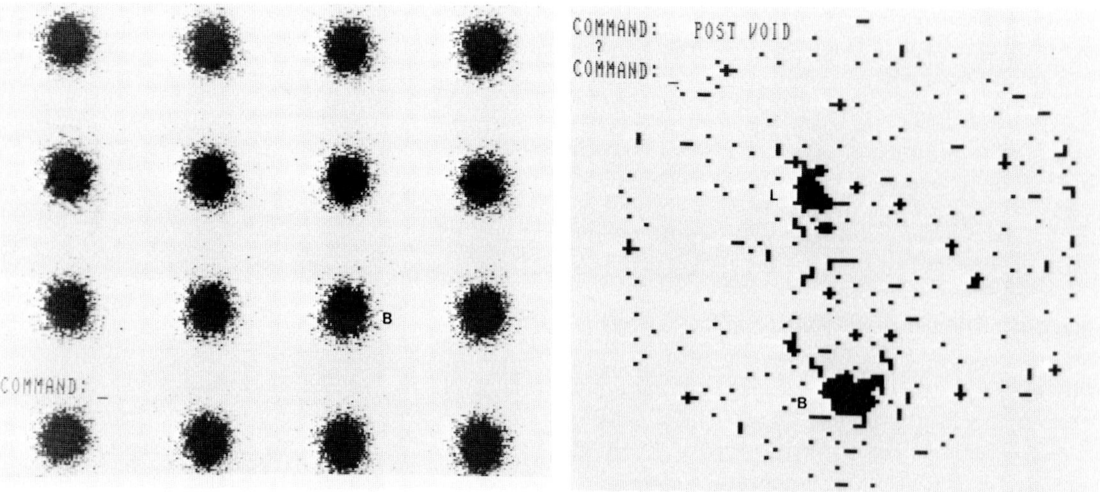

Figure 5-13. Left vesicoureteric reflux detected only after voiding *(right)*. During the filling phase *(left)*, no reflux is demonstrated. This study was done in a 5-year-old female with a left refluxing duplex system.

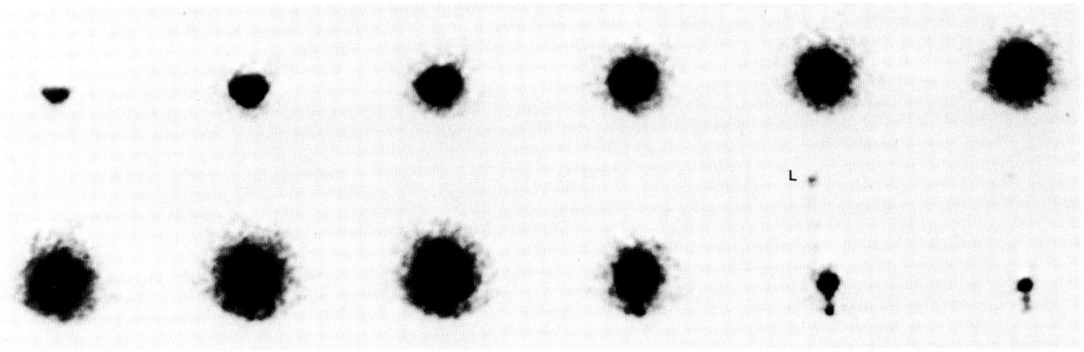

Figure 5-14. Small left vesicoureteric reflux during voiding only, in a 9-year-old female with a previously demonstrated bilateral grade II reflux.

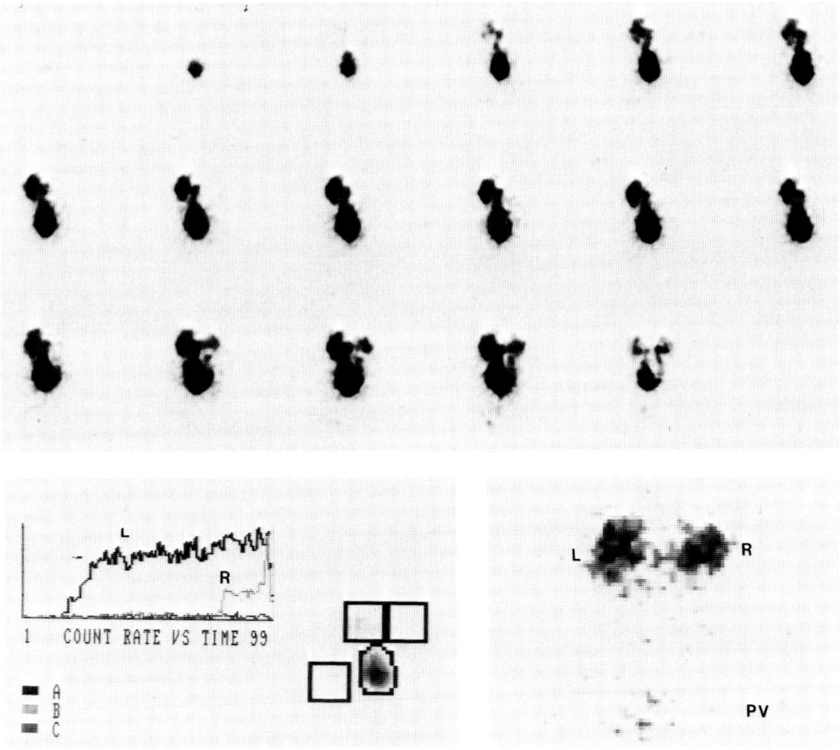

Figure 5-15. Bilateral vesicoureteric reflux beginning at different bladder volumes *(below left)* with retention of radiotracer within both renal pelves after voiding *(below right)*.

bladder contraction. The intravesical pressure at the initiation of voiding is not significantly higher than at the end of filling.

Bladder Emptying

We calculated the voiding flow rates in 75 patients.[44,48] The average flow rate in 26 normal children was 10.2 ml/sec (range, 2–21 ml/sec ± 4.5 SD). In 49 abnormal patients (reflux with or without infection or previous surgery), the voiding flow rates averaged 10.5 ml/sec (range, 1.4–31 ml/sec ± 5.7 SD). In all 75 patients, the average voiding flow rate was 10.4 ml/sec (range, 1.4–31 ml/sec ± 5.3 SD). The average voiding flow rate seemed to relate to the initial bladder volume and thus to age.

The greater the initial bladder volume, the higher the voiding flow rate. The presence of an indwelling catheter did not seem to reduce the voiding flow rate significantly. In patients with an indwelling catheter, it averaged 10.7 ml/sec (range, 2.0–31 ml/sec), while in those without a catheter, the average flow rate was 9.8 ml/sec (range, 1.4–25 ml/sec). The voiding time was 10–116 sec with an average of 35 sec. With the exception of a few extreme values, the voiding time in normal patients is comparable to that in patients with reflux.

Gierup observed that children usually do not use abdominal straining during voiding.[14] When they do, the urinary flow either increases or decreases, probably in relation to whether or not the external sphincter is being contracted along with the abdominal muscles.[54] Thus, urging the child to strain in order to void may be counterproductive.

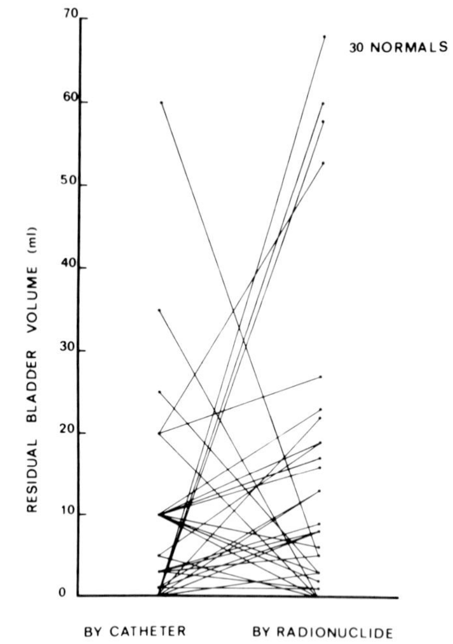

Figure 5-16. Residual bladder volumes measured in the same patients by catheterization and by radionuclide cystography in 30 normal children.

Residual Bladder Volume

Residual volumes measured by catheterization and by radionuclide cystography may or may not be the same (Fig. 5-16), and in many instances, there is gross discrepancy between these two measurements. The reasons for such inconsistency are many. The patient may not adequately empty the bladder because of some underlying abnormality such as aberrant micturition, as in some cases of reflux, or dysuria.[20,55] The bladder may not be properly drained due to the placement of the tip of the catheter against the bladder wall,[25] or the patient may simply be unwilling or unable to void due to the unnatural situation.[32]

We have observed more complete emptying of the bladder in patients who have had their bladder filled to a maximum or optimal volume during cystography. Apparently a high tonicity of the bladder wall induced adequate contraction and more complete emptying. A large residual volume in children either at the beginning or at the end of the study does not necessarily mean that the patient has a significant abnormality. Demonstration of an empty bladder on the other hand is useful.[5]

Urine Cultures

We reviewed the results of urine cultures in 113 consecutive children referred for radionuclide cystography. Urinary infection with *Escherichia coli* or *Streptococcus fecalis* was found in 11% of our patients in spite of their allegedly being on continuous antibiotic treatment and carefully followed by their physicians. There was a nearly equal incidence of urinary infection in patients on antibiotic treatment and in those who had undergone surgery. Our experience agrees with that of other workers indicating that reflux and infection are independent of one another.[8,11,13,15,46,47]

Dosimetry

For children undergoing radionuclide cystography who are between 1 and 10 years of age, the absorbed radiation dose estimates for the bladder are 18–27 mrad and for ovaries 1–2 mrad. The testicular dose is less than the dose to the ovaries. The dose to the kidneys is estimated to be 0.02–0.04 mrad/ml of reflux per minute of residence in the collecting system. The estimated dose to the ureter in reflux is 1.3 mrad/min, which is the same as the dose to a sphere of 1 ml filled with Tc-99m at a concentration of 2 mCi/liter.[9,27,43]

Comparing our results with those published by Conway et al.,[5] the dose to the bladder is similar. With regard to the doses to which the gonads of a girl are exposed during conventional voiding cystourethrography, there is approximately 50–200 times less radiation with computerized radionuclide voiding cystography.[12,26]

The residence time for the activity in the bladder was determined from the duration of the study in patients of various age groups. The average bladder capacities were taken from the data of Fig. 5-2. The empty bladder mass was estimated by extrapolation from data in adults using growth curves.[42] The specific activity of the solution of Tc-99m in saline was 2 mCi/liter.

References

1. Apperson JW, Atkins H, Fleming R. The value of the isotope cystogram in determining pressure and volume at which ureteral reflux occurs. J Urol 1963; 89:405–13.
2. Bailey RR. Sterile reflux: is it harmless? In: Hodson J, Kinkaid-Smith P, eds. Reflux nephropathy New York: Masson, 1979.
3. Blaufox MD, Gruskin A, Sandler P, Goldman H. Radionuclide scintigraphy for detection of vesicoureteral reflux in children. J Pediatr 1971; 79:239–46.
4. Conway JJ, Kruglik GD. Effectiveness of direct and indirect radionuclide cystography in detecting vesicoureteral reflux. J Nucl Med 1976; 17:81–83.
5. Conway JJ, King LR, Belman AB, Thorson T. Detection of vesicoureteral reflux with radionuclide cystography. AJR 1972; 115:720–7.
6. Conway JJ, Belman AB, King LR. Direct and indirect radionuclide cystography. Semin Nucl Med 1974; 4:197–211.
7. Conway JJ, Belman AB, King LR, Filmer RB. Direct and indirect radionuclide cystography. J Urol 1975; 113:689–93.
8. Cremin BJ. Observations on vesico-ureteric reflux and intrarenal reflux: a review and survey of material. Clin Radiol 1979; 30:607–21.
9. Dilman LD, Van der Lage FC. Radionuclide decay schemes and nuclear parameters for use in radiation dose estimation. In: MIRD pamphlet no. 10. New York: Society of Nuclear Medicine, September 1975.
10. Dodge EA. Vesico-ureteric reflux, diagnosis with iodine-131 sodium ortho-iodohippurate. Lancet 1963; 303–4.
11. Faure C. Le reflux vesico-ureteral. In: Lefebvre J, ed. Traite de radiodiagnostic, XVIII. Paris: Masson et Cie, Paris, 1973.
12. Fendel H. Radiation exposure due to urinary tract disease. In: Progress in pediatric radiology, Vol. 3: Genitourinary tract. Basel: Karger 1970.
13. Friedland GW. Recurrent urinary tract infections in infants and children. Radiol Clin North Am 1977; 15:19–35.
14. Gierup P. Micturition studies in infants and children. Scand J Urol Nephrol 1970; 4:191–207.
15. Gross GW, Lebowitz RL. Infection does not cause reflux. AJR 1981; 137:929–32.
16. Handmaker H, McRae J, Buck EG. Intravenous radionuclide voiding cystography (IRVC). Radiology 1973; 108:703–5.
17. Hass EA, Solomon DJ. Telling children about diagnostic radiology procedures. Radiology 1977; 124:521.
18. Hodson CJ, Edwards D. Chronic pyelonephritis and vesicoureteric reflux. Clin Radiol 1960; 11:219–31.
19. Hutch JA. Theory of maturation of the intravesical ureter. J Urol 1961; 86:534–8.
20. Hutch JA. Aberrant micturition. J Urol 1966; 96:743–5.
21. Jerkins GR, Noe HN. Familial vesicoureteral reflux: a prospective study. J Urol 1982; 128:774–8.
22. King LR. Vesicoureteral reflux: history, etiology, and conservative management. In: Kelalis PD, King LR, Belman AB, eds. Clinical pediatric urology. Philadelphia: WB Saunders, 1976.
23. Lattimer JK, Apperson JW, Gleason DM, Baker D, Fleming SS. The pressure at which reflux occurs, an important indicator of prognosis and treatment. J Urol 1963; 89:395–404.
24. Lebowitz RL. Voiding cystourethrography in children. Contemp Diagn Radiol 1978; 5:1–6.
25. Lebowitz RL, Avni FE. Misleading appearances in pediatric uroradiology. Pediatr Radiol 1980; 10:15–31.
26. Leibovic SJ, Lebowitz RL. Reducing patient dose in voiding cystourethrography. Urol Radiol 1980; 2:103–7.
27. Loevinger R, Berman M. A revised schema for calculating the absorbed dose from biologically distributed radionuclides. In: MIRD pamphlet no. 1 (revised). New York: Society of Nuclear Medicine, January 1975.
28. Lyon RP, Marshall S, Tanagho EA. Theory of maturation: a critique. J Urol 1970; 103:795–800.
29. Nasrallah PF, Conway JJ, King LR, Belman AB, Weiss S. Quantitative nuclear cystogram. Urology 1978; 12:654–8.
30. Normand ICS, Smellie J. Vesicoureteric reflux: the case for conservative management. In: Hodson J, Kincaid-Smith P, eds. Reflux nephropathy. New York: Masson 1979.
31. Orr WA, Kimbrough H, Gillenwater JY. Alterations in renal blood flow with voiding in the presence of vesicoureteral reflux. J Urol 1971; 106:214–9.
32. Poznanski E, Poznanski A. Psychogenic influences

on voiding: observations from voiding cystourethrography. Psychosomatics 1969; 10:339–42.
33. Ransley PG. Vesicoureteral reflux: continuing surgical dilemma. Urology 1978; 12:246.
34. Ransley PG. Vesicoureteric reflux. In: Williams DI, Johnston JH, eds. Pediatric urology, 2nd ed. London: Butterworth Medical, 1982.
35. Report of the International Reflux Study Committee. Medical versus surgical treatment of primary vesicoureteral reflux. Pediatrics 1981; 67:392–400.
36. Rolleston GL, Shannon FT, Utley WLF. Relationship of infantile vesicoureteral reflux to renal damage. Br Med J 1970; 70:460–3.
37. Rolleston GL, Maling TMJ, Hodson CJ. Intrarenal reflux and the scarred kidney. Arch Dis Child 1974; 49:531–9.
38. Rolleston GL, Shannon FT, Utley WLF. Follow-up of vesicoureteric reflux in the newborn. Kidney Int 1975; 8:S59–S64.
39. Rosenthall L. Residual urine determination by roentgenographic and isotope means. Radiology 1963; 80:454–9.
40. Smellie J, Edwards D, Hunter N, Normand ICS, Prescod N. Vesicoureteral reflux and renal scarring. Kidney Int 1975; 8:S65–S72.
41. Smith JC. Urethral resistance to micturition. Br J Urol 1968; 40:125–55.
42. Snyder WS, Cook MJ, Nasset ES. Report of the task group on reference man. Oxford: Pergammon Press, by The International Commission on Radiological Protection, 1975.
43. Snyder WS, Ford MR, Warner GG. Estimates of specific absorbed fractions for photon sources uniformly distributed in various organs of heterogenous phantom. In: MIRD pamphlet no. 5 (revised). New York: Society of Nuclear Medicine, January 1978.
44. Spencer RP, Treves S. Bladder emptying flow rates as a function of bladder volume. Yale J Biol Med 1971; 44:199–205.
45. Starfield B. Functional bladder capacity in enuretic and nonenuretic children. J Pediatr 1974; 111:167–72.
46. Stephens FD. Urologic aspects of recurrent urinary tract infections in children. J Pediatr 1972; 80:725–37.
47. Stephens FD, Lenaghan D. The anatomical basis and dynamics of vesicoureteral reflux. J Urol 1962; 87:669–80.
48. Strauss BS, Blaufox MD. Estimation of residual urine and urine flow rates without urethral catheterization. J Nucl Med 1970; 11:81–84.
49. Tanagho EA, Meyers FH, Smith DR. Urethral resistance: its components and implications. I. Smooth muscle component. Invest Urol 1969; 7:136–49.
50. Tanagho EA, Meyers FH, Smith DR. Urethral resistance: its components and implications. II. Striated muscle component. Invest Urol 1969; 7:195–205.
51. Timmermans L, Merchie G. Les radionuclides dans le diagnostic de maladies des reins et des voies urinaires: E reflux vesicoureterorenaux. Acta Urol Belg 1967; 35:254–9.
52. Timmermans L, Merchie G. Une nouvelle methode d'exploration des reflux vesico-uretero-renaux. Acta Urol Belg 1969; 37:105–10.
53. Timmermans L, Collard M, Merchie G. Le diagnostic des reflux vesicoureteraux par la cystometrie associee au radio-cinema et aux radioisotopes. Acta Clin Belg 1964; 19:23–37.
54. Whitaker J, Johnston GS. Urinary flow rate with two techniques of bladder pressure measurement. Invest Urol 1966; 4:235–8.
55. Willi UV, Lebowitz RL. The so-called megaureter-megacystis syndrome. AJR 1979; 133:409–16.
56. Winter CC. A new test for vesicoureteral reflux: an external technique using radioisotopes. J Urol 1959; 81:105–111.
57. Winter CC. Pediatric urological tests using radioisotopes. J Urol 1966; 95:584–7.

Chapter 6 Scrotal Scintigraphy

George Taylor
S. T. Treves

General Considerations

The use of scrotal scintigraphy has dramatically improved our ability to evaluate children with acute testicular pain. Before the introduction of this technique in 1973 by Nadel et al.,[25] the differentiation between testicular torsion and epididymitis was frequently impossible on purely clinical grounds.[17] It often required scrotal exploration for definitive diagnosis.

Although surgical exploration is a relatively benign and very reliable method of diagnosis, scrotal scintigraphy offers a noninvasive and highly reliable means of differentiating inflammatory processes that do not require surgery, from surgical ischemic conditions of the scrotum. Scintigraphy of the scrotum, however, has not been as reliable in the differential diagnosis of pathologic conditions such as tumors, abscess, hydrocele, and missed torsion.

Normal Anatomy

The testes descend to their usual position in the scrotum during the seventh month of fetal life. As they descend, they become invested by the peritoneal and muscular layers of the abdominal wall which elongate and become the scrotal coverings. The processus vaginalis, which is an extension of the peritoneal cavity, is obliterated above the testis. The scrotal portion remains as a peritoneum-lined cavity, the tunica vaginalis, around the anterior surface of the testis. Posteriorly, the testis and epididymis are attached directly to the scrotal wall.[14,15]

The major blood supply to the testis and epididymis is provided by the testicular artery, a branch of the aorta. It passes through the inguinal canal and accompanies the remaining components of the spermatic cord to the mediastinum testis. The scrotum and the vas deferens are fed by branches of the pudendal and inferior epigastric arteries which anastomose with the testicular artery within the scrotum.[14]

Testicular Torsion

Torsion of the spermatic cord has been recognized as a clinical entity since its first description by Delasieuve in 1840.[6] The condition is caused by a sudden twisting of the spermatic cord, which constricts the blood vessels of the cord causing acute vascular compromise and ischemia of the testicle. The twisting initially occludes the veins but not the arteries, which causes edema of the testis and cord up to the point of occlusion. If occlusion is allowed to persist, it will lead to hemorrhagic infarction of the testis. The age range of patients with testicular torsion is extremely broad. Skoglund et al.[28] in a review of the literature were able to find patients ranging from the newborn to 78 years of age. Most cases, however, occur between the ages of 12 and 18 years, coinciding with the rapid growth of genitalia.[13] The incidence of torsion in published series ranges from 21 to 33%.[7,23,28] Presenting symptoms are varied. Typically, affected children have a sudden onset of scrotal pain, nausea, and vomiting. Occasionally, these attacks are intermittent. Examination usually reveals a swollen, tender, and elevated testis, with a variable degree of scrotal edema and discoloration. Secondary hydrocele may develop rapidly, making palpation of the scrotum more difficult. Pain and discomfort are characteristically absent in neonates, who often present with a smooth, firm, painless mass in a discolored scrotum.[3,26,32]

An anatomic anomaly is found in the majority of cases that predisposes the testis to intravaginal torsion. In the normal situation, the tunica vaginalis covers only the testis and anterolateral aspect of the epididymis. This allows the posterior aspect of the epididymis to attach to the posterior scrotal wall. In an abnormal situation, the tunic vaginalis completely surrounds both the testis and the epididymis such that there are no scrotal attachments. The tunica vaginalis may also cover a portion of the distal spermatic cord so that the testis, epididymis, and cord form a long, freely moveable pedicle likened to a "bell-clapper." Less common anatomic variations associated with torsion include various degrees of separation of the testis and epididymis with an elongated mesorchium (defined as that portion of the tunica vaginalis reflected from the fixed posterior surface of the testis) as well as a spiral insertion of the cremasteric muscle fibers extending down the spermatic cord.[19,24,26,28,30] The anatomic anomaly is almost invariably bilateral. Although trauma or rapid movement may be the precipitating event, the mechanism for the initiation of a torsion remains unclear. Extravaginal torsion (torsion of the entire spermatic cord and scrotal contents at the external inguinal ring) is found only in newborns. It is thought to be related to a lack of fixation of the testis and its membranes through the scrotum. Often this torsion has occurred in utero.[39]

The importance of prompt diagnosis and subsequent surgical intervention is shown by the salvage rate of up to 80% in patients operated upon within 5 h and only 20% in those operated upon having symptoms for more than 10 h.[28,39] Preservation of hormonal and spermatogenic function, however, is usually possible only within 6–10 h after the onset of ischemia.[5,26,29,33,40] If testicular ischemia is allowed to continue, the symptoms gradually resolve, leaving only a hard shrunken testicular remnant.

Epididymitis

Epididymitis in children is most commonly encountered during adolescence. The etiology may be gonorrheal, tuberculous, or related to reflux of urine, infected or sterile, into the ejaculatory duct.[24] Associated underlying urologic problems are seen in infancy but are rare in older boys. Urethroejaculatory duct reflux does not occur normally. In children it is seen in mainly in those who have had instrumentation, chronic infection, or urinary outlet obstruction.[2,8,18,38] Example of these situations include posterior urethral valves, uretheral strictures, duplicated urethral stenosis, neurogenic bladder, and imperforate anus. Epididymitis has also been seen in association with Henoch-Schonlein purpura. Biopsy in some of these patients has shown necrosis of the vascular walls with sparing of the ductular epithelium.[16] Typically, children present with a swollen, tender epididymis and/or testis, with the epididymis in its normal posterior location. A history of fever and evidence of urinary tract infection on urinalysis frequently accompany this diagnosis. Treatment includes appropriate antibiotics as well as rest, scrotal support, and observation for abscess formation. The prognosis in boys appears to be more favorable than in adults in whom subsequent testicular atrophy is more common.[12,13,20]

Appendix Testis Torsion

The appendix testis is a vestigial remnant of the Müllerian duct, attached to the upper pole of the testis by a small stalk. Torsion occurs most often in preadolescent boys and is usually a self-limited process with little morbidity except for pain. Symptoms tend to be less severe than those with torsion of the spermatic cord. Patients may present with a palpable tender nodule along the upper pole of the testis, and if infarction has occurred, the overlying skin may be discolored (blue dot).

Miscellaneous Conditions

Other entities that occasionally enter into the differential diagnosis of a painful or enlarged scrotum include trauma, testicular tumors, secondary involvement in patients with leukemia or lymphoma, and hydrocele.

Method

Radiopharmaceutical

An intranvenous bolus injection of 200 μCi/kg of Tc-99m sodium pertechnetate (with a minimum dose of 2 mCi) is used for this examination.

Technique of Examination

A dose of 6 mg/kg of potassium perchlorate is given orally prior to the examination in order to block the uptake of pertechnetate by the thyroid gland. The patient is placed in a supine position. The penis is taped away from the scrotal region, usually over the symphysis pubis. In older children, the scrotum may be supported by tape across the thighs or a towel wedged between the thighs. Veins of the upper extremities are preferred for injection. Use of lower extremity veins is discouraged since this route may lead to asymmetric activity in the region of the groin, making it more difficult to assess subtle changes in blood flow.

Scrotal scintigraphy consists of two phases: radionuclide angiography (flow phase) and static scrotal scintigraphy (tissue phase). We obtain the radionuclide angiogram without lead shielding over the thighs in order to preserve anatomic orientation. Images are recorded at a rate of 1 frame/3 sec for 60 sec using a low-energy, converging collimator. Subsequent static images of 300,000 counts are obtained 3–5 min after injection with lead shielding placed underneath the scrotum in order to reduce background activity from the thighs. One of these images is recorded with a cobalt line source delineating the (median) raphe of the scrotum. We use a converging collimator in most cases. Infants and small children are imaged using a pinhole collimator for improved spatial resolution. Images of 150,000 counts are obtained. Although there are many acceptable variations of this technique, we have found the above routine to provide excellent imaging results in children of all ages.

The importance of correlation between the radionuclide examination and clinical history as well as physical examination cannot be overemphasized. Questioning the patient (or parents) and examination of the scrotum should be considered mandatory parts of the study. The above, together with clinical experience and attention to detail, contribute greatly to the accuracy of interpretation.

Clinical Applications

Normal Scintigraphic Appearance

Blood flow to the scrotum and its contents is relatively small such that in the normal patient only an ill-defined area of activity is appreciated over the testes on radionuclide angiography. The most intense activity in the regions represents iliac and femoral activity in the pelvis and thighs (Fig. 6-1a).[19,30] During the static or tissue phase, the testes appear as intense as the tissues in the adjacent thighs when no lead shielding is used. Without shielding, since radioactivity is cumulative, the testes and cord structures may appear slightly more intense than the surrounding thighs (Fig. 6-1b). In normal patients under 5 years of age the radioactivity in cord structures is similar to that of the thighs.[32]

Scintigraphic patterns seen in various scrotal conditions are listed in Table 6-1.

Testicular Torsion

In acute torsion (less than 24 h duration) decreased perfusion to the affected side results in decreased uptake of traces in the entire hemiscrotum when compared with the opposite normal side. Perfusion (and hence activity) is not typically increased on the twisted side in acute torsion. The static images reveal a central "cold" area in the area of the testicle, sometimes with a surrounding rim of normal or slightly increased activity (Fig. 6-2).[11,17,19] The age of the torsion affects the scan appearance. Torsion present longer than 24 h (missed torsion) usually has normal or slightly decreased radionuclide angiogram activity to the affected side and a variable peripheral rim or halo of hyperemia surrounding the testicle (Fig. 6-3). The increased peritesticular activity is thought to be secondary to a reactive hyperemic response in scrotal tissues to an ischemic testis. Blood flow in this situation is probably provided by branches of the pudendal artery supplying the scrotum. Although the involved testis may not be salvageable, it is important to recognize missed torsion on scintigraphy, since it identifies

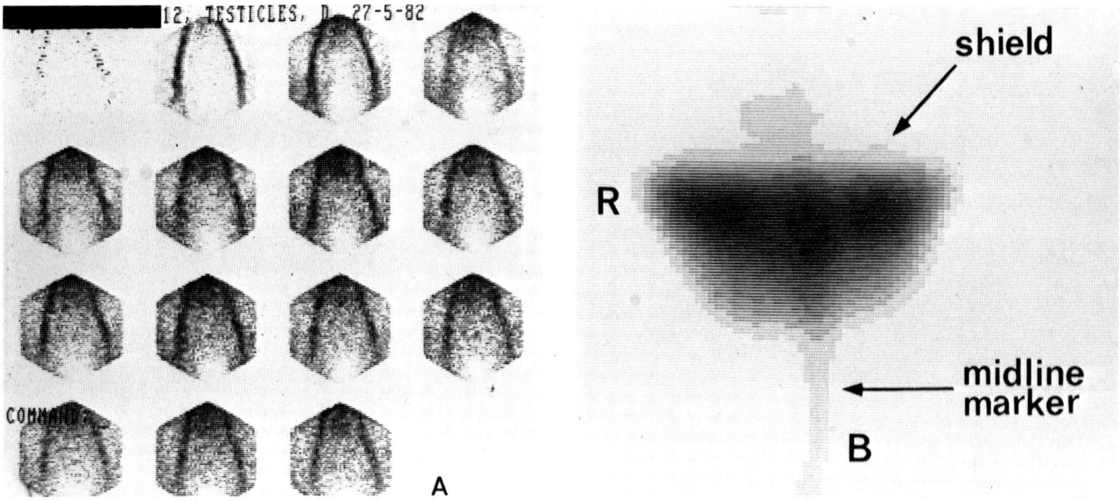

Figure 6-1. Normal scintigram. Twelve-year-old male with 15 h of left testicular pain. History of similar episodes in the past. **A:** Radionuclide angiogram (flow phase). There is symmetrical flow demonstrated in both iliac vessels. Note the apparent lack of activity in the region of the scrotum. **B:** Static image (tissue phase) 5 min following injection. There is symmetric and homogeneous uptake of the tracer in each hemiscrotum.

who should have a prophylactic contralateral orchiopexy.[9,19]

The current literature suggests that testicular scanning is a highly reliable technique in differentiating acute testicular torsion from epididymoorchitis if the examination is performed within 24 h of the onset of symptoms.[1,21,27,31,34,37] The technique is not as reliable if pain and swelling have been present for longer than 48 h. The "rim sign" of peripheral hyperemia is nonspecific and may be seen with several other conditions such as tumor, trauma, hematoma, hydrocele, or varicocele (Fig. 6-4).[4,22,35]

In our experience with 75 patients with sus-

Table 6-1. Scintigraphic Appearance

Condition	Flow Phase (Angiogram)	Static Image
Acute torsion (< 24 h)	Decreased or normal	Central cold area
Missed torsion (< 24 h)	Variable: normal or decreased	Central cold area, peripheral rim of hyperemia
Epididymoorchitis	Increased	Hot area
Abscess	Increased	Central "cool" area or cold area with intense peripheral hyperemia
Hydrocele	Normal	Peripheral crescentic cool area
Tumor	Normal or increased	Variable: irregular or homogeneous increased uptake central cold area peripheral hyperemia
Torsion appendix testis	Normal or increased	Normal

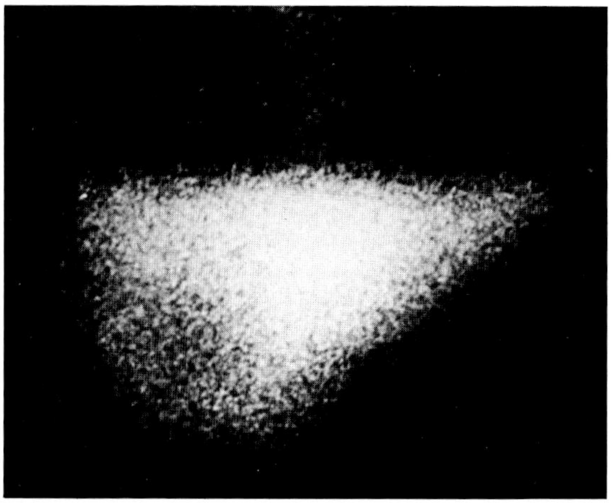

Figure 6-2. Acute testicular torsion. Eleven-year-old with sudden onset of right testicular pain lasting 6 h. Static images show replacement of the right testis by a rounded "cold" area. The flow phase showed vascular activity indistinguishable from normal (not shown).

pected testicular torsion who had scintiscan and adequate clinical followup, the scintiscan diagnosed 12/13 cases of (on surgical exploration) missed torsion and 3/3 cases of acute complete torsion. The scans successfully distinguished all 35 cases of epididymoorchitis, 14 cases of torsion of the appendix testis, and 8 other miscellaneous conditions from testicular torsion.

Epididymoorchitis

Conditions associated with inflammation of the scrotum or any of its contents are usually depicted as areas of increased blood flow on radionuclide angiography proportional to the extent and degree of involvement. Occasionally, the hyperemic flow is sufficient to delineate the territory of pudendal or inferior epigastric arteries on the affected side. On static scans, the inflammed scrotum appears as an intense area of increased radiotracer uptake (Fig. 6-4). If the infection is complicated by abscess formation, the scan may have an appearance similar to that of missed torsion and differentiation between these two entities may be impossible. The scrotum exhibits increased tracer uptake but may have focal areas that are "cool" representing the nonperfused abscess.[10,19,36] These abnormally perfused areas are often eccentrically located in the scrotum, not as rounded as the expected shape of the testicle, and not completely surrounded by a rim of hyperemia. In either case, the treatment involves surgical exploration of the scrotum.

Torsion of the Appendix Testis

Infarction of the appendix testis is undetectable scintigraphically because of its size. When inflammation occurs, increased uptake may be seen that is indistinguishable from epididymoorchitis (Fig. 6-5). Precise differentiation is clinically unimportant

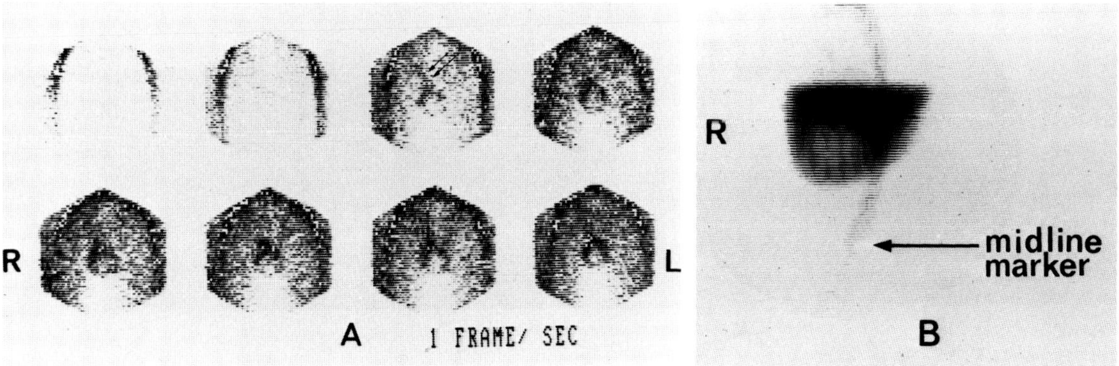

Figure 6-3. Missed testicular torsion. Thirteen-year-old with 5 days of right scrotal pain and swelling. **A:** Angiogram (flow phase). Increased radioactivity is seen in the territory of the right pudendal artery *(arrow)*. A peripheral rim of hyperemia surrounds the testicle. **B:** Static phase. Diffuse hyperemia of the scrotum is seen surrounding a rounded "cold" area representing the ischemic rich testis.

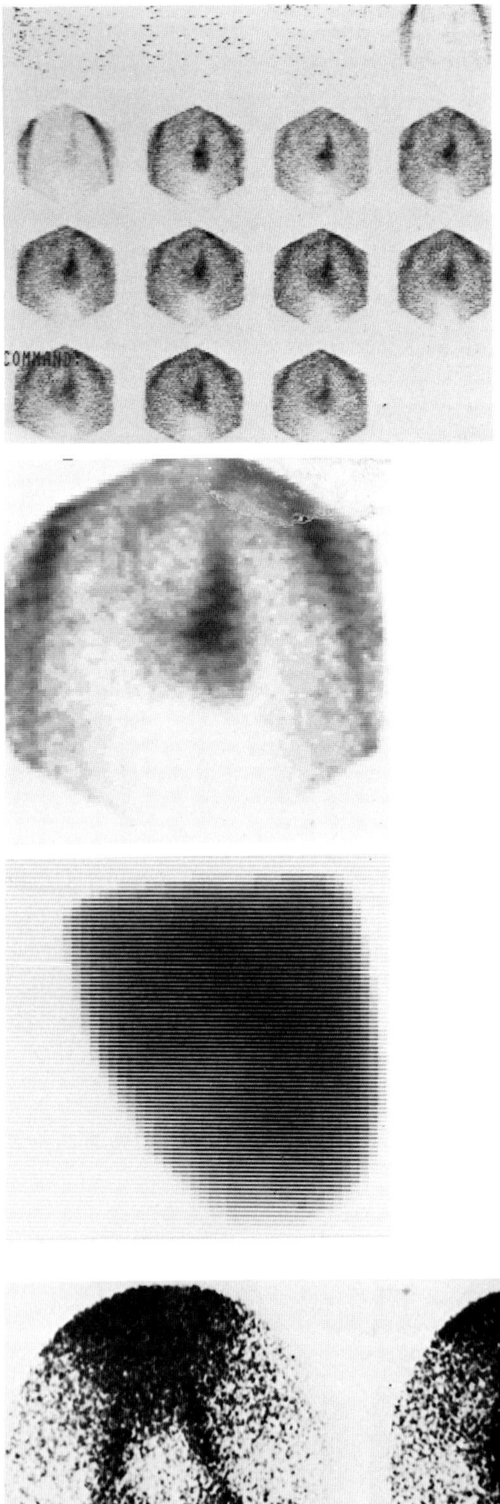

since both diseases usually respond to nonoperative management. Of greater importance is the ability of scintiscans to distinguish torsion of the appendix testis from testicular torsion, frequently a difficult clinical judgment.[1,19,32]

Miscellaneous Conditions

Hydrocele

Typically, the radionuclide angiogram is normal and the static images show a lucency, often crescentic in shape, surrounding a normal testicle (Fig. 6-6).[1,19,34] If the hydrocele is large, the lucency may encompass most of the hemiscrotum and superficially mimic torsion.

Testicular Tumors

Primary malignancies of the testes are usually encountered in male teenagers and young men. Scintigraphic patterns seen with these neoplasms are very nonspecific. They may be confused with inflammation or torsion, depending on the degree of inflammatory response generated by the tumor and areas of necrosis within the mass.[4,35]

◁ **Figure 6-4.** Epididymoorchitis. Eighteen-year-old kicked in left scrotum 2 weeks previously. Increasing pain and swelling occurred over the last 24 h. *Top:* Radionuclide angiogram shows markedly increased flow to the left scrotum. *Center:* Composite image of the radionuclide angiogram. *Bottom:* Static image. Diffuse tissue hyperemia is present on the affected side.

▽ **Figure 6-5.** Torsion of the appendix testis. Five-year-old with sudden right scrotal pain lasting 12 h. Radionuclide angiogram shows minimally increased flow to the right scrotum. The static tissue phase was normal.

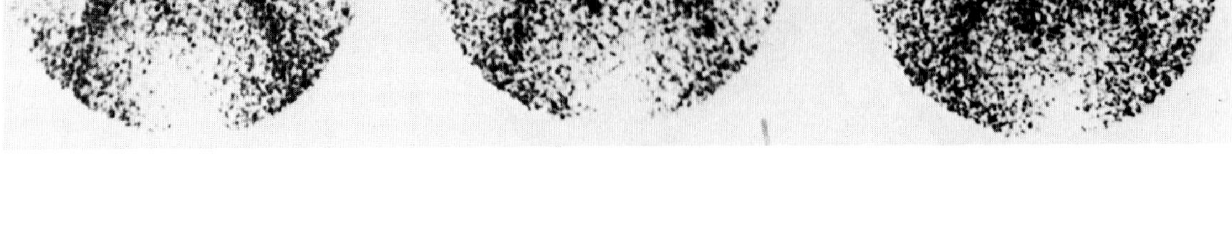

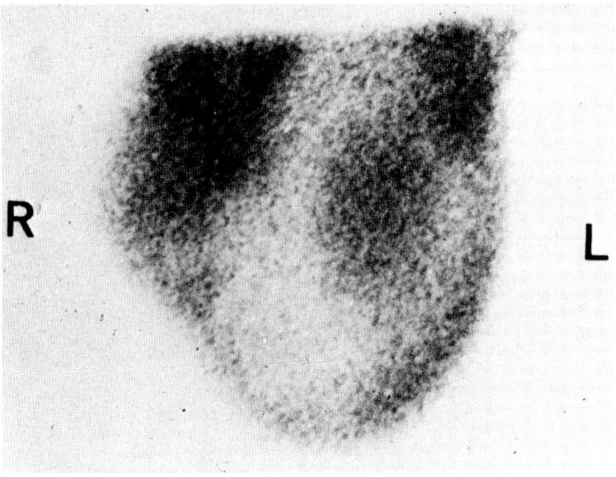

Figure 6-6. Hydrocele. Twelve-year-old with trauma to the scrotum and increasing swelling over a 2-day period. Static image shows a lucency surrounding a normal left testis that encompasses the entire hemiscrotum.

References

1. Abu-Sleiman R, Ho JE, Gregory JG. Scrotal scanning. Present value and limits of interpretation. Urology 1973; 13:326–30.
2. Amar AD, Kamla C. Epididymitis in prepubertal boys. Presenting manifestation of vesicoureteral reflux. JAMA 1969; 207:2397–400.
3. Behrman RE, Vaughan VC, eds. In: Nelson textbook of pediatrics, 12th ed. Philadelphia: WB Saunders, 1983.
4. Boedecker RA, Glicklich M, Sty JR. Rim sign in endodermal sinus tumor. Clin Nucl Med 1979; 4:130–1.
5. Boedecker RA, Sty JR, Jona FJ. Testicular scanning as a diagnostic aid in evaluating scrotal pain. J Pediatr 1979; 94:760–2.
6. Delasieuve L. Descente tardive dutesticle gauche, prise pour une hernie etranglee. Rev Med Fra Etrang 1840; 1:363.
7. DelVillar RG, Ireland GW, Cass A. Early exploration in acute testicular conditions. J Urol 1972; 108:887–8.
8. Doolittle KH, Smith JP, Saylor ML. Epididymitis in the prepubertal boy. J Urol 1966; 96:364–6.
9. Dunn EKI, Macchia RJ, Solomon NA. Scintigraphic pattern in missed testicular torsion. Radiology 1981; 139:175–80.
10. Dymus L, Mishkin F. Radionuclide imaging in epididymo-orchitis. J Urol 1974; 112:387–9.
11. Falkowski WS, Firlit CF. Testicular torsion: the role of radiosotope scanning. J Urol 1980; 124:886–8.
12. Gierup J, von Hedenberg C, Osterman A. Acute nonspecific epididymitis in boys. Scand J Urol Nephrol 1975; 9:5–7.
13. Gislason T, Noronha R, Gregory J. Acute epididymitis in boys: a 5-year retrospective study. J Urol 1980; 124:533–4.
14. Gray H. Anatomy of the human body. Goss CM, ed. Philadelphia: Lea & Febiger, 1973.
15. Gray SW, Skandalakis J. The ovary and testis. In: Embryology for surgeons. The embryological basis for the treatment of congenital defects. Philadelphia: WB Saunders, 1972.
16. Haahr J, Sparrevbhn S. Epididymitis in children (abstract). Acta Paediat Scand 1970; 60:248.
17. Hahn LC, Nadel NS, Gitter MH, Vernon AR. Testicular scanning: a new modality for the preoperative diagnosis of testicular torsion. J Urol 1975; 113:60–62.
18. Harrison JH, Nickel WR, Plumb RT, eds. Other infections and inflammations of the external genitalia. In: Cambells Urology, 4th ed. Philadelphia: WB Saunders, 1978.
19. Holder LE, Martire JR, Holmes ER. Testicular radionuclide angiography and static imaging: anatomy, scintigraphic interpretation and clinical indications. Radiology 1977; 125:739–52.
20. Kaplan GW, King LR. Acute scrotal swelling in children. J Urol 1970; 104:219–23.
21. Kogan SJ, Lutfker LG, Perez LA et al. The value of the negative radionuclide scrotal scan in the management of the acute inflamed scrotum in children. J Urol 1979; 122:223–5.
22. Mishkin FS. Differential diagnostic features of the radionuclide scrotal image. Am J Roentgen 1977; 128:127–9.
23. Moharib NH, Krahn HP. Acute scrotum in children with emphasis on torsion of the spermatic cord. J Urol 1970; 104:601–3.
24. Muschat M. The pathological anatomy of testicular torsion. Surg Gynecol Obstet 1932; 54:758–63.
25. Nadel NS, Gitter MH, Hahn LC et al. Preoperative diagnosis of testicular torsion. Urology 1973; 1:478–9.
26. Parker RM, Robison JR. Anatomy and diagnosis of torsion of the testicle. J Urol 1971; 106:243–7.
27. Riley TW, Mosbaugh PG, Coles JL, Newman DM, Van Hove ED, Heck LL. Use of radioisotope scan in evaluation of intrascrotal lesions. J Urol 1976; 116:472–5.
28. Skoglund RW, McRoberts JW, Ragde H. Torsion of testicular appendages: presentation of 43 new cases and a collective review. J Urol 1970; 104:598–600.
29. Smith GI. Cellular changes from graded testicular ischemia. J Urol 1955; 73:355–62.
30. Smith SP, King LR. Torsion of the testis. Techniques of assessment. Urol Clin North Am 1979; 6:429–43.

31. Stage KH, Schoenvogel R, Lewis S. Testicular scanning: clinical experience with 72 patients. J Urol 1981; 125:334–7.
32. Sty JR, Starshak RJ, Miller JH, eds. In: Pediatric nuclear medicine. Norwich: Appleton-Century-Crofts, 1983.
33. Thomas WE, Williamson RC. Diagnosis and outcome of testicular torsion. Br J Surg 1983; 70:213–6.
34. Valvo JR, Caldamone AA, O'Mara R, Rabinowitz R. Nuclear imaging in the pediatric acute scrotum. Am J Dis Child 1982; 136:831–5.
35. Vieras F, Kuhn CR. Nonspecificity of the "rim sign" in the scintigraphic diagnosis of missed testicular torsion. Radiology 1983; 146:519–22.
36. Vordermark JS, Buck AS, Brown SR, Tuttle WK. The testicular scan. Use in diagnosis and management of acute epididymitis. JAMA 1981; 245:2512–4.
37. Wasnick RJ, Pobutsky KR, Macchia RJ. Testicular torsion and usefulness of radionuclide scanning. Urol 1980; 15:318–320.
38. Williams CB, Litvak AS, McRoberts JW. Epididymitis in infancy. J Urol 1979; 121:125–6.
39. Williamson RC. Torsion of the testis and allied conditions. Br J Surg 1976; 63:465–476.
40. Wright JE. Torsion of the testis. Br J Surg 1977; 64:274.

Chapter 7 Liver

S. T. Treves
John A. Markisz

Hepatic scintigraphy in children presents certain special problems because of the types of diseases usually encountered and the wide range of body sizes in the pediatric population. The principles, technique, and interpretation of hepatic scintigraphy using technetium-99m (Tc-99m) sulfur colloid are presented in this chapter. Hepatobiliary scintigraphy and splenic scintigraphy are discussed in other chapters.

Reticuloendothelial scintigraphy with Tc-99m sulfur colloid provides information on the size, location, morphology, structure, and function of the liver and spleen. This simple and relatively noninvasive procedure is suitable for studying a variety of pediatric conditions: masses or lesions displacing or replacing normal hepatic or splenic tissue, infectious processes (focal or diffuse), trauma, congenital malformations, accessory spleens, and diffuse parenchymal disease.[7,19,20,25]

Like other studies in nuclear medicine, hepatic scintigraphy does not generally yield a specific diagnosis, and findings must be carefully interpreted in light of the patient's medical history and physical examination. Currently, evaluation of hepatic lesions may be carried out using one or more of the following methods: scintigraphy, ultrasonography, and computed tomography (CT). In the future, nuclear magnetic resonance (NMR) may also play a role.

Ultrasonography and CT have inherently high spatial resolution but do not provide information on regional hepatic function. Certain lesions, such as metastatic neuroblastoma, have an echodensity similar to that of normal liver substance so that they may not be detectable by ultrasonography (Fig. 7-1).

Hepatic scintigraphy provides views of the entire organ in multiple projections. This overall map of the liver often can aid selection of hepatic regions for evaluation by CT or ultrasonography. These three modalities, although competitive at times, tend to be complementary when a logical approach to diagnosis is used. Changes in the distribution of radiocolloid within the liver, spleen, or bone marrow often give a clue about normal and altered liver function. A limitation of hepatic scintigraphy is its spatial resolution: only lesions of 1.5–2 cm or larger may be detected, depending on their location.

Method

Radiopharmaceuticals

In our institution the usual dose of Tc-99m sulfur colloid is 30 μCi/kg of body weight with a minimum dose of about 300 μCi. Absorbed dose estimates for children are shown in Table 7-1.

After intravenous injection, Tc-99m sulfur colloid is rapidly absorbed by cells of the reticuloendothelial system in the liver, spleen, and bone marrow. The normal circulating half-time of this radiotracer in adults is approximately 2.5 min. The size of colloidal particles is 0.01–1.0 μm. Once absorbed, these particles have an effective half-life equal to the physical half-life of Tc-99m. Approximately 80–90% of the radiocolloid is taken up by the liver, about 5–10% by the spleen, and the remainder by the bone marrow. The principal mechanism of uptake of Tc-99m sulfur colloid is phagocytosis by Kupffer cells.[2]

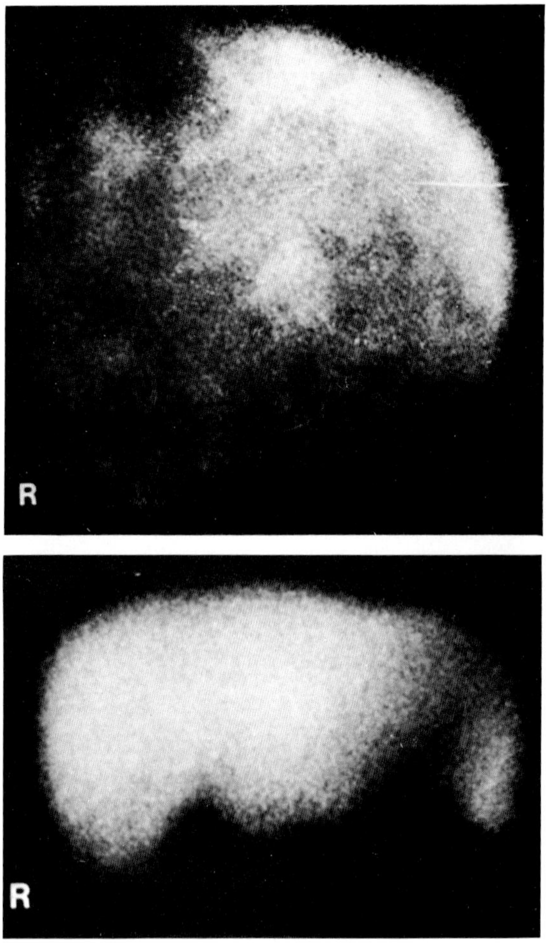

Radiopharmaceuticals that may be used to complement Tc-99m sulfur colloid in evaluation of the liver include gallium-67 citrate or indium-111 white blood cells for the diagnosis of infection, Tc-99m heat-damaged red blood cells for identification of the spleen, and Tc-99m red blood cells or human serum albumin to define intrahepatic or parahepatic lesions with large blood pools.

Imaging Technique

Static imaging of the liver with Tc-99m sulfur colloid is begun about 15 min after intravenous injection. In patients with severe heaptic insufficiency, blood disappearance of the tracer is prolonged and relatively high background will be present at the normal time for imaging. Therefore, waiting a few more minutes before imaging allows for further

◁ **Figure 7-1.** Metastatic neuroblastoma. Tc-99m sulfur colloid hepatic scintigram obtained from a 6-month-old male at presentation showing a massively enlarged liver with multiple intrahepatic defects *(top)*. A scan on the same patient following therapy at 15 months of age shows a marked reduction in the size of the liver and no evidence of intrahepatic defects *(bottom)*. Ultrasonography at presentation did not reveal the focal hepatic lesions, probably because they had echodensity similar to that of the liver. R, right.

Table 7-1. Radiation Dose from Tc-99m Sulfur Colloid for Liver-Spleen Imaging

Age (years)	Newborn	1	5	10	15	Adult
Weight (kg)	3.5	12.1	20.3	33.5	55.0	70.0
Usual administered dose (mCi)	0.3	0.6	1.0	1.7	2.7	5.0
Absorbed dose (rad)						
Total body	0.036	0.057	0.066	0.073	0.059	0.095
Liver	0.960	0.840	0.820	1.139	1.323	1.700
Spleen	0.840	0.720	0.650	0.833	0.891	1.050
Red marrow	0.174	0.108	0.110	0.1377	0.0972	0.135
Ovaries	0.043	0.0384	0.038	0.0272	0.0224	0.0280
Testes	0.012	0.0126	0.019	0.0238	0.0062	0.0055

The biologic data of MIRD Dose Estimate Report No. 3, J Nucl Med 16:1, P 108A–B were used.

The age-dependent *S* values of Henrichs et al. (Heinrichs K, Kaul A, Krause M. Age Dependant Values of Specific Absorbed Dose. Klinikum Steglity Physik unk Strahlenschutz (Biophysiks). Freie Universitat, Berlin, Germany, 1980.), were used, except for the 1-year-old *S* values, which were taken from preliminary phantom work of the Metabolism and Dosimetry Group at ORNL.

Note that administered and absorbed doses are higher in bone marrow images (see dosage and administration).

blood clearance and leads to images with better contrast.

A high-resolution, parallel-multihole collimator is recommended for imaging the liver and spleen. Anterior, posterior, and right lateral views are obtained for 500,000 counts as a minimum routine schedule. Additional views are required in certain instances. For example, after abdominal trauma images are obtained in the right anterior oblique, left anterior oblique, right posterior oblique, left posterior oblique, and left lateral projections. Magnification with a pinhole collimator is used to help detect or improve delineation of small lesions.

It is important to ensure that all photon-absorbing objects are removed from clothing before imaging. Tc-99m sulfur colloid imaging of the liver should not be attempted in the presence of barium within the abdomen because it may cause artifacts on the scintigram. In children who are crying or breathing deeply, the liver will move significantly with each respiratory cycle and degrade the hepatic and splenic images. Although not generally used at present, respiratory gating devices may be useful in these patients in order to obtain images of greater clarity.

Radionuclide angiography with Tc-99m sulfur colloid may be performed prior to static liver scintigraphy in order to determine the vascularity of abdominal masses.[8,26,27] Also, radionuclide venography may be useful to determine the course and patency of the inferior or superior vena cava in abdominal or thoracic masses or in the heterotaxia syndrome (Fig. 7-2).[7]

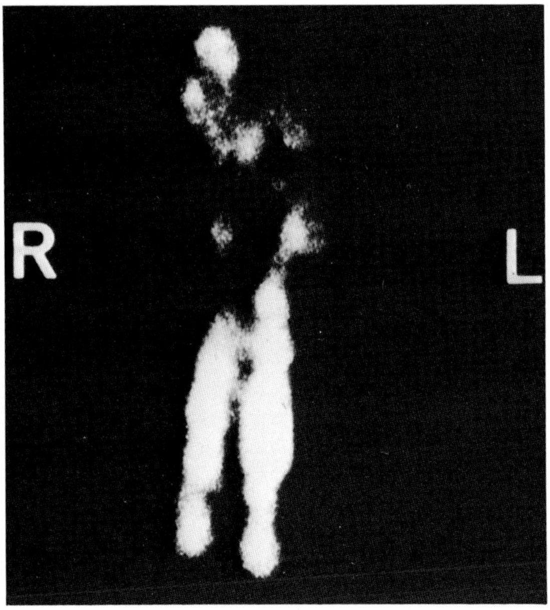

Figure 7.2. Double inferior vena cava. Simultaneous intravenous injection of Tc-99m sulfur colloid in veins of the feet reveal two inferior venae cavae with apparent interruption at the hepatic level and azygos continuation.

Clinical Applications

Liver Size

Comments on the scan size of the liver and spleen must be evaluated with caution because in children these organs grow and change size relatively rapidly. Further, it is difficult to establish precise normal hepatic and splenic sizes in children. In practice, estimates of the size of these organs are made by the physician after physical examination with consideration of the patient's overall size and body proportions and sometimes with the aid of hepatic scintigraphy. Information on hepatic and splenic sizes by scintigraphy must be refined in terms of distribution by sex, weight percentile, age, body surface area, nutritional status, and other factors.

The maximum vertical dimension (*MVD*) in centimeters of the hepatic silhouette on liver scans has been related to age (*A*) in years in 66 children from 0 to 19 years of age by the formula:

$$MVD = 8.8 + 0.46A$$

The correlation coefficient was 0.89. Similarly the maximum splenic dimension (*MSD*) on posterior splenic scintigraphy was related to age (*A*) in 45 children by the formula:

$$MSD = 5.7 + 0.31A$$

The liver/spleen ratio of the lengths was essentially independent of age: 1.55 at birth, 1.52 at 10 years of age, and 1.52 at 18 years of age.[22,24] It may be possible to compare the calculated weights or dimensions of the liver or spleen (from height, weight, body surface area, or other measurements) with that suggested by the scans.[4,18] Markisz and others from our institution found a reasonably good correlation between the maximum vertical dimension on the liver scan and the age and body weight in children with normal liver function. Good correlation was also found between liver volume and patient weight (Fig. 7-3) (Markisz, Treves, et al., unpublished data, 1983).

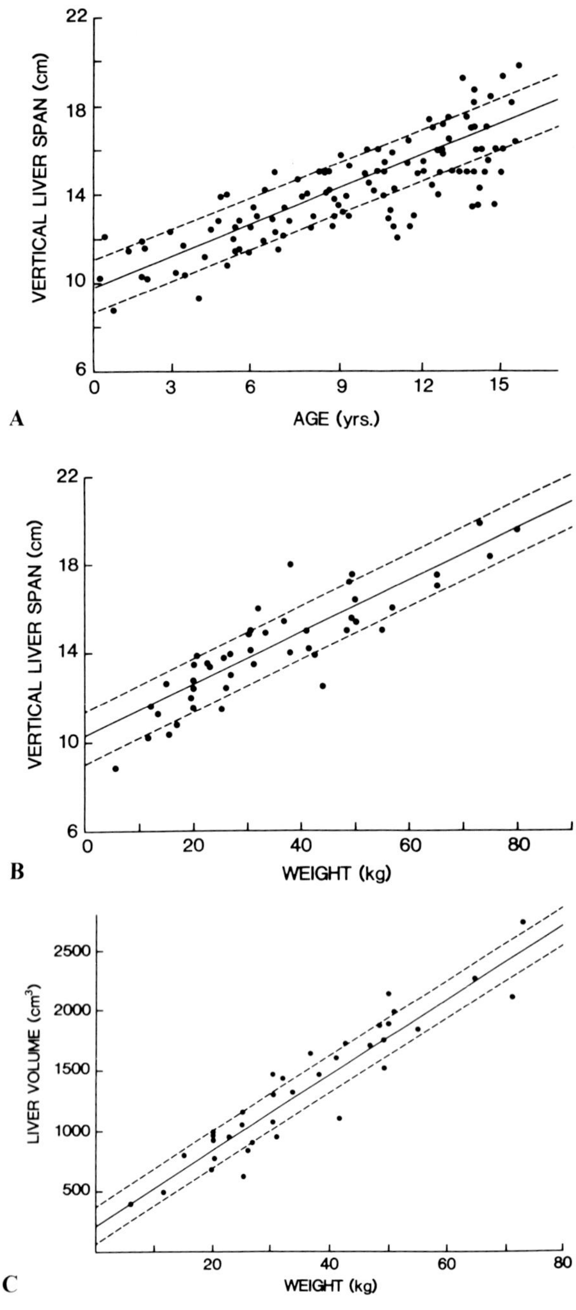

Figure 7-3. Hepatic size in children. **A:** Vertical liver span versus age. **B:** Vertical liver span versus weight. **C:** Liver volume versus weight.

Normal Variants

Recognition of normal variants on liver and spleen scintiscans is difficult at times. Prominent notches or separation of the left and right lobes of the liver or impressions by surrounding organs or the costal margins may produce irregularities in the radiotracer distribution. An accentuated porta hepatis may simulate intrahepatic disease. A kidney situated in a high position can produce impressions on either the liver or the spleen. Gastric dilatation may produce an impression on the splenic silhouette and/or on the left lobe of the liver that may mimic a lesion.[25]

Congenital Abnormalities

Congenital abnormalities such as organ malposition, symmetric liver, asplenia, polysplenia, and accessory spleens can be readily diagnosed by radiocolloid scintigraphy.

The heterotaxia syndrome, which includes complex congenital heart disease, visceral heterotaxia, bronchopulmonary abnormalities, and often asplenia or polysplenia, may be accompanied by abnormalities such as double inferior vena cava or absence of the hepatic portion of the inferior vena cava. The liver may have a symmetric, so-called horizontal appearance or it may be located in the left upper quadrant. This syndrome lends itself to study by a combination of radionuclide venography using Tc-99m sulfur colloid followed by conventional liver/spleen scintigraphy. By injecting this tracer simultaneously into veins of the lower or upper extremities, assessment of the patency or morphologic abnormalities of the venae cavae is possible. Radionuclide venography may serve to establish the patency of the vena cava prior to cardiac catheterization. In this syndrome, the spleen may be normal or abnormal due to asplenia, polysplenia, or malposition.[7]

If there is a difference in the concentration of Tc-99m sulfur colloid in the liver compared with the spleen or if the spleen is clearly distinguishable, radiocolloid imaging may suffice. If the apparent concentrations of the Tc-99m sulfur colloid in the liver and the spleen are similar and/or these organs are not clearly distinguishable from one another, selective splenic imaging using Tc-99m heat-damaged red blood cells may be useful.[5]

Diffuse and Focal Liver Disease

Diffuse liver disease, enlargement of the liver and/or the spleen, as well as the presence of abdominal mass or tumor are probably the most common indications for hepatic scintigraphy. Enlargement of the liver can be due to homogeneous involvement such as in glycogen storage disease (Fig. 7-4),[6] biliary obstruction (Fig. 7-5), congestive heart failur infection, leukemia, Hodgkin's disease or diffuse

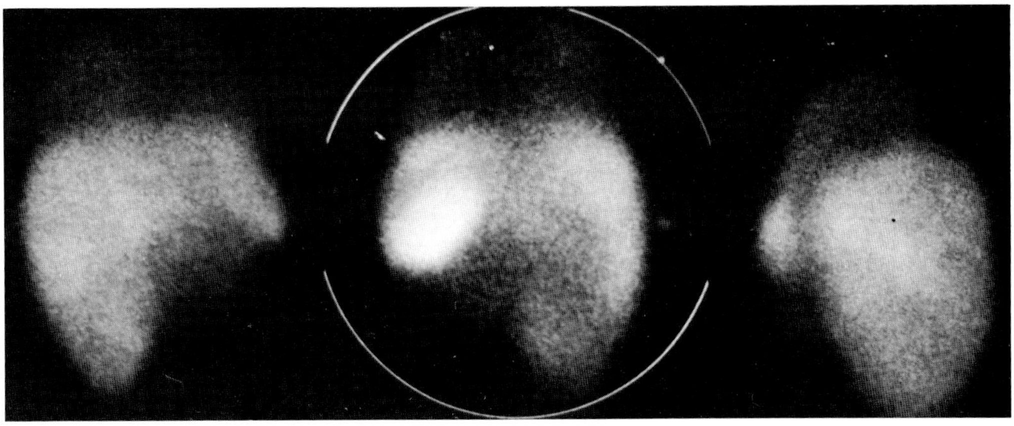

Figure 7-4. Glycogen storage disease. Tc-99m sulfur colloid liver-spleen scan showing massive, diffuse enlargement of the liver. The spleen is of normal size and is displaced inferiorly by the liver. *Left:* anterior view; *center:* posterior view; *right:* right lateral view.

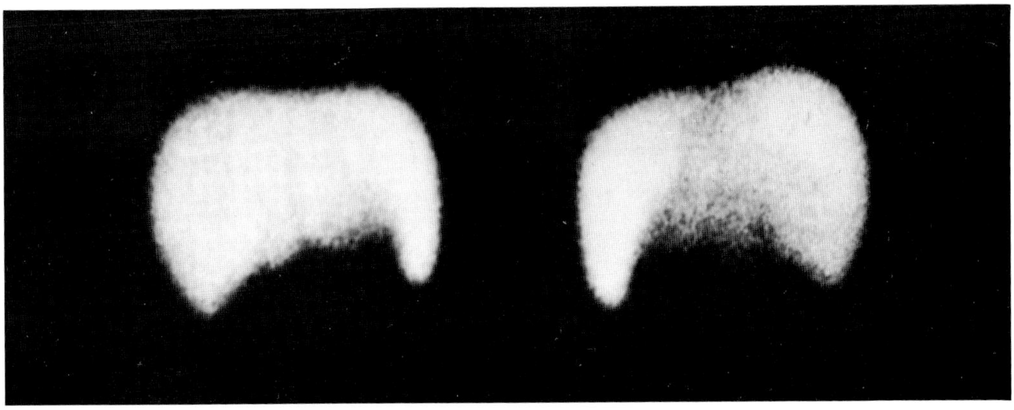

Figure 7-5. Biliary obstruction. Tc-99m sulfur colloid liver-spleen scan in a 2-year-old male with a tumor of the pancreas involving the common bile duct and producing obstructive jaundice. The scan reveals hepatosplenomegaly presumably due to obstruction.

tumor. The usual appearance in glycogen storage disease is a diffuse reduction in the concentration of activity within the liver. Diffuse parenchymal processes, such as cirrhosis (α_1-antitrypsin deficiency, congenital hepatic fibrosis, cyctic fibrosis) may show depending on the stage of the disease the degree of severity, and the increased or decreased size of the liver. Often these patients have increased uptake of radiocolloid in the spleen and vertebral marrow (Figs. 7-6–7-8). In diffuse lung disease (cystic fibrosis, asthma), the hepatic silhouette may be depressed inferiorly by the expanded lungs (Fig. 7-9).

Single or multiple space-occupying lesions of the liver can also occur with or without hepatomegaly, for example, abscess (Fig. 7-10), cyst, tumors (hepatoma, hepatoblastoma, metastatic Wilm's tumor, neuroblastoma, hemangioma, lymphoma), and cirrhosis (primary, cystic fibrosis, α_1-antitrypsin deficiency) (Figs. 7-9 and 7-11–7-17). Liver metastases from lymphoma, leukemia, or neuroblastoma can be diffuse and infiltrative and can cause hepatomegaly without defects. Focal space-occupying lesions will appear on the liver scan as areas of reduced to absent radiocolloid activity. A scintiscan using a Tc-99m-labelled hepatobiliary agent may demonstrate increased uptake in a functional hepatoma. Areas of increased normal or decreased radiocolloid uptake within the liver may be detected in focal nodular hyperplasia.[3,21]

Enlargement, tumors, or abscesses of neighboring structures will produce abnormal scintiscans. For example, a gallbladder cyst, renal mass or enlargement (Fig. 7-18), pancreatic tumors or cysts,

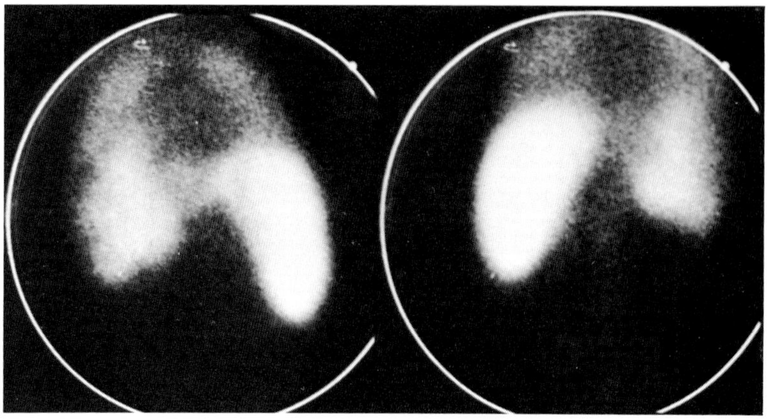

Figure 7-6. α_1-Antitrypsin deficiency. Tc-99m sulfur colloid liver-spleen scan. The hepatic silhouette is small and irregular. The spleen is massively enlarged, and there is a shift of radiocolloid concentration to the spleen, bone marrow, and lungs. *Left:* anterior view; *right:* posterior view.

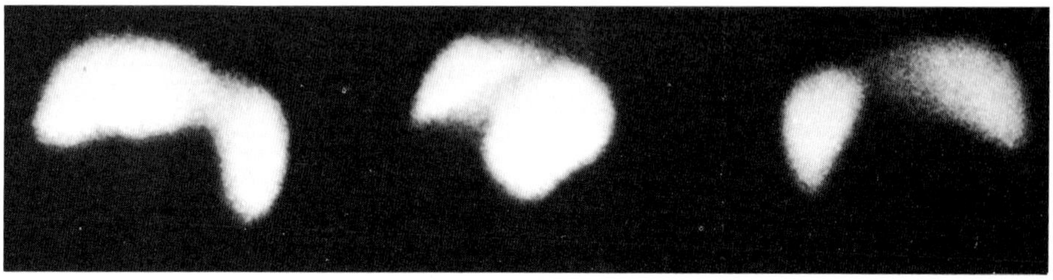

Figure 7-7. Congenital hepatic fibrosis. There is splenomegaly with a relatively small liver. Tc-99m sulfur colloid scan. *Left:* anterior view; *center:* left lateral view; *right:* posterior view.

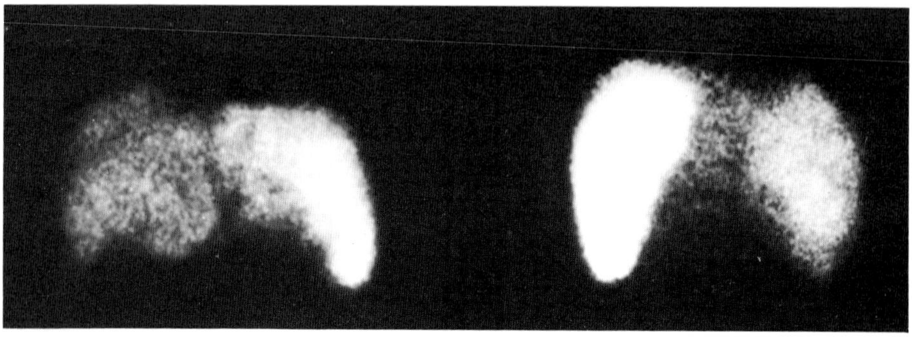

Figure 7-8. Cirrhosis of the liver. Tc-99m sulfur colloid liver-spleen scan on a 19-year-old female with advanced cystic fibrosis and portal hypertension. The liver is small and shows poor and irregular distribution of radiocolloid. The spleen is enlarged. *Left:* anterior view; *right:* posterior view.

gastric or mesenteric tumors or cysts, the diaphragm, the aorta, the paraaortic nodes, as well as pulmonary pathology, may all cause impressions on the hepatic or splenic image that can be indistinguishable from true intrahepatic or intrasplenic disease.[9,19]

The course of hepatic regeneration after partial hepatectomy or radiation therapy can be followed by means of hepatic scintigraphy. Radiotherapy directed to an area of normal hepatic tissue will produce a defect with well-defined margins corresponding to the radiotherapy portal.[1,22,23] Sometimes radiation injury to the liver is reversible and the liver scan returns to normal. In others, fi-

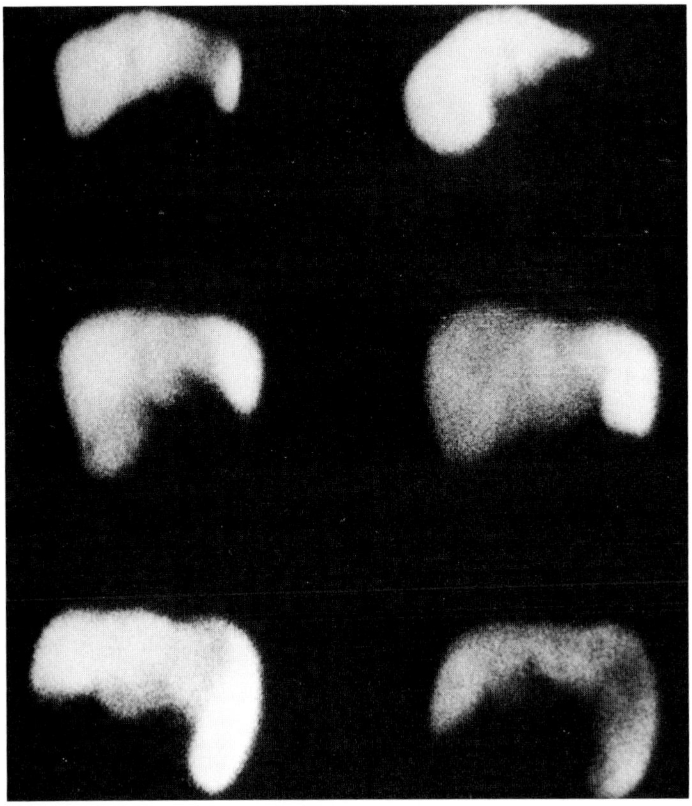

Figure 7-9. Six patients with cystic fibrosis. Tc-99m sulfer colloid liver-spleen scans show a variety of findings including inferior displacement of the liver and the spleen by the expanded lungs.

brosis leads to atrophy of the involved area of the liver (Fig. 7-19). The intact portion of the liver hypertrophies in these patients, and the normal portion of the liver rapidly becomes hyperplastic and assumes a globular shape. Portions of the liver within a radiation therapy portal may not be visible by Tc-99m sulfur colloid scintigraphy, but they may be delineated with Tc-99m-labelled hepatobiliary agents.[11]

The liver usually undergoes rapid regeneration following partial hepatectomy and resumes a normal size and shape.

Focal defects can be seen in intrahepatic gallbladder, choledochal cysts, and Caroli's disease. Hepatobiliary scintigraphy will confirm the biliary nature of these lesions.

Reticuloendothelial scintigraphy can be very helpful in the diagnosis of eventration or herniation of the liver (Fig. 7-20).

Multiple intrahepatic defects can be found in polycystic disease and are associated with renal cysts. Single or multiple focal defects may be seen in patients with hydatid cysts.

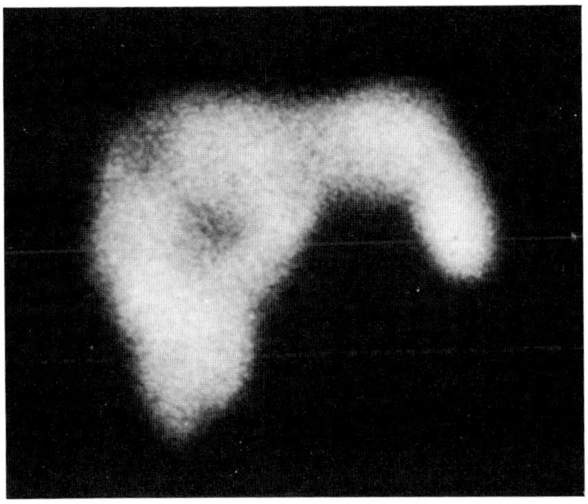

Figure 7-10. Chronic granulomatous disease. Tc-99m sulfur colloid liver-spleen scan with multiple defects corresponding to abscesses.

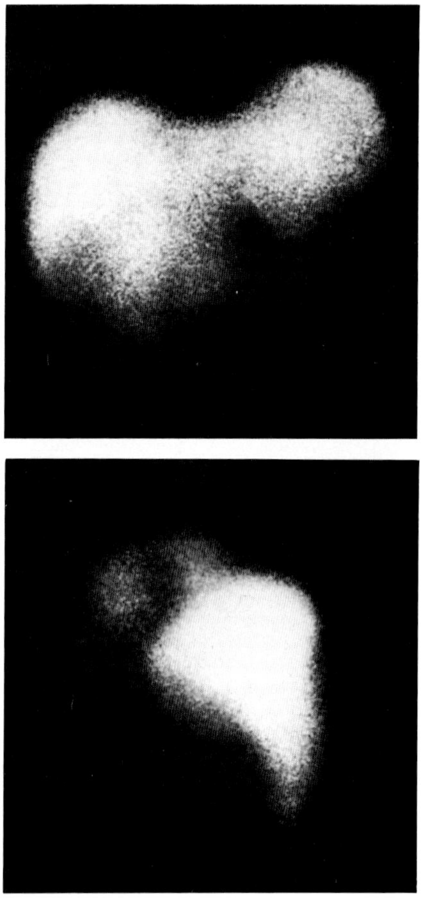

Figure 7-11. Metastatic testicular tumor. Tc-99m sulfur colloid scan showing intrahepatic defects. *Top:* anterior view; *bottom:* right lateral veiw.

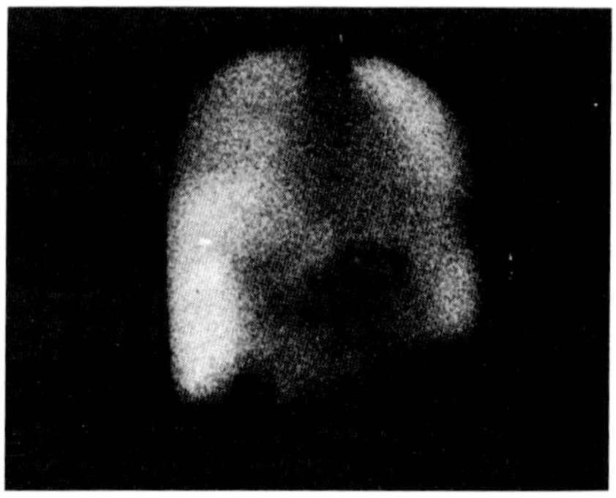

Figure 7-12. Hepatoma. Tc-99m sulfur colloid liver-spleen scan showing a massive intrahepatic defect and increased pulmonary radiocolloid uptake.

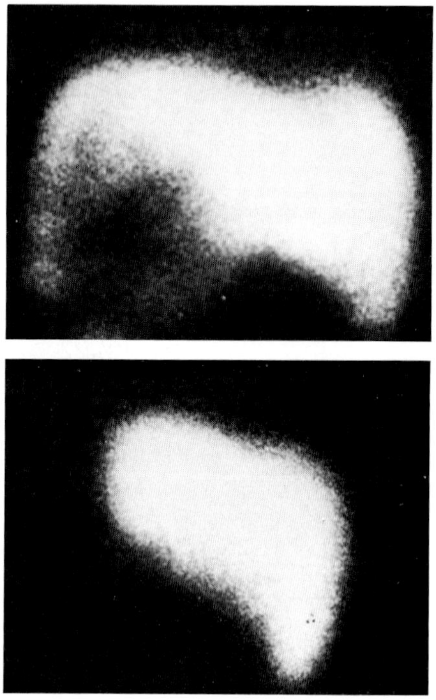

Figure 7-13. Hepatoblastoma. Tc-99m sulfur colloid liver-spleen scans. Scan at presentation *(top)* shows a massive intrahepatic defect occupying most of the left lobe of the liver with enlargement of the left lobe. After surgical excision and local radiotherapy, there has been no regeneration of the right lobe of the liver *(bottom)*.

Primary tumors of the liver may be solitary or multifocal, avascular or hypervascular. Scintigraphy does not permit differentiation of malignant and benign lesions of the liver. Tumors with high blood flow within the liver may show a so-called arterial blush on radionuclide angiography. Conventional hepatic scintigraphy will reveal those tumors as areas of decreased to absent radiotracer uptake (Figs. 7-12 and 7-14).

Liver abscesses are uncommon in children. When they occur, they are usually a complication of an underlying process. For example, abscesses can be seen in chronic granulomatous disease, leukemia, and other diseases. These lesions show no radiocolloid concentration and can be seen on gallium-67 scintigraphy as areas of increased or decreased uptake.

Trauma to the liver can be effectively detected by reticuloendothelial scintigraphy. Multiple projections and awareness of anatomic variants are essential for correct interpretation. Hematoma or rupture of the liver will appear as an area of re-

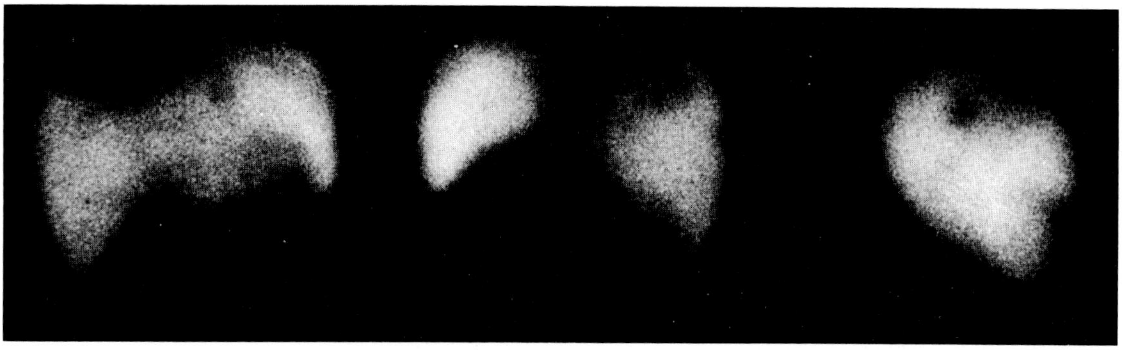

Figure 7-14. Metastatic gastric carcinoma. Tc-99m sulfur colloid liver-spleen scan shows multiple intrahepatic defects. *Left:* anterior view; *center:* posterior view; *right:* right lateral view.

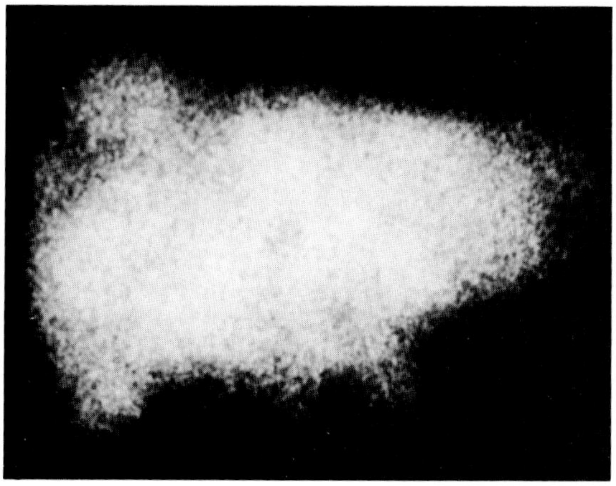

Figure 7-15. Multiple intrahepatic abscesses in a 3-year-old female with leukemia.

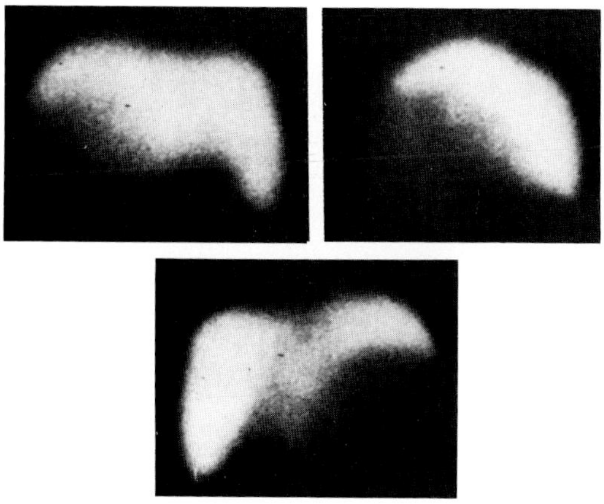

Figure 7-16. Metastatic Wilm's tumor. Tc-99m sulfur colloid liver-spleen scan showing a large defect in the right lobe of the liver. *Top left:* anterior view; *top right:* right lateral view; *bottom:* posterior view.

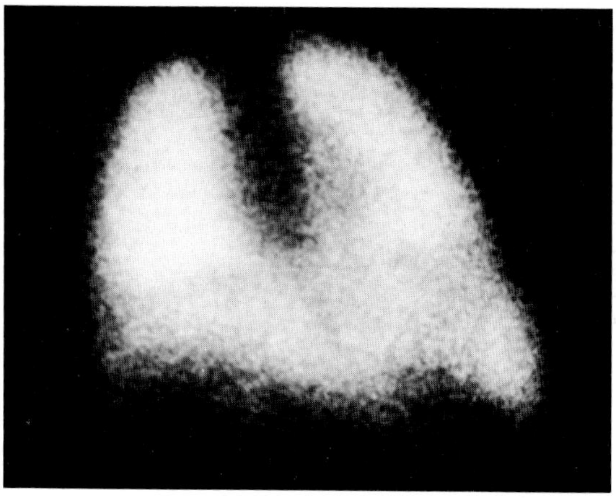

Figure 7-17. Bilateral Wilm's tumor. Tc-99m sulfur colloid liver-spleen scan showing upward displacement of the liver and spleen and focal defects within these organs. There is also high uptake of radiocolloid within the lungs.

duced or absent uptake of variable size or shape within the organ (Figs. 7-21 and 7-22). Hepatosplenic scintigraphy could be the primary screening examination for liver-spleen trauma.[10]

Patients with superior vena caval obstruction and the Budd-Chiari syndrome[17] may exhibit increased focal uptake of radiocolloid within the liver. In superior vena caval obstruction, systemic-to-portal venous shunting occurs through the internal thoracic and periumbilical venous channels.[14] After intravenous injection (within a vein of an upper extremity), part of the radiotracer reaches the liver in high concentrations, bypassing the systemic circulation. This results in an area of increased radiocolloid concentration in the mid-anterior portion of the liver. If the injection is done in

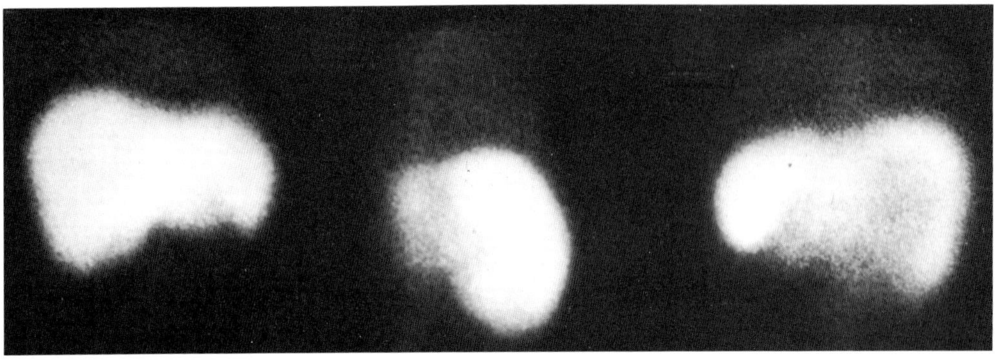

Figure 7-18. Hypertrophy of the right kidney. Tc-99m sulfur colloid liver-spleen scan shows a defect in the posterior aspect of the right lobe of the liver corresponding to a hypertrophied right kidney. *Left:* anterior view; *center:* right lateral view; *right:* posterior view.

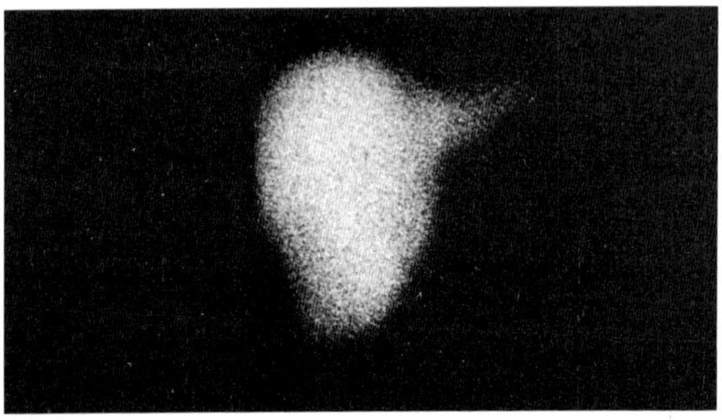

Figure 7-19. Radiation damage of the left lobe of the liver. Tc-99m sulfur colloid liver-spleen scan from an 18-year-old male with Hodgkin's disease following splenectomy and radiation therapy. The left lobe of the liver appears small while the right lobe is enlarged.

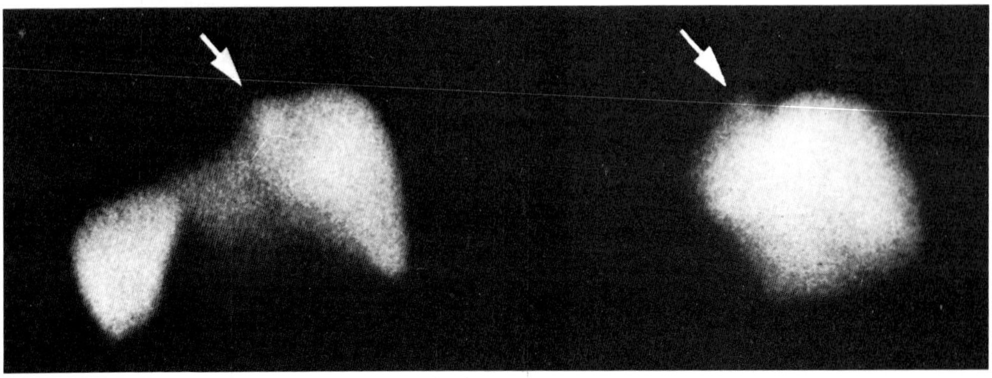

Figure 7-20. Herniation of the liver through the diaphragm. Tc-99m sulfur colloid liver-spleen scan. The herniated portion of the liver is clearly visible *(arrow)*. *Left:* posterior view; *right:* right lateral view.

a vein of the lower extremities, the tracer reaches the liver through the normal pahtways and the distribution of colloid in the liver is normal. In inferior vena caval obstruction, the reverse will be true.[12]

Hepatic scintigraphy in lymphoma and leukemia usually reveals hepatosplenomegaly without focal defects, although sometimes these are also found. Hepatotoxicity due to chemotherapy in leukemia and other disorders may result in hepatomegaly with or without uniform distribution of tracer within the spleen and with or without splenomegaly. If severe hepatocellular damage occurs, an apparent shift of the colloid deposition to the liver may be apparent. In other cases, when chemother-

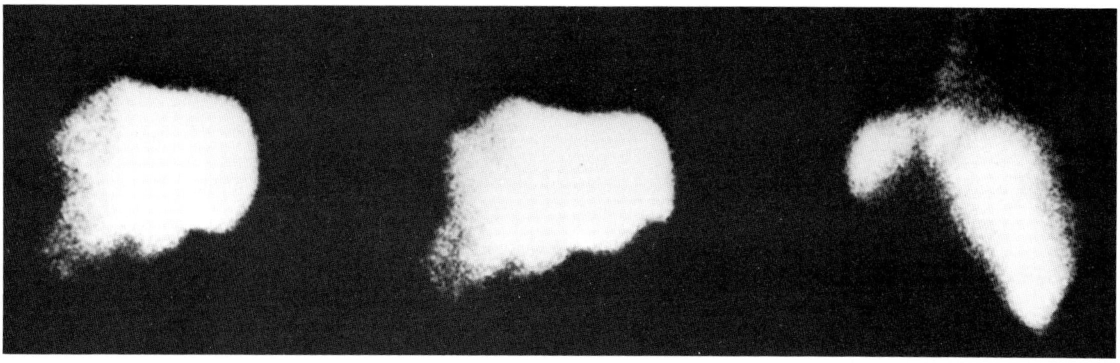

Figure 7-21. Blunt abdominal trauma resulting in a large hematoma located in the right lateral aspect of the liver and extending superiorly under the diaphragm. Tc-99m sulfur colloid. *Left:* right anterior oblique view; *center:* anterior view; *right:* right posterior oblique view.

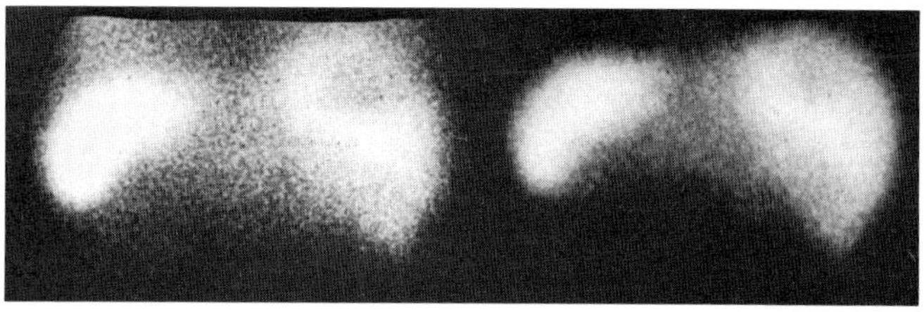

Figure 7-22. Blunt abdominal trauma resulting in an intrahepatic hematoma in the superior and posterior aspects of the right lobe of the liver. Tc-99m sulfur colloid liver-spleen scan on the *left* obtained the day of trauma. The image on the *right,* obtained several days later, shows a decrease in size of the intrahepatic hematoma.

apeutic agents are given together with radiation therapy, multiple focal defects can be detected within the liver. These defects are not necessarily metastatic tumors, and they may represent local congestion, atrophy, or necrosis.

Children with Wilm's tumor treated with radiation therapy and chemotherapy may develop sudden enlargement of the liver with intrahepatic defects resembling metastases. Temporary withdrawal of chemotherapy may result in resolution of the intrahepatic abnormalities and normalization of the liver size. Awareness of this effect of chemotherapy and irradiation on the liver may prevent diagnostic errors in metastatic disease.

References

1. Antar MA, Spencer RP, Lange RE, Kligerman MM. Radionuclide studies on effects of different doses of focal radiation on the function of the liver (abstract). J. Nucl Med 1970; 11:296.
2. Atkins HL, Richards P, Schiffer L. Scanning of the liver, spleen, and bone marrow with colloidal Tc-99m. Nucl Appl 1966; 2:27.
3. Atkinson GO, Kodroff M, Sones PJ, Gay BB. Focal nodular hyperplasia of the liver in children: a report of thre new cases. Radiology 1980; 137:171–4.
4. Deland FH, North WA. Relationship between liver size and body size. Radiology 1968; 91:1195–8.
5. Ehrlich CP, Papanicolaou N, Treves S, Hurwitz RA, Richards P. Splenic scintigraphy using Tc-99m labelled heat denatured red blood cells in pediatric patients. J Nucl Med 1982; 23:209–13.
6. Folkman J, Philippart A, Tze WJ, Crigler J Jr. Portacaval shunt for glycogen storage disease: value of prolonged intravenous hyperalimentation before surgery. Surgery 1972; 72:306–14.
7. Freedom RM, Treves S. Splenic scintigraphy and radionuclide venography in the heterotaxy syndrome. Radiology 1973; 107:381–6.
8. Freeman LM, Mandell CH. Dynamic scintiphotography of the liver. Semin Nucl Med 1972; 2:133–8.
9. Freeman LM, Meng CH, Johnson PM, Bernstein RG, Bosniak MA. False positive liver scans caused

by disease processes in adjacent organs and structures. Br J Radiol 1969; 42:651–6.
10. Froelich JW, Simeone JF, McKusick KA, Winzelberg GG, Strauss HW. Radionuclide imaging and ultrasound in liver-spleen trauma: a prospective comparison. Radiology 1982; 145:457–61.
11. Gelfand MJ, Saha S, Aron BS. Imaging of irradiated liver with Tc-99m sulfur colloid and Tc-99m IDA. Clin Nucl Med 1981; 6:399–402.
12. Gooneratne NS, Buse MG, Quina LL. "Hot spot" on hepatic scintigraphy and radionuclide venacavography. Am J Roentgenol 1977; 129:447–50.
14. Johnson FL, Balis FM. Hepatopathy following irradiation and chemotherapy for Wilm's tumor. Am J Pediatr Hematol Oncol 1982; 4:217–21.
15. Lee KR, Preston DF, Martin NL, Robinson RG. Angiographic documentation of systemic portal venous shunting as a cause of a liver scan "hot spot" in superior vena caval obstruction. Am J Roentgenol 1976; 127:637–9.
16. Milder MS, Larson SM, Bagley CM Jr, DeVita VT Jr, Johnson RE, Johnston GS. Liver-spleen scan in Hodgkin's disease. Cancer 1973; 31:826–34.
17. MIRD Dose Estimate Report No. 3. Summary of current radiation dose estimates to humans with various liver conditions from Tc-99m sulfur colloid. J Nucl Med 1975; 16:108A–B.
18. Neindok H, Langer B. Liver scan Budd-Chiari syndrome. J Nucl Med 1976; 17:365–8.
19. Rollo RD, Deland FH. The determination of liver mass from radionuclide images. Radiology 1968; 91:1191–5.
20. Rosenfield N, Treves S. Liver-spleen scanning in pediatrics. Pediatrics 1974; 53:692–701.
21. Rosenthall L. Gastrointestinal imaging: imaging the liver in pediatrics. In: James AE, Wagner HN, Cooke RE, eds. Pediatric nuclear medicine. Philadelphia: WB Saunders, 1974.
22. Slavo AF, Schiller A, Athanasoulis C, Goldabini, J, McKusick KA. Hepatoadenoma and focal nodular hyperplasia: pitfalls in radiocolloid imaging. Radiology 1977; 125:451–5.
23. Spencer RP, Benever C. Growth of the human liver; a preliminary scan study. J Nucl Med 1970; 11:660–2.
24. Spencer RP, Kligerman MM. Scan evidence of hepatic refunction after tumor radiation. J Nucl Med 1970; 11:140–1.
25. Spencer RP, Pearson HA, Lange RC. Human spleen: scan studies on growth and response to medications (abstract). J Nucl Med 1971; 12:466.
26. Treves S, Spencer RP. Liver and spleen scintigraphy in children. Semin Nucl Med 1973; 3:137–50.
27. Waxman AD, Apau R, Siemsen JK. Rapid sequential liver imaging. J Nucl Med 1972; 13:522–4.
28. Yeh SH, Wei-Jen S, Liang JC. Intravenous radionuclide hepatography in differential diagnosis of intrahepatic mass lesions. J Nucl Med 1973; 14:565–7.

Chapter 8 Spleen

S. T. Treves

After the liver, the spleen is the next major site of phagocytosis. This function of the spleen causes the organ to take up intravenously administered technetium-99m (Tc-99m) sulfur colloid. In addition, the spleen is the principal site for red cell sequestration. As a consequence, selective splenic imaging is possible after intravenous administration of Tc-99m heat-damaged red blood cells.

Indications for splenic scintigraphy include evaluation of abdominal trauma, splenomegaly, tumors, and left upper quadrant mass; search for accessory spleen(s) and diaphragmatic eventration or herniation; and assessment of infarction, functional asplenia, polysplenia, and the heterotaxia syndrome.

Method

Radiopharmaceuticals

Tc-99m sulfur colloid is given in the same dose as for hepatic scintigraphy. A usual dose is 30 μCi/kg of body weight with a minimum total dose of 300 μCi. See Table 8-1 for absorbed radiation dose estimates and usual administered doses.

Tc-99m heat-denatured red blood cells are usually prepared in vitro from the patient's own red blood cells. We employ a scaled-down version of the Brookhaven National Laboratory kit for labelling of red blood cells. After 1 ml of the patient's blood is obtained, the procedure is as shown in Fig. 8-1.

After intravenous injection, a variable amount of Tc-99m damaged red cells concentrate in the spleen (30–90% has been reported in the literature). The usual dose of Tc-99m damaged red blood cells at Children's Hospital in Boston is 100–500 μCi depending on the patient's age (see Table 8-2). Absorbed dose estimates for children are also shown in Table 8-2.

Tc-99m methylene diphosphonate (MDP) has been found to localize in the spleen of patients with sickle-cell disease.

Method of Imaging

Tc-99m Sulfur Colloid

The same method and instrumentation described under hepatic scintigraphy are used for splenic scintigraphy. Magnification using the pinhole collimator is employed when higher resolution is needed. Anterior, posterior, left lateral, and oblique views are obtained.

Tc-99m Heat-Denatured Red Blood Cells

Scintigraphy is begun approximately half an hour after intravenous injection of the red cells using the same technique as described for Tc-99m sulfur colloid.

Table 8-1. Radiation Dose from Tc-99m Sulfur Colloid for Liver-Spleen Imaging[a]

Age (years)	Newborn	1	5	10	15	Adult
Weight (kg)	3.5	12.1	20.3	33.5	55.0	70.0
Usual administered dose (mCi)	0.3	0.6	1.0	1.7	2.7	5.0
Absorbed dose (rad)						
Total body	0.036	0.057	0.066	0.073	0.059	0.095
Liver	0.960	0.840	0.820	1.139	1.323	1.700
Spleen	0.840	0.720	0.650	0.833	0.891	1.050
Red marrow	0.174	0.108	0.110	0.1377	0.0972	0.135
Ovaries	0.043	0.0384	0.038	0.0272	0.0224	0.0280
Testes	0.012	0.0126	0.019	0.0238	0.0062	0.0055

Based on the biologic data of MIRD Dose Estimate Report No. 3, J Nucl Med 16:108A–B.

Except for the 1-year-old *S* values, which were taken from preliminary phantom work of the Metabolism and Dosimetry Group at ORNL, the age-dependent *S* values were taken from Henrichs K, Kaul A, Krause M. Age-dependent values of the specific absorbed dose. Klinikum Steglitz, Physik und Strahlenschutz (Biophysik). Berlin, West Germany: Freie Universitat, 1980.

[a]Note that administered and absorbed doses are higher for bone marrow images (see dosage and administration).

Table 8-2. Radiation Absorbed Dose for Tc-99m Heat-Denatured Red Blood Cells

Age (years)	Newborn	1	5	10	15
Administered dose (mCi)	0.1	0.2	0.3	0.4	0.5
Absorbed dose (rad)					
Spleen	4.0	3.0	2.6	2.4	2.0
Whole body	0.0036	0.025	0.019	0.017	0.012

It is assumed that 90% of the administered activity was in the spleen.

From the Radiopharmaceutical Internal Dosimetry Information Center, Oak Ridge Tennessee (J. Coffey).

Figure 8-1. A modification of the Brookhaven National Laboratory kit for Tc-99m labelling of red blood cells (RBCs).

1. Add 4 ml of saline for intravenous injection to standard Brookhaven kit[+] and mix.
2. Add 1 ml from step #1 to a small sterile tube (Vacutainer tube B-D #6495, 5 ml).
3. Draw 1 ml of patient's blood into a heparinized syringe and add to the tube from step #2. Mix (rotate) gently for 10 minutes at room temperature.
4. Add 0.5–1 ml of Tc-99m pertechnetate in a dose appropriate to the study into a sterile vial. Use of more than 3 mCi is not recommended. Do not use the first eluent on a new generator or from a generator that has not been eluted for 24 hours.
5. After incubation of the blood (from step #3 above), add 2–3 ml of normal saline. Remove air so that there is some negative pressure within the tube. Mix gently and centrifuge for 5 minutes at 1300 x g.
6. Withdraw approximately 0.3 ml of packed RBCs from tube using a long needle without disturbing cells and without withdrawing plasma. Add to vial containing Tc-99m pertechnetate (from step #4 above).
7. Incubate approximately 10 minutes with gentle mixing (rotate). Heat-damaged cells may be prepared by eliminating the 10-minute incubation and substituting gentle mixing in a water bath at 49°C for 12–15 minutes.
8. Draw suitable portion of the well-mixed labelled RBC suspension for determining labelling efficiency (should exceed 96%).

Prepared by Powell Richards of the Brookhaven National Laboratory, Upton, New York.

[+]Standard kit contains: 2.0 ug tine, 3.67 mg trisodium citrate dihydrate, 5.50 mg dextrose (anhydrous), 0.11 mg sodium chloride.

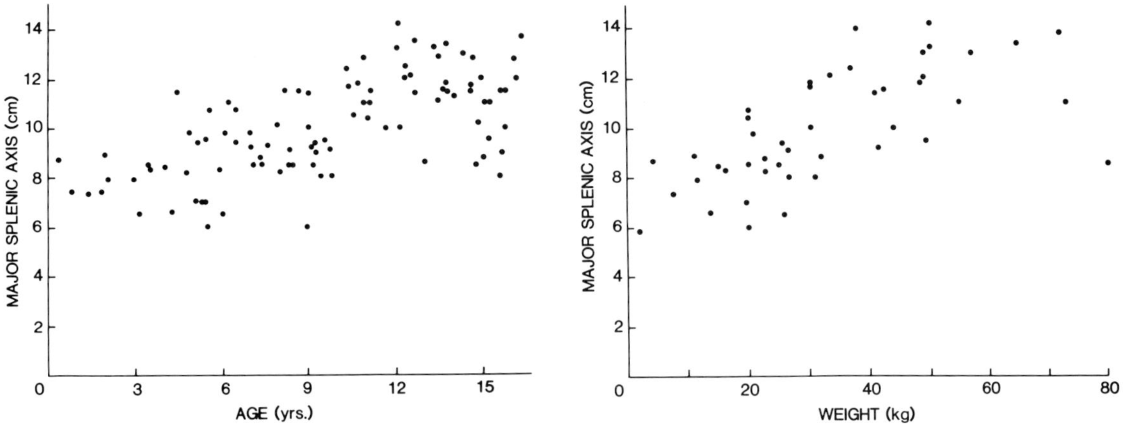

Figure 8-2. Normal splenic size as a function of age *(left)* and weight *(right)* in children.

Tc-99m MDP

Imaging is begun 2–4 h after intravenous injection of Tc-99m MDP. Posterior, left posterior, oblique, and lateral projections using a high-resolution, low-energy, parallel-hole collimator usually suffice to outline the spleen.

Clinical Applications

Normal Spleen Size

The spleen increases in size with age. Spencer et al.[44] have reviewed splenic scintigrams in children and found that the maximum splenic dimension (*MSD*) correlates with age (*A*) by the formula:

$$MSD = 5.7 + 0.31A$$

Markisz, Treves, and Davis in our institution measured the spleens of normal children of various ages. A good correlation with age and weight was found (Fig. 8-2) (unpublished information).

Splenomegaly

Enlargement of the spleen can be seen in a variety of conditions including portal hypertension (cirrhosis, cystic fibrosis, α_1-antitrypsin deficiency), Gaucher's disease, leukemia, lymphoma, anemia, congestive heart failure, bacterial endocarditis, pyelonephritis, metastatic disease, hepatitis, granulomatous disease, hemolytic disease, glycogen storage disease, and systemic infections.

Increased Uptake of Sulfur Colloid

Increased uptake of Tc-99m sulfur colloid in the spleen without increase in size of the organ can be found in children suffering from any of a large variety of infectious diseases or in children with splenic congestion following trauma. Relatively increased Tc-99m sulfur colloid uptake in the spleen with or without splenomegaly is found in severe liver dysfunction including hepatic cirrhosis, chemotoxicity, trauma with edema of the liver, and storage disease of the liver.

Focal Splenic Defects

Focal splenic defects can be found in the presence of splenic rupture, subcapsular hematoma, tumor, lymphoma, abscess, cyst, leukemia, infarction, and histiocytosis. Positional changes may affect the shape of the spleen or may simulate focal splenic defects (Fig. 8-3). It is important to remember that gastric dilatation due to food and/or carbonated liquids may change the shape of the spleen (Fig. 8-4). This appearance must not be confused with a space-occupying lesion. Sometimes it is difficult to separate the image of the left lobe of the liver from that of the spleen. In these cases, one may consider using oral carbonated beverges to induce gastric dilatation in the hope of obtaining better separation of these organs.[29,34] In their review of 2000 Tc-99m sulfur colloid liver/spleen scans, Freeman and Tonkin et al.[23] found focal defects on 18 of them (six infarcts, six metastases, five lymphomas, one inflammation).

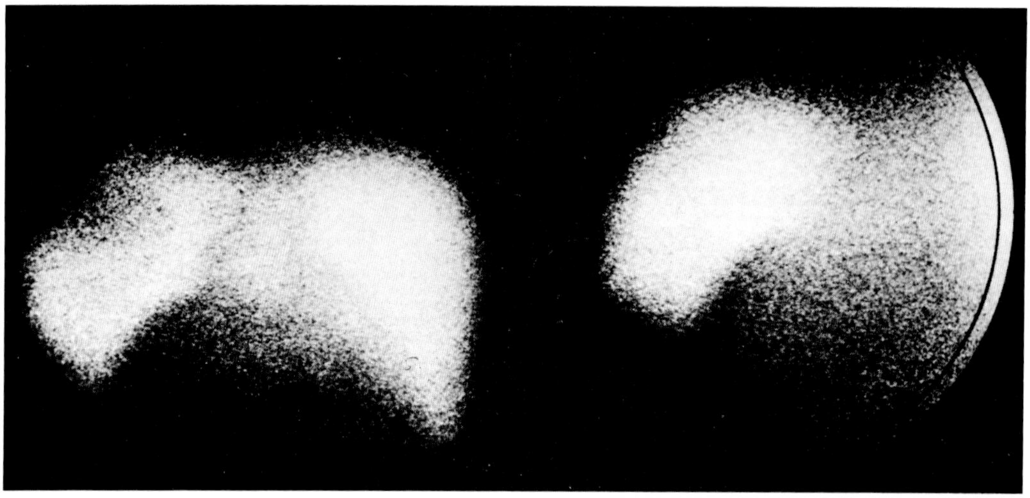

Figure 8-3. An apparent focal defect of the spleen caused by unusual position of the organ *(left)*. This artefactual defect disappears when the patient is scanned while upright. Posterior views.

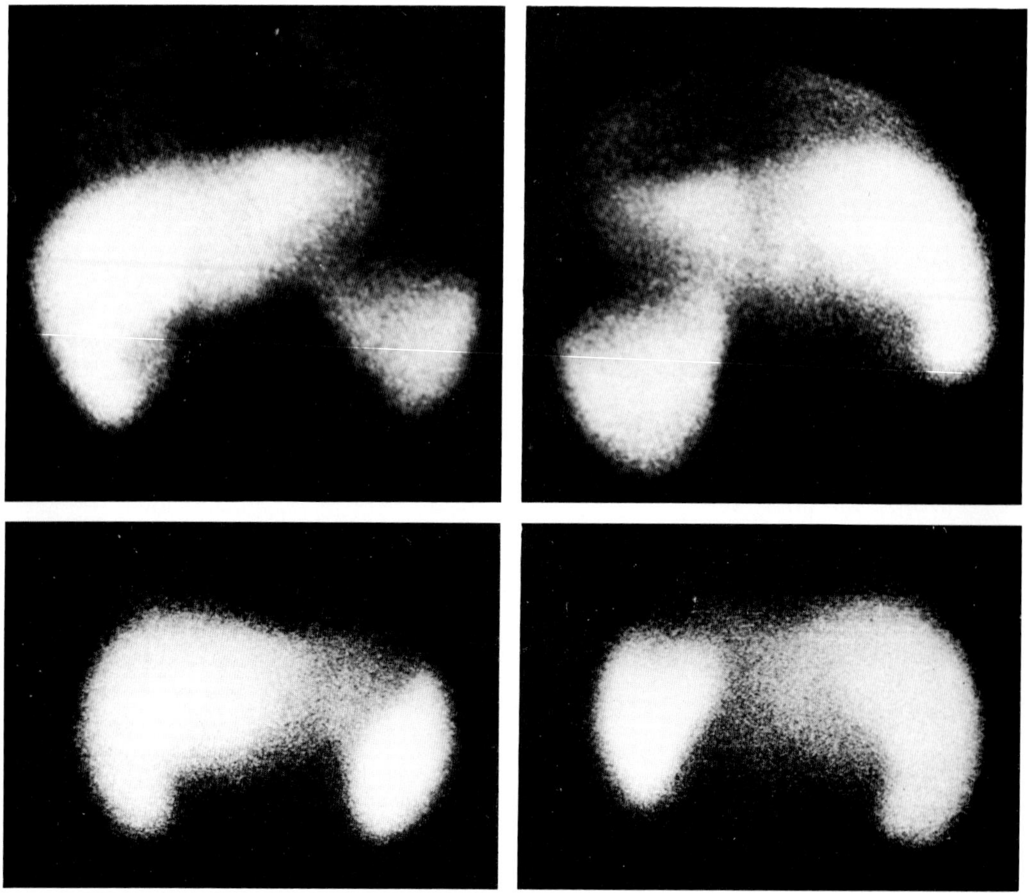

Figure 8-4. An artefactual focal defect in the splenic contour caused by gastric dilatation in an infant *(top)*. Following evacuation of the gastric content the scan appears normal *(bottom)*. *Left, top and bottom:* anterior view; *right, top and bottom:* posterior view.

Splenic Trauma

The spleen comprises 25% of the total lymphoid mass of the body and functions to clear the body of particulate antigens. In the past years, several investigators have reported an increased risk of septicemia, often fatal in children, following splenectomy.[19,28,40,41,46,47] The risk of overwhelming sepsis is greatest in patients who require splenectomy as part of the therapy for an underlying disease. Otherwise healthy children who undergo splenectomy because of trauma are also susceptible.[40,46] At present, whenever possible, splenectomy for splenic trauma has been replaced by nonsurgical treatment. If surgery is required, alternatives to total splenectomy include oversewing splenic lacerations or partial splenectomy (Fig. 8-5).[16,32]

The risk of overwhelming and lethal infection following splenectomy is about 0.1% in otherwise normal individuals.[12] This risk is considerably greater if the patient has an underlying debilitating disease such as portal hypertension or thalassemia. The total incidence of postsplenectomy mortality from sepsis in all groups is estimated to range from 0.25% to 0.58%.[40,46]

This risk appears to be greatest in children, especially those under the age of 1 year. Approximately 75% of infections occur within 2 years after operation.[47] Fifty percent of these infections are due to *Diplococcus pneumoniae* and the remainder are due to *Haemophilus influenzae, Staphylococcus aureus,* group A streptococci, and *Neisseria meningitidis.* The exact explanation for the increased incidence of infection is not known. One theory attributes the susceptibility to the low serum opsonin levels and defective production of IgM.[30]

Potential risks or complications associated with failure to excise a damaged spleen include delayed rupture and the development of a splenic pseudocyst. Delayed rupture of the spleen is a controversial subject.[3,4,33] We have not seen a single case of delayed rupture of the spleen among our patients. Splenic pseudocysts are nonepithelial lined cystic structures containing bloody material.[45,48] These can present as an abdominal mass at a time when the episode of trauma may not even be remembered.

With Tc-99m sulfur colloid and multiple projections, splenic scintigraphy is a reliable, simple, safe, and convenient method for diagnosing splenic injury and following its anatomic resolution.[21,24,42] In one large series,[24] 134 (98.5%) of 136 patients with splenic trauma had abnormal scans. In that series there were also 7% false-positives, but multiple views were not taken.

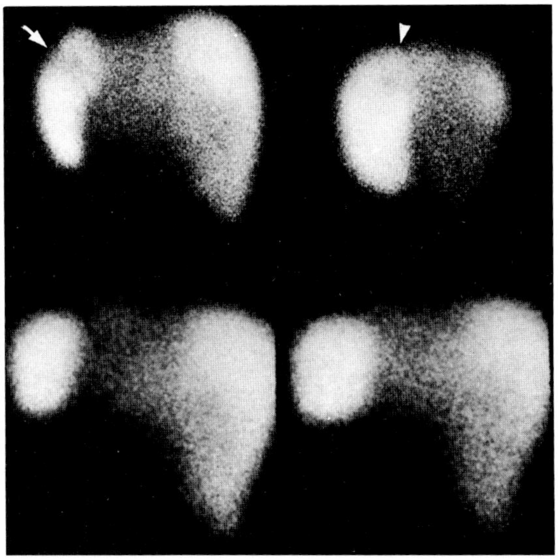

Figure 8-5. Splenic trauma followed by partial splenectomy. Before surgery *(top)* the posterior and left posterior oblique projections (Tc-99m sulfur colloid) demonstrate a focal defect in the superior aspect of the spleen After partial splenectomy *(bottom)*, the spleen appears smaller and well perfused.

Splenic injury may be seen on scintigraphy as a focal defect, a band of decreased to absent activity, apparent amputation of a portion of the spleen, a T- or Y-shaped defect or band, or a very small or absent spleen (Figs. 8-6–8-10).

After the diagnosis of splenic trauma has been made, scintigraphy can show that the laceration and/or hematoma is resolving and that no posttraumatic cyst is developing. Scintigraphic followup should be mandatory if pain develops or if a left upper quadrant mass appears.[21] Fischer et al.[21] from our institution followed 20 patients with splenic trauma from 2 months to 1 year. The majority of their patients showed persistent defects that became smaller with time. In no case did the scan defect enlarge with time. Only three of the 20 patients examined showed scintigraphic healing or total disappearance of the scan defect. Thus the presence of a residual defect on followup scintigraphy is probably no reason for keeping the patient on restricted activity.

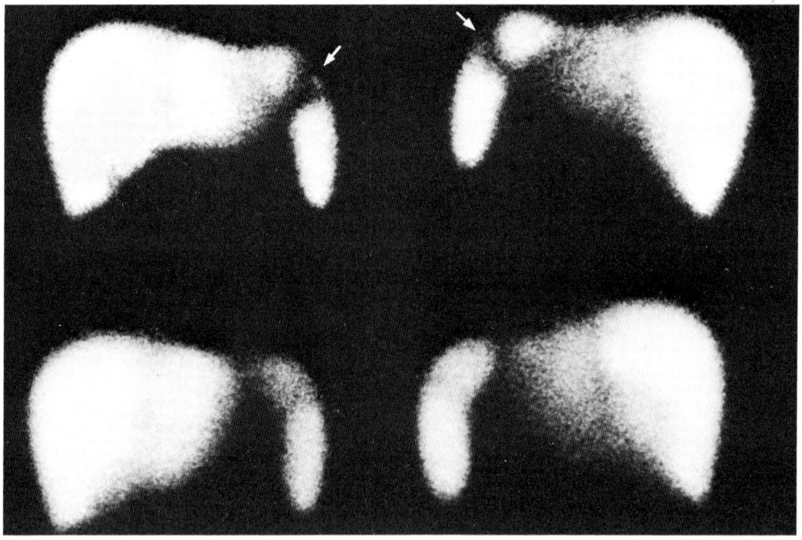

Figure 8-6. Splenic trauma. Nonsurgical treatment. Images on the *top* are anterior *(left)* and posterior *(right)* views. These Tc-99m sulfur colloid scintiscans were taken a few hours after blunt abdominal trauma. A well-defined band without radiocolloid uptake extends across the splenic silhouette *(arrows)*. Similar images obtained 2 months later (*bottom*) reveal only a minimal decrease in radiocolloid uptake in the upper third of the spleen.

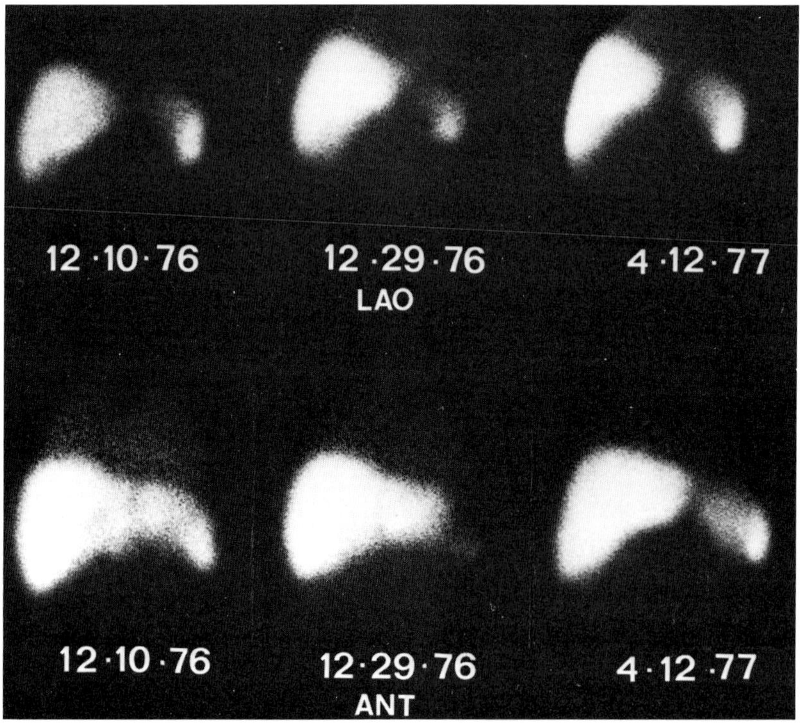

Figure 8-7. Splenic trauma. Tc-99m sulfur colloid images obtained from 1-year-old battered child. Initial anterior (ANT) and left anterior oblique (LAO) views reveal a suspicious area of decreased activity in the left lobe of the liver, but the spleen appears normal. A second study at a later admission for further trauma shows decreased activity in the spleen. Repeat study at 3 months shows normal distribution of radiocolloid. (Reproduced with permission from Fischer et al. J Nucl Med 1978; 19:3–9.)

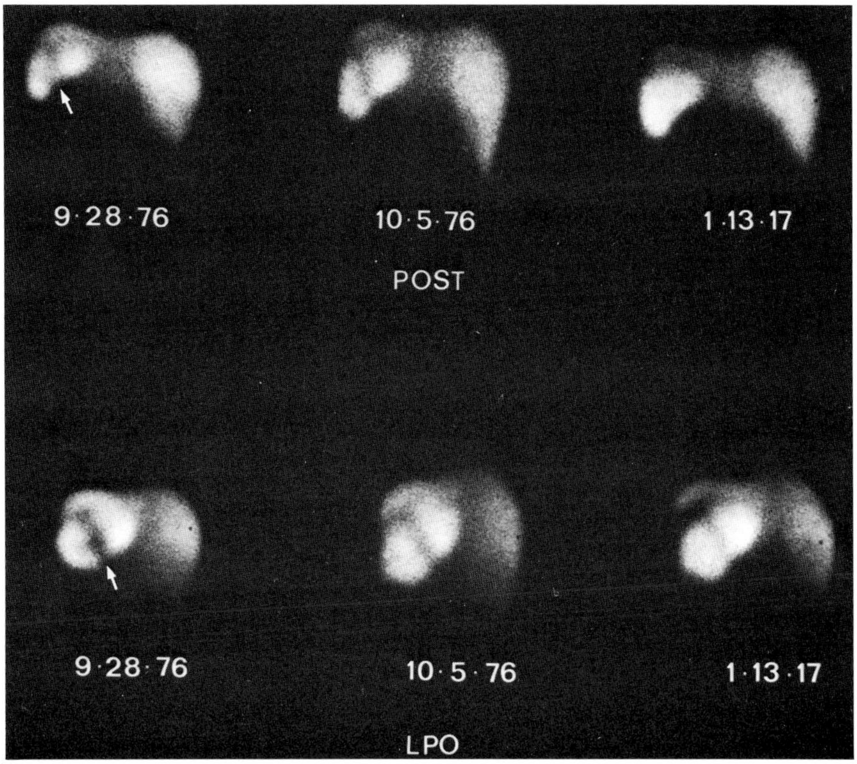

Figure 8-8. Splenic trauma. Serial Tc-99m sulfur colloid scans taken over a 20-month period. A splenic defect clearly visible on the first images diminishes in size with time. POST, posterior; LPO, left posterior oblique.

Splenosis

Splenosis is autotransplantation of splenic tissue following splenic trauma.[1,2,8,26] It does not have a characteristic clinical picture and is not a common occurrence. In the past the diagnosis of splenosis has been made at laparotomy. Splenic scintigraphy is a useful method for nonoperative identification of abnormally placed splenic tissue.

When evaluating liver/spleen scans in patients with previous abdominal trauma who may or may not be splenectomized, the possibility of splenosis should be kept in mind. Splenosis can also occur in the thorax.[1,15] The uptake of radiocolloid in the splenic tissue in splenosis may be minimal in relation to the liver uptake. In order to recognize splenosis, it may be necessary to overexpose the hepatic image or use contrast enhancement (Figs. 8-11 and 8-12).

Intrathoracic splenosis may present on radiographs as a chest film density that is indistinguishable from lung carcinoma. Tc-99m sulfur colloid or Tc-99m denatured red blood cell scans are useful in making the diagnosis of splenosis and should be performed before considering thoracotomy.

Accessory Spleen

Accessory spleens (one or more) are found in about 10–15% of autopsies in children.[9,18] They can be found anywhere in the abdomen but are most frequently seen in the left upper quadrant. Usually accessory spleens are not visible on routine imaging with Tc-99m sulfur colloid or Tc-99m damaged red blood cells. Accessory spleens are more likely to be seen by scintigraphy following splenectomy[17] (Figs. 8-13 and 8-14).

Splenic Torsion and Wandering Spleen

Torsion of the spleen, which is a rare condition, can present with a varied clinical picture. In one reported patient, the abnormality caused acute intestinal obstruction.[5] Radiographically, torsion of the spleen may not be apparent or it may appear as a mass lesion on plain films. Scintigraphically,

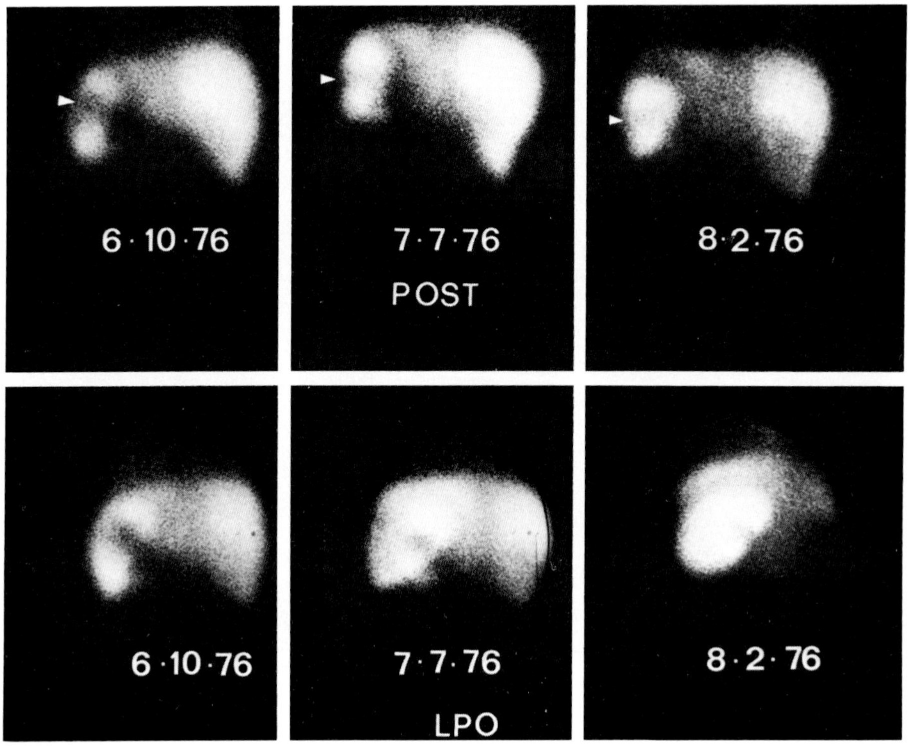

Figure 8-9. Splenic trauma slowly resolving on conservative treatment. POST, Posterior, LPO, left posterior oblique.

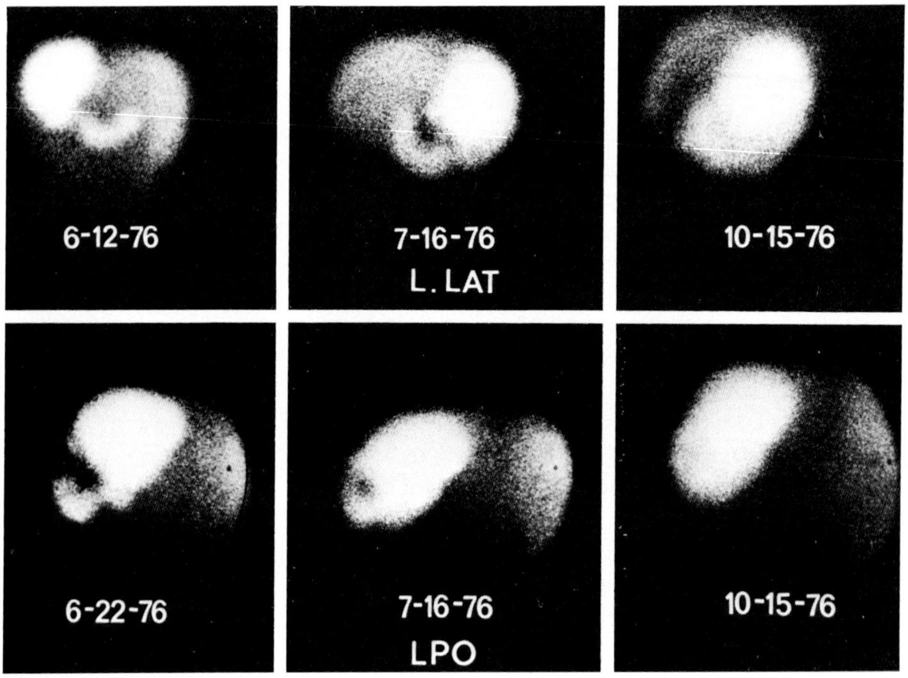

Figure 8-10. Splenic trauma in a 13-year-old male after a fall. Left lateral scan shows a defect in the inferior portion of the spleen. One month after trauma, the defect has decreased in size. Four months after trauma, only a suggestion of the defect remains. (Reproduced with permission from Fischer et al. J Nucl Med 1978; 19:3–9.)

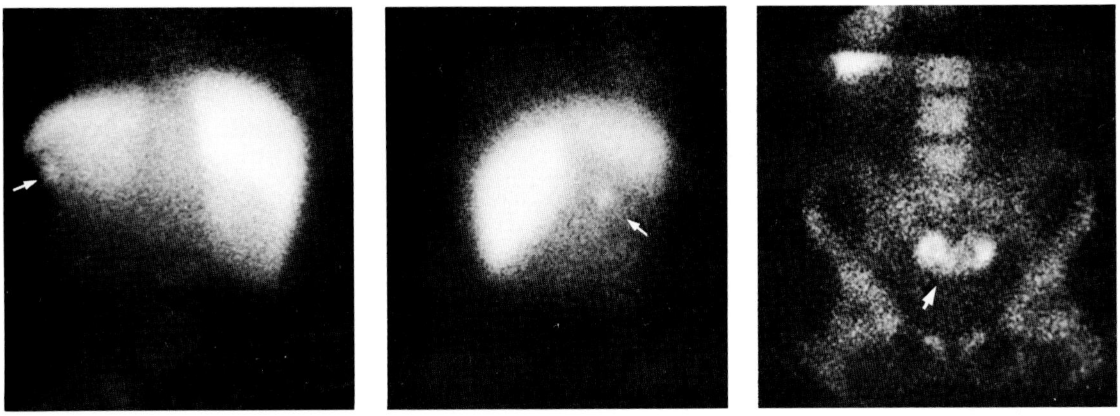

Figure 8-11. Splenosis. Tc-99m sulfur colloid scan shows two foci of splenic tissue. One is next to the left lobe of the liver, posteriorly, and the other is in the midline within the pelvis. The marrow of the pelvic bones is visible. *Left:* anterior view; *center:* left lateral view; *right:* anterior view of the pelvis.

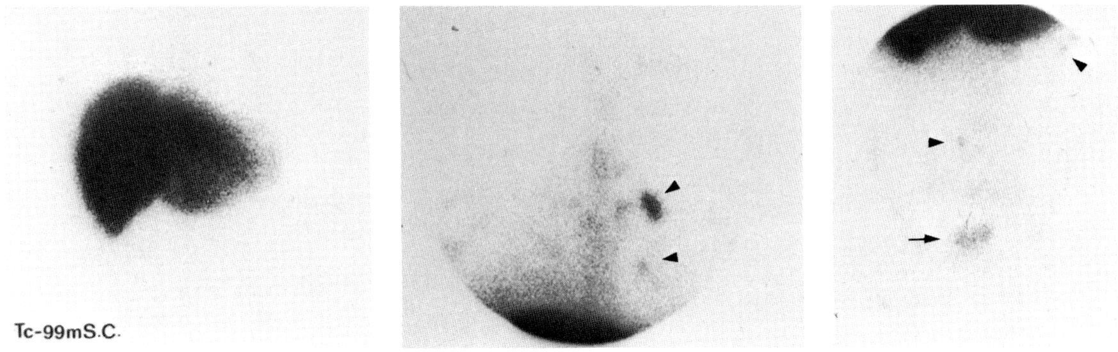

Figure 8-12. Splenosis. Tc-99m sulfur colloid scan (anterior view). The spleen is not visible *(left)*. There are at least three foci of selective radiocolloid concentration in the left hemithorax *(arrows, center)*. In addition, there are three or more additional foci of colloidal uptake in the abdomen *(arrows, right)*.

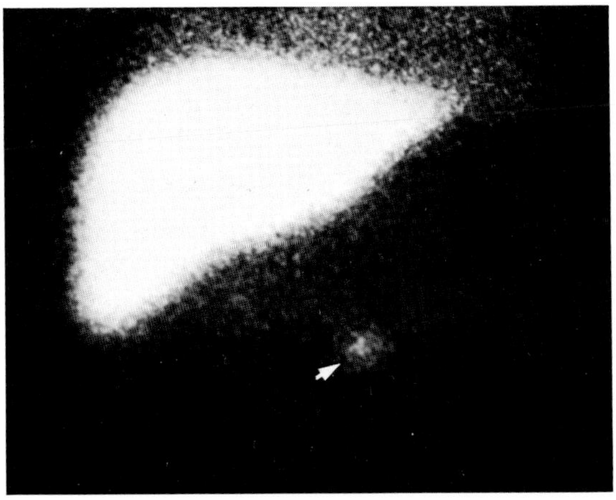

Figure 8-13. Accessory spleen. This overexposed Tc-99m sulfur colloid scan, anterior view, shows evidence of an accessory spleen below the hepatic silhouette *(arrow)*.

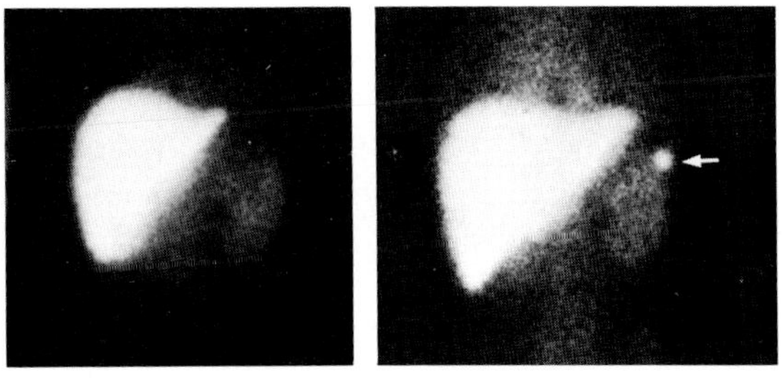

Figure 8-14. Accessory spleen. Recurrent idiopathic thrombocytopenic purpura after splenectomy in a 13-year-old female. A Tc-99m sulfur colloid scan *(left)* shows no evidence of residual splenic tissue. A repeat scan (not shown) with Tc-99m sulfur colloid taken 7 months later suggested a small accessory spleen. A scan done with Tc-99m heat-damaged red blood cells shows the accessory spleen very clearly *(right)*. (Anterior views) (Adapted with permission from Ehrlich et al. J Nucl Med 1982; 23:209–13.)

splenic torsion will cause nonvisualization of the spleen.

The main support of the spleen is believed to be provided by its various ligaments and vessels. The surrounding organs and the intraabdominal pressure also help to keep the spleen in its normal position and to limit its mobility. Wandering spleen is a rare condition that is characterized by unusual mobility of this organ and is usually discovered when torsion of the splenic pedicle occurs. The patient usually presents with an acute abdomen. On scintigraphy, the spleen may appear in its normal position or displaced inferiorly and/or medially. Repeated views with the patient in various positions may help diagnose the unusual mobility of the spleen.[6]

Acute torsion of the spleen reportedly has caused gastric varices that subsequently bled.[43] In this instance chronic splenic vein occlusion probably led to retrograde filling of the short gastric and gastroepiploic veins that ruptured in response to the increased pressure.

Asplenia, Polysplenia, and Nonvisualization of the Spleen

Asplenia is usually associated with other congenital abnormalities, including complex cardiac anomalies, isomerism of the liver and lungs, bowel malrotation, and dextroposition of the stomach.[10,22,25,38,39] Most patients with asplenia have Howell-Jolly and Heinz bodies in their blood and siderocytes in the peripheral erthrocytes. Occasionally the erythrocytes of a normal premature or term infant also demonstrate these abnormalities, possibly due to splenic immaturity. Documentation of splenic hypofunction in patients with congenital cyanotic heart disease by hematologic findings is highly suggestive of the congenital asplenia syndrome and the associated cardiac anomalies.

Patients with the heterotaxia syndrome frequently have asplenia or polysplenia and present difficult therapeutic problems. In heterotaxia, anomalies of the abdominal viscera include abnormal hepatic symmetry, a common gastrointestinal mesentery (often with malrotation), nonretroperitoneal location of the pancreas, and abnormal position of the spleen. These patients often exhibit complex cardiovascular disease and bronchopulmonary abnormalities as well.

The specific diagnosis of polysplenia with normal splenic function can be made by scintigraphic demonstration of multiple spleens (Figs. 8-15–8-19).

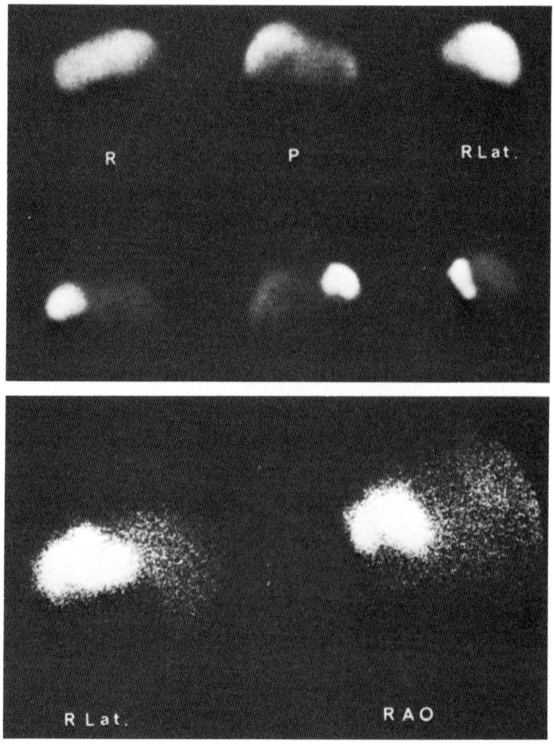

Figure 8-15. Polysplenia and heterotaxia. **A:** *Upper panel:* Tc-99m sulfur colloid scans. The distribution of radiocolloid is rather uniform along both upper quadrants. No spleen is visible, and the majority of the reticuloendothelial mass is in the right upper quadrant. *Lower panel:* Tc-99m heat denatured red cells scan demonstrating the spleen in the right upper quadrant. **B:** Pinhole magnification with Tc-99m heat denatured red cells showing polysplenia. R, right; P, posterio; R.Lat., right lateral; RAO, right anterior oblique.

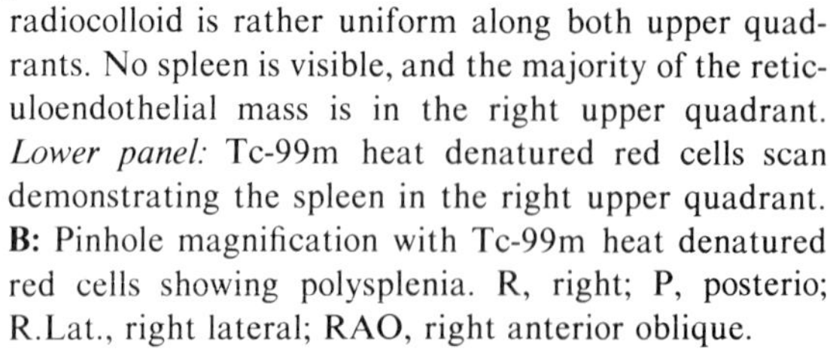

Figure 8-16. Heterotaxia. Anterior scintigrams with Tc-99m sulfur colloid *(left)* and I-131 rose bengal *(right)*. The image with radiocolloid does not permit identification of the spleen. Most of the reticuloendothelial mass is in the right upper quadrant. The image with rose bengal demonstrates a void or lack of tracer concentration in the right upper quadrant corresponding to the spleen.

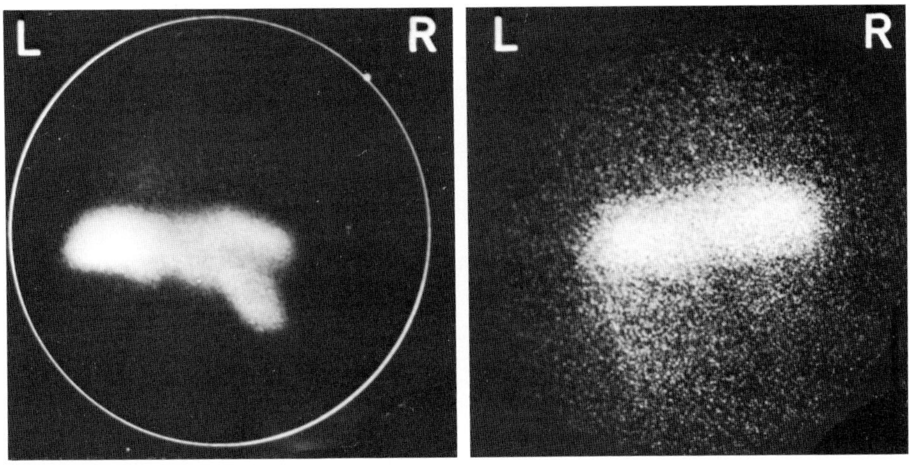

Figure 8-17. Splenic malposition and symmetric liver. *Left:* A symmetric hepatic silhouette. The spleen seems to be in the right upper quadrant. *Right:* Selective labelling of hepatocytes with rose bengal confirms the finding of a right-sided spleen. Posterior views. (Reproduced with permission from Freedom and Treves. Radiology 1973; 107:381–6.)

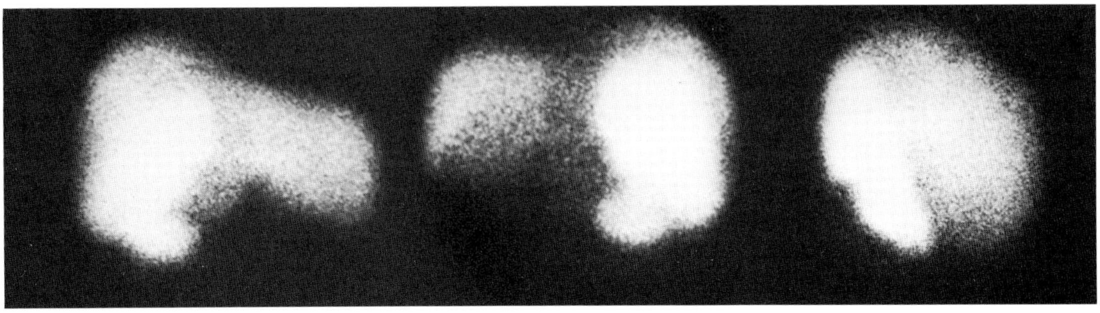

Figure 8-18. Polysplenia and heterotaxia. Tc-99m sulfur colloid scan. The spleens are located in the right upper quadrant posteriorly. *Left:* anterior view; *center:* posterior view; *right:* right lateral view.

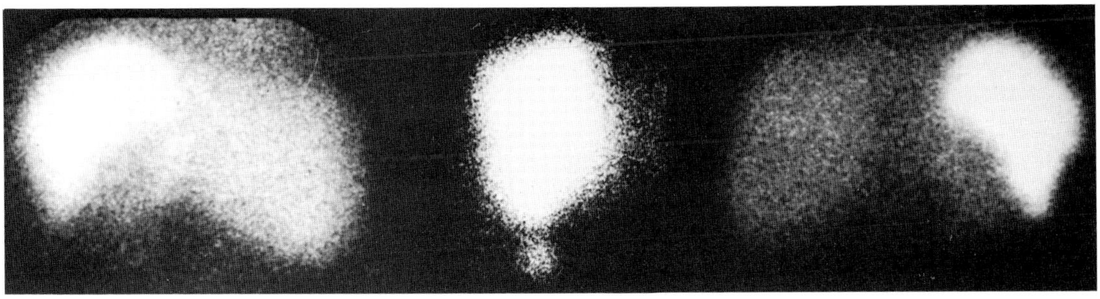

Figure 8-19. Polysplenia and heterotaxia. Tc-99m heat-denatured red blood cell scan. The spleens are in the right upper quadrant. *Left:* anterior; *center:* right lateral; *right:* posterior.

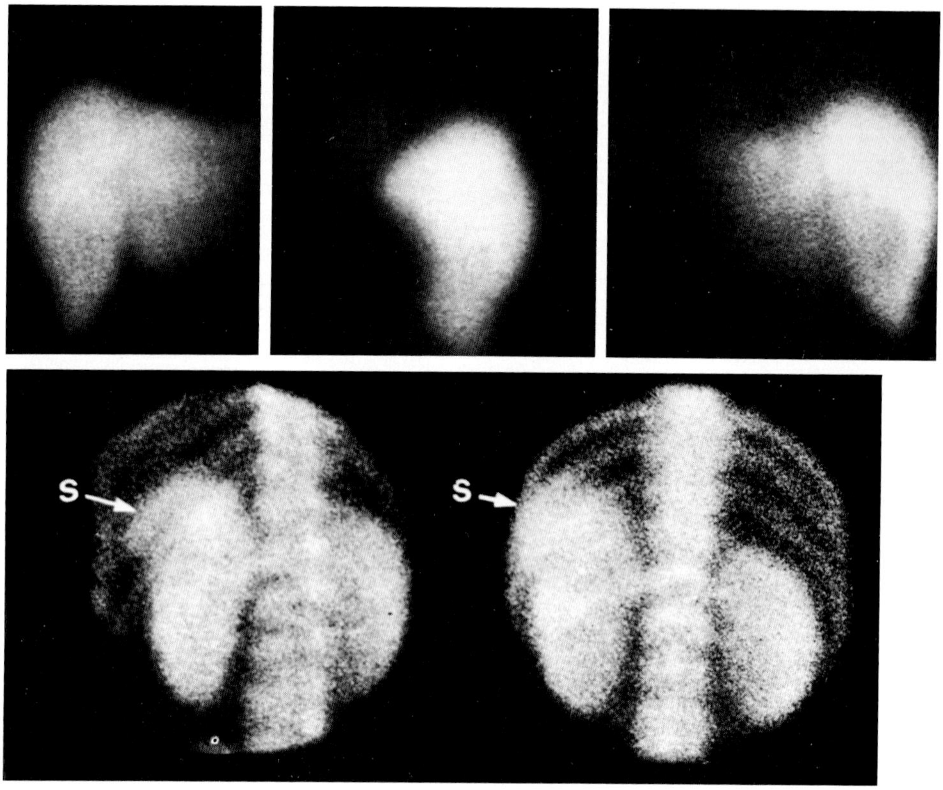

Figure 8-20. Sickle-cell disease. Tc-99m sulfur colloid scan of a 16-year-old male with sickle-cell disease. There is no evidence of splenic uptake of radiocolloid (*top; left:* anterior view; *center:* right lateral; *right:* posterior). Tc-99m MDP scan shows splenic uptake of this tracer (*bottom; left:* left posterior oblique; *right:* posterior view). Reproduced with permission from Fischer et al. Radiology 1977; 122:398.

Associated abnormalities include absence of the proximal portion of the inferior vena cava and bilateral hyperarterial bronchi viewed on chest radiographs. Radionuclide venography can detect patency of the inferior vena cava and facilitate cardiac catheterization. Polysplenia can occur without significant heart disease. Absence of the renal-to-hepatic portion of the inferior vena cava is accompanied by azygos or hemiazygos extension.[22] (See Chapter 7 for a fuller account of this variation.) In some cases, these patients also have a double superior vena cava.

Nonvisualization of the spleen on Tc-99m colloid images was first described in patients with sickle-cell disease.[35,36,37] The spleen in these patients can be identified with a Tc-99m bone-seeking radiopharmaceutical (Figs. 8-20–8-22).

Reversible functional asplenia in a 61-year-old man with chronic hepatitis was reported by Dhawan et al.[14] The same authors published a tentative classification of disorders associated with reversible functional asplenia including certain cyanotic congenital heart diseases (treated), sickle-cell disease, hemoglobin sickle-cell disease, and combined immunodeficiency.

Functional asplenia of patients with sickle-cell disease can be reversed by transfusion of normal red blood cells. The circulating level of normal red blood cells required for visualization of the spleen is about 50%. Functional asplenia can be observed in some patients with no circulating Howell-Jolly bodies.[13] Kevy et al.[27] reported a small number of children with hereditary splenic hypoplasia. These children had extraordinary susceptibility to infec-

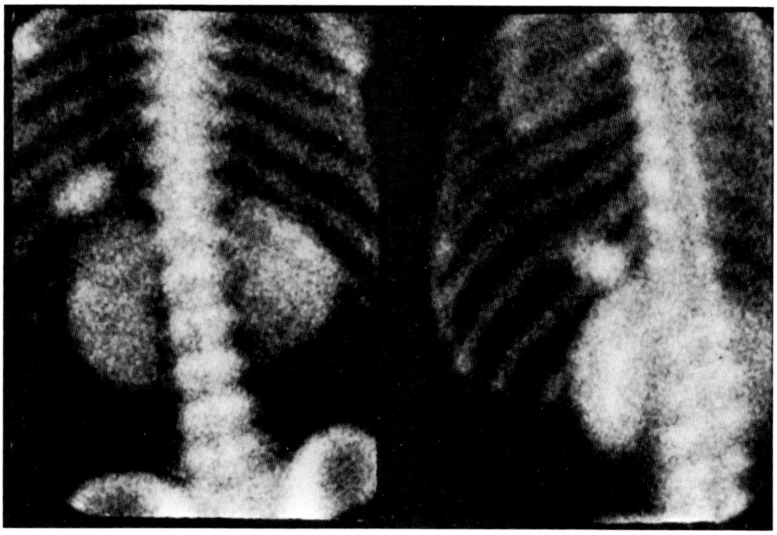

Figure 8-21. Sickle-cell disease. Visualization of a small spleen using Tc-99m MDP. *Left:* posterior view; *right:* left posterior oblique view. Tc-99m sulfur colloid scan (not shown) failed to reveal an image of the spleen.

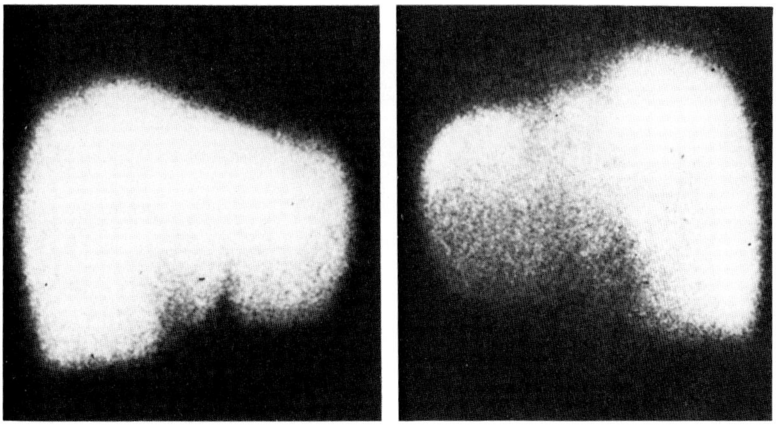

Figure 8-22. Sickle-cell disease. Tc-99m sulfur colloid scan demonstrates the so-called functional asplenia. *Left:* anterior view; *right:* posterior view.

tion and showed little or no evidence of significant splenic function by scintigraphy.

Candidiasis of the Spleen

Miller et al.[31] studied four children with leukemia and candidiasis in their spleens; three of the children also had candidiasis in their livers. The infection produced focal defects within the spleen and the liver. Uptake of gallium-67 (Ga-67) in these lesions was variable.

Splenic Abscess

Abscesses of the spleen are very rare. They are found most often in patients with a preexisting hematologic disorder, primary infection elsewhere, or trauma to the spleen (Fig. 8-23). Trauma is responsible for about 15% of cases of splenic abscess. Brown et al. Reported a *Salmonella* splenic abscess detected on the Tc-99m sulfur colloid scan and also shown as a defect surrounded with a halo of increased uptake on Ga-67 scans.[7]

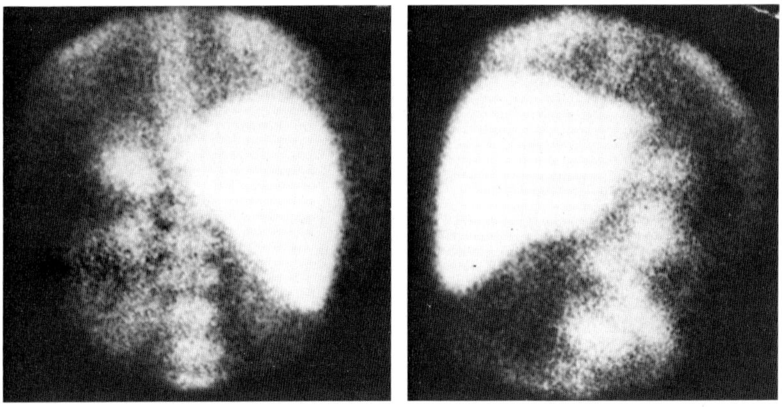

Figure 8-23. Multiple abscesses in the spleen in a patient with leukemia. Grossly enlarged spleen with multiple defects shows little or no uptake of Tc-99m sulfur colloid. *Left:* posterior view; *right:* anterior view.

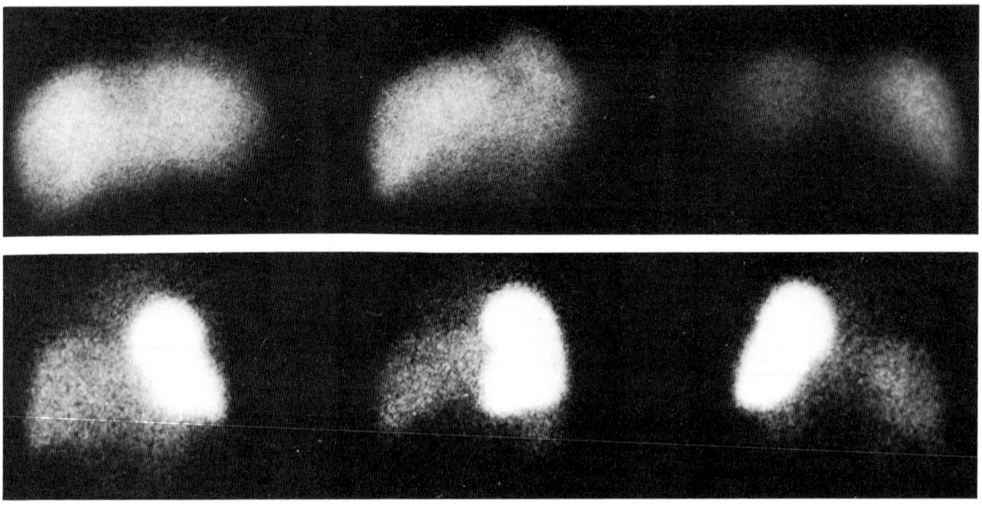

Figure 8-24. Herniation of the spleen. *Top row:* Tc-99m sulfur colloid scans reveal reticuloendothelial activity in the lower chest. It is difficult to ascertain whether the activity is liver or spleen. *Bottom row:* Tc-99m damaged red cells scan shows unequivocally that this is new herniation of the spleen. *Left:* anterior view; *center:* left lateral view; *right:* posterior view.

Splenic Infarction

Splenic infarcts occur in association with cyanotic congenital heart disease and in sickle-cell disease. They appear as wedge-shaped defects on scintiscans.

Herniation of the Spleen

In the presence of a mass in the lower left lung field, splenic scintigraphy with Tc-99m sulfur colloid or, better, Tc-99m damaged red cells is a rapid and specific procedure to identify misplaced splenic tissue (Fig. 8-24).

Splenic Artery Ligation

Crass et al.[11] report that Tc-99m sulfur colloid scans show a decrease in splenic size and function after splenic artery ligation in patients with hypersplenism. Immediately following splenic artery ligation, these authors report little or no splenic concentration of radiocolloid. After 4 days to 2 weeks, however, there is a gradual return of radiocolloid uptake in the spleen, eventually becoming a normal appearance in many cases (Fig. 8-25). Collateral vessels dilated over time. In some cases, focal intrasplenic defects (infarcts) were revealed.

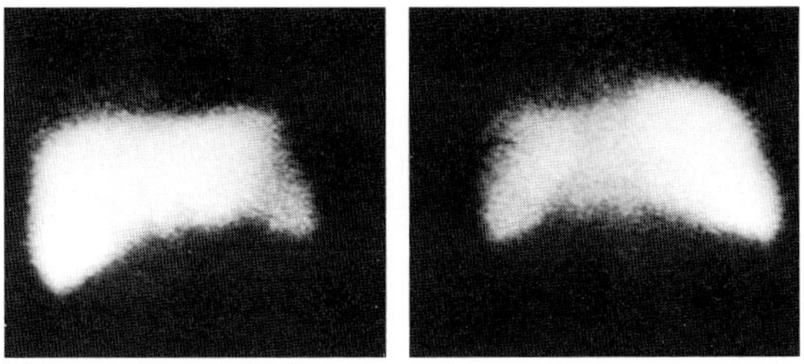

Figure 8-25. Splenic artery ligation with return of Tc-99m sulfur colloid uptake in the spleen after 1 week. *Left:* anterior view; *right:* posterior view.

References

1. Ahmadi A, Faber LP, Milloy F, Jensik RJ. Intrathroacic splenosis. J Thorac Cardiovasc Surg 1968; 55:667–81.
2. Albrecht H. Ein Fall von schr Zahlreichen uber ganze Peritoneum versprentgen nebenmilzen. Beitr Pathol Anat 1896; 20:513–27.
3. Ayala LA, Williams LF, Widrich WL. Occult rupture of the spleen. Ann Surg 1974; 179:472–8.
4. Benjamin CI, Engrav LH, Perry JF. Delayed rupture or delayed diagnosis of rupture of the spleen. Surg Gynecol Obstet 1976; 142:171–2.
5. Broker FH, Khettry J, Filler RM, Treves S. Splenic torsion and accessory spleen: a scintigraphic demonstration. J Pediatr Surg 1975; 10:913–7.
6. Broker FHL, Fellows K, Treves S. Wandering spleen in three children. Pediatr Radiol 1978; 6:211–4.
7. Brown JJ, Sumner TE, Crowe JE, Shaffner L. Preoperative diagnosis of splenic abscess by ultrasonography and radionuclide scanning. South Med J 1979; 72:575–7.
8. Buchbinder JH, Lipkoff CJ. Splenosis: multiple peritoneal splenic implants following abdominal injury. Surgery 1939; 6:927–34.
9. Cahalane SF, Kiesselbach N. The significance of accessory spleen. J Pathol 1970; 100:139–44.
10. Chandra RS. Biliary atresia and other structural anomalies in the congenital polysplenia syndrome. J Pediatr 1974; 85:649–55.
11. Crass JR, Frick MP, Loken MK. The scintigraphic appearance of the spleen following splenic artery resection. Radiology 1980; 136:737–9.
12. Dawer CC, Korns RF, Schuman LM. Infectious diseases. Cambridge, Massachusetts: Harvard University Press, 1968.
13. Dhawan VM, Spencer RP, Pearson HA, Sziklas JJ. Functional asplenia in the absence of circulating Howell-Jolly bodies. Clin Nucl Med 1977; 2:395–6.
14. Dhawan VM, Spencer RP, Sziklas JJ. Reversible functional asplenia in chronic aggressive hepatitis. J Nucl Med 1979; 20:34–36.
15. Dillon ML Jr, Koster JK, Coy J, Utley JR, Vasquez M, Canlas M. Intrathoracic splenosis. South Med J 1977; 70:112–4.
16. Douglas GJ, Simpson JS. The conservative management of splenic trauma. J Pediatr Surg 1971; 6:565–70.
17. Enrlich CP, Papanicolaou N, Treves S, Hurwitz RA, Richards P. Splenic scintigraphy using Tc-99m labelled heat denatured red blood cells in pediatric patients. J Nucl Med 1982; 23:209–13.
18. Eraklis AJ, Filler RM. Splenectomy in childhood: a review of 1413 cases. J Pediatr Surg 1972; 7:382–8.
19. Eraklis AJ, Kevy SV, Diamond LK, Gross RE. Hazard of overwhelming infection after splenectomy in childhood. N Engl J Med 1967; 276:1225–9.
20. Fischer KC, Shapiro S, Treves S. Visualization of the spleen with a bone-seeking radionuclide in a child with sickle-cell anemia. Radiology 1977; 122:398.
21. Fischer KC, Eraklis A, Rosello P, Treves S. Scintigraphy in the followup of pediatric splenic trauma. J Nucl Med 1978; 19:3–9.
22. Freedom RM, Treves S. Splenic scintigraphy and radionuclide venography in the heterotaxia syndrome. Radiology 1973; 107:381–6.
23. Freeman MH, Tonkin AK. Focal splenic defects. Radiology 1976; 121:689–92.
24. Gilday D, Alderson PO. Scintigraphic evaluation of liver and spleen injury. Semin Nucl Med 1974; 4:357–70.
25. Ivemark BI. Implications of agenesis of the spleen on the pathogenesis of conotruncus anomalies in childhood; an analysis of the heart malformations in the splenic agenesis syndrome, with fourteen new cases. Acta Paediatr Upps 1955; 44(Suppl 104):7–110.
26. Jacobson SJ, De Nardo GL. Splenosis demonstrated by splenic scan. J Nucl Med 1971; 12:570–2.
27. Kevy SV, Tefft M, Vawter GF, Rosen FS. Hereditary splenic hypoplasia. Pediatrics 1968; 42:752–7.
28. King H, Schumaker HB. Splenic studies. I. Susceptibility to infection after splenectomy performed in infancy. Ann Surg 1952; 136:239–42.
29. Landgarten, S, Spencer RP. Splenic displacement due to gastric dilatation. J Nucl Med 1972; 13:223.
30. Likhite VV. Immunological impairment and susceptibility to infection after splenectomy. JAMA 1976; 236:1376–7.

31. Miller JH, Greenfield LD, Wald BR. Candidiasis of the liver and spleen in childhood. Radiology 1982; 142:375–80.
32. Mishalany H. Repair of the ruptured spleen. J Pediatr Surg 1974; 9:175–8.
33. Olsen WR. Delayed rupture of the spleen as an index of diagnostic accuracy (editorial). Surg Gynecol Obstet 1974; 138:82.
34. Parker JD, Bennett LR. Effect of water ingestion on spleen size as determined by radioisotope scans. Acta Radiol [Diagn] (Stockh) 1971; 11:385–92.
35. Pearson HA, Spencer RP, Cornelius EA. Functional asplenia in sickle-cell anemia. N Engl J Med 1969; 281:923–6.
36. Pearson HA, Cornelius EA, Schwartz AD, Zelson JH, Wolfson SL, Spencer RP. Transfusion-reversible functional asplenia in young children with sickle-cell anemia. N Engl J Med 1970; 283:334–7.
37. Pearson HA, Schiebler GL, Spencer RP. Functional hyposplenia in cyanotic congenital heart disease. Pediatrics 1971; 48:277–80.
38. Roberts WC, Berry WB, Morrow AG. The significance of asplenia in the recognition of inoperable congenital heart disease. Circulation 1962; 26:1251–53.
39. Rose V, Izukawa T, Moses CAF. Syndromes of asplenia and polysplenia. A review of cardiac and non-cardiac malformations in 60 cases with special reference to diagnosis and prognosis. Br Heart J 1975; 37:840–52.
40. Singer DB. Postsplenectomy sepsis. In: Rosenberg HS, Bolande RP, eds. Perspectives in pediatric pathology. Chicago: Yearbook Medical Publishers, 1973.
41. Smith CH, Erlindson, M, Schulman I, Stern G. Hazard of severe infections in splenectomized infants and children. Am J Med 1957; 22:390–404.
42. Solheim K, Nerdrum HJ, Radionuclide imaging of splenic laceration and trauma. Clin Nucl Med 1979; 4:528–33.
43. Sorgen RA, Robbins DI. Bleeding gastric varices secondary to wandering spleen. Gastrointest Radiol 1980; 5:25–27.
44. Spencer RP, Pearson HA, Lange RC. Human spleen: scan studies on growth and response to medications (abstract). J Nucl Med 1971; 12:466–7.
45. Topilow AA, Steinhoff NG. Splenic pseudocyst: a late complication of trauma. J Trauma 1975; 15:260–3.
46. Walker W. Splenectomy in childhood: a review in England and Wales, 1960–1964. Br J Surg 1976; 63:36–43.
47. Winter ST. Trauma, splenectomy and the risk of infection (editorial). Clin Pediatr (Phila) 1974; 13:1011–2.
48. Wright RW, Williams EW. Large posttraumatic splenic cyst diagnosed by radiology, isotope scintigraphy and ultrasound. Br J Radiol 1974; 47:454–6.

Chapter 9 Hepatobiliary Scintigraphy

S. T. Treves
Alun Jones

Relatively noninvasive methods for the evaluation of the biliary system (such as ultrasonography, computed tomography, oral cholangiography, and intravenous cholecystography) provide excellent anatomic information. Hepatobiliary scintigraphy adds information on regional hepatic function, biliary flow, and drainage. The specific *indications* for hepatobiliary scintigraphy in children include the following: differentiation between biliary atresia and hepatitis in jaundiced newborns; evaluation of older children with right upper quandrant pain; postoperative evaluation of patients after the Kasai procedure and other abdominal interventions; and evaluation of right upper quadrant masses (Table 9-1).

In a review of the indications for hepatobiliary scintigraphy during 1981 and 1982 at Children's Hospital in Boston, there were two distinct age groups. The first consisted of neonatal patients with an average age of 2 months (range: premature to 5 months of age). The majority of these neonates were evaluated because of jaundice in order to determine patency of the biliary tract (neonatal hepatitis vs. biliary atresia) or status after the Kasai procedure. The other group included older children and young adults with an average age of 12 years (range 1–22 years of age). In this group, the most frequent indications were right upper quadrant pain, question of cholestasis or obstruction, cholecystitis, right upper quadrant mass, and postoperative evaluation.

Table 9-1. Indications for Hepatobiliary Scintigraphy at Children's Hospital Medical Center, Boston over 2 Years (1981–1982).

Biliary atresia versus neonatal hepatitis	39%
Cholestasis: right upper quadrant pain	37%
Postoperative evaluation	14%
Mass: choledochal cyst	10%

Another use of Tc-99m hepatobiliary agents is in the identification of hepatoma. Utz et al.[58] demonstrated uptake of Tc-99m pyridoxylidene glutamate in the hepatoma that showed no uptake on a conventional Tc-99m sulfur colloid liver/spleen scan.

Method

Radiopharmaceuticals

Taplin et al.[55] introduced iodine-131 (I-131) rose bengal for functional studies of the liver and for differentiation of hepatocellular disease from common bile duct obstruction. Following their work, many new agents labelled with I-131 or technetium-99m (Tc-99m) were proposed, but none had properties as favorable as those of rose bengal.* All of these agents have been extensively considered in recent review articles.[16,46]

Since the mid-1970s, cholescintigraphy has been principally performed using hepatobiliary agents

*References 1, 2, 4, 5, 7, 8, 9, 11, 12, 15, 18, 22, 28, 31, 49, 54, 56, 57, 59, 69.

based on iminodiacetic acid (IDA), a class of Tc-99m-labelled complexes developed by Loberg and his colleagues.[44,45] An initial IDA substance to be used clinically was Tc-99m *N*(2,6)-dimethylphenylcarbamoylmethy-IDA (Tc-99m HIDA), which showed short hepatic transit times and bolus excretion into the bile with relatively low levels of urinary excretion. Further adding to the appeal was the capability for routine preparation of the complex using the existing stannous ion kit technology originally developed by Eckelman and Richards.[24]

Today a variety of IDA derivatives are used clinically, and the original HIDA preparation is probably the least commonly used of them all. The clinical differences among these radiopharmaceuticals are variations in hepatic time, percentage of the compound that is excreted through the kidney, and bilirubin level at which optimal visualization of biliary structures takes place. More important than any of the IDA differences, however, is the examiner's personal preference and experience with one or another preparation. Modification of technique can usually ensure comparable quality from each of the agents regardless of the clinical situation. Thus the following discussion of the IDA derivatives is provided for those who are interested but it should not be construed to overshadow the greater number of similarities among these IDA derivatives.

Chemical Characteristics of IDA Agents

Loberg[44,46] and Nunn[48] have reviewed both the theoretical and pharmacologic effects of structural changes in the IDA module. Further, Nunn et al.[48,49] have developed the use of in vitro parameters to the point where these can be used to predict the route of elimination of different members of the class, emphasizing the increasing understanding in general of the relationship between the nature of the ligand and the eventual biodistribution of a material.

Useful as these results are, however, they do not benefit from an exact knowledge of the stereochemical form of the complexes being injected. The HIDA complex itself has now been chemically, although not structurally, characterized as being a singly charged anionic complex of technetium in the (+3) oxidation state with two HIDA ligands bound to the central technetium atom.[20] It is assumed to have an octahedral configuration with one nitrogen and two oxygen atoms from each ligand coordinating the metal. The result confirms the hypothesis put forward originally by Harvey et al.[32] and by Burns.[10] It is interesting to note that this is the first time that a commercially available radiopharmaceutical, apart from pertechnetate itself, was chemically identified by direct means.

After entering a liver sinusoid, a radiolabelled substrate may be bound to membrane-bound carriers. There are separate carriers for anions, cations, neutral substrates, and bile salts.[53] Further subdivisions have been described in the anion and bile salts substrates.[43,60] These carriers appear to compete with serum proteins for the free drug. Inside the hepatocyte the radiotracer may undergo binding and/or may be metabolized before being excreted into the bile. A series of enzymes, which are glutathione *S*-transferases, called *ligandins*,[3] are recognized as the major binding sites. These ligandins catalyze the conjugation of glutathione to hydrophobic compounds such as bromsulphalein (BSP). These enzymes also bind bilirubin, which is a hydrophobic compound. This binding is accomplished in a noncatalytic manner.

The speed of transheptatic transit of Tc-99m hepatobiliary agents decreases with increased lipophilicity.[17] An active transport system in the biliary canaliculi is presumed to be involved in excretion of these agents into the bile. In jaundiced patients, saturation of bilirubin uptake, storage, and excretion sites will inhibit not only elimination of bilirubin but also any hepatobiliary agent whose transport depends on the same carrier and storage sites.[44,46,52]

Lengthening the alkyl chain on the benzene ring of the IDA molecule results in relatively longer hepatic transit time, enhances liver uptake (in hyperbilirubinemia), and reduces renal excretion of the radiocompound. Therefore the IDA derivatives with longer chains improve hepatobiliary visualization in hyperbilirubinemia. As shown in Figure 9-1, the differences among the most commonly used IDA derivatives lie in the choice of alkyl group at positions R_1, R_3, and R_4. The latest variant, mebrofenin, is unique in that it has four substituent groups, including bromine atom at R_2.

Tc-99m HIDA

Biliary visualization with Tc-99m HIDA is obtained at normal or slightly elevated bilirubin levels and is acceptable at 5–8 mg/100 ml. Normally about 85% of this tracer is excreted in the hepatobiliary system and about 15% in the urine. With increasing hepatocellular dysfunction, a greater

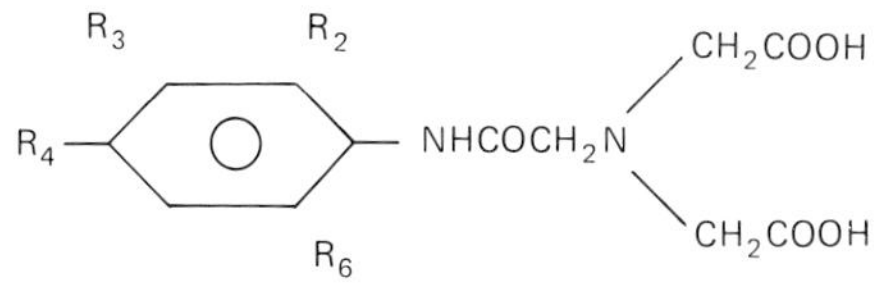

Ligand	R_2	R_3	R_4	R_6
HIDA (Lidofenin)	$-CH_3$	-H	-H	$-CH_3$
DIDA	$-C_2H_5$	-H	-H	$-C_2H_5$
DISIDA (Disofenin)	$-CH(CH_3)_2$	-H	-H	$-CH(CH_3)_2$
PIPIDA	-H	-H	$-CH(CH_3)_2$	-H
BIDA	-H	-H	$-C_4H_9$	-H
MEBROFENIN	$-CH_3$	-Br	$-CH_3$	$-CH_3$

Figure 9-1. Derivatives of phenylcarbamoylmethyl-iminodiacetic acid: the HIDA class of ligands.

proportion of the activity appears in the urine and less in the biliary system. This characteristic makes Tc-99m HIDA less optimal in the evaluation of neonatal jaundice than IDA derivatives that exhibit less renal excretion.

Tc-99m PIPIDA

Compared with HIDA, the *p*-isopropyl IDA derivative has relatively poorer visualization of the extrahepatic biliary system at lower bilirubin levels, but it offers increased delineation of the biliary system when the bilirubin level reaches the teens.[51,67]

It has been suggested that more accurate differentiation of biliary atresia from neonatal hepatitis can be obtained by two serial Tc-99m PIPIDA scans. The second study is done after 3–7 days of treatment with oral phenobarbital, 5 mg/kg daily.[47] There is no doubt that phenobarbital may enhance hepatic excreation of Tc-99m IDA derivatives, but it is important to take into account the time element. Neonates with hepatitis who do not demonstrate radiotracer in the intestine during an early examination tent to show passage of radiotracer into the bowel if the study is repeated a week or so later even without the administration of phenobarbital.

Tc-99m BIDA

When bilirubin levels exceed 10 mg/100 ml, Tc-99m p-bityl-IDA (BIDA) permits good visualization of the liver with minimal renal excretion. The diminished hepatic uptake and slower hepatic transit may be limiting factors in patients with a low bilirubin level,[35] but we have not found these characteristics to be a major problem in our pediatric population. In patients with higher bilirubin levels (>10 mg/100 ml), the diminished renal concentration permits recognition of small amounts of radiotracer that may appear in the intestine, especially in neonates with hyperbilirubinemia. Radiotracer in the intestine indicates a patent biliary system.

The short physical half-life of Tc-99m BIDA also may limit differentiation between biliary atresia from neonatal hepatitis with this agent. Collier et al.[19] found that in the initial examination, Tc-99m BIDA identified neonatal hepatitis in two of five infants. On the other hand, I-131 rose bengal identified intestinal activity in all five of the same infants. Activity in the three additional patients was recorded at 48 h in two and at 178 h in the third. I-131 rose bengal is no longer used in our institution, and we have had good results with Tc-99m IDA derivations.

Tc-99m PRIDA

Tc-99m PRIDA appears to have a combination of the most desirable properties of the current IDA derivatives. Its capacity to collect in the biliary tract at low bilirubin levels is as good as or even better than that of HIDA. It also appears superior to the other agents at bilirubin levels of 20–30 mg/100 ml.[29,35,66]

Biokinetics of IDA Agents

Bobba et al.[6] determined the biokinetics of four Tc-99m hepatobiliary scintigraphic agents in 34 normal humans. These workers measured blood clearance, urinary excretion, hepatic peak time, and urinary excretion half-time. They also evaluated imaging parameters with these agents including the time of appearance in the common bile duct, gallbladder, and duodenum. The radiopharmaceuticals tested in that study included Tc-99m diethyl- (EIDA or DEIDA), Tc-99m dimethyl- (HIDA), Tc-99m *p*-isopropyl (PIPIDA), and Tc-99m *p*-butyl- (BIDA) iminodiacetic acid derivatives. The fastest blood disappearance rate was found with DEIDA followed by HIDA, PIPIDA, and BIDA. Within the first hour, the blood level of BIDA was as high as that of DEIDA. By 1 h, the blood level of the four tracers was below 5% of the injected activity. BIDA showed the lowest excretion in the urine, with 5.6% ± 1.7 of the activity recovered in the urine at 24 h. There were no major differences in renal excretion among the other three agents (DEIDA, 17.1 ± 5.0%; HIDA, 15.5 ± 4.2%; PIPIDA, 14.3 ± 1.7% at 24 h). The hepatic peak time was earliest with DEIDA (14.0 ± 1.8 min) followed by HIDA (20.0 ± 0.9 min), PIPIDA (20.7 ± 1.2 min), and finally BIDA (26.3 ± 0.8 min).

The hepatic excretion half-times of these agents were DEIDA, 37.3 ± 11.8 min; HIDA, 42.3 ± 5.4 min; PIPIDA, 59.3 ± 5 min; and BIDA, 107.6 ± 14.1 min. The differences in hepatic excretion of DEIDA, PIPIDA, and HIDA are not statistically different from each other. The pharmacokinetics of DISIDA appear similar to those of DEIDA. Administered doses and absorbed dose estimates for Tc-99m DISIDA are shown on Table 9-2.

Method of Imaging

The patient should fast for at least 4 h before the examination. An injection of 100–200 μCi/kg of body weight of one of the Tc-99m hepatobiliary agents is given intravenously. Serial, 1-min images of the anterior abdomen are obtained for 1 h with the gamma camera-computer system while the patient lies supine. Additional images are obtained at 2, 4, and 24 h or until activity is detected in the intestine. Lateral and posterior views are obtained as necessary in order to define the nature of any extrahepatic activity in the abdomen. Cholecystokinin or a fatty meal may be given during the study to evaluate gallbladder contraction.

Clinical Applications

Neonatal Hepatitis and Biliary Atresia

Neonatal hepatitis is difficult to differentiate from biliary atresia because these two entities have similar clinical, biochemical, and histologic features (Figs. 9-2–9-4). Early diagnosis of biliary atresia is important, however, because surgical intervention (Kasai procedure) is most successful during the first 2 weeks of life[37,38] whereas surgery is not desirable in patients with neonatal hepatitis (Figs. 9-5–9-8).

Clinical Characteristics

Odell and Boitnott[50] have reported that neonatal hepatitis is almost four times more common in male infants and that biliary atresia is encountered twice as often in females. These authors describe clinical criteria that provide some help in differentiation of neonatal hepatitis and biliary atresia although the wide variation and overlap of these two diseases must always be kept in mind. Biliary atresia is accompanied by familial incidence, low birth weight for gestational age, associated anomalies, hemolytic anemia, and splenomegaly.

These factors are not usually encountered in patients with neonatal hepatitis, which tends to occur in otherwise healthy infants between 1 and 4 weeks of age.[50] Hepatitis patients do have splenomegaly and jaundice, and with time cirrhosis may develop. The pathologic findings vary, but in general multinucleated giant cells are present (as they are in some other liver diseases). The canaliculi are free of bile, and there is parenchymal disorganization.

Table 9-2. Estimated Absorbed Dose (rad) from Intravenous Injection of Tc-99m-DISIDA

Age (years)	Newborn	1	5	10	15
Body weight (kg)	3.5	9.4	19.1	32.1	54.5
Administered dose (mCi)	0.18	0.47	0.95	1.6	2.7
Bladder wall	0.22	0.21	0.24	0.27	0.3
Gallbladder wall	0.43	0.52	0.36	0.37	0.46
Wall of small intestine	0.4	0.56	0.64	0.67	0.7
Wall of upper large intestine	0.95	1.0	1.1	1.2	1.2
Wall of lower large intestine	0.72	0.75	0.81	0.85	0.86
Liver	0.059	0.08	0.089	0.099	0.10
Ovary	0.10	0.16	0.20	0.22	0.26
Testes	0.012	0.026	0.28	0.029	0.027
Total body	0.025	0.035	0.043	0.048	0.051

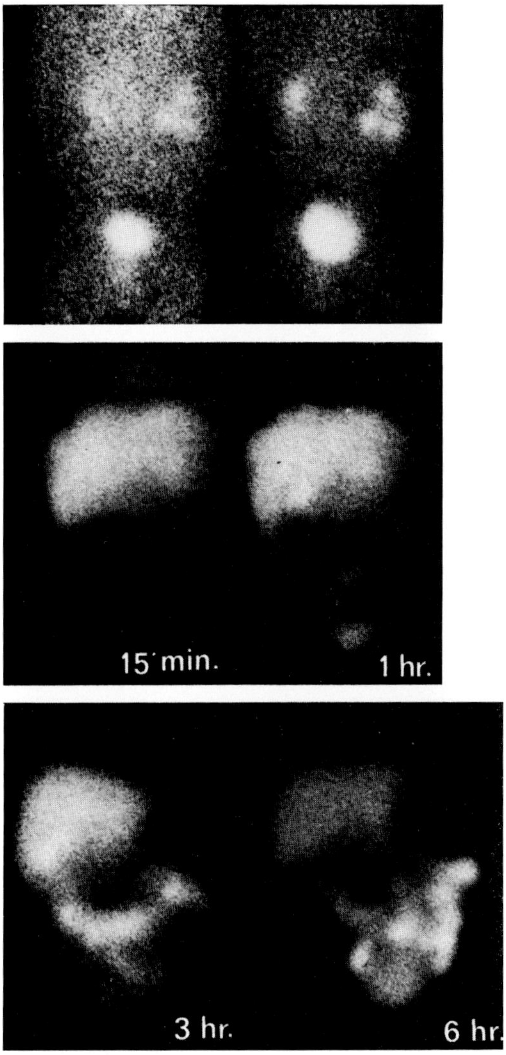

Figure 9-2. Neonatal hepatitis in a 1-month-old infant. Tc-99m HIDA *(top)* and Tc-99m BIDA *(middle and bottom)* studies were done 2 days apart. The HIDA study reveals very poor liver uptake and significant renal excretion of the tracer. The BIDA study shows relatively adequate liver uptake and demonstrates patency of the biliary tree.

Etiology

Neonatal hepatitis has been associated with a number of entities affecting the liver during the neonatal period: infectious agents (cytomegalovirus, hepatitis A and B, rubella, toxoplasmosis, spirochetes) and metabolic factors (α_1-antitrypsin deficiency, inborn errors of matabolism). Bilary atresia and neonatal hepatitis may represent variations of the same process, or, in some patients hepatitis may deteriorate into biliary atresia.[34]

In biliary atresia, there is sclerosing cholangitis of the extrahepatic biliary system[26] and sometimes progressive occlusion of bile ducts after birth. In patients with biliary atresia, there is partial or total absence of the major biliary ducts. Periportal fibrosis and intrahepatic proliferation of small bile ducts are characteristic, but there is no dilation of these intrahepatic ducts. Cirrhosis of the liver ultimately develops in biliary atresia unless surgical correction is successful.[33]

In neonatal hepatitis the intrahepatic and extrahepatic biliary system is patent but small.

Differential Diagnosis

Clinical and laboratory diagnosis of biliary atresia is difficult and often impossible. Ultrasonography and computed tomography are not very useful unless a patent biliary tree can be demonstrated. After attempting to delineate the biliary tree with ultrasonography, we perform a hepatobiliary study with one of the Tc-99m IDA compounds (Tc-99m DISIDA). Biliary atresia is ruled out if the hepatobiliary study demonstrates passage of the radiotracer into the bowel. If there is no demonstration

▽ **Figure 9-3.** Newborn baby boy with neonatal hepatitis. I-131 rose bengal study shows delayed hepatic transit time with activity in the bowel at 4 h and later.

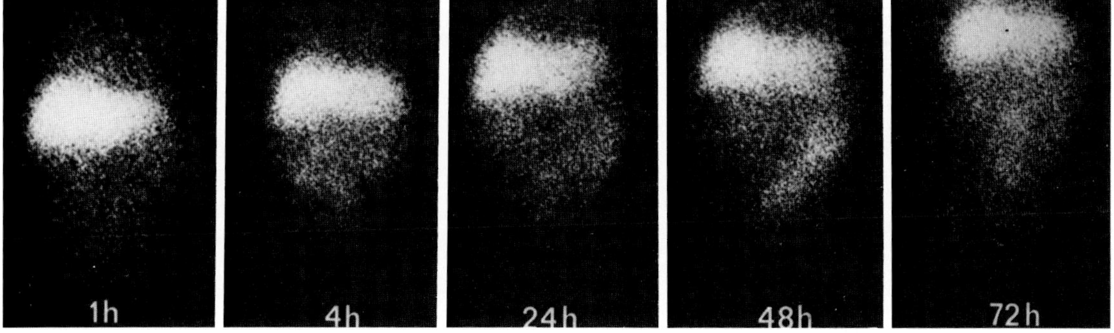

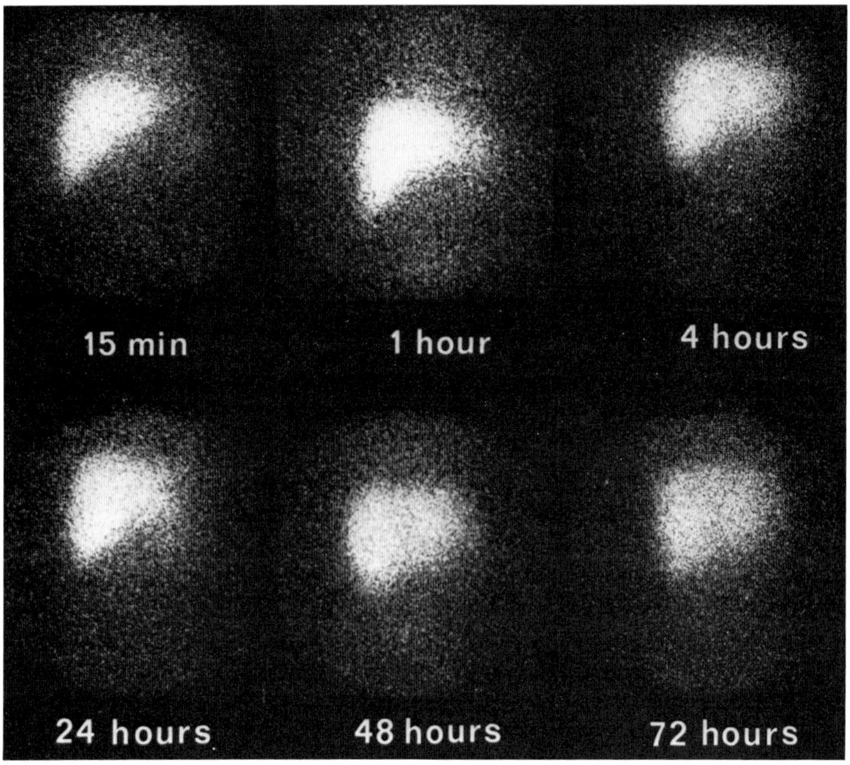

Figure 9-4. One-month-old male with biliary atresia. I-131 rose bengal study shows no elimination of tracer into the intestine up to 72 h.

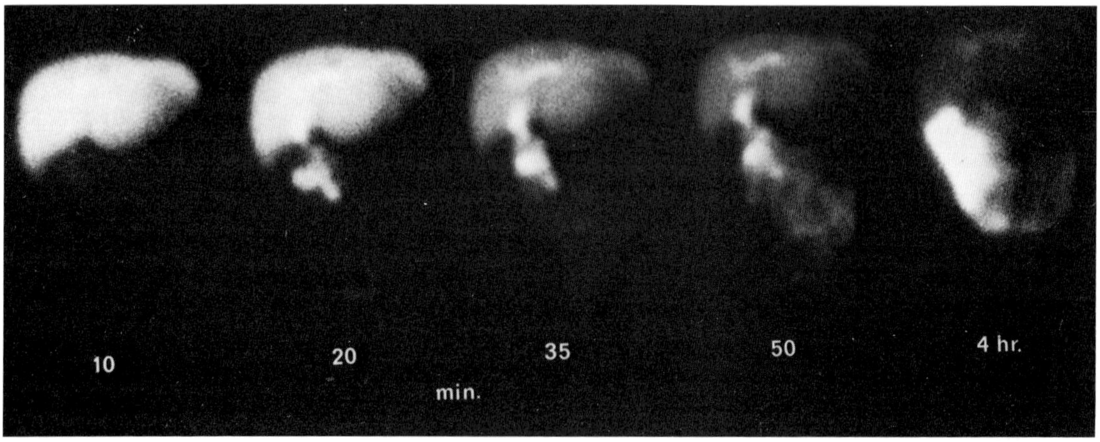

Figure 9-5. Tc-99m BIDA study after Kasai anastomosis showing adequate hepatic transit time with patency and dilation of intrahepatic ducts.

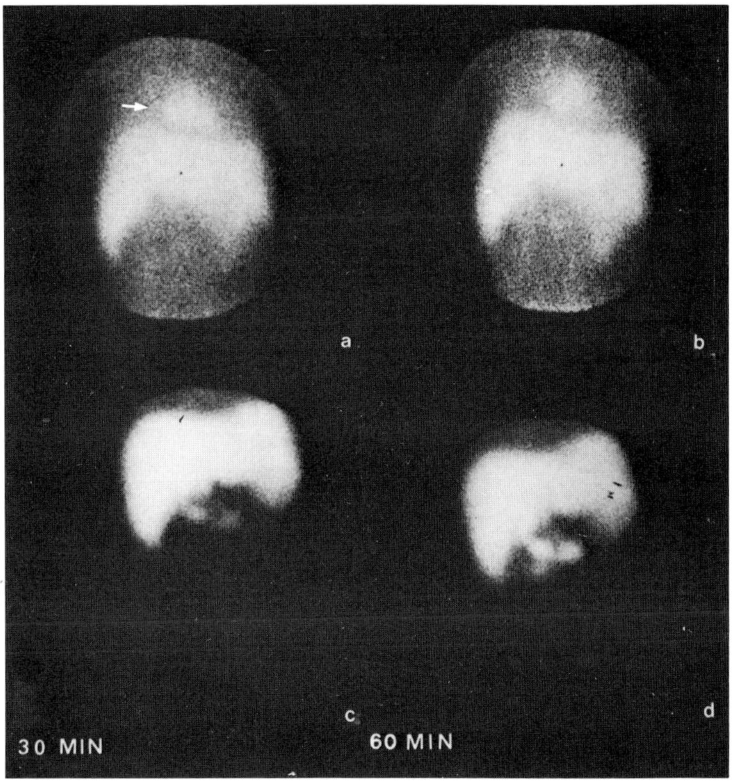

Figure 9-6. Biliary atresia. Tc-99m BIDA studies before (**a** and **b**) and after (**c** and **d**) Kasai procedure. The first study (**a** and **b**) reveals poor blood clearance of the tracer as evidenced by the high levels of activity in the body and within the cardiac blood pool *(arrow)*. After surgery, there is better blood clearance and evidence of biliary drainage of the tracer.

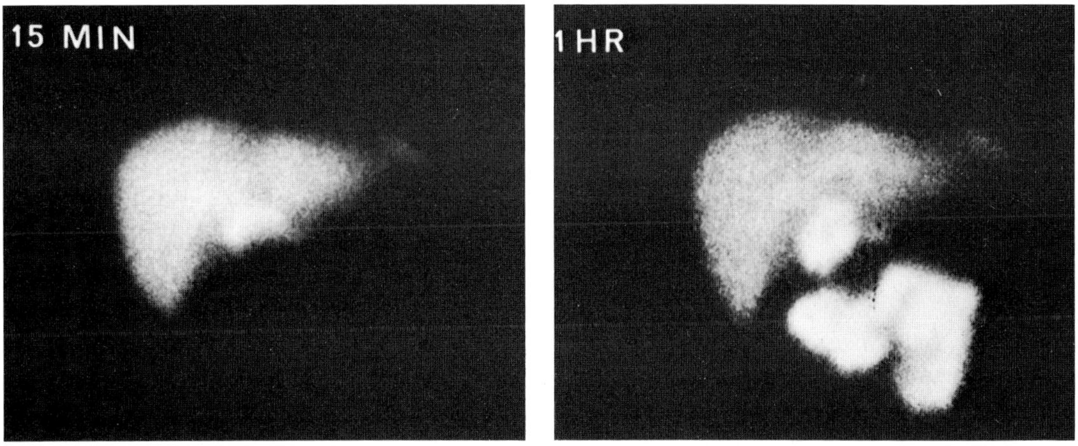

Figure 9-7. Tc-99m BIDA study. Several months after Roux-en-Y choledochojejunostomy, this patient presented with right upper quadrant pain. Evidence of rapid hepatic transit time with an area of partial retention of the radiotracer suggests a partial obstruction to the flow of bile.

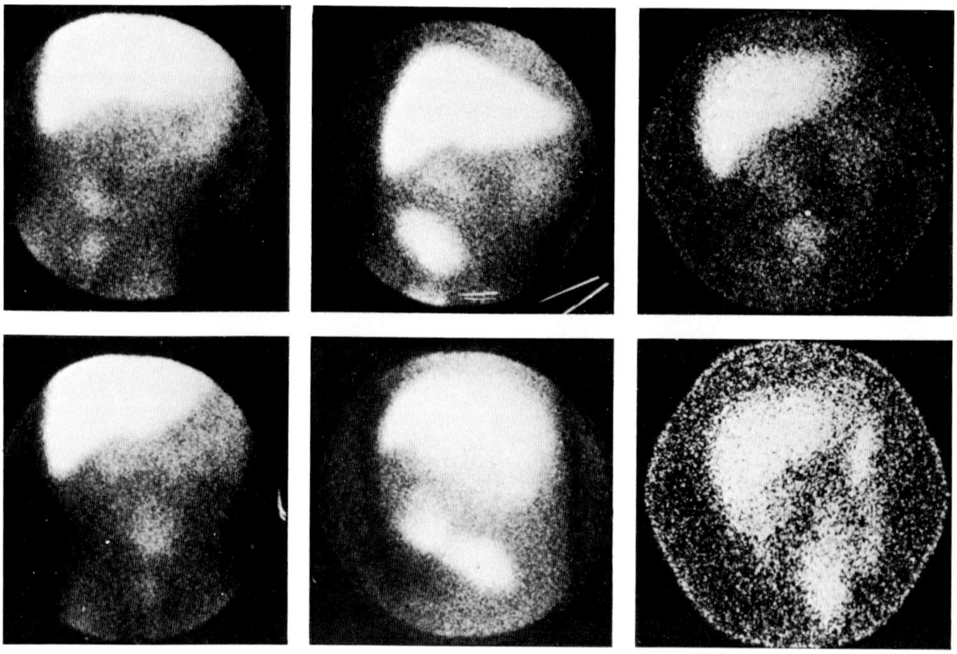

Figure 9-8. Neonatal hepatitis. Two Tc-99m BIDA studies done 11 days apart. In the first study there is no evidence of biliary patency, but in the second study radiotracer is visible within the bowel.

of radiotracer in the bowel, the distinction between biliary atresia and severe hepatocellular disease cannot be made with certainty. Definitive differential diagnosis may then be made by percutaneous transhepatic cholangiography, laparotomy, laparoscopy, or analysis of duodenal fluids.[25,30,33,36]

Gerhold et al.[27] have demonstrated the accuracy (91%), sensitivity (97%), and specificity (82%) of hepatobiliary imaging in the diagnosis of biliary atresia. These authors employed Tc-99m diethyl-IDA (DEIDA) and Tc-99m diisopropyl-IDA (DISIDA).[40–42,68] They used an interesting visual grading that includes the assessment of hepatocyte clearance and timing the appearance of radiotracer in the intestine or in the extrahepatic biliary system. Hepatocyte clearance was graded by visually comparing hepatic activity with cardiac blood pool activity on the 5-min image.

The studies were categorized as normal when hepatocyte clearance was normal and radiotracer appeared in the biliary tract and/or intestine in 15 min after injection. The diagnosis was biliary atresia when there was no intestinal activity through 24 h and hepatocyte clearance was relatively preserved. Studies were interpreted as neonatal hepatitis when there was similar impairment in hepatocyte clearance and hepatobiliary transit time and the radiotracer reached the intestine. The interpretation was intrahepatic cholestasis when hepatocyte clearance was relatively preserved compared with hepatobiliary transit time but radiotracer eventually reached the intestine. Indeterminate studies were those in which there was no intestinal radiotracer and hepatocellular function was severely impaired.

In another study of 22 neonates with jaundice, Majd et al.[47] concluded that scintigraphy using Tc-99m PIPIDA after 3–7 days of phenobarbital therapy is highly accurate for differentiating biliary atresia from other causes of neonatal jaundice. These authors administered 5 mg/kg/day phenobarbital orally divided into two equal doses.

Biliary Obstruction

Obstruction of the cystic duct is a major factor in the development of acute cholecystitis. The obstruction may be partial or complete and may or may not be associated with cholelithiasis.

Visualization of the gallbladder on the scintiscans rules out the diagnosis of acute cholecystitis with a high degree of accuracy in adults. Weissmann and others[64,65,67] have also reported that nonvisualization of the gallbladder was diagnostic of

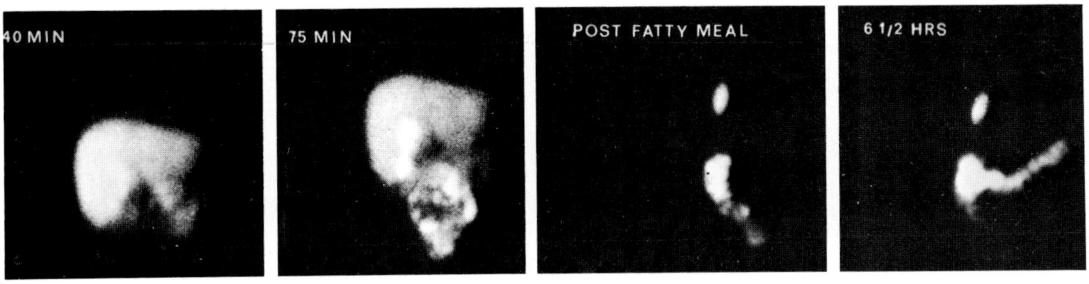

Figure 9-9. Acalculus cholecystitis. Tc-99m BIDA study obtained on a 17-year-old female after several episodes of right upper quadrant pain. The gallbladder filled slowly, and raiotracer was evident in the bowel as early as 10 min after injection (not shown). Following a fatty meal, the gallbladder fails to empty significantly. An image at 6.5 h still reveals substantial amounts of tracer within the gallbladder. This failure to empty suggests inflammation or infection of the gallbladder without cystic duct obstruction.

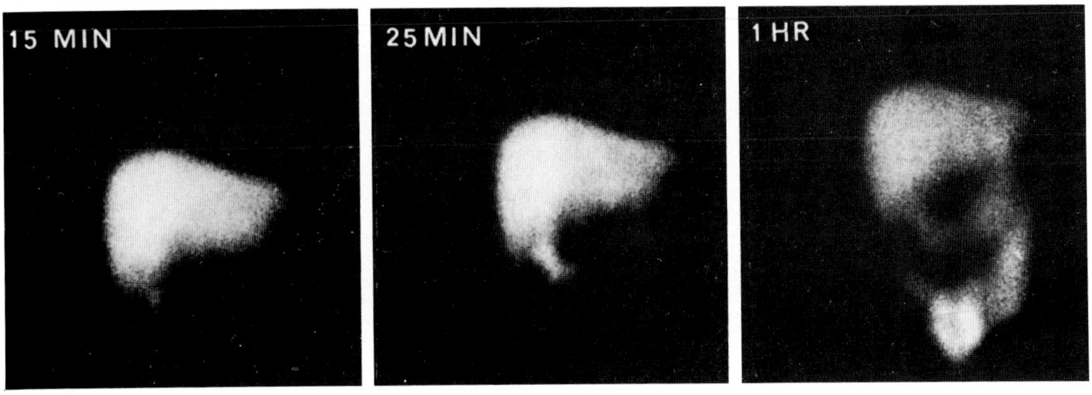

Figure 9-10. Eleven-year-old female with recent onset of right upper quadrant pain. Tc-99m BIDA images reveal prompt liver uptake with passage of radiotracer into the bowel at 15 min. The patient had fasted for 8 h prior to the study. The gallbladder is not visible up to 1 h after injection of the tracer. This study suggests cholecystitis with cystic duct obstruction.

acute cholecystitis in their patients, who also showed scintigraphic evidence of patency of the common bile duct. Among their 296 patients, these authors found an accuracy of 98%, a specificity of 100%, a false-negative rate of 5%, and a false-positive rate of 0% for hepatobiliary scintigraphy in the diagnosis of acute cholecystitis.[67]

The gallbladder can be visualized in acalculus cholecystitis or in toxic cholecystitis. Patients affected by these conditions may have only partial obstruction of the cystic duct and the gallbladder may not visualize due to edema of the cyctic duct. When acalculus cholecystitis is present, a fatty meal or injection of cholecystokinin usually results in failure of the gallbladder to contract completely. This failure of the gallbladder to contract suggests partial cystic duct obstruction, chronic cholecystitis, or acalculus cholecystitis. In chronic cholecystitis there may be a delay in gallbladder filling in the presence of normal liver function (Figs. 9-9–9-12).

Hepatobiliary scintigraphy cannot determine the presence of cholelithiasis. Ultrasonography is an essential diagnostic modality in evaluation of the biliary tract and should be performed in conjunction with hepatobiliary imaging. Cholecystitis in pediatric patients is infrequently associated with cholelithiasis and is usually a complication of another infection (such as scarlet fever, other streptococcal infections, Kawasaki, or others).[21,23,61] Children with acute cholecystitis generally present with abdominal pain localized to the right upper quadrant several days after a systemic infection or a streptococcal pharingitis. The gallbladder may be enlarged and palpable and jaundice may be present. A large gallbladder with a thickened wall may be apparent on ultrasound images. Usually there is no concomitant dilatation of the biliary tree.

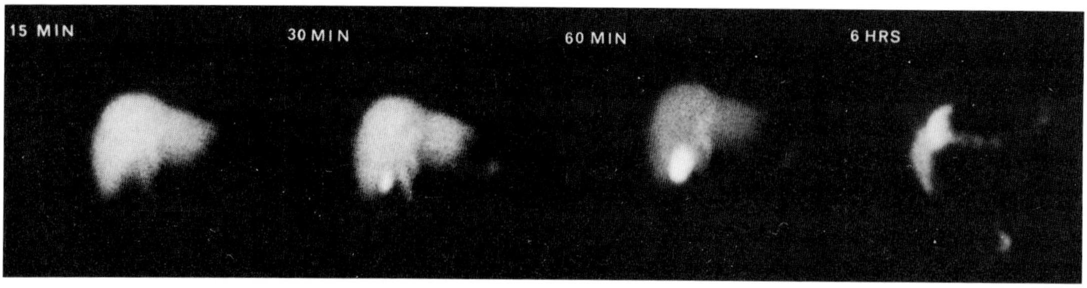

Figure 9-11. Tc-99m BIDA series on a 16-year-old female with right upper quadrant pain for 3 days. The study shows slow passage of tracer into the bowel with failure of the gallbladder to contract at 60 min (following a fatty meal). The gallbladder is visualized clearly at 6 h following another fatty meal. Dismotility? Acalculus cholecystitis?

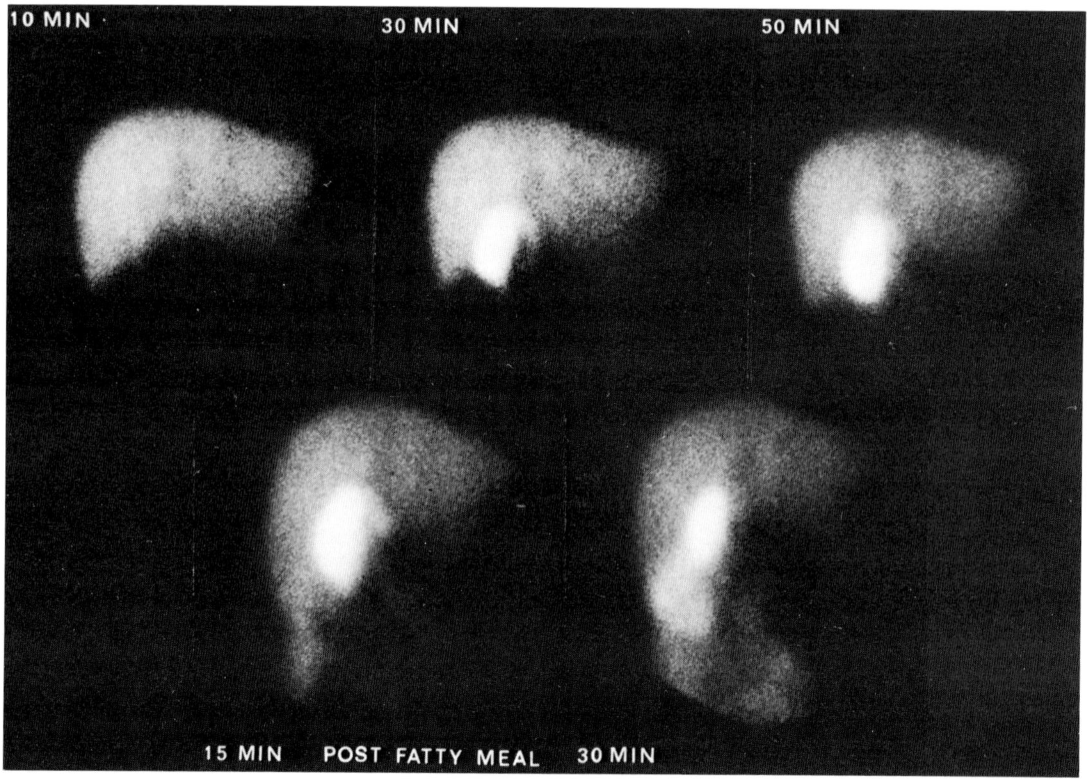

Figure 9-12. Tc-99m *p*-butyl-IDA scintigraphy on a 19-year-old male with right upper quadrant pain and no evidence of stones by ultrasound. There is adequate uptake of the tracer in the liver and rapid filling of an apparently large gallbladder. There was no evidence of passage of the tracer into the bowel up to 50 min. After the fatty meal, the gallbladder does not empty completely and only a little tracer passes into the bowel. This study suggests inflammation with partial obstruction of the choledochus.

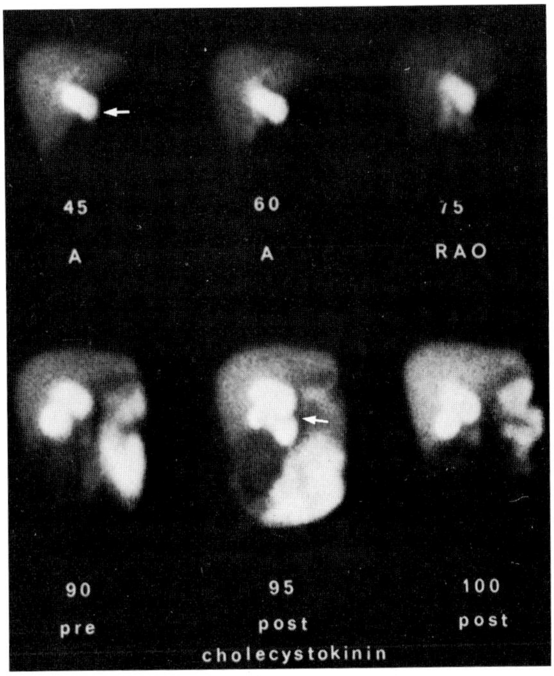

Figure 9-13. Choledochal cyst. Prompt delineation of a dilated common bile duct *(arrow)*. The gallbladder contracts after administration of cholecystokinin while the choledochal cyst shows retention of tracer.

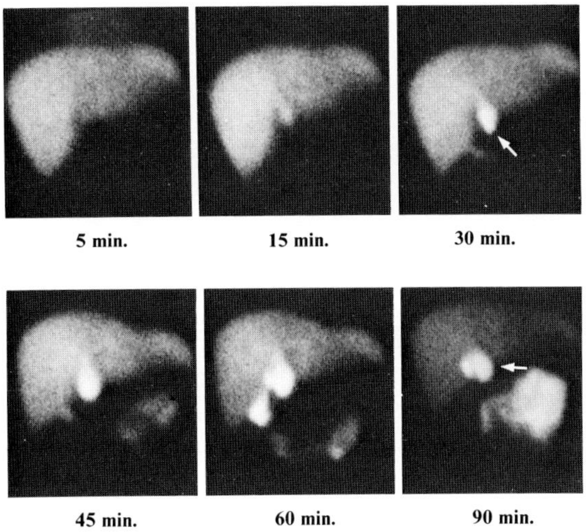

Figure 9-14. Choledochal cyst in a 12-year-old male. Tc-99m BIDA series reveals adequate liver uptake of the tracer with delineation of a dilated common duct *(arrow)* on the images at 15, 30, and 45 min. At 60 min, the gallbladder can be seen with the dilated bile duct superiorly and medially from it. The image at 90 min demonstrates complete drainage of the gallbladder with radiotracer retention within the choledochal cyst *(arrow)*.

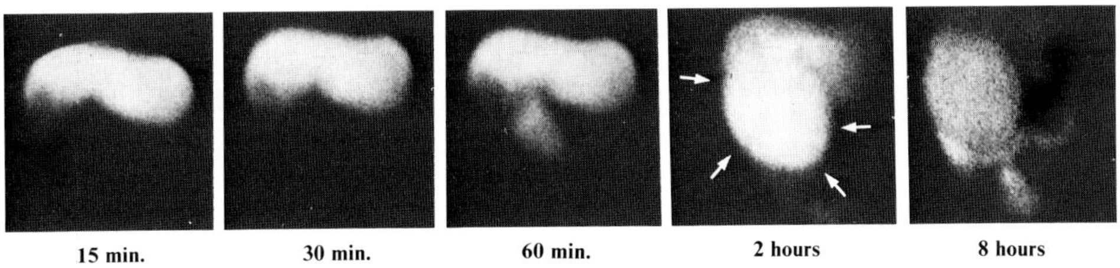

Figure 9-15. Choledochal cyst. Tc-99m BIDA series reveal defect on the inferior aspect of the right lobe of the liver. This defect corresponds to a large choledochal cyst that fills with the radiotracer *(arrows)*.

Choledochal Cyst

Choledochal cyst is a congenital dilatation of the extrahepatic biliary tree (Figs. 9-13–9-15). There are three types of choledochal cyst. The most common one is a dilatation of the common bile duct, which may be accompanied by dilatation of the hepatic ducts. In this type of cyst, the cystic duct and the gallbladder are usually not dilated. About 15% of these patients also have biliary atresia. In a review by Kim,[39] dilatation of the common bile duct accounted for 93% of 188 cases of choledochal cyst reviewed. The second type of choledochal cyst is a diverticulum of the common bile duct with the biliary tree being otherwise normal (diverticulum). The third type is a dilatation of the duodenal intramural portion of the common bile duct (choledochocele).

Ninety percent of the patients with choledochal cyst present before 12 years of age and 70% of them present before 6 years of age, with about 40% presenting before 1 year of age. The lesion occurs 2–3 times more frequently in females than in males. The symptoms of presentation in order of decreasing frequency include jaundice (70%), abdominal pain (55%), dark urine (50%), hepatomegaly (45%), acholic stools (45%), abdominal mass (40%), and fever (35%). Other symptoms include splenomegaly, anemia, cholecystitis, and vomiting.

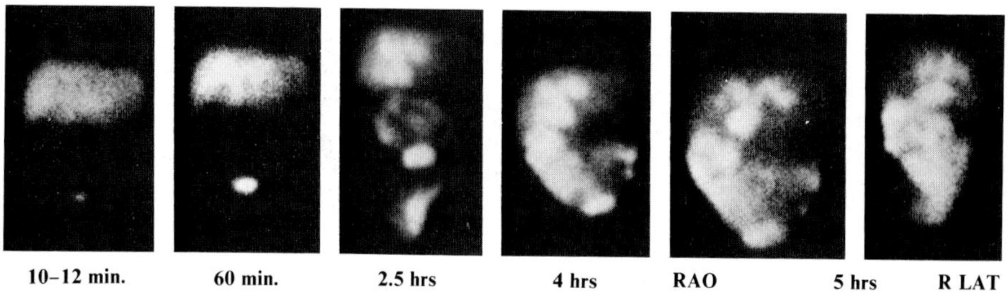

Figure 9-16. Caroli's disease. Tc-99m BIDA series showing marked dilatation of the biliary ducts and delayed hepatic transit time without obstruction.

Caroli's Disease

In Caroli's disease, there is a saccular dilatation of the intrahepatic biliary ducts but no evidence of obstruction of the biliary tract.[13,14] This rare disease is sometimes associated with congenital hepatic fibrosis.[62] Infection of the dilated ducts may result in cholangitis, calculus formation, and cirrhosis. Ultrasonography and transhepatic cholangiography will diagnose this rare disease by demonstrating widespread dilatation of the biliary ducts. Hepatobiliary scintigraphy will also demonstrate dilatation of the ducts and sometimes delay in transit time without obstruction (Fig. 9-16).

Biliary Leak

Biliary leak secondary to trauma or surgical complication can be readily demonstrated with hepatobiliary scintigraphy. This technique can demonstrate leakage of radiotracer into the peritoneal cavity or confined to the hepatic capsule.

Advantages of the tracer method over routine radiographic studies include its inherent higher contrast and lack of interference from bowel gas. Ultrasonography and computed tomography can define biliary collections within the heptic capsule but they cannot determine whether there is an active leak. A radiotracer study can establish the integrity of the capsule and determine the presence of an active leak.[63]

References

1. Anghileri LJ. Preparation of bilirubin labeled with I-131. Int J Appl Radiat Isot 1963; 14:630–3.
2. Ansari AN, Atkins HL, Lambrecht RM. I-123 indocyanine green (I-123 ICG) as an agent for dynamic studies of the hepatobiliary system. In: Dynamic studies with radioisotopes in medicine I. Vienna: IAEA, 1975.
3. Awasthi YC, Dao DD, Saneto RP. Interrelationships between anionic and cationic forms of glutathione *S*-transferases of human liver. Biochem J 1980; 191:1–10.
4. Baker RJ, Bellen JC, Ronai PM. Tc-99m pyridoxylideneglutamate: a new rapid cholescintigraphic agent (abstract). J Nucl Med 1974; 15:476.
5. Bastomsky CH, Horton PW, Shimmins J. Gamma camera study of the hepatobiliary excretion of I-131-thyroxine glucuronide and I-131-rose bengal in the rat. J Nucl Med 1973; 14:34–39.
6. Bobba VVR, Krishnamurthy GT, Kingston E, Brown PH, Eklem M, Turner FE. Comparison of biokinetics and biliary imaging parameters of four Tc-99m iminodiacetic acid derivatives in normal subjects. Clin Nucl Med 1983; 8:70–75.
7. Brent RL, Geppert LJ. The use of radioactive rose bengal in the evaluation of infantile jaundice. J Dis Child 1959; 98:720–30.
8. Burns D, Marzilli L, Sowa D, Baum D, Wagner HN Jr. Relationship between molecular structure and biliary excretion of Tc-99m HIDA and HIDA analogs (abstract). J Nucl Med 1977; 18:624.
9. Burns HD, Sowa DT, Marzilli LG. Improved synthesis of *N*-(2,6-dimethyl-phenyl-carbamoylmethyl) iminodiacetic acid and analogs. J Pharm Sci 1978; 67:1434–6.
10. Burns HD, Sowa DT, Worley P, Vaum R, Marzilli LG. Electrophoretic determination of charge on carrier-free ^{99m}Tc-labeled complexes. J Pharm Sci 1981; 70:436–9.
11. Butterman G, Wolf I, Pabst HW. Quantitative analysis of hepatograms using a gamma camera and labeled contrast media. In: Dynamic studies with radioisotopes in medicine I. Vienna: IAEA, 1975.

12. Callery P, Faith WC. Loberg MD, Fields AT, Harvey EB, Cooper MD. Tissue distribution of Tc-99m and C-14 labeled *N*-(2,6-dimethylphenylcarbamoylmethyl) iminodiacetic acid. J Med Chem 1976; 19:962–4.
13. Caroli J. Diseases of intrahepatic bile ducts. Isr J Med Sci 1968; 4:21–35.
14. Caroli J, Soupault R, Kossakowski J, Plocker L, Paradowska M. La dilatation polykystique congenitale des voies biliaires intrahepatiques. Essai de classification. Semin Hop Paris 1958; 34:488–95.
15. Chaberek S, Martell AE. Stability of metal chelates I. Iminodiacetic and iminodipropionic acids. J Am Chem Soc 1952; 74:5052–6.
16. Chervu LR, Nunn AD, Loberg MD. Radiopharmaceuticals for hepatobiliary imaging. Semin Nucl Med 1982; 12:5–17.
17. Chiotellis E, Varvarigou A. Tc-99m labelled N-substituted carbamoyl iminodiacetates: relationship between structure and biodistribution. Int J Nucl Med Biol 1980; 7:1–7.
18. Christy B, King G, Smoak WM. Preparation of iodine-123 labeled rose-bengal and its distribution in animals (abstract). J Nucl Med 1974; 15:484.
19. Collier BD, Treves S, Davis MA, Heyman S, Subramanian G, McAfee JG. Simultaneous Tc-99m *p*-butyl-IDA and I-131 rose-bengal scintigraphy in neonatal jaundice. Radiology 1980; 134:719–22.
20. Costello CE, Brodack JW, Jones AG, Davison A, Johnson DL, Kasina S, Fritzberg AR. The investigation of radiopharmaceutical components by fast atom bombardment mass spectrometry: the identification of Tc-HIDA and the epimers of Tc-CO_2DADS. J Nucl Med 1983; 24:353–5.
21. Crystal RF, Fink RL. Acute acalculous cholecystitis in childhood. Clin Pediatr 1971; 10:423–6.
22. Czerniak P, Boruchowsky S, Yarshova A, et al. Use of radioactive toludine blue for cholescintigraphy. In: Medical radioisotope scintigraphy II. Vienna: IAEA, 1972.
23. Dickinson SJ, Corley G, Santulli TV. Acute cholecystitis as a sequel of scarlet fever. Am J Dis Child 1971; 121:331–3.
24. Eckelman W, Richards P. Instant ^{99m}Tc-DTPA. J Nucl Med 1970; 11:761.
25. Franken EA, Smith WL, Smith JA, Fitzgerald JR. Percutaneous cholangiography in infants. AJR 1978; 130:1057–8.
26. Gellis SS. Biliary atresia. Pediatrics 1975; 55:8–9.
27. Gerhold JP, Klingensmith WC, Kuni CC, Lilly JR, Silverman A, Fritzberg AR, Nixt TL. Diagnosis of biliary atresia with radionuclide hepatobiliary imaging. Radiology 1983; 146:499–504.
28. Goris ML. I-123-iodo-bromosulphtalein as a liver and biliary scanning agent. J Nucl Med 1973; 14:820–5.
29. Green A. Rosenberg N, Sheahan M. Multicenter trial of Tc-99m disofenin (diisopropylphenylcarbamoylmethyl iminodiacetic acid): a new hepatobiliary agent for imaging jaundiced and unjaundiced patients (abstract). J Nucl Med 1980; 21: 18.
30. Greene HL, Helinek GL, Moran R, O'Neill J. A diagnostic approach to prolonged obstructive jaundice by 24-hour collection of duodenal fluid. J Pediatr 1979; 95:412–4.
31. Hallaba E, Abdullah E. Preparation of diiodo-I-131 fluorescein and tetraiodo-I-131 phenolphthalein for diagnostic purposes. Int J Appl Radiat Isot 1966; 17:424–6.
32. Harvey E, Loberg MD, Cooper M. Tc-99m-HIDA: a new radiopharmaceutical for hepatobiliary imaging (abstract). J Nucl Med 1975; 16:533.
33. Hashimoto T, Yura J. Percutaneous transhepatic cholangiography (PTC) in biliary atresia with special reference to the structure of the intrahepatic bile ducts. J Pediatr Surg 1981; 16:22–25.
34. Hays DM, Woolley MM, Snyder WH Jr, Reed GB, Gwinn JL, Landing BH. Diagnosis of biliary atresia: relative accuracy of percutaneous, liver biopsy, open liver biopsy, and operative cholangiography. J Pediatr 1967; 71:598–607.
35. Hernandez M, Rosenthal L. A cross-over study comparing the kinetics of Tc-99m-labeled diisopropyl and para-butyl IDA analogs in patients. Clin Nucl Med 1980; 5:159–65.
36. Hirsig J, Rickham PP, Early differential diagnosis between neonatal hepatitis and biliary atresia. J Pediatr Surg 1980; 15:13–15.
37. Hitch DC, Shikes RH, Lilly JR. Determinants of survival after Kasai's operation for biliary atresia using actuarial analysis. J Pediatr Surg 1979; 14:310–4.
38. Kasai M, Watanabe I, Ohi R. Follow-up studies of long-term survivors after hepatic portoenterostomy for "noncorrectable" biliary atresia. J Pediatr Surg 1975; 10:173–82.
39. Kim SH. Choledochal cyst: survey by the surgical section of The American Academy of Pediatrics. J Pediatr Surg. 1981; 16:402–7.
40. Klingensmith WC, Fritzberg AR, Koep LJ. Comparison of Tc-99m diethyl-iminodiacetic acid and I-131 rose bengal for hepatobiliary studies in liver transplant patients. J Nucl Med 1979; 20:314–8.
41. Klingensmith WC, Fritzberg AR, Spitzer VM, Koep LJ. Clinical comparison of ^{99m}Tc-diethyl-IDA and ^{99m}Tc-PIPIDA for evaluation of the hepatobiliary system. Radiology 1980; 134:195–9.
42. Klingensmith WC, Fritzberg AR, Spitzer VM, Kuni CC, Shanahan WSM. Clinical comparison of Tc 99m diisopropyl-IDA and diethyl-IDA Tc 99m for evaluation of the hepatobiliary system. Radiology 1981; 140:791–5.
43. Laperche Y, Graillot C, Arondal J, Berthelot P.

Uptake of rifampicin by isolated rat liver cells. Interaction with sulfobromophthalein uptake and evidence for separate carriers. Biochem Pharmacol 1979; 28:2065–9.
44. Loberg MD. Radiotracer distribution by active transport: the implication of non-linear kinetics. In: Colombetti LG, ed. Principles of Radiopharmacology. Boca Raton Fla: CRC Press, 1979.
45. Loberg MD, Cooper M, Harvey E, Callery P, Faith W. Development of new radiopharmaceuticals based on N-substitution of iminodiacetic acid. J Nucl Med 1976; 17:633–8.
46. Loberg MD, Nunn AD, Porter DW. Development of hepatobiliary imaging agents. In: Freeman LM, Weissmann HS, eds. Nuclear medicine annual. New York: Raven Press, 1981.
47. Majd M, Reba RC, Altman RP. Hepatobiliary scintigraphy with Tc-99m PIPIDA in the evaluaton of neonatal jaundice. Pediatrics 1981; 67:140–5.
48. Nunn AD. Structure-distribution relationships of radiopharmaceuticals. Correlation between the reversed-phase capacity factors for Tc-99m phenylcarbamoylmethyliminodiacetic acids and their renal elimination. J Chromatogr 1983; 255:91–100.
49. Nunn AD, Loberg MD, Conley RA. A structure-distribution relationship approach leading to the development of Tc-99m mebroferin: an improved cholescintigraphic agent. J Nucl Med 1983; 24:423–430.
50. Odell GBN, Boitnott JK. Evaluation of jaundice. In: James AE, Wagner HN, Cook RE, eds. Pediatric nuclear medicine. Philadelphia: W.B. Saunders, 1974.
51. Porter DW, Loberg MD, Eacho PI, Weiner M. Comparison of hepatobiliary radiopharmaceuticals in an in-vitro model (abstract). J Nucl Med 1979; 20:642.
52. Reyes H, Levi AJ, Gatmaitan Z, Arias IM. Studies of Y and Z, two hepatic cytoplasmic organic anion-binding proteins: effect of drugs, chemicals, hormones and cholestasis. J Clin Invest 1971; 50:2242–52.
53. Schwenk M. Transport systems of isolated hepatocytes. Studies on the transport of biliary compounds. Arch Toxicol 1980; 44:113–26.
54. Spenney JG, Tobin MM, Mihas AA, Gibson RG, Hirschowitz BI, Johnson BJ, Tauxe WN. Utilization of a radioiodinated bile salt for kinetic studies and hepatic scintigraphy. Studies in nonhuman mammals. Gastroenterology 1979; 76:272–8.
55. Taplin GV, Meredith OM, Kade H. The radioactive I-131 tagged rose bengal uptake excretion test for liver function using eternal gamma ray scintillation counting techniques. J Lab Clin Med 1955; 45:665–78.
56. Tubis M, Blahd DW, Nordyke RA. The preparation and use of radioiodinated congo red in detecting amyloidosis. J Am Pharm Assoc Sci Ed 1960; 49:422–5.
57. Tubis M, Nordyke RA, Posnick E, Blahd WH. Preparation and use of ^{131}I labeled sulfobromophtalein in liver function testing. J Nucl Med 1961; 2:282–8.
58. Utz JA, Lull RJ, Anderson JH, Lambrecht RW, Brown JM, Henry W. Hepatoma visulaization with Tc-99m pyridoxylidene glutamate. J Nucl Med 1980; 21:747–9.
59. Van Rijk PP, DeGraff CN. I-131 asialo-1-acid-glycoprotein. A new radiopharmaceutical for dynamic liver function studies. In: Dynamic studies with radioisotopes in medicine I. Vienna: IAEA, 1975.
60. Vonk RJ, Danhof M, Coenraads T, Van Doorn ABD, Keulmans K, Scaf AHJ, Meijer DKF. Influence of bile salts on hepatic transport of dibromosulphthalein. Am J Physiol 1979; 237:524-34
61. Walker CHM. Aetiology of cholelithiasis in childhood. Arch Dis Child 1957; 32:293–7.
62. Wechsler RL. Van Thiel D. Fibropolycystic disease of the hepatobiliary system and kidneys. Am J Dig Dis 1976; 21:1058–69.
63. Weissmann HS, Chun KH, Frank MS, Koenigsberg M, Milstein DM, Freeman LM. Demonstration of traumatic bile leakage with cholescintigraphy and ultrasonography. AJR 1979; 133:843–7.
64. Weissmann HS, Frank M, Bernstein LM, Freeman LM. Rapid and accurate diagnosis of acute cholecystitis with Tc-99m HIDA cholescintigraphy. AJR 1979; 132:523–8.
65. Weissmann HS, Rosenblatt R, Sugarman LA, Freeman LM. The role of nuclear imaging in evaluating the patient with cholestasis. Semin Ultrasound 1980; 1:134–42.
66. Weissmann HS, Sugarman LA, Freeman LM. The clinical role of technetium-99m iminodiacetic acid cholescintigraphy. In: Freeman LM, Weissmann HS, eds. Nuclear medicine annual. New York: Raven Press, 1981.
67. Weissman HS, Badia J, Sugarman LA, Kluger L, Rosenblatt R, Freeman LM. Spectrum of cholescintigraphic patterns in acute cholecystitis. Radiology 1981; 138:167–75.
68. Wistow BW, Subramanian G, Van Heertum RL, Henderson RW, Gagne GM, Hall RC, McAfee JG. An evaluation of ^{99m}Tc-labeled hepatobiliary agents. J Nucl Med 1977; 18:455–61.
69. Yokoyama A, Terauchi Y, Horiuchi K, Tanaka H, Odori T, Morita R, Mori T, Torizuka K. Technetium-99m kethoxal-bis(thiosemicarboxone), an uncharged complex with a tetravelant ^{99m}Tc state, and its excretion into the bile. J Nucl Med 1976; 17:816–19.

Chapter 10 Gastroesophageal Reflux and Gastric Emptying

Paul Rosen
S. T. Treves

Gastroesophageal reflux (GER) may be defined as a dysfunction of the distal esophagus causing return of gastric contents into the esophagus.[13] GER is a rather common problem during infancy, with an incidence estimated as 1 in 500 infants. The common clinical manifestations of GER can be attributed to the regurgitation of acidic gastric contents into the esophagus. In reviewing the symptomatology associated with GER, Weissbluth[28] summarized the clinical features in 1070 children with GER. Vomiting occurred in two-thirds of the children, usually beginning at birth, and frequently associated with loss of appetite resulting in weight loss or failure to thrive. Twenty-eight percent of the children exhibited bleeding secondary to esophagitis caused by erosion of the lower esophageal mucosa. Nineteen percent of the patients had associated respiratory symptomatology.[27] Symptoms frequently will mimic those of allergic bronchitis, asthma, or recurrent episodes of pneumonitis. The findings of airway disease in association with reflux do not suggest a causal relationship. However, a series reported by Berquist et al.[3] revealed a significant improvement in respiratory symptomatology upon medical or surgical therapy for GER.

There are some rare complications of GER that are not such obvious consequences of reflux. These include a "pseudoneurologic syndrome" with unusual posturing manifested by dystonia associated with dysphagia, irritability, and developmental retardation.[5] Some infants with GER may present with apnea, cyanosis, and what appears to be near-miss sudden infant death syndrome.[14,19] The contribution of GER to the etiology of sudden infant death syndrome is unclear at this point. Finally, Herbst et al.[15] reported a group of 14 patients with severe prolonged lung disease in the neonatal period. In these infants, GER was implicated as a major problem contributing to the patient's difficult course. However, there is no clear data concerning the frequency of complications of GER contributing to chronic lung disease in premature infants.

Carre[7] has evaluated the natural history of GER. He notes that almost all infants with GER will have symptoms by 6 weeks of age, and indeed, 97% of patients will exhibit symptoms by 3 months of age. In the absence of therapy approximately 60% of patients will be symptom-free by 18 months of age, with the greatest improvement occurring when the child starts to sit up at 8–10 months of age. A remaining 30% will continue to have symptoms until 4 years of age. In the absence of therapy, approximately 5% will develop esophageal strictures. Knowledge of the above natural history suggests that only a small percentage of children have or will develop complications warranting aggressive surgical intervention. In addition, medical therapy may be more confidently prolonged in an infant in whom the natural history suggests a favorable outcome.

Several methods are available to diagnose and quantitate GER. These include fluoroscopy after barium feedings, in conjunction with an upper gastrointestinal series; esophageal manometry; endoscopy; pH probe monitoring, in conjunction with a Tuttle Test; and extended pH probe evaluation for a 24-h period. Gastroesophageal scintigraphy has been advocated as an alternative noninvasive study requiring no sedation.[16,21] Scintigraphy offers the advantages of prolonged observation, high sensitivity, and low radiation exposure.

Data concerning gastric emptying are frequently recorded simultaneously with examination for GER. Interest in these associated data in infants and children has increased. This is a result of descriptions of GER associated with delayed gastric emptying[2,17] and recent reports of antral dysmotility causing chronic vomiting and GER in infants.[6] Gastric emptying studies are occasionally performed in patients who have experienced abdominal surgery, or who have required gastrostomies to maintain an adequate caloric intake and nutritional state.

Method

Radiopharmaceuticals

The radiopharmaceutical utilized for the gastric esophageal scintigraphy, as well as for gastric emptying studies, is Tc-99m sulfur colloid. Studies by Heyman et al.[16] demonstrated the stability of a milk-sulfur colloid mixture in an acidic medium. The use of Tc-99m pertechnetate is not appropriate due to its absorption through the gastric mucosa and its solubility in the lungs.

Heyman et al.[16] estimated the absorbed radiation dose in infants as 300–500 mR to the stomach, 17–36 mrad to the gonads and a total body dose of 33–65 mrad. These estimates were predicted on a feeding of 5 μCi/ml of Tc-99m sulfur colloid in volumes of 30 ml–200 ml for up to 1 year of age. Siegel et al.[25] calculated the radiation burden for 1 mCi of oral Tc-99m DTPA administered to an adult. Absorbed dose was highest for the upper large intestine—520 mrad. An ovarian dose of 98 mrad and a total body burden of 20 mrad were estimated.

Technique of Examination

Patients are studied in the fasting state, after either having missed their previous feeding or having fasted for a minimum of 4 h. The volume of the patient's usual meal is administered as 5% glucose and water, milk, or formula. The dose of Tc-99m sulfur colloid is dissolved in a small volume of feeding, administered to the patient, and followed by a second, tracer-free, volume to complete the feeding.

The usual activity administered is 5 μCi/ml, with a minimum of 200 μCi and a maximum of 1 mCi.

After completion of feeding, the infants are burped and placed supine with the gamma camera positioned anteriorly or posteriorly (Fig. 10-1). A low-energy, high-sensitivity collimator is utilized. The infant is positioned to include the stomach, the thorax, and the mouth in the field-of-view. Analog images are generated every 2 min for 1 h. Data are recorded in the computer at a rate of one frame/30 sec for 1 h (Fig. 10-2). At the conclusion of the first hour, the patient is released to resume normal feeding and activities. Two to three hours later, a computerized anterior image of the chest is obtained.

Computer analysis includes contrast enhancement to improve visualization of low levels of activity representing small volumes of gastric activity in either the esophagus or the lungs (Figs. 10-3 and 10-4). The frames of the study are also displayed in a cinematographic mode which is helpful to trace the temporal course of reflux and gastric emptying. Regions of interest (ROIs) are drawn over the esophagus and stomach followed by calculation of time-activity curves to determine the duration and amount of esophageal reflux as well as the pattern and amount of gastric emptying

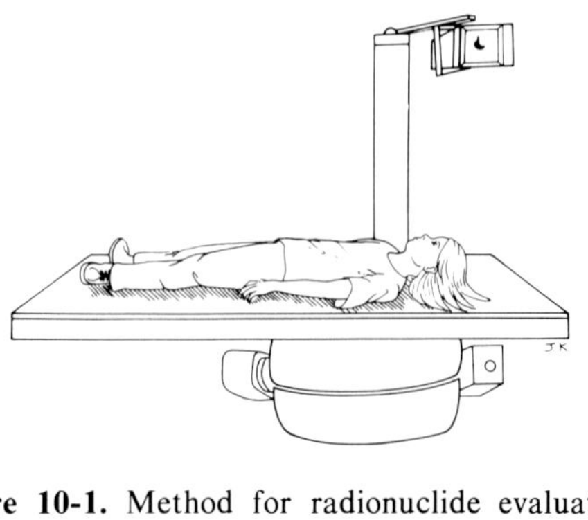

Figure 10-1. Method for radionuclide evaluation of GER and gastric emptying. The patient lies supine on the examining table and the gamma camera views the upper abdomen, thorax, and mouth.

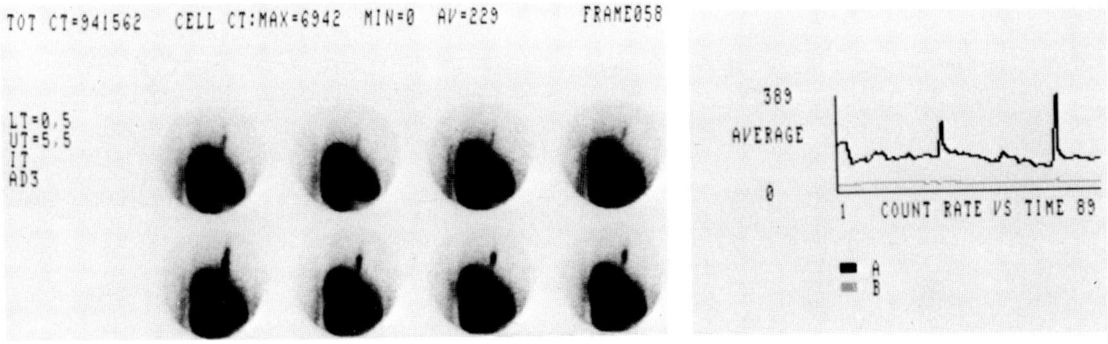

Figure 10-2. *Left:* Series of images after oral administration of Tc-99m sulfur colloid showing intermittent GER (each frame represents 120 sec). The images are processed so that the lowest count rates are represented more vividly. *Right:* Time-activity curve over the esophagus showing two episodes of reflux. The patient was a 1-month-old who had apneic spells and frequent vomiting.

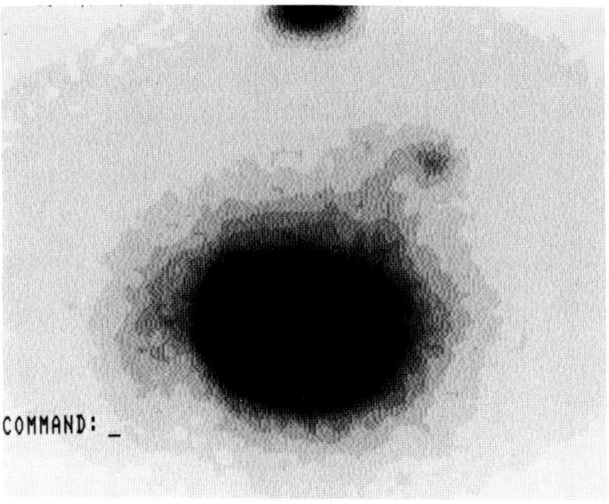

Figure 10-3. Aspiration of Tc-99m sulfur colloid in the right lower lung field. The image was obtained 5 min after ingestion of the tracer.

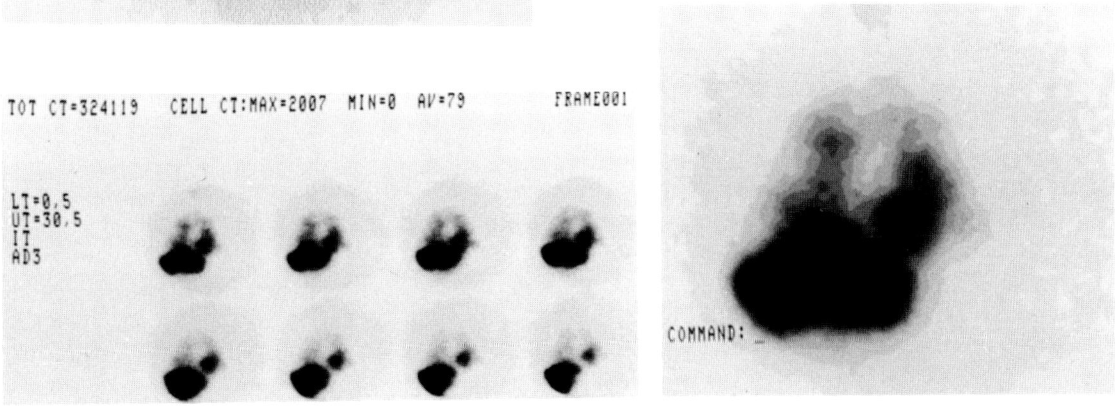

Figure 10-4. Massive aspiration of Tc-99m sulfur colloid during feeding. The tracer is seen widely throughout both lungs.

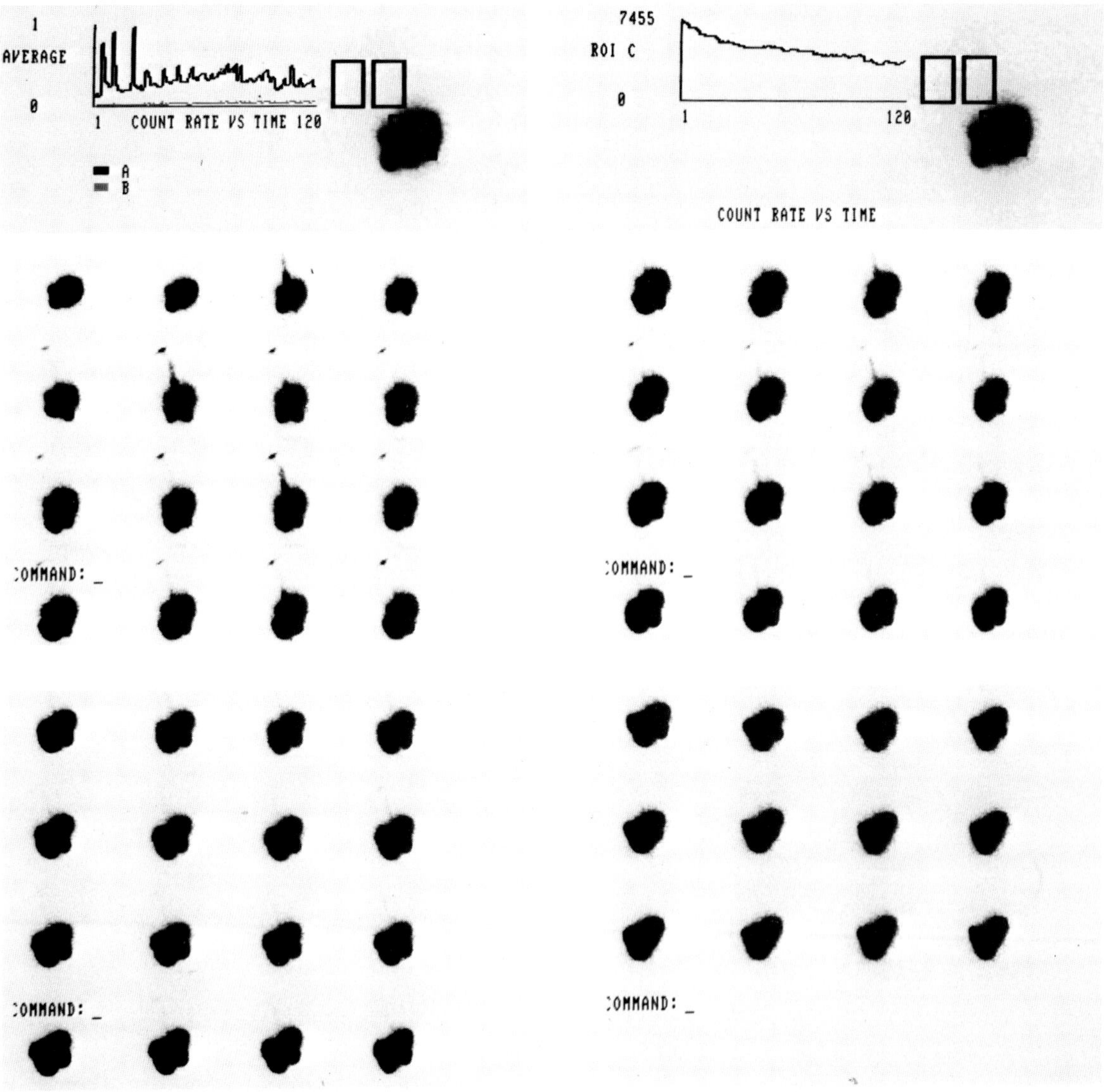

Figure 10-5. Series of computer images showing multiple episodes of GER. Esophageal time-activity curves show several peaks during the hour of observation *(top, left)*. The gastric emptying curve *(top, right)* shows normal gastric emptying.

(Fig. 10-5). If movement of the patient or superimposition of small intestinal activity occurs, gastric emptying is determined using the total activity in the gastric region for the initial and final frames of the study.

The percent gastric residual is simply calculated as follows:

$$\% \text{ Gastric residual} = \frac{\text{Gastric counts at 60 sec} \times 100}{\text{Initial gastric counts}}$$

Clinical Applications: Interpretation

No single method has emerged as the best for evaluation of children for GER. Blumhagen et al.[4] compared the acid reflux test, barium esophagography with water-siphon testing, and gastroesophageal scintigraphy. They questioned the importance of one or two episodes of reflux in the first 5 min on radionuclide studies, and therefore graded patients as the following grades: 0; none; 1; less than two episodes in the first 5 min; 2, up to four episodes; and 3, greater than five episodes. A study with grades 0 or 1 was considered negative. This grading resulted in a radionuclide sensitivity of 75% and a specificity of 71%, using the acid reflux study as the standard. The barium study exhibits considerably less specificity.

Arasu et al.[1] performed a similar prospective study, adding esophageal manometry and endoscopy to the procedures evaluated. Demonstration of any esophageal activity was considered indicative of GER, and no attempt was made to grade severity. A group of 30 patients with symptoms of GER were studied in conjunction with 15 "control" patients with no such symptomatology. The control group experienced no positive tests with the upper gastrointestinal series, radionuclide study, or the acid reflux test. In the group with GER symptomatology, 15 patients had positive barium examination, 17 positive radionuclide examinations (sensitivity of 56.6%), and 29 experienced a positive acid Tuttle test. Using the acid reflux test, a single episode of reflux was considered a negative test. Arasu et al.[1] concluded that the acid reflux test correlates best with GER symptomatology, and that the upper gastorintestinal and radionuclide studies complement each other with respect to the identification of patients with GER.

Finally, Seibert et al.,[22] using 24-h pH probe as the "gold standard," compared radionuclide gastroesophageal scintigraphy and simultaneous 1-h pH probe, as well as upper gastrointestinal barium studies. Their results demonstrated a sensitivity for scintigraphy of 79% and a specificity of 93%, compared with barium upper gastrointestinal study sensitivity of 86% and a specificity of 21%. If the 24-h study was used as the "gold standard," only one episode of reflux was considered necessary for scintigraphy to be positive. Reflux was significant anytime during the 1-h monitoring. This group recommended on the basis of their results that all patients who are evaluated for vomiting have an upper gastrointestinal series to ensure that the vomiting is not caused by anatomic conditions such as duodenal or antral webs. In addition, radionuclide gastroesophageal scintigraphy is used, which if positive for reflux results in medical treatment, i.e., freqent small feedings and upright positioning. If delayed gastric emptying is identified in conjunction with the gastroesophageal scintigraphy, they recommend metoclopramide or bethanechol. A lack of response to medical treatment results in the evaluation being extended to a 24-h pH probe. This is the approach that we ascribe to at this time, with any episode of reflux during the 1 h considered as a positive study.

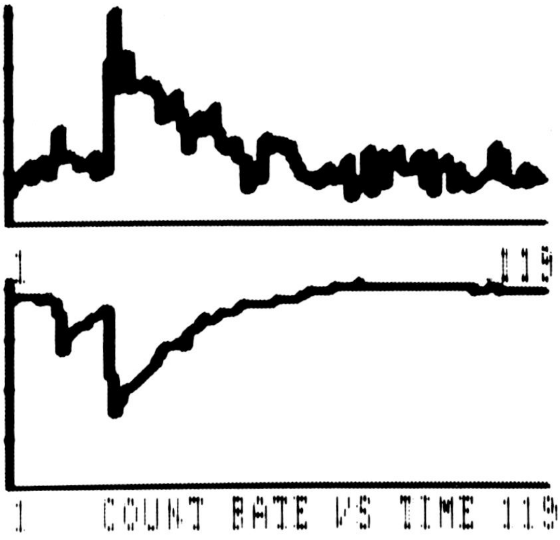

Figure 10-6. Simultaneous record of esophageal pH *(bottom)* and radionuclide activity *(top)* demonstrates an increase in count rate in the esophagus concomitant with a decrease of esophageal pH.

In additon to the initial 1-h record, patients return for static images of the chest 2–4 h following the initial study. If this portion of the study is positive, it certainly provides direct evidence of reflux and pulmonary aspiration. Heyman et al.[16] reported that 2 of 39 patients exhibited positive delayed chest images. Volumes as small as 0.25 ml should be detectable.

Comparison of the determination of GER by radionuclides and by simultaneous esophageal pH probe monitoring are favorable. We have recorded simultaneously the computer tracings of esophageal activity and pH in a small number of patients (Fig. 10-6). In some instances lack of correlation (i.e., reflux by radionuclide and lack of pH lowering) was probably due to the buffering of stomach content by the milk or formula. In our studies we find GER to be highly variable in the same patient (Treves S, Winter H, Heyman S, Abramson S, Papanicolaou N, unpublished observations).

The reported incidence for GER in children with chronic pulmonary disease varies from 16 to 75%.[12]

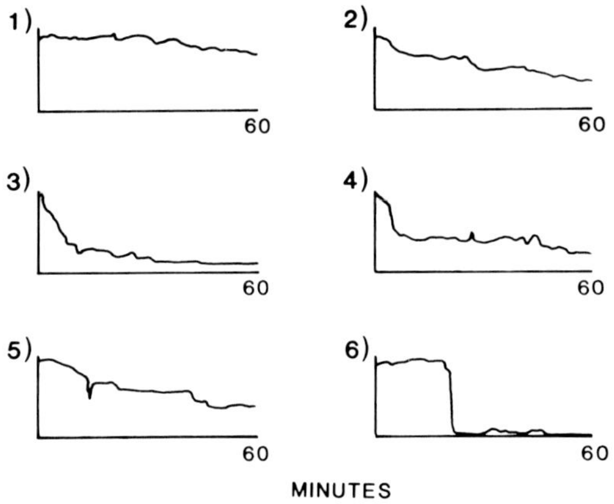

Figure 10-7. Various patterns of gastric emptying. Each curve represents the counts from the gastric area during 1 h of observation.

Several clinical features have been noted as more apparent in patients with GER and pulmonary disease and may serve as guidelines in the selection of patients for GER studies. A significant number of patients with GER have a history of recurrent pneumonitis and nocturnal cough. Although an association between acid reflux and pulmonary disease has been demonstrated in numerous studies, this does not establish a causal relationship. Berquist et al.[3] reported the results of fundoplication in 24 patients with GER and associated recurrent pneumonia and chronic asthma. Twenty-two of these 24 patients improved dramatically and indeed became asymptomatic following fundoplication. This would seem to establish that at least in some patients, GER is associated with recurrent pulmonary disease in a causal manner. Identical difficulties arise in evaluation of the role of GER in infants with apnea and cyanosis. The presence of an association of these two entities may simply reflect a higher degree of physiologic immaturity in these infants. Indeed, the temporal association of reflux with episodes of apnea has not been confirmed.

The interpretation of gastric emptying in conjunction with GER is exceedingly difficult. The patterns of gastric emptying are quite variable (Fig. 10-7). This difficulty reflects the complex nature of the physiologic event being measured. Comparison of studies should be made keeping in mind the variability introduced by alterations in volumes fed, nature of the feeding, and the age of the subjects. When this is combined with variable methods of data recording and analysis, it is even more difficult to establish comparable normal values. This difficulty in the establishment of normal values for infants and children is compounded by the lack of normal controls. We feel that it is not appropriate to subject normal infants who do not have any symptoms of reflux to either barium swallows, invasive monitoring, or radioisotope gastric emptying studies.

Expressing gastric emptying as percent gastric residual at 60 min analysis of the data acquired at Children's Hospital revealed no difference in gastric emptying between those with and without GER. Values obtained did seem to be age-related, with the group <2 years of age exhibiting a mean percent residual of 53, and the group >2 years of age having a mean percent residual of 30.[20] This agrees with Seibert et al.[23] who were also unable to demonstrate a relationship between GER and gastric emptying, thereby disagreeing with Hillemeier, whose work showed a distinct delay of gastric emptying rates in those with GER.

The above studies all exhibit a wide range and standard deviation of data, resulting in unclear delineation of normal and abnormal values for gastric emptying. Further, as clinicians develop a greater interest in gastric emptying, the adequacy of the percent residual as a valid expression of gastric emptying may be questioned.[10,11] Numerous studies in the literature on adults express gastric emptying data as $T_{1/2}$, using the work by Hunt et al.[18] which demonstrated a monoexponential pattern for this physiologic function. There are numerous recent studies showing that the pattern of gastric emptying is frequently multiexponential in form, with early phases of either rapid or slower emptying.[8,9,24,26] We question the applicability of simple and rigid models to the analysis of gastric emptying (Fig. 10-7). Although we continue to report the percent residual gastric contents at 60 min, reporting the entire time-activity curve for the course of study and examining other statistical parameters may enable comparison of sequential studies in patients prior to and following therapy, as well as between groups. Regardless of the method of analysis, gastric emptying should be recorded in a rigorous, standardized manner, particularly if sequential studies are being performed. Interpretation of gastric emptying data should be performed with caution and after statistical analysis of the patient population being studied.

References

1. Arasu TS, Wyllie R, Fitzgerald JF, Franken EA, Siddiqui AR, Lehman GA, Eigen H, Grosfeld JL. Gastroesophageal reflux in infants and children. Comparative accuracy of diagnostic methods. J Pediatr 1980; 96:798–803.
2. Behar J, Ramsby G. Gastric emptying and antral motility in reflux esophagitis. Gastroenterology 1978; 74:253–6.
3. Berquist WE, Rachelefsky GS, Kadden M, Siegel SC, Katz RM, Fonkalsrud EW, Ament ME, Gastroesophageal reflux-associated recurrent pneumonia and chronic asthma in children. Pediatrics 1981 68:29–35.
4. Blumhagen JD, Rudd TG, Christie DL. Gastroesophageal reflux in children: radionuclide gastroesophagography. AJR 1980; 135:1001–4.
5. Bray PF, Herbst JJ, Johnson DG, Book LS, Ziter FA, Condon VR. Childhood GER. Neurologic and psychiatric syndromes mimicked. JAMA 1977; 237:1342–5.
6. Byrne WJ, Kangarloo H, Ament ME, Lo CW, Berquist W, Foglia R, Fonkalsrud EW. "Antral dysmotility": an unrecognized cause of chronic vomiting during infancy. Ann Surg 1981; 193:521–4.
7. Carre IJ. The natural history of the partial thoracic stomach ("hiatal hernial") in children. Arch Dis Child 1959; 34:344.
8. Cavell B. Gastric emptying in preterm infants. Acta Paediatr Scand 1979; 68:725–30.
9. Cavell B. Gastric emptying in infants fed human milk or infant formula. Acta Paediatr Scand 1981; 70:639–41.
10. Dugas MC, Schade RR, Lhotsky D, Van Theil D. Comparison of methods for analyzing gastric isotopic emptying. Am J Physiol 1982; 243:G237–G242.
11. Elashoff JD, Reedy TJ, Meyer JH. Analysis of gastric emptying data. Gastroenterology 1982; 83:1306–12.
12. Euler AR, Byrne WJ, Ament ME, Fonkalsrud EW, Strobel CT, Siegel SC, Katz RM, Rachelefsky GS. Recurrent pulmonary disease in children: a complication of GER. Pediatrics 1979; 63:47–51.
13. Herbst JJ. Gastroesophageal reflux. J Pediatr 1981; 98:859–70.
14. Herbst JJ, Book LS, Bray PF. GER in the "near miss" sudden infant death syndrome. J Pediatr 1978; 92:73–75.
15. Herbst JJ, Minton SD, Book LS. Gastroesophageal reflux causing respiratory distress and apnea in newborn infants. J Pediatr 1979; 95:762–8.
16. Heyman S, Kirkpatric JA, Winter HS, Treves S. An improved method for the diagnosis of gastroesophageal reflux and aspiration in children (milk scan). Radiology 1979; 131:479–82.
17. Hillemeier AC, Lange R, McCallum R, Seashore J, Gryboski J. Delayed gastric emptying in infants with gastroesophageal reflux. J Pediatr 1981; 98:190–3.
18. Hunt JN. Gastric emptying and secretion in man. Physiol Rev 1959; 39:491–533.
19. Leape LL, Holder TM, Franklin JD, Amoury RA, Ashcraft KW. Respiratory arrest in infants secondary to GER. Pediatrics 1977; 60:924–8.
20. Rosen PR, Treves S. The relationship of gastroesophageal reflux and gastric emptying in infants and children: Concise communication. J Nucl Med 1984; 25:571–574.
21. Rudd TG, Christie DL. Demonstration of GER in children by RN gastroesophagography. Radiology 1979; 131:483–6.
22. Seibert JJ, Byrne WJ, Euler AR. Gastric emptying in children. AJR 1983; 141:49–51.
23. Seibert JJ, Byrne WJ, Euler AR, Latture T, Leach M, Campbell M. Gastroesophageal reflux—the acid test. AJR 1983; 140:1087–90.
24. Siegel M, Lebenthal E. Development of gastrointestinal motility and gastric emptying during the fetal and newborn periods. In: Lebenthal E, ed. Textbook of gastroenterology and nutrition in infancy. New York: Raven Press, 1981.
25. Siegel JA, Wu RK, Knight LC, Zelac RE, Stern HS, Dalnud LS. Radiation dose estimates for oral agents used in upper gastrointestinal disease. J Nucl Med 1983; 24:835–7.
26. Signer E, Fridrich R. Gastric emptying in newborns and young infants. Acta Paediatr Scand 1975; 64:525–30.
27. Weissbluth M. Gastroesophageal reflux. Clin Pediatr 1981; 20:7–14.

Chapter 11 Meckel's Diverticulum

S. T. Treves
Richard Grand

The primary application of technetium-99m (Tc-99m) pertechnetate scintigraphy of the abdomen is in the diagnosis of Meckel's diverticulum. Abdominal scintigraphy with the pertechnetate anion (Tc-99mO_4^-) was initially proposed for identifying Meckel's diverticula containing gastric mucosa by Harden et al.[21] and was subsequently introduced into clinical practice for this purpose by Jewett et al.[30] in 1970. Since then, many reports have demonstrated the safety and effectiveness of the examination. An excellent two-part review of the subject has been written by Sfakianakis and Conway.[63,64] Because Meckel's diverticulum cannot be diagnosed reliably by other imaging methods,[6,14,17,46] radiopertechnetate scintigraphy is currently the best nonoperative method of definitive diagnosis for this condition. The radiation exposure is approximately equivalent to 20 sec of radiographic fluoroscopy.[12]

Meckel's (or ileal) diverticulum is a noninherited congenital abnormality of the antimesenteric side of the small intestine resulting from incomplete closure of the embryonic vitelline or omphalomesenteric duct. Meckel's diverticuli may measure 1–56 cm in length and 1–50 cm in diameter. Most Meckel's diverticula are found within the ileum approximately 90 cm proximal to the ileocecal valve.[15]

The first recorded observation of an ileal diverticulum has been attributed to Fabricius Hildamus in 1650,[24] and the first comprehensive embryologic and pathologic description of the lesion was made by Johan Friedrick Meckel, the younger, in 1809.

A Meckel's diverticulum usually contains ileal mucosa, but it has been found to contain gastric mucosa, duodenal mucosa, jejunal mucosa, colonic mucosa, or pancreatic tisuue. Heterotopic tissue in a diverticulum of the pancreatic type was reported by Zonkel in 1861 and of the gastric type by Tillmans in 1882. The relationship of aberrant gastric mucosa to ulcer of a diverticulum was considered by Deetz in 1907. Gastric mucosa is present in Meckel's diverticuli in about 50% of cases.[2,57]

Meckel's diverticulum is the most common cause of lower gastrointestinal hemorrhage in previously healthy infants, and more than 50% of infants with the remnant have symptoms before the second year of life.[58] Clinical symptoms occur in 25–30% of all the patients. Estimates of the probable incidence of Meckel's diverticulum in the general population range from about 1 to 3%, with a frequency 3 times greater in males than in females.[2] The most common symptom of Meckel's diverticulum is rectal bleeding with or without associated abdominal symptoms. The bleeding apparently results from mucosal ulceration in the diverticulum or in the adjacent ileum caused by hydrochloric acid secreted by the ectopic gastric mucosa. Nearly all diverticula of patients with symptoms of gastrointestinal bleeding contain ectopic gastric mucosa.[2,35,36,43,48,58] Other pathologic conditions associated with Meckel's diverticulum include intestinal obstruction due to bands, knots, volvulus, or intussusception; regional enteritis; hernia; enterolith; calcification; diverticulitis; tuberculosis; and foreign body.[8,58]

Some years ago we reviewed the records of all

patients with Meckel's diverticulum under 2 years of age undergoing operation at the Children's Hospital in Boston between 1951 and 1972. Among 60 infants under 2 years of age, 32 had painless rectal bleeding. Of these 32, 56% presented before reaching 1 year of age and the remaining 44% before 2 years of age. Among those symptomatic patients, 91% (29 of 32 patients) had ectopic gastric mucosa in their Meckel's diverticula.[46]

The differential diagnosis of rectal bleeding in infants <2 years of age includes Meckel's diverticulum, anal fissure, volvulus, intussusception, peptic ulcer, and colonic polyp. Of these, only colonic polyp and Meckel's diverticulum usually cause painless bleeding. Radiologic studies using barium by mouth or by rectum only exceptionally demonstrate Meckel's diverticula, as this contrast material rarely enters the lesion.

Indications

A pediatric patient who presents with rectal bleeding suspected to be caused by ulceration of Meckel's diverticulum should have a complete physical examination which may include a careful examination of the anal area, rectoscopy, or sigmoidoscopy in order to exclude distal colonic disease and, where indicated, a hematologic examination to exclude a generalized bleeding disorder. A Tc-99m pertechnetate abdominal survey should then be performed.

Method

Radiopharmaceuticals

Abdominal scintigraphy does not detect a Meckel's diverticulum per se but will reveal uptake of radiopertechnetate by functioning ectopic gastric mucosa within the diverticulum. Normally about 25% of the intravenously administered dose of Tc-99m sodium pertechnetate localizes in the wall of the stomach.

A number of workers have investigated the cellular localization of Tc-99m pertechnetate in the stomach. Kerzmidas et al.[33] found no significant differences in the concentration of pertechnetate in the body and antrum of the stomach in dogs. Meier-Ruge and Freidrich, using microautoradiography, demonstrated that Tc-99m as sodium pertechnetate is selectively taken up by the parietal cells of the stomach whereas I-131 as sodium iodine is absorbed and secreted by the gastric chief and mucosal cells.[47] Wine et al.,[74] using Heidenhain pouches and denervated antral pouches in dogs, suggested that parietal cells are not essential for Tc-99m pertechnetate concentration and that both acid output and volume output relate to the amount of Tc-99m output. Priebe et al.[55] found that contact radioautographs of canine gastric mucosa demonstrated Tc-99m concentrated in surface mucous cells of the gastric pits but not in the gastric glands. Berquist et al.[4,5] showed, by autoradiography, pertechnetate concentration in the superficial cells only. These authors also had six cases of histologically proven Barrett's esophagus, in all of whom the radionuclide scans were abnormal. Biopsy material revealed complete absence of parietal cells in all but one. In contrast, the gastric type of surface epithelial cells were present in every case.

The pertechnetate anion is now believed to be accumulated selectively by surface cells of gastric mucosa and then secreted into the bowel lumen, although the mechanism of secretion is not clear.[9,10,69,75]

Approximately 20% of the injected dose of Tc-99m sodium pertechnetate is rapidly eliminated by the kidneys. Organs that also normally concentrate radiopertechnetate include the choroid plexus, the thyroid, and the salivary glands.[22,23,37,39] The blood disappearance rate of Tc-99m pertechnetate may be prolonged in small infants due to renal immaturity, a normally low gastric mucosal uptake, or both. Slow blood disappearance and low gastric uptake of pertechnetate in older children who have normal renal function may be caused by hormonal, vascular, or stress-related factors.

A variety of drugs and hormones affect the gastric uptake of pertechnetate. Perchlorate suppresses uptake of pertechnetate by the gastric mucosa two- to fourfold.[34,42,51,62,73] Although administration of perchlorate has not actually been known to result in failure to identify a Meckel's diverticulum, this is theoretically possible. Consequently, we do not recommend premedication with perchlorate in patients undergoing radiopertechnetate abdominal scintigraphy.

Pentagastrin increases gastric mucosal uptake of pertechnetate and it has been used to enhance imaging on patients and animals.[28,31,32,34,70]

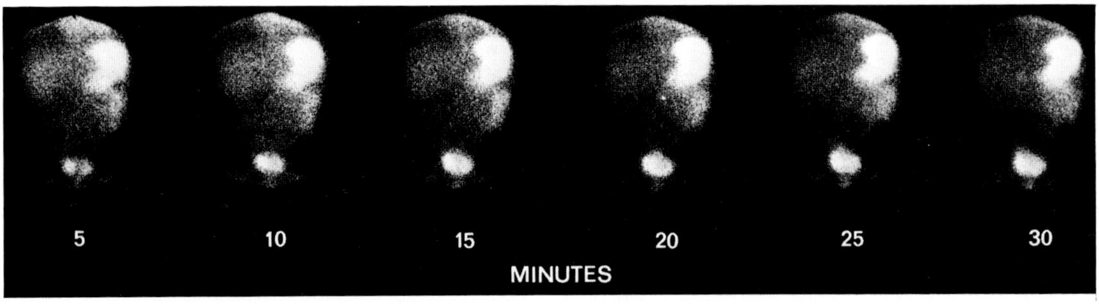

Figure 11-1. Normal abdominal scintigraphy. A 25-month-old boy was evaluated because of abdominal pain and reddish stools. The patient had a history of intussusception 3 months prior to this study. Sigmoidoscopy, barium enema, an air contrast study, and an upper gastrointestinal series with small bowel follow through had been normal. The radiopertechnetate abdominal survey is normal, and at 5 min, the cardiac and hepatic blood pools can be seen. There is also activity in the stomach and urinary bladder as well as in the small bowel. The series of images over time demonstrate lowering blood background, increasing gastric uptake, and increasing activity in the bladder.

Cimetidine and glucagon show promise for clinical use. Cimetidine, a histamine H_2-receptor antagonist, inhibits release of pertechnetate by the intraluminal cells.[52,59] Glucagon, however, reduces slightly gastric activity of pertechnetate, suppresses peristaltic activity,[50] and has been shown to improve imaging in animals.[1]

Other agents that have been investigated include histalog,[34,55] which had lesser effect than pentagastrin, and secretin.[34] Secretin has little effect on pertechnetate localization.

A case report has shown the failure of intravenous pertechnetate to leave the intravascular space in the presence of hyperaluminemia. Normal uptake returned 2 months after the aluminum hydroxide medication was discontinued.[71]

Examination Technique

Patient Preparation

The patient should fast for about 4 h prior to the study to reduce the apparent size of the stomach. Infants who have been fed recently may require nasogastric aspiration.[18,53,67] No sodium or potassium perchlorate should be administered before the test, but perchlorate may be given after the completion of the study in order to wash the radiotracer from the thyroid.[63,64] Barium studies (barium enema, barium swallow) should not be performed within 3–4 days before abdominal scintigraphy because the contrast material can prevent detection of a Meckel's diverticulum by shielding the gamma rays of Tc-99m.[5,46]

Concentration of the radiotracer in ectopic gastric mucosa can be increased with one of several drugs. Pentagastrin (6 μg/kg of body weight subcutaneously) is given 5–15 min before administering the tracer to stimulate uptake in gastric mucosa.[70] Because of the potential of this drug to cause further bleeding, the patient should be carefully observed. In our experience, we have not encountered such complication, however. Cimetidine (300 mg/day for 2 days before the study) has been used in patients also.[52]

Images

During imaging, the patient lies supine with the gamma camera viewing the abdomen from the xyphoid to the symphysis pubis. A parallel-hole or diverging collimator designed for low energies is used. Tc-99m as sodium pertechnetate is injected intravenously in a dose of 100 μCi/kg of body weight. A radionuclide angiogram (1–5-sec frames for 60 sec) is obtained to evaluate for vascular malformations. A series of images are then taken in the anterior projection at 5-min intervals for 30–60 min (Fig. 11-1). Each image is obtained for 200,000 to 500,000 counts. Right lateral and/or posterior views are obtained at any time after the injection to help identify potentially confusing concentration of the tracer, particularly in the kidneys and/or in the ureter. The lateral image is helpful in determining the anterior position of uptake in a

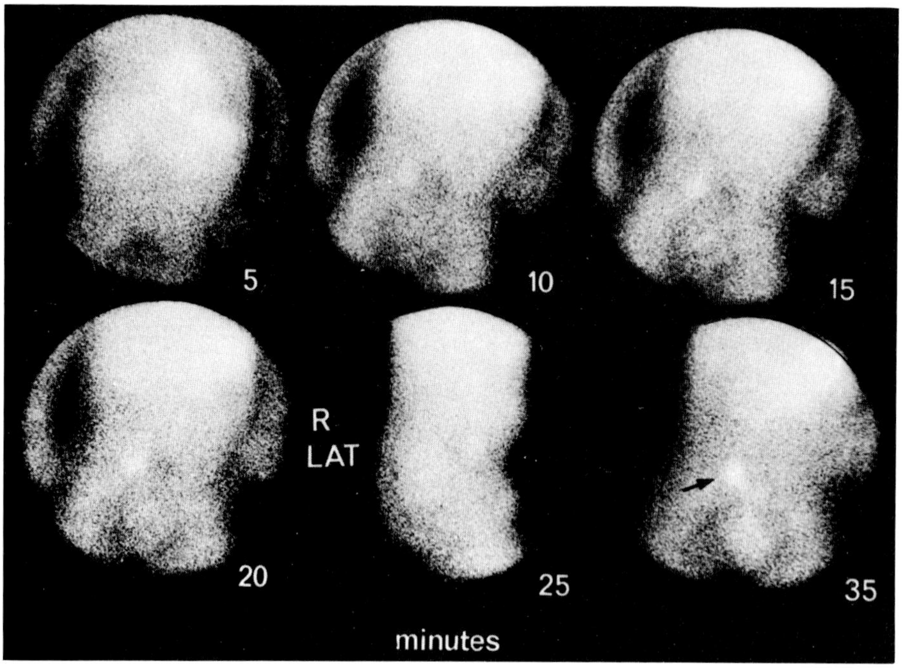

Figure 11-2. Meckel's diverticulum. This 6-month-old boy had two maroon-colored jelly bowel movements 1 day before this examination. The patient was pale and the hematocrit was 27%. On the abdominal scintiscan a focal accumulation of radiotechnetium in the right lower quadrant became visible at about 10 min after injection and continued to be visible for the entire observation period. In the right lateral projection, the abnormal focus of activity can be seen anteriorly. Note that the slow blood disappearance of radiopertechnetate is evident by the high background, the small amount accumulated in the bladder within 35 min, and the relatively low concentration of radionuclide in the stomach. At surgery on the same day, a Meckel's diverticulum was found 3 feet proximal to the ileocecal valve.

Meckel's diverticulum. Renal and ureteral activities appear posteriorly. The lateral view should be obtained as soon as a suspicious area of increased activity is visualized on the anterior view. Prompt timing of the lateral view is important in order to avoid the possibility of not being able to define the abnormal uptake in three dimensions at a later time, due to superimposed radiopertechnetate in the intestine.

If the right renal pelvis contains radioactivity its appearance may confuse some observers, especially if the left renal pelvis is obscured by the gastric outline, as it often is. Moving the patient to the upright position to help empty the renal pelves may allow a subsequent scan that will clarify the images.[64] Serial images in multiple projections and after voiding are useful to eliminate or define radioactivity within a localized portion of the ureter that may mimic the appearance of a Meckel's.[67] Upright anterior and oblique images may assist differentiation of duodenal activity, which will not change position, from ectopic gastric mucosa, which may move more in response to the altered direction of gravitational pull.

Background activity in the abdomen reflecting blood levels of pertechnetate decreases with time, and in most cases allows for identification of ectopic gastric mucosa within 30 min after injection of pertechnetate. If blood disappearance and gastric uptake of the tracer are slow, as in infants or anemic patients, the scanning time should be prolonged in order to increase the chance for identification of a lesion not visible early on the study.

Clinical Applications

Normal Abdominal Scan

A normal Tc-99m pertechnetate abdominal series reveals a gradual increase of tracer in the wall of the stomach. Tc-99m is eliminated into the gastric

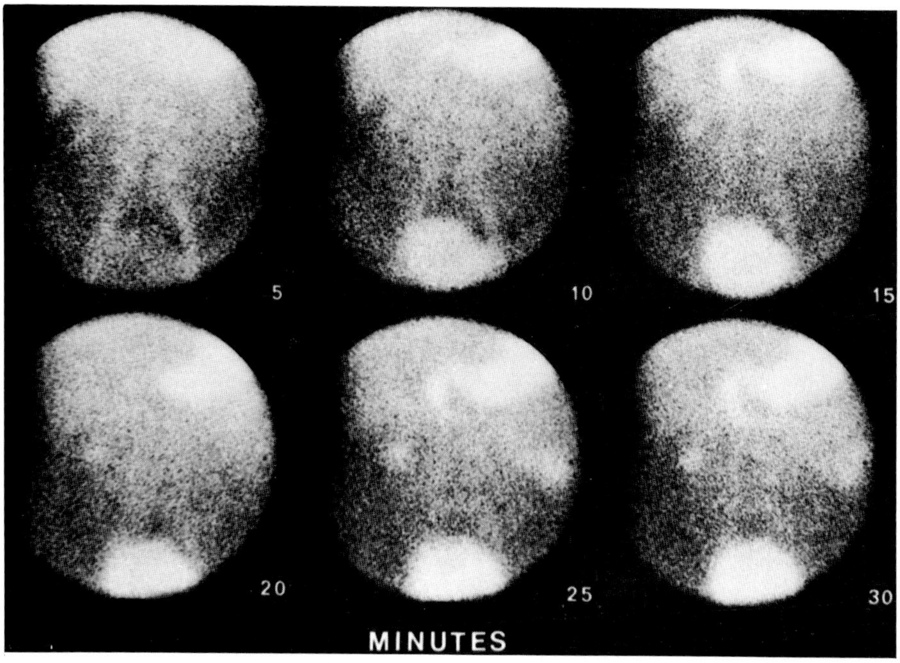

Figure 11-3. Meckel's diverticulum. This radiopertechnetate abdominal series was obtained on the second admission of a 6-year-old boy with rectal bleeding. Two days prior to admission he had complained of abdominal pain. On the day of admission, he had bright red blood with clots in his underwear. The hematocrit was 31%. On the radionuclide study a well-defined focal accumulation of activity about the junction of the right upper and lower quadrants appeared at 5 min along with gastric activity and persisted for the observation period. Activity within the major vessels on the 5-min frame disappear in the later frames. The stomach continued to concentrate the radiopertechnetate, the bladder gradually filled with radioactivity, and the background decreased during the observation period. The duodenum and a portion of the proximal bowel were also seen. At surgery, a Meckel's diverticulum was found and resected.

cavity and transported into the lumen of the duodenum and small intestine (Fig. 11-1). The speed of this transit is variable. In some patients with rapid gastric emptying, activity in the duodenum and intestine may be substantial and interfere with interpretation. The gastric outline usually shows a central area of relatively lower concentration of pertechnetate corresponding to the gastric cavity. This area of decreased uptake can be quite large if the patient has eaten before the examination. The bladder (if full) initially contains less activity than background. As radiopertechnetate is eliminated by the kidneys, progressively increasing levels of activity are evident in the bladder.

Meckel's Diverticulum

A scintigraphic abdominal survey revealing ectopic gastric mucosa is almost unmistakable: in addition to the normal uptake pattern, there is a small and well-defined area of increased radiopertechnetate uptake usually in the right lower quadrant that appears at the same time as the stomach which persists and increases in intensity throughout the study (Figs. 11-2–11-9). Activity in the lesion may occasionally fluctuate due to intestinal secretions or hemorrhage carrying the radiotracer away from the diverticulum.[64] In addition, a right lateral view reveals the abnormal uptake to be anterior (Figs. 11-2 and 11-4–11-8). Observation for 30 min after injection of the radiopertechnetate is usually sufficient to detect most cases of Meckel's diverticulum containing functioning gastric mucosa.

In questionable cases or when the gastric uptake or the gastric-to-background ratio is low, one should prolong the imaging time to 1 or more hours later (Fig. 11-9). A problem with delayed images is that radioactive gastric contents may have migrated into the duodenum, small bowel, and even large bowel and thus obscure uptake within the ec-

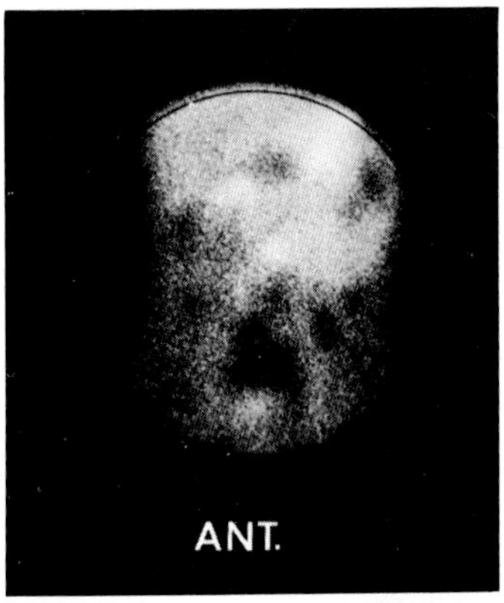

Figure 11-4. Effect of intraintestinal barium in the scintigraphic detection of Meckel's diverticulum. This 4-year-old boy presented with lower abdominal cramps and guaiac-positive stools. A barium enema showed no evidence of intussusception or polyp. **A:** The first abdominal scintigraphic series, done less than 24 h after the barium enema, reveals radiotechnetium in the stomach, small bowel, urinary bladder, and other soft tissues. In addition, several areas of very low radionuclide concentration throughout the abdomen correspond to barium within the large bowel from the examination performed previously. There is no scintigraphic evidence to suggest the presence of functioning ectopic gastric mucosa.

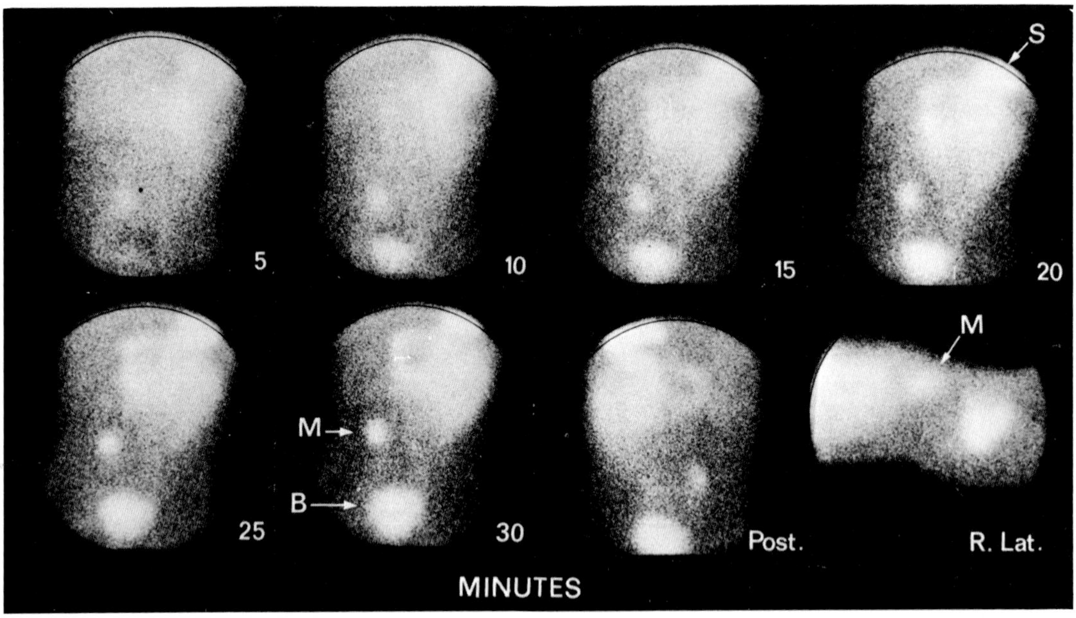

Figure 11-4. B. A second Tc-99m sodium pertechnetate abdominal survey conducted 2 days later, after the patient was cleared of barium, reveals an accumulation of radiotechnetium in the right lower quadrant (M) that persisted throughout the examination and appeared at the same time as the gastric activity (S). The urinary bladder (B) is visible at 5 min and remained visible for the observation period. The posterior view also shows the area of increased uptake and the cross-table right lateral projection reveals the abnormal accumulation of radioactivity to be anterior. At surgery, a Meckel's diverticulum containing gastric mucosa was removed.

topic gastric mucosa. An alternative is to restudy the patient on another day using pentagastrin (and perhaps cimetidine) in order to enhance mucosal uptake.

A Meckel's diverticulum may move caudally if the patient is raised or has voided. Very rarely, more than one area of ectopic gastric mucosa may occur in the intestine, or the ectopic mucosa may extend beyond the diverticulum, producing a larger area of uptake on the scan.[5,64]

Abnormal Uptake Due to Other Causes

Other conditions in the abdomen that accumulate pertechnetate include intestinal obstruction or intussusception,[16] inflammation,[16,19,26,40] vascular malformations,[7,11,66] ulcers,[26] some tumors,[54,68] and various urinary tract abnormalities that interrupt urinary excretion of the pertechnetate. Certain drugs, such as ethosuximide (Zarontin®) or laxatives, may also cause unpredictable uptake of

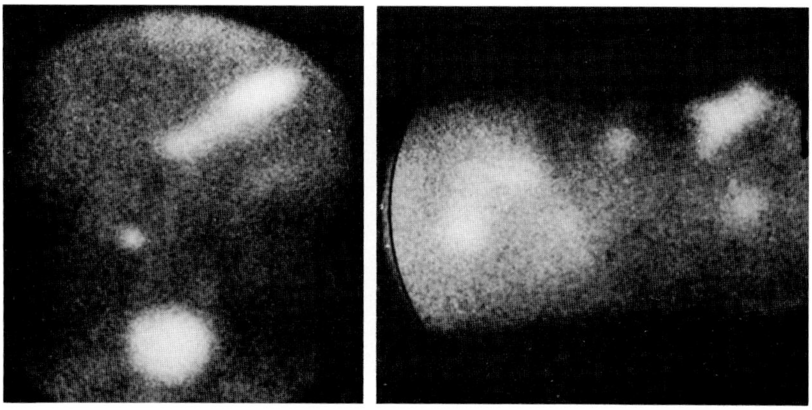

Figure 11-5. Meckel's diverticulum. This 2-year-old boy had a 3-month history of blood in the stools. The clearly abnormal scintiscan demonstrates a small, well-localized area of increased radiopertechnetate uptake in the right lower quandrant anteriorly. *Left:* 10 min., anterior view; *right:* 15 min., right lateral view.

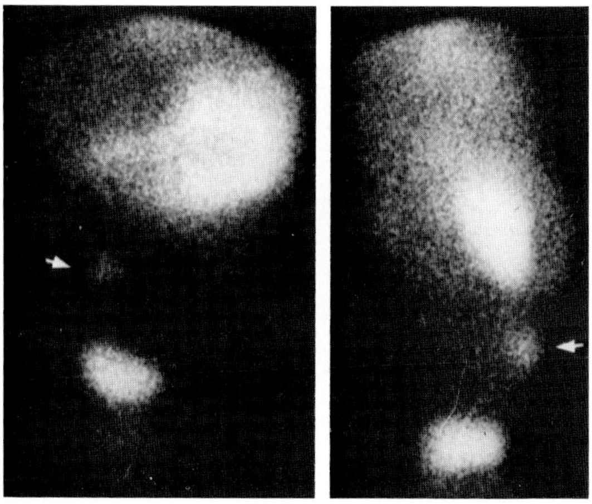

Figure 11-6. Meckle's diverticulum. This radiopertechnetate abdominal survey was performed on a 10-month-old boy who was admitted for evaluation of rectal bleeding for 2 days. The appearance of the stools ranged from melena to bright red blood. A barium enema, upper gastrointestinal series, and proctoscopy were normal. The hemoglobin was 9 g/100 ml. The hematocrit at admission was 27%. The scintiscan is abnormal, showing a well-circumscribed area of increased uptake in the right lower quandrant anteriorly *(arrows)*. At surgery the next day, a Meckel's diverticulum with bleeding gastric mucosa was found.

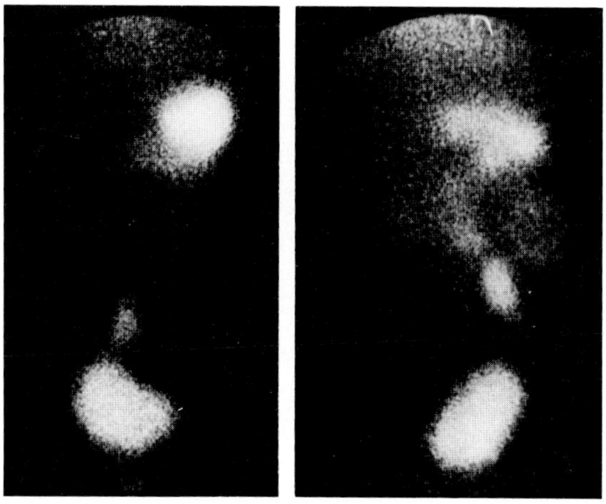

Figure 11-7. Meckel's diverticulum. This 13-month-old boy had a 2-day history of tarry black stools. The mother noted that the baby was fussy and had less appetite than normally; there were no other complaints. At admission, the hematocrit was 20%. The day after admission, a radiopertechnetate abdominal scintigraphic survey was obtained. *Left:* On the anterior projection at 10 min, an abnormal accumulation of radioindicator in the right lower quandrant projects just above the urinary bladder. *Right:* The right lateral projection reveals the same abnormal areas of uptake above the urinary bladder and anteriorly. This was interpreted as evidence of functioning ectopic gastric mucosa, probably in a Meckel's diverticulum. A laparotomy done within a few hours after the scintigram revealed a Meckel's diverticulum with gastric mucosa and an ulcer.

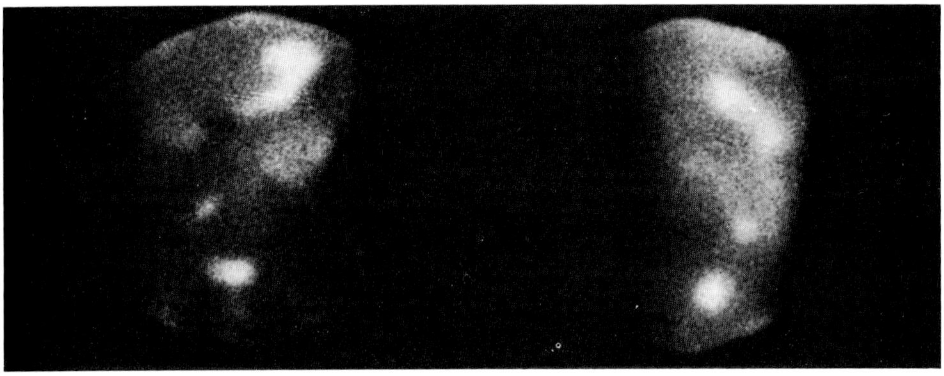

Figure 11-8. Meckel's diverticulum. This 13-month-old boy passed dark red blood in his diaper and 2 h later had another large bowel movement of dark red blood. The hematocrit was 29%. A barium enema and anoscopy were normal. The radiopertechnetate abdominal survey reveals an anterior focus of abnormal accumulation of activity within the right lower quandrant. The patient was taken immediately to the operating room, where a Meckel's diverticulum containing ectopic gastric mucosa was found. *Left:* Anterior view; *right:* right lateral view. Images obtained at 10 and 15 minutes after injection.

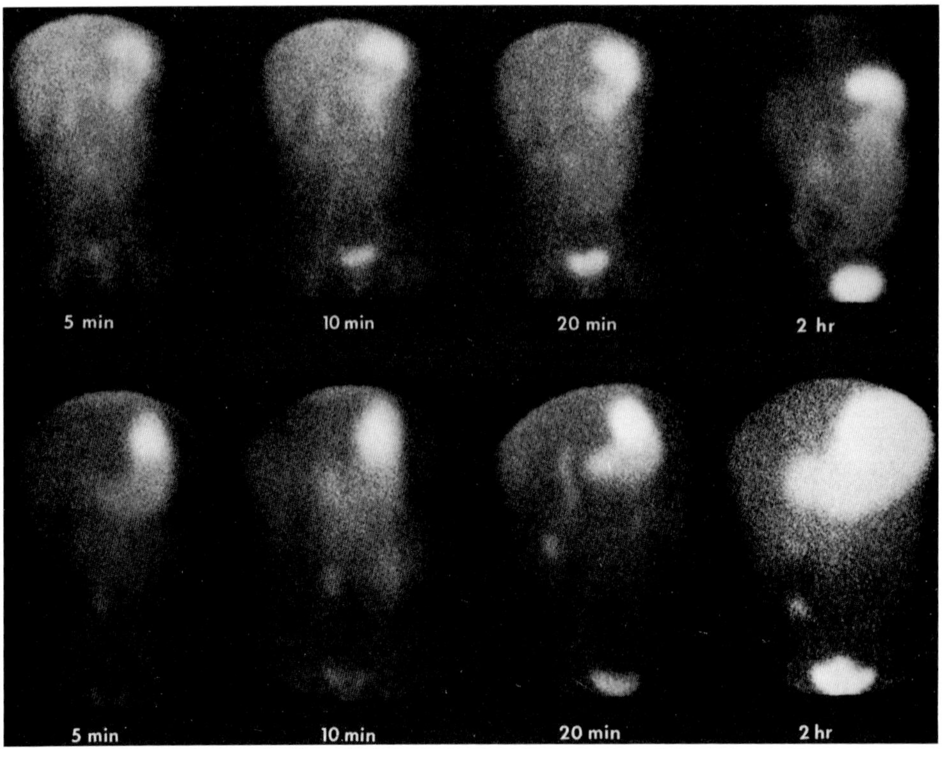

Figure 11-9. Pentagastrin stimulation of radiopertechnetate uptake in a Meckel's diverticulum. This 3-year-old girl had three episodes of gastrointestinal bleeding within the past 2 years. Multiple radiographic examinations and two radiopertechnetate abdominal series in another hospital were normal. In the present admission a repeat abdominal survey with radiopertechnetate was interpreted as normal or minimally suspicious *(top row)*. Two days later, on another study with pentagastrin stimulation, a well-defined area of increased uptake in the right lower quadrant changes in position but remains clearly visible for the 2 h of observation *(bottom row)*. This was interpreted as a high probability of Meckel's diverticulum containing ectopic gastric mucosa. At surgery, a Meckel's diverticulum was found 2 feet from the ileocecal valve. The diverticulum contained gastric mucosa at its tip with an ulcer at the junction of the gastric and ileal mucosa. There was no evidence of active bleeding at that time.

tracer in the intestine. The nature of these findings should be recognized during evaluation of the images. Therefore such findings should not be considered falsely positive. They are true abnormalities in the distribution of radiopertechnetate in the abdomen and they usually have a different appearance than Meckel's.

Blood pool uptake, as in vascular malformations or hemangiomas, will be apparent on the radionuclide angiogram and on the initial images and may or may not fade with time.[63,64] However, these lesions do not exhibit a response to pentagastrin.

Other abnormalities that may contain ectopic gastric mucosa include otherwise normal bowel,[5] enteric duplication,[25,44,72] duplication cysts,[26,56,76] and gastrogenic cysts.[41] As in Meckel's the complications and symptoms in these conditions are due to hydrochloric acid secretion by the gastric mucosal cells. The treatment is also surgical excision, as in Meckel's.

In Barretts's esophagus, the esophageal mucosa is lined with gastric epithelium rather than normal squamous epithelium and takes up pertechnetate, yielding scans with uptake above the stomach.[3]

False-Negative Studies

A normal pertechnetate study does not rule out the presence of a Meckel's diverticulum for a variety of reasons. Low pertechnetate uptake by gastric mucosa in infants may be a cause of false-negative examinations. As the child matures normal Tc-99m pertechnetate uptake will allow detection of ectopic gastric mucosa. Drug effects and normal structures may obscure uptake by the gastric mucosa in the diverticulum. Because peptic ulceration of the intestinal mucosa is usually responsible for the bleeding, most of the Meckel's diverticula that bleed contain some ectopic gastric mucosa. Experiments on animals show that at least 1–2 cm^2 of such tissue may be required for the lesion to be visible on the scintiscans.[1,13,55,65] One reported patient whose scan was negative had considerable scarring of the diverticulum and little intact gastric mucosa.[5]

The ectopic gastric mucosa must be functioning in order to take up pertechnetate. Hypofunction due to necrosis, fibrosis, ischemia, or other causes will reduce or even prevent scintigraphic detection.[34,48,74] In one of our patients, the pertechnetate survey was normal in the presence of a cystic Meckel's diverticulum with fluid within the cyst and with atrophic gastric mucosa.

Accuracy

Among the surgically proven cases of Meckel's diverticulum in the literature, the accuracy of Tc-99m pertechnetate scintigraphy is 90%.[63] The overall sensitivity among published accounts is 85% and the specificity has risen to 95%.[63] Prior to use of pertechnetate scintigraphy for Meckel's diverticulum, the lesion was diagnosed at laparotomy in approximately 60% of the symptomatic patients.[29,61]

References

1. Anderson GF, Sfakianakis GN, King DR, Boles ET Jr. Hormonal enhancement of technetium-99m pertechnetate uptake in experimental Meckel's diverticulum. J Pediatr Surg 1980; 15:900–5.
2. Berquist TH, Nolan NG, Adson MA, Shutt AJ. Diagnosis of Meckel's diverticulum by radioisotope scanning. Mayo Clin Proc 1973; 48:98–102.
3. Berquist TH, Nolan NG, Carlson HC, Stephens DH. Diagnosis of Barrett's esophagus by pertechnetate scintigraphy. Mayo Clin Proc 1973; 48:276–9.
4. Berquist TH, Nolan NG, Stephens DH, Carlson HC. Radioisotope scintigraphy in diagnosis of Barrett's esophagus. AJR 1975; 123:401–11.
5. Berquist TH, Nolan NG, Stephens DH, Carlson HC. Specificity of Tc-99m pertechnetate in scintigraphic diagnosis of Meckel's diverticulum: review of 100 cases. J Nucl Med 1976; 17:465–9.
6. Bree RL, Reuter SR. Angiographic demonstration of a bleeding Meckel's diverticulum. Radiology 1973, 108:287–8.
7. Broca M, Bach CH, Sedgrez A. Hemorragies intestinales: contribution a la detection des heterotopies de muqueuse gastrique et du diverticule de Meckel: interet de scintigramme gastrinque. Chirurgie 1972; 98:649–52.
8. Canty T, Meguid MM, Eraklis AJ. Perforation of Meckel's diverticulum scan (letter to the editor). Surgery 1972; 71:313.
9. Chaudhuri TK. Cellular site of secretion of $^{99m}TcO_4$ in the stomach—a controversial point (letter to the editor). J Nucl Med 1975; 16:1204–5.
10. Chaudhuri TK, Polak, JJ. Autoradiographic studies of distribution in the stomach of Tc-99m pertechnetate. Radiology 1977; 123:223–4.
11. Chaudhuri TK, Chaudhuri TK, Christie JH. False positive Meckel's diverticulum scan (letter to the editor). Surgery 1972; 71:313.
12. Conway JJ. Radionuclide diagnosis of Meckel's diverticulum. Gastrointest Radiol 1980; 5:209–13.
13. Conway JJ, and the Pediatric Nuclear Club of the

Society of Nuclear Medicine. The sensitivity, specificity and accuracy of radionuclide imaging of Meckel's diverticulum (abstract). J Nucl Med 1976; 17:553.
14. Dalinka MK, Wunder JF. Meckel's diverticulum and its complications, with emphasis on roentgenologic demonstration. Radiology 1973; 106:295–8.
15. DeBartolo HM, van Heerden JA. Meckel's diverticulum. Ann Surg 1976; 183:30–33.
16. Duszynski DO, Jewett TC, Allen JE. ^{99m}Tc pertechnetate scanning of the abdomen with particular reference to small bowel pathology. AJR 1971; 113:258–62.
17. Faris JC, Whitley JE. Angiographic demonstration of Meckel's diverticulum. Radiology 1973; 108:285–6.
18. Feggi LM, Bighi SM. Technical notes for scintigraphy of Meckel's diverticulum. J Nucl Med 1979; 20:888–9.
19. Gelfand MJ, Silberstein EB, Cox J. Radionuclide imaging of Meckel's diverticulum. Angiographic demonstration. Radiology 1976; 120:327–8.
20. Gershater R. Enterolith causing bleeding in a patient with Meckel's diverticulum. Angiographic demonstration. Radiology 1976; 120:327–8.
21. Harden RMG, Alexander WD, Kennedy I. Isotope uptake and scanning of stomach in man with Tc-99m pertechnetate. Lancet 1967; i:1305–7.
22. Harper PV, Andros G, Lathrop K. Preliminary observations on the use of six hour Tc-99m as a tracer in biology and medicine. Argonne Cancer Research Hospital Semiannual Report to the AEC, No. 18, Office of Technical Services, Dept. of Commerce, Washington, D.C. 1962; 76–88.
23. Harper PV, Lathrop KA, Jiminez F, Fink R, Gottschalk A. Technetium-99m as a scanning agent. Radiology 1965; 85:101–8.
24. Hildamus F. Cited by Neff G. Sas Meckelsche Divertikel. Ergeb Chir Orthop 1937; 30:227–315.
25. Ho JE, Konieczny KM. The sodium pertechnetate Tc-99m scan: an aid in the evaluation of gastrointestinal bleeding. Pediatrics 1975; 56:34–40.
26. Ho JE, Gleason WA, Thompson JS. The expanding spectrum of disease demonstrable by Tc-99m pertechnetate abdominal imaging (abstract). J Nucl Med 1978; 19:691.
27. Hofmeyr NG. Stomach scanning after intravenous Tc-99m administration. A preliminary report. South Afr Med J 1967; 41:572–5.
28. Holder LE, Ashare AB, Smith W, Saenger E. Pentagastrin: a new drug for stimulating gastric secretion of pertechnetate (abstract). J Nucl Med 1975; 16:535–6.
29. Jaros R, Schussheim A, Levy LM. Preoperative diagnosis of bleeding Meckel's diverticulum utilizing technetium-99m pertechnetate scintiimaging. J Pediatr 1973; 82:45–49.
30. Jewett TC Jr., Duszynski DO, Allen JE. The visualization of Meckel's diverticulum wiht Tc-99m-pertechnetate. Surgery 1970; 68:567–70.
31. Jewett TC Jr., Lebowitz R, Treves S. Search for Meckel's diverticulum (letter to the editor and response). Surgery 1972; 72:492–3.
32. Johnson LR. The trophic action of gastrointestinal hormones. Gastroenterology 1976; 70:278–88.
33. Keramidas DC, Coran AG, Zaleska RW. An experimental model for assessing the radiopertechnetate diagnosis of gastric mucosa in Meckel's diverticulum. J Pediatr Surg 1974; 9:879–83.
34. Khettry J, Effmann E, Grand RJ, Treves S. Effect of pentagastrin, histalog, glucagon, secretin and perchlorate on the gastric handling of Tc-99m-pertechnetate in mice. Radiology 1976; 120:629–31.
35. Kilpatrick JM. Scanning in diagnosis of Meckel's diverticulum. Hosp Pract 1974; 9:131–8.
36. Kilpatrick ZM, Aseron CA. Radioisotope detection of Meckel's diverticulum causing acute renal hemorrhage. N Engl J Med 1972; 287:653–4.
37. Lathrop KA, Harper PV. Biologic behavior of ^{99m}Tc from ^{99m}Tc pertechnetate ion. Prog Nucl Med 1972; 1:145–62.
38. Leonidas JC, Germann DR. Technetium-99m pertechnetate imaging in diagnosis of Meckel's diverticulum. Arch Dis Child 1974; 49:21–26.
39. Loken MK, Telander GT, Salmon RJ. Technetium-99m compounds for visualization of body organs. JAMA 1972; 194:152–6.
40. Lunia S, Lunia C, Chandramouly B, Chodos RB. Radionuclide meckelogram with particular reference to false-positive results. Clin Nucl Med 1979; 4:285–8.
41. Mark R, Young L, Ferguson C, Sutherland JB. Diagnosis of an intrathoracic gastrogenic cyst using Tc-99m-pertechnetate. Radiology 1973; 109:137–8.
42. Marsden DS, Priebe CJ. Preliminary appraisal of present Tc-99m-pertechnetate techniques for detecting ectopic gastric mucosa. Radiology 1974; 113:459–60.
43. Martin GI, Kutner FR, Moses L. Diagnosis of Meckel's diverticulum by radioisotope scanning. Pediatrics 1976; 57:11–12.
44. Case records of the Massachusetts General Hospital. Case 16-1980: duplication of ileum with ectopic gastric mucosa and peptic ulceration with perforation. N Engl J Med 1980; 302:958–62.
45. Meckel JF. Veber die Diverticel am darmkanal. Arch Physiol 1809; 9:421.
46. Meguid MM, Wilkinson RH, Canty T, Eraklis AJ, Treves S. Futility of barium sulfate in diagnosis of bleeding Meckel diverticulum. Arch Surg 1974; 108:361–2.
47. Meier-Ruge W, Fridrich R. Die Verteilung von Technetium-99m und Jod-131 in der Magen-

schleimhaut. Ein Beitrag sur Methodik der Mikrohistoautoradiographie wasserloslicher Isotope. Histochemie 1969; 19:147–54.
48. Moss AA, Kressel HY. Intestinal infarction: current problems and new methods of diagnosis using radionuclide scans. Appl Radiol Nucl Med 1976; 156–60.
49. Muroff LR, Casarella WJ, Johnson PM. Preoperative diagnosis of Meckel's diverticulum: angiographic and radionuclide studies in an adult. JAMA 1974; 229:1900–2.
50. Necheles H, Sporn J, Walker L. Effect of glucagon on gastrointestinal motility. Am J Gastroenterol 1966; 45:34–39.
51. Oldendorf WH, Sisson WB, Iisaka Y. Compartmental redistribution of ^{99m}Tc-pertechnetate in the presence of perchlorate ion and its relation to plasma protein binding. J Nucl Med 1970; 11:85–88.
52. Petrokubi JR, Baum S, Rohrer GV. Cimetidine administration resulting in improved pertechnetate imaging of Meckel's diverticulum. Clin Nucl Med 1978; 3:385–8.
53. Polga JP. Nasogastric suction to improve gastrointestinal scanning. J Nucl Med 1974; 15:374.
54. Polga JP, Sargent J, Dickinson P. Positive intestinal scan caused by carcinoid tumor. J Nucl Med 1974; 15:365–6.
55. Priebe CJ Jr., Marsden DS, Lazarevic B. The use of ^{99m}technetium pertechnetate to detect transplanted gastric mucosa in the dog. J Pediatr Surg 1974; 9:605–12.
56. Rodgers BM, Youssef S. "False positive" scan for Meckel diverticulum. J Pediatr 1975; 87:239–40.
57. Rosenthall L, Henry JN, Murphy DA, Freeman L. Radiopertechnetate imaging of the Meckel's diverticulum. Radiology 1972; 105:371–3.
58. Rutherford RB, Akers DR. Meckel's diverticulum: a review of 148 pediatric patients with special reference to the pattern of bleeding and to mesodiverticular vascular bands. Surgery 1966; 59:618–26.
59. Sagar VV, Piccone JM. The gastric uptake and secretion of Tc-99m pertechnetate after H_2 receptor blockage in dogs (abstract). J Nucl Med 1980; 21:P67.
60. Sailer JF, Janeway CM. Pertechnetate demonstration of a Barrett's esophagus involving the length of the esophagus (letter to the editor). J Nucl Med 1978; 19:1366–7.
61. Seitz W, Keim HJ, Hahn K. Abdominal scintigraphy for diagnosis of intestinal bleeding. World J Surg 1978; 2:613–9.
62. Seltzer MH, Conte PJ Jr, Rickert RR, Singer M. Diagnosis of a bleeding Meckel's diverticulum using radiopertechnetate. Am J Gastroenterol 1977; 67:235–9.
63. Sfakianakis GN, Conway JJ. Detection of ectopic gastric mucosa in Meckel's diverticulum and in other aberrations by scintigraphy: I. Pathophysiology and 10-year clinical experience. J Nucl Med 1981; 22:647–54.
64. Sfakianakis GN, Conway JJ. Detection of ectopic gastric mucosa in Meckel's diverticulum and in other aberrations by scintigraphy: II. Indications and methods. A 10-year experience. J Nucl Med 1981; 22:732–8.
65. Sfakianakis GN, Anderson GF, King DR, Boles ET Jr. The effect of gastrointestinal hormones on the pertechnetate imaging of ectopic gastric mucosa in experimental Meckel's diverticulum. J Nucl Med 1981; 22:678–83.
66. Siddiqui A, Ryo UY, Pinsky SM. Arteriovenous malformation simulating Meckel's diverticulum on Tc-99m-pertechnetate abdominal scintigraphy. Radiology 1977; 122:173–4.
67. Singh PR, Russel CD, Dubovsky EV, Bridges WM. Technique of scanning for Meckel's diverticulum. Clin Nucl Med 1978; 3:188–92.
68. Tauscher JW, Bryant DR, Gruenther RC. False-positive scan for Meckel diverticulum. J Pediatr 1978; 92:1022–3.
69. Taylor AT Jr, Alazraki N, Henry JE. Intestinal concentration of ^{99m}Tc-pertechnetate into isolated loops of rat bowel. J Nucl Med 1976; 17:470–2.
70. Treves S, Grand RJ, Eraklis AJ. Pentagastrin stimulation of technetium 99m uptake by ectopic gastric mucosa in a Meckel's diverticulum. Radiology 1978; 128:711–2.
71. Wang TST, Fawwaz RA, Esser PD, Johnson PM. Altered body distribution of (^{99m}Tc) pertechnetate in iatrogenic hyperaluminemia. J Nucl Med 1978; 19:381–3.
72. Wilson JP, Wenzel WW, Campbell JB. Technetium scans in the detection of gastrointestinal hemorrhage. Preoperative diagnosis of enteric duplication in an infant. JAMA 1977; 237:265–6.
73. Wine CR, Nahrwold DL, Waldhausen JA. Role of the technetium scan in the diagnosis of Meckel's diverticulum. J Pediatr Surg 1974; 9:855–88.
74. Wine CR, Nahrwold DL, Rose RC, Miller KL. Effect of histamine on technetium-99m excretion by gastric mucosa. Surgery 1976; 80:591–4.
75. Winter PF. Cellular site of $^{99m}TcO_4$ secretion in the stomach (letter to the editor). J Nucl Med 1976; 17:756.
76. Winter PF. Sodium pertechnetate Tc-99m scanning of the abdomen. Diagnosis of an ileal duplication cyst. JAMA 1977; 237:1352–3.

Chapter 12 Thyroid

S. T. Treves
Reed Larsen
Roger Pezzuti

Although precise measurements of circulating thyroid hormones and thyrotropin have reduced substantially the need for radioiodine thyroid uptake, this test still has some useful applications. Scintigraphy, however, remains a unique method for the evaluation of the thyroid gland, providing information on its anatomy and function simultaneously. The use of iodine-131 (I-131) has always been limited in the evaluation of disorders of the thyroid in children because of concern over the rather excessive radiation absorbed dose from this tracer. With the introduction of technetium-99m (Tc-99m) and of iodine-123 (I-123), both of which result in much lower radiation doses than I-131, the applications of scintigraphy of the thyroid in pediatric patients have been expanded.[3]

Indications for scintigraphy of the thyroid in children include the evaluation of thyroid nodules, evaluation of nodules or masses in the neck, detection of ectopic thyroid, and in some situations diagnosis of hyper- and hypothyroidism. Also, scintigraphy is employed for the detection of metastatic disease in thyroid cancer. Determination of thyroid uptake is useful in the evaluation of iodine kinetics, including evaluation of iodine turnover before radioiodine therapy.

Method

Radiopharmaceuticals

Iodine-123

The radiopharmaceutical of choice for scintigraphy of the thyroid in children is I-123. This cyclotron-produced radionuclide has a physical half-life of 13.3 h and emits a 159 KeV gamma ray which is ideally suited for imaging with the gamma camera. The radiation absorbed dose resulting from administration of I-123 is considerably lower than with I-131 or I-125 and almost as low as with Tc-99m. The radiation absorbed dose to the thyroid for a newborn is 0.160 rad/μCi, and for an adult 0.015 rad/μCi administered.[41] Although I-123 has been commercially available for some time, it has usually been produced by the Te-124(*p,2n*)I-123 reaction using enriched Te-123 as the target material. This method leads to the presence of small but significant amounts of I-124. The presence of I-124 results in an increase in the radiation exposure to the patient. Because the physical half-life of I-124 is 4.18 days, its relative contribution increases with time after production. In addition I-124 produces high-energy photons that, by causing septal penetration in collimators designed for low energies, results in significant image degradation. This method of production has the advantage of requiring only a relatively low-energy cyclotron. A more satisfactory source of I-123 is either via the I-127(*p,5n*)Xe-123 → I-123, or Cs-133(*p,spal*)Xe-123 → I-123 reactions using high-energy cyclotrons or linear accelerators.[1,5,18,34,39] Both of these routes provide a product free of I-124, containing a very small amount of I-125, and utilize target materials naturally abundant. Disadvantages with this tracer are relatively high production costs, and the need for an efficient distribution system. Imaging with I-123 is usually carried out at 4 h, and up to 24 h after the administration of the tracer. A usual administered dose of I-123 is from 25 to 100 μCi.

Technetium-99m

Technetium-99m (Tc-99m) as sodium pertechnetate (NaTc-99mO_4^-) is trapped by the thyroid in the same manner as iodine by an active transport system. This tracer, unlike isotopes of iodine, is not organified. Therefore, visualization of the gland depends on the presence of a high thyroid/plasma gradient for pertechnetate. The scintigraphic image must therefore be obtained while the pertechnetate is in relatively high concentration in the plasma. Propylthiouracil and tapazole do not affect the TcO_4^- scan as they do the iodine scan. Only about 1.8–4.0% of the administered activity of Tc-99m is taken up by the thyroid gland 20 min after intravenous administration. Petechnetate is released from the thyroid gland after trapping, and it can be washed out from the thyroid by administration of sodium or potassium perchlorate. Tc-99m petechnetate may be administered intranveously or orally. Since this tracer is trapped by the thyroid rapidly, imaging may begin within 5 min after administration. Tc-99m pertechnetate is also taken up by the salivary glands and is eliminated in the saliva. This is an important factor that must be kept in mind when interpreting images of the thyroid, particularly in the diagnosis of lingual or sublingual thyroid. These ectopic thyroids are usually hypofunctioning. Activity in the saliva may be intense enough to overshadow uptake by a midline hypothyroid gland. Imaging immediately after the injection of Tc-99m is recommended in order to avoid this problem. Advantages with this tracer are that it is conveniently available, and that radiation exposure to patients is relatively small. The radiation absorbed dose to the thyroid from Tc-99m NaO_4^- ranges from 3.4 to 0.35 rad/mCi administered. The gut, receives from 2.0 to 0.2 rad/mCi administered. The usual administered doses of Tc-99m pertechnetate for imaging of the thyroid range from 0.200 in a newborn to 3.0 mCi in an adult. Disadvantages are the relatively low thyroid uptake and the lack of specificity for thyroid tissue. Images with Tc-99m will have high background as compared with images obtained with I-123. Discrepant results may be found with Tc-99m and radionuclides of iodine in the evaluation of thyroid nodules. Occasionally, an adenoma or carcinoma of the thyroid may take up Tc-99m, and appear as a "cold" lesion on iodine scanning.

Iodine-131

Iodine-131 (I-131) has been available for imaging of the thyroid for the past 30 years. The cost of this tracer is reasonably low, and it is widely available. I-131 has a physical half-life of 8.1 days and it decays by beta emission. This beta radiation contributes to a relatively high radiation to the thyroid gland, even when it is administered for diagnostic purposes. The energy of its major gamma emission, 364 keV, is higher than ideal for imaging with gamma cameras. The radiation absorbed dose to the thyroid with I-131 for an adult is about 1.5 rad/μCi of tracer administered. In the newborn, the radiation absorbed dose to the thyroid gland per microcurie of I-131 administered is about 16 rad.[41] We do not recommend the use of I-131 for diagnostic imaging of the thyroid in children or adults. The high radiation dose from I-131 is useful for the treatment of hyperthyroidism and carcinoma of the thyroid. Therapy with I-131 to the thyroid gland for hyperthyroidism in children is used by some centers as the standard treatment, while others feel it should be employed only in exceptional circumstances in this age group.[35,36] The long physical half-life of this tracer is useful when searching for metastases from thyroid carcinoma. Images of high contrast between metastases and body background can be obtained 2–3 days after administration of the radionuclide.

Iodine-125

Iodine-125 (I-125), once used widely for imaging of the thyroid, is no longer recommended. Its physical half-life is 60 days and it decays with x-ray and gamma emissions of 27 and 35 keV. The radiation absorbed dose with I-125 is lower than with I-131 but is considerably higher than with I-123 or Tc-99m. The absorbed radiation dose to the thyroid for a newborn is about 11.0 rad/μCi and to an adult about 1.0 rad/μCi administered.[41]

Examination Technique

We use the gamma camera equipped with the pinhole collimator for routine scintigraphy of the thyroid in all patients. The patient is examined supine with the gamma camera viewing the anterior aspect of the hyperextended neck. The pinhole collimator is advanced toward the neck until the image of the thyroid occupies about two-thirds of the field-of-view of the camera. With I-123 we obtain images of the thyroid of 25,000 to 150,000 counts. Imaging time varies from 5 to 15 min depending on age, thyroid uptake, and dose administered. Oblique views are obtained, in order to identify relationships between the thyroid and nodule(s).

In addition to those obtained with the pinhole collimator, other images using a high-resolution parallel-hole collimator are recorded in the computer at 4.0 h and at 24.0 h in order to measure the percentage uptake of the administered dose of iodine in the thyroid. Images of a carefully measured standard of the administered dose are recorded at 4.0 and 24.0 h. An image of a radioactive ruler is also obtained using the same collimator. This view is also used to obtain a panoramic view of the neck in order to evaluate the size of the gland, and to establish anatomic relationships between the thyroid and nodules in the neck, or to reveal any extrathyroidal uptake of the tracer. The thyroid gland and the neck are palpated by the physician while the patient is on the examining table. When thyroid or neck nodules are present, we use a small source of Tc-99m or cobalt-57 to identify the limits of thyroid and/or neck nodules and their location relative to thyroid tissue. These and other landmarks, such as the suprasternal notch, are superimposed on another image of the thyroid.

Imaging of the thyroid using Tc-99m is begun 5–10 min after the administration of the tracer. The technique is the same as that described for I-123.

TSH Stimulation Test

At present this test is probably used only in defining hemiatrophy (Fig. 12-12). The response of the thyroid to the administration of exogenous TSH (thyroid-stimulating hormone) was used in the past to differentiate primary from secondary (pituitary or hypothalamic) hypothyroidism. In primary hypothyroidism the thyroid gland does not respond to the administration of TSH with an increase in activity. The gland in this case is already under maximal stimulation by endogenous TSH. In secondary hypothyroidism the thyroid gland responds with an increase in activity to exogenous TSH. The etiology of hypothyroidism is much more easily determined by measuring serum TSH concentrations, which are elevated in patients with primary hypothyroidism.

TSH Suppression Test (T3)

The purpose of this test is to establish whether the thyroid gland is functioning autonomously. It may be used either in patients suspected of having Graves' disease or those with functioning nodules. A radioiodine uptake is performed first. Then triidothyronine (T3) is given for 6–8 days at 25–50 μg per day depending on the age of the patient. In normal patients, suppression of endogenous TSH reduces thyroid uptake by at least 50%. Children with thyrotoxicosis show no significant suppression of the thyroidal uptake of I-123. This test is valuable in establishing the presence of "autonomy" of the thyroid gland in patients with mild thyrotoxicosis, when other studies are equivocal. It may supplement the use of the thyrotropin-releasing hormone (TRH) infusion test in those patients with functioning nodules. In patients with thyroid autonomy due to any thyroid disease, pituitary TSH synthesis is inhibited, and there is no increase in serum TSH 20–30 min after intravenous infusion of 200 μg of TRH.

Clinical Applications

Normal Study

The normal thyroid weight at birth is about 1 g. The thyroid grows at a rate of 1 g per year until the age of 15–16 years. The mean thyroid weight in 762 normal adult individuals in New York City was determined by Mochizuky et al. to be 16.7 ± 6.9 g.[25] The radioactive silhouette of the thyroid is located in the normal position in the neck. I-123 uptake in the thyroid is much higher than background compared with images obtained with Tc-99m pertechnetate. The thyroid lobes are of approximately the same size. Each lobe in the adult measures approximately 5.0 cm in maximum length. The pyramidal lobe is rarely visualized in children (Fig. 12-1). The isthmus may be visualized and it has a variable appearance. The right lobe may be normally lower than the left lobe. The normal observed thyroid uptake of iodine varies widely, partly due to diet, medications, iodine in the diet, place of residence, previous administration of iodinated contrast agents, etc. Normal values of thyroid uptake of iodine are believed to be 5–12% at 4 h, and 10–40% at 24 h after administration of the tracer.

In scintigraphs with Tc-99m the contrast between thyroid and background will be lower than

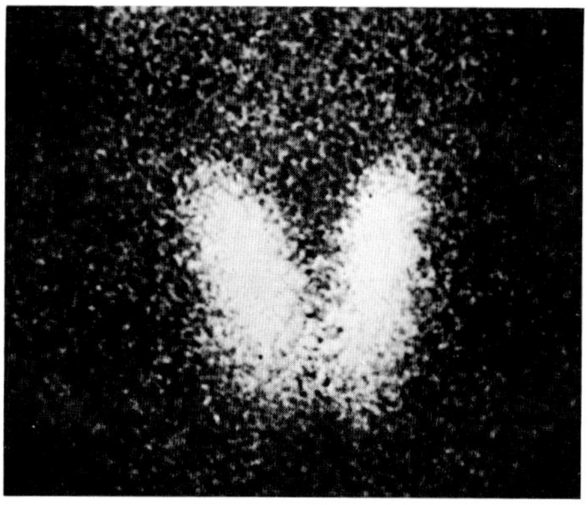

Figure 12-1. Normal thyroid scan obtained with Tc-99m sodium pertechnetate.

with I-123. Activity in the salivary glands, saliva in the mouth, and sometimes in the esophagus, may be visualized. This is due to the fact that pertechnetate images must be obtained while there is considerable blood activity (within about 60 min after administration).

Ectopic Thyroid

In some patients the only functioning thyroid tissue is located in the posterior aspect of the tongue or in the midline, between the tongue and the thyroid cartilage. Children with congenital hypothyroidism due to ectopic thyroid may have a lower risk of intellectual impairment than do athyreotic infants. Categorization of the anatomic thyroid defect may be of some prognostic value for hypothyroidism. Initiation of treatment should not be delayed for this study since the elevated TSH will persist for at least several days after T4 treatment is begun.[27]

Imaging using I-123 is useful in the evaluation of ectopic thyroid and masses in the base of the tongue (Figs. 12-2 and 12-3) in older children as well. Etiologies for masses at the base of the tongue include lingual thyroid, cyst, teratoid tumor, hypertrophic lingual tonsil, lipoma, adenoma, angioma, and fibroma. A nodule in the base of the tongue is present frequently in lingual thyroid.[32]

Thyroid and Neck Nodules

Management of solitary thyroid nodules remains controversial. Nodules in the thyroid or the neck may or may not be composed of thyroid tissue. Scintigraphy is helpful to establish the relationship of such lesions to the thyroid gland. It has been customary to classify thyroid nodules as "hot" or "cold," depending on their avidity for radioiodine (Figs. 12-4–12-13). This division is not completely justified from the clinical or histologic point of view. Nodules with greater concentration of radioiodine than the thyroid gland ("hot" nodules) may be due to an autonomous thyroid tissue (toxic or nontoxic) (Figs. 12-10 and 12-11), hyperfunction-

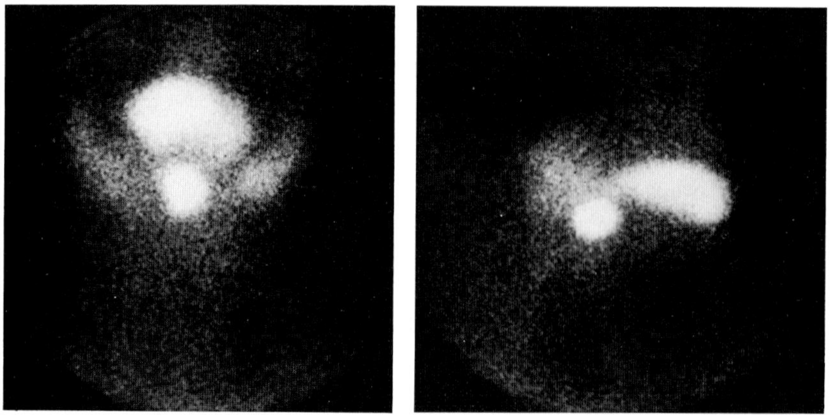

Figure 12-2. Lingual thyroid. Tc-99m pertechnetate scan. Anterior view *(left)* shows a central, well-defined area of radiopertechnetate uptake corresponding to a lingual thyroid. In addition activity is seen in the mouth and in the salivary glands. On the right lateral view *(right)* the level of the ectopic glandular tissue and its relation to the oropharynx can be appreciated. This image was from a mentally retarded female child. Her tests of thyroid function were depressed and the thyroid could not be palpated.

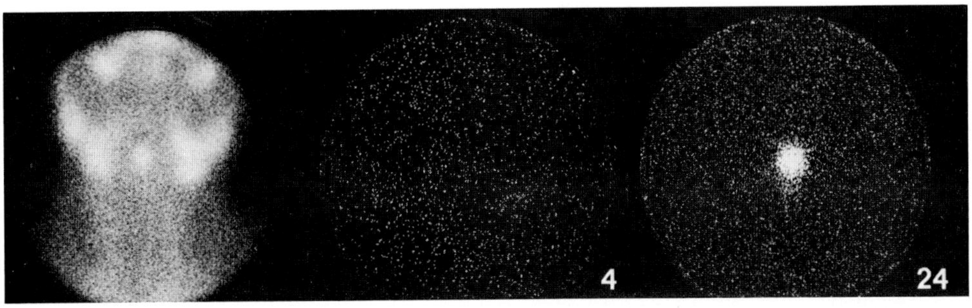

Figure 12-3. Lingual thyroid. An anterior Tc-99m sodium pertechnetate scan *(left)* obtained 5 min after injection of the tracer shows a small, well-defined area of uptake high in the neck. The salivary glands and body background are relatively high. On the *right* are two I-123 thyroid scintigraphs obtained at 4 and 24 h after adminstration of the tracer. There is no visualization of the lingual thyroid at 4 h, but this is visualized on the scan at 24 h.

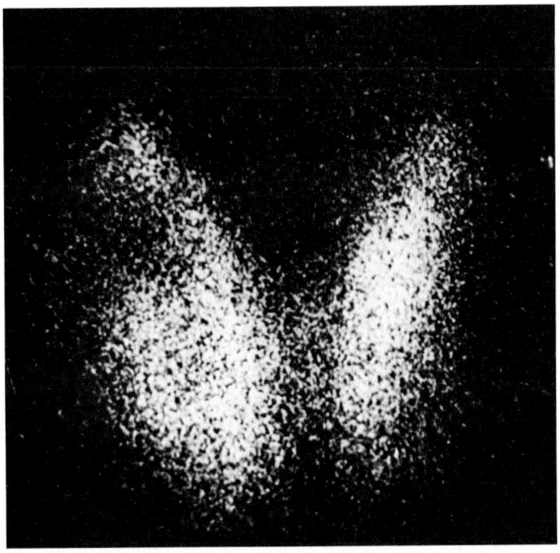

Figure 12-4. Adenoma of the thyroid. Anterior I-123 scan of the thyroid demonstrates a well-defined area of absent radioiodine uptake in the lateral and superior aspects of the right lobe of the thyroid gland.

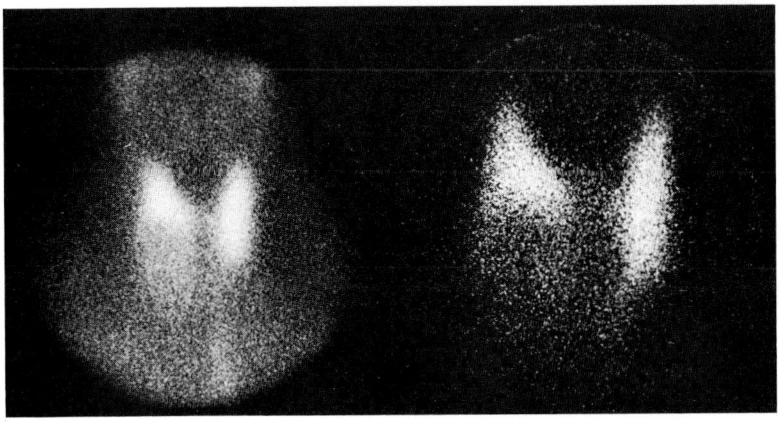

Figure 12-5. Microfollicular adenoma of the thyroid. Tc-99m pertechnetate *(left)* and I-123 *(right)* thyroid scans. The Tc-99m scan reveals an area of decreased uptake in the right lower lobe corresponding to a soft palpable nodule in the same location. The scan performed with I-123 reveals lower tissue background and almost absent radiotracer uptake in the right lower lobe.

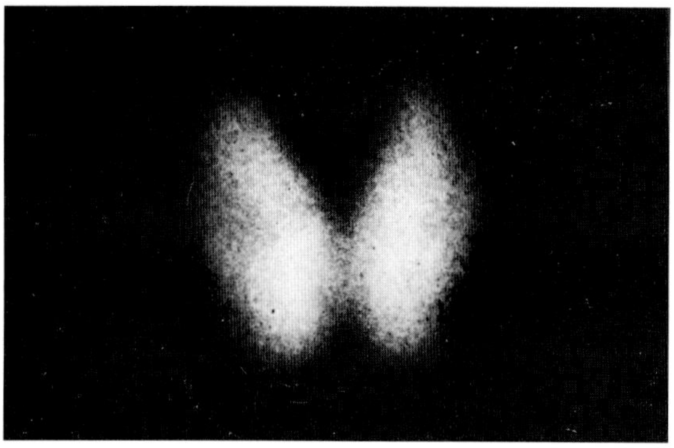

Figure 12-6. Papillary carcinoma of the thyroid. I-123 thyroid scan of the thyroid from a 13-year-old female. Her right thyroid lobe was tender to palpation. The scan reveals an area of decreased uptake in the lateral aspect of the right lobe. The patient was treated with a right lobectomy. Anterior view.

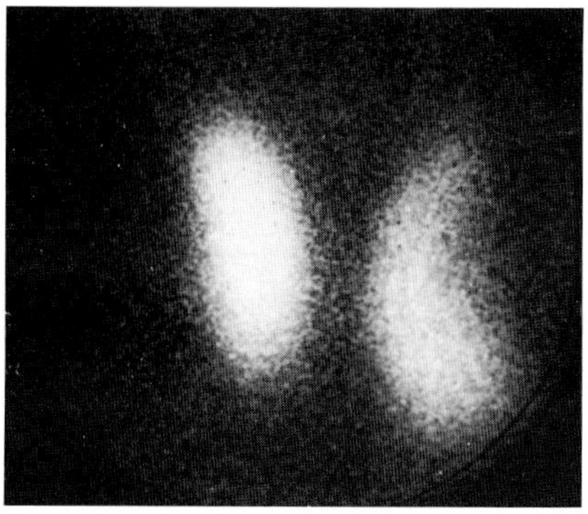

Figure 12-8. Branchial cleft cyst. Tc-99m pertechnetate thyroid scan. This 11-year-old male had a mass in the left side of the neck felt by palpation to be within the thyroid gland. His thyroid function tests were normal. The scintiscan reveals a concave-shaped lesion in the lateral aspect of the left lobe of the thyroid. At surgery a branchial cleft cyst adjacent to the thyroid was removed. Anterior view.

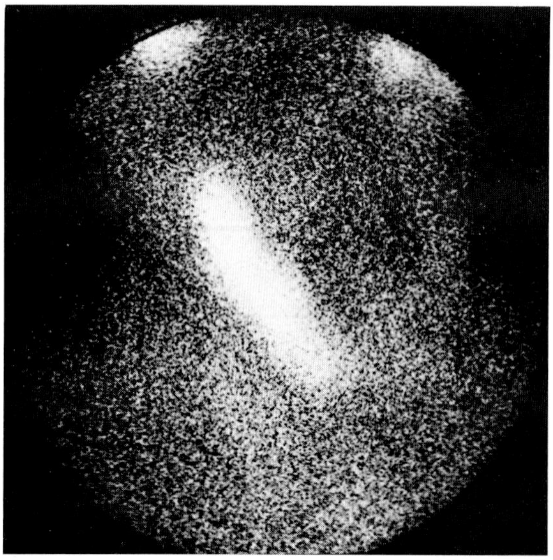

Figure 12-7. Lipoblastoma. Tc-99m pertechnetate scan. This study is from a 13-year-old male who presented with a mass in the left side of his neck. This mass was not tender and had been present for several weeks before his examination. Thyroid function tests were normal. An elongated area of uptake is visualized in the right side of the neck that appears too large for a single lobe of the thyroid and may represent the normal right lobe and a displaced left lobe overlying the lower lobe of the right lobe. There is a large area of decreased tracer uptake in the left side of the neck corresponding to a lipoblastoma not connected to the thyroid gland. Anterior view.

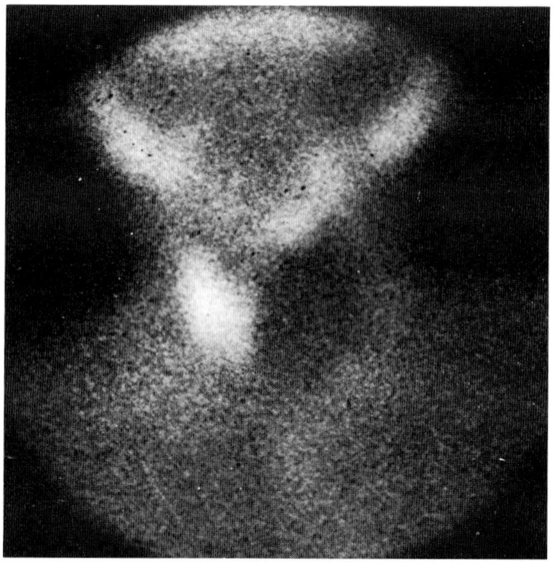

Figure 12-9. Thyroglossal duct cyst. Tc-99m sodium pertechnetate scan. This was a 4-year-old male who presented with a mass in the left side of his neck for about 6 months. This mass had grown in size very slowly. A radiograph of the chest revealed deviation of the trachea to the right. Thyroid function tests were normal. The mass was fluctuating and not tender and measured about 2 × 1.5 cm. The scintiscan reveals the thyroid gland displaced to the right side of the neck. There is a "cold" area in the left side of the neck corresponding to the palpable mass which appears to compress and displace the small left lobe of the thyroid. A cyst was removed from the left side of the neck. It contained clear, colorless fluid. The cyst was not attached to the thyroid.

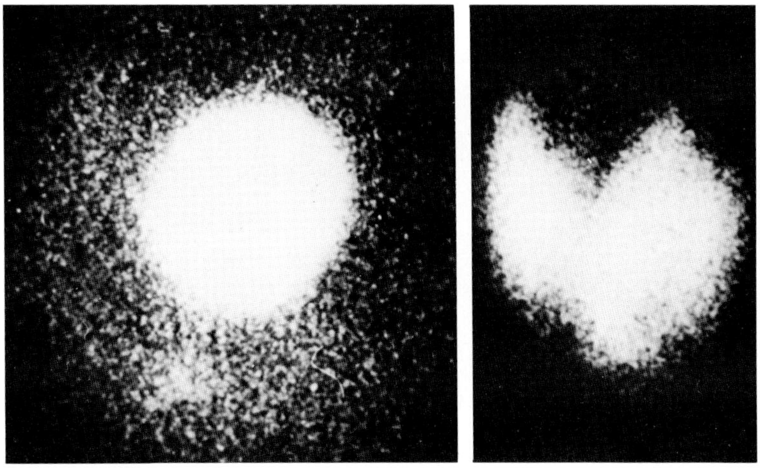

Figure 12-10. Autonomous nodule. This patient with a palpable nodule was treated with T3 for 14 days. A Tc-99m thyroid scan revealed a single area of uptake within the thyroid gland corresponding to the palapble mass. No other functioning thyroid tissue could be identified at this time *(left)*. A repeat Tc-99m scan was done after administration of TSH and the remainder of the thyroid gland was visualized *(right)*.

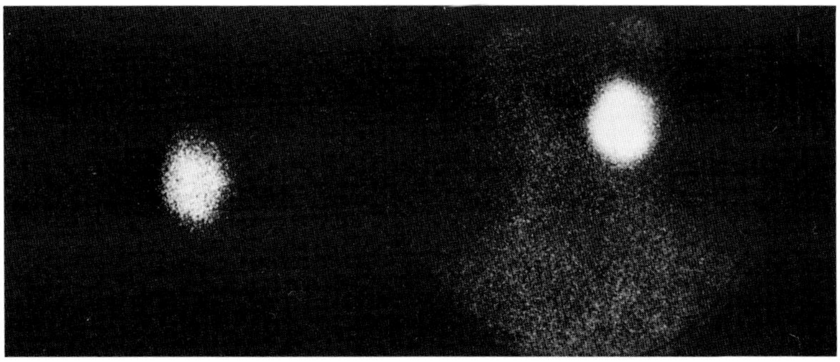

Figure 12-11. Autonomous nodule. I-123 *(left)* and Tc-99m *(right)* scans from a 12-year-old female patient. These scans were obtained following suppression with T3 and demonstrate a well-defined area of increased uptake of the tracer in the left lobe of the thyroid corresponding to a palpable nodule.

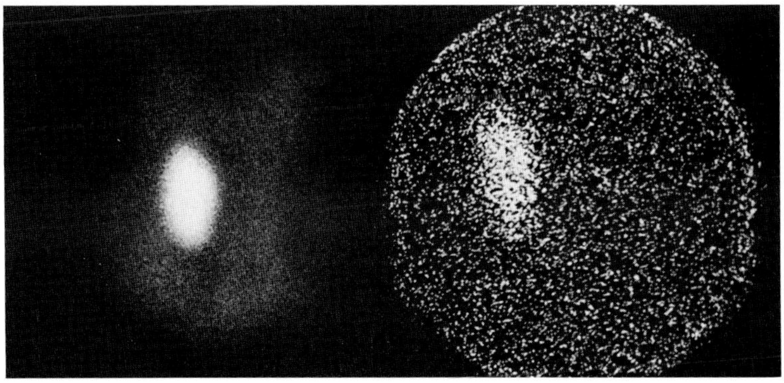

Figure 12–12. Thyroid hemiatrophy. Tc-99m pertechnetate and I-123 thyroid scans from a 4-year-old clinically euthyroid female who presented with painless swelling of the right side of her neck for about 1 year. A firm thyroid nodule measuring about 1.7 × 1.5 cm was palpated. Repeated scans were performed with stimulation; however, they failed to demonstrate functioning thyroid tissue in the left side of the neck.

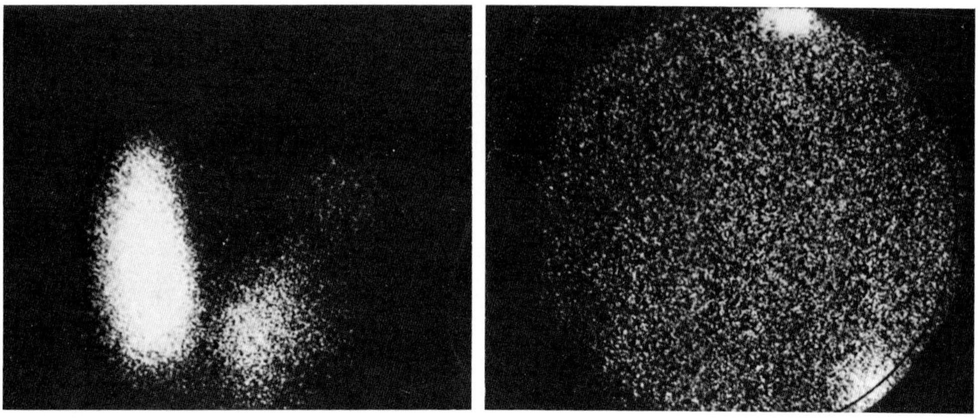
A

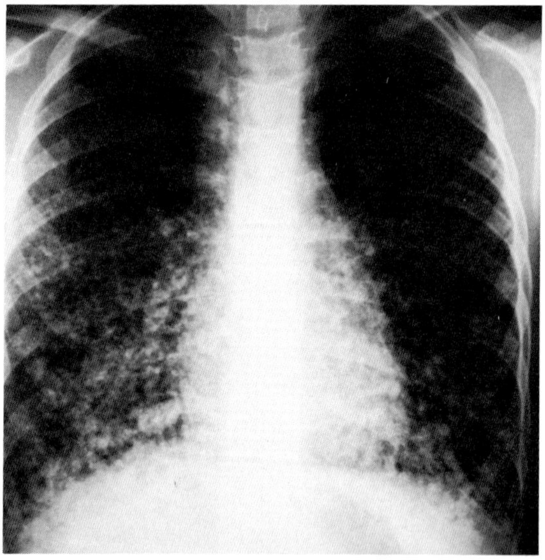
B

Figure 12-13. Papillary carcinoma of the thyroid in a 9-year-old female. She had a palpable mass in the left side of the neck. **A:** Selected images of her initial I-131 scan following stimulation with TSH. The right thyroid lobe appears normal in size, shape, and configuration. The left lobe shows absent radioiodine uptake in the upper pole corresponding to the palpable mass with reduced uptake of the tracer in a distorted lower pole. The scan of the chest shows no selective uptake of radioiodine. **B:** Initial radiograph of the chest showing a diffuse infiltrate. The patient had restrictive pulmonary disease at the time. **C:** I-131 scan a few days following total thyroidectomy. There is uptake of radioiodine generally within the thyroid bed and beyond, particularly on the left side. There is abundant uptake of radioiodine throughout the lungs.

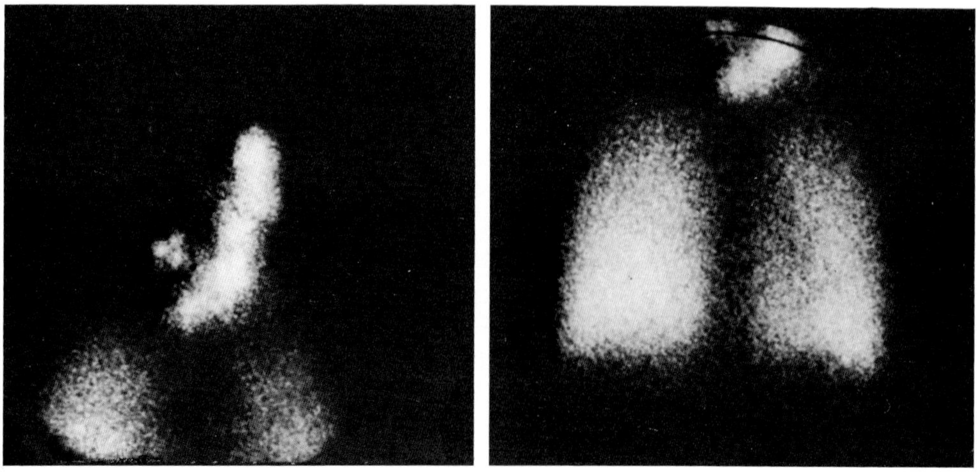
C

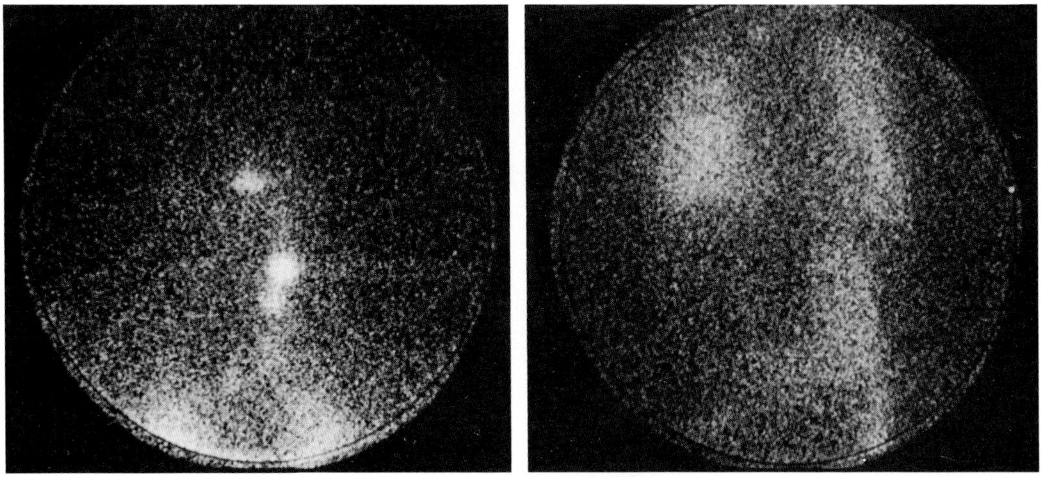

D

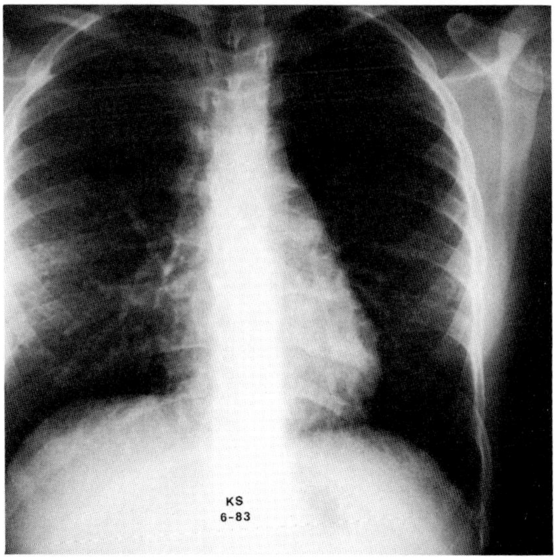

E

Figure 12-13. D: Followup I-131 scan 5 years following administration of two doses of 100 mCi of I-131 revealing some residual uptake of radioiodine in two areas in the neck and much diminished uptake of radioiodine in the lungs. **E:** Radiograph of the chest also obtained 5 years after radioiodine therapy showing a marked reduction of the diffuse infiltrate seen on the initial examination.

ing tissue in cases of previous surgery, irradiation or infection, and finally to anatomic variation. They are defined scintigraphically as scans in which tracer is exclusively localized in nodular tissue. Hot nodules are rare in children, being found in <5% of all solitary palpable nodules in children. By our criteria "warm nodules" are those nodules that contain more activity than normal thyroid tissue, but are not functioning to such a great extent as to suppress TSH secretion and therefore, nonnodular thyroid tissue. Warm nodules may also be associated with cancer of the thyroid. Nodules that contain minimal or no radioiodine ("cold" nodules) on radioiodine scans may be found in association with a variety of lesions including cyst, adenoma, dermoid cyst or tumor, lymph node, carcinoma, hemorrhage, edema, and thyroiditis (Figs. 12-4–12-8). A "warm" nodule on a Tc-99m scan may appear as a "cold" nodule on a radioiodine scan. Most significant nodules are palpable. Occasionally a nonpalpable nodule may be detected by scintigraphy. In all patients presenting with nodule(s) it is imperative that scintigraphic and palpatory findings are evaluated together.

Nodules of the neck that exhibit no selective uptake of radioiodine include lymph nodes, cysts, hemorrhage, dermoid cyst or tumor, infection, and metastatic disease. Ectopic thyroid tissue such as sublingual thyroid will frequently concentrate radioiodine. It is important to perform a thyroid scintigram in children with thyroid nodules in order to identify the presence and distribution of functioning thyroid tissue, especially before contemplating surgery. This will avoid accidental excision of an ectopic thyroid gland, which may be the only thyroid tissue that the patient may have. In a small proportion of nodules there is a discordant appearance between findings on radioiodine and technetium scintigraphy.

Solitary nodules of the thyroid gland in the pediatric age group are rare (1–2%). Wellington et al. evaluated 39 children and adolescents with a solitary nodule of the thyroid. Thirty-five of these patients had their nodules removed surgically. Twenty-seven of the 39 patients had a cold nodule on scintigraphy. The most common cause of solitary thyroid nodule in this group was follicular adenoma. Five of the 27 cold nodules were malignant. No malignancies were present in either the warm or the hot nodules.[42] In a series of 120 patients operated for solitary thyroid nodules, neoplasia was found in about 30% of the cases and the malignancy rate was about 12%.[29] Some workers advocate the use of thallium-201 (Tl-201) for the evaluation of thyroid nodules that are "cold" on I-123 scans. Ochi and coworkers report that Tl-201 is taken up in about 95% of malignant tumors both on early (5–15 min) and late (3–5 h) images. On the other hand, delayed Tl-201 scans demonstrated no uptake of the tracer in about 90% of benign tumors.[28] Experience in children is limited with this technique. For radiation absorbed doses with Tl-201 refer to Chapter 16.

Hyperthyroidism

The majority of children with thyrotoxicosis have a diffuse goiter, usually due to Graves' disease. The levels of thyroid hormone in blood are elevated, and there is often mild exophthalmus. When the iodine turnover is very rapid, only the early uptake of iodine will be high, and 24-h values may be normal. Nonsuppressibility of the thyroid uptake after administration of thyroid hormone is characteristic. It has been suggested that Graves' disease is due to an autoimmune disorder. Circulating immunoglobulins that bind to TSH receptors of thyroid cells have been demonstrated in most patients. Presumably these stimulate the thyroid cell. Another form of hyperthyroidism is toxic nodular goiter (uninodular or multinodular). In these cases there is autonomous hyperfunction of the thyroid nodule(s) leading to hyperthyroidism. TSH secretion by the pituitary and the function of extranodular thyroid tissue are suppressed. These nodules are adenomas or adenomatous nodules. A scan of the thyroid is indicated when hyperthyroidism is associated with a nodular thyroid in order to rule out the possibility of a toxic adenoma, or rarely a toxic functional thyroid carcinoma. In these cases, which are extremely rare in children, the normal thyroid is suppressed and may not be visualized on the scan. Exogenous TSH (10 units, intramuscular, about 24 h before scanning) stimulation will help outline the remainder of the thyroid gland to prove the existence of suppressed, but potentially functioning tissue (Figure 12-10).

Hypothyroidism

Hypothyroidism without goiter may be caused by primary thyroid disease, as in congenital anatomic abnormality (aplasia), or destructive disorders (thyroiditis, irradiation, surgery). Hypothyroidism may be caused by TSH deficiency (pituitary insufficiency, hypothalamic causes). Hypothyroidism with goiter may be present in thyroiditis, secondary to drugs such as iodine and propylthiouracil, in inborn errors of thyroid hormonogenesis, and in iodine deficiency.

In primary hypothyroidism, TSH levels in blood are elevated. In secondary hypothyroidism the serum TSH is low and exogenous TSH causes an increase in serum thyroid hormones and radioiodine uptake.

Neonatal hypothyroidism has an incidence of approximately 1:4000.[13] I-123 thyroid uptake and scintigraphy differentiate athyreotic or ectopic hypothyroidism from other causes of decreased thyroid function in the newborn. Normal or increased uptakes can be seen in newborns with biochemical hypothyroidism who have no palpable goiter but require treatment. In newborn patients with primary nongoitrous hypothyroidism the incidence of ectopic thyroid gland is high, and it has been reported to be from 22 to 75%.[20] We found an incidence of ectopic thyroid of 50% in a small group of patients. In two of 10 patients with abnormal thyroid scintigraphy there was no demonstrable uptake of I-123. The incidence of ectopic thyroids in these patients is greater in females than in males with a female-to-male ratio of 2:1–5:1. The finding of ectopic thyroid tissue rather than athyreosis may favor a better prognosis for mental development in these individuals. Thyroid evaluation with I-123 adds useful information in the clinical evaluation of infants suspected of hypothyroidism as a result of neonatal screening.[16]

Thyroiditis

Chronic lymphocytic thyroiditis (Hashimoto's thyroiditis) is a common cause of acquired hypothyroidism in children.[45] It presents most typically as an euthyroid goiter. Chronic thyroiditis in children younger than 5 years of age is unusual, and its incidence increases during puberty. Chronic thyroiditis is thought to be an autoimmune disorder. The goiter is usually of modest size, diffuse, and moderately firm. Nodular goiters may sometimes occur, and may be a result of scarring or asymetric hyperplasia. Clinical and biochemical tests during the acute stage may indicate only normal or low thyroid function. The 4- and 24-h radioiodine uptake may be low, normal, or even elevated in this condition. The demonstration of significant titers of thyroid antibodies usually suffices to make the diagnosis. Thyroid scans with I-123 vary in appearance, depending on the stage of evolution of the disease. A relatively large radioactive thyroid silhouette may be seen in the acute stages. Radioiodine uptake may be abnormally high. Images later on may show a pattern of diffuse or patchy distribution of the tracer. Hyperthrophic nodules may be present causing discrete areas of increased radionuclide uptake in the thyroid. Due to deficient production of thyroid hormone, elevated values of TSH are maintained. Discrete or poorly defined areas of decreased or absent uptake of the tracer may be seen in subacute or chronic thyroiditis.

Subacute thyroiditis (acute simple thyroiditis, giant-cell thyroiditis, granulomatous thyroiditis, de Quervain thyroiditis) is rare in children. It is a self-limiting inflammatory disease of the thyroid. The etiology of this disease is unknown, but it may be due to a viral infection.[11,14,40] Characteristically, the patient may present with pain and tenderness in the thyroid, fever, and systemic manifestations. However, the presentation may vary and cases of painless thyroiditis are not uncommon. Transient hyperthyroidism may be present, and it may be followed by a period of hypothyroidism. Scintigraphy reveals poor or even absent uptake of radioiodine. Patchy distribution of the tracer may be seen also. Later on, the thyroid scan usually returns to normal. Scintigraphy may be useful to separate hyperthyroidism due to Graves' disease from that caused by subacute painless thyroiditis.

Other Nonneoplastic Causes of Goiter

Iodine ingestion in the form of expectorants is a very frequent cause of goiter in patients with chronic respiratory diseases such as cystic fibrosis. These goiters may be quite firm. Other disorders causing thyromegaly include acute bacterial thyroiditis, iodine deficiency, and colloid goiter.

Head and Neck Irradiation

Hypothyroidism is sometimes a sequela of external radiation therapy directed to the face and neck. There is also an increased incidence[31] of thyroid carcinoma secondary to irradiation of head and neck.[10,12,21,31,33] In a large series of children with thyroid carcinoma, 76% of 496 patients for whom appropriate history was available were found to have had prior irradiation to the head and neck.[44] Multicentric foci have been found in about 50% of the cases and in 30% both lobes were involved. The latent period between irradiation and the occurrence of thyroid carcinoma extends from about 3 years to an apparent peak at 25–35 years; however, thyroid carcinoma will probably appear beyond this peak time.[31]

Thyroid Carcinoma

Carcinoma of the thyroid is an unusual neoplasm in children, accounting for <3.0% of cancer from all sites in patients under 15 years of age.[9] About 90% of all thyroid carcinomas in children are well-differentiated and consist of papillary and/or follicular cells.[44] In most cases a mixed pattern of papillary and follicular elements is present, particularly in those patients under 40 years of age. These tumors usually concentrate iodine. Metastatic dissemination of these tumors is mostly via lymphatics to local lymph nodes, with pulmonary and bony metastases less frequent. In a series of 58 children with thyroid carcinoma who were followed over a 40-year period 88% developed cervical metastases, including 63% at the time of initial diagnosis, and 19% had pulmonary metastases when first seen.[15] Adult patients with extrathyroidal papillary carcinoma have a 10-year survival rate of about 60%, and those with papillary carcinoma limited to the thyroid found only at microscopy a 10-year survival rate of about 90%.[4] Winship and Rosvoll, in their worldwide survey of thyroid carcinoma in children, reported a 14% mortality with papillary and/or follicular histology. Others report mortality rates of 2–8% in children with thyroid cancer.[7,15,17,19] The prognostic significance of cervical metastases is controversial.[4,43] Patients with pulmonary metastases have a far worse prognosis. However, in these individuals, longterm survival, even for decades, is not uncommon.[4] In follicular carcinoma of the thyroid, metastatic disease to the lungs is more common than with papillary carcinoma.[8] Follicular carcinoma accounts for about 20% of the cancers of the thyroid. This tumor is slow-growing and frequently concentrates radioiodine.

A tumor of the thyroid that does not concentrate radioiodine is the anaplastic carcinoma. This tumor grows and invades very rapidly. Anaplastic carcinoma of the thyroid is one of the most malignant tumors found in humans. Another tumor that does not concentrate iodine is the medullary carcinoma of the thyroid. This rare neoplasm is of parafollicular or C-cell origin and accounts for 5–10% of all thyroid malignancies. This tumor can be associated with various paraneoplastic syndromes and may be part of one of the multiple endocrine neoplasia (MEN) syndromes. Both sporadic and familial forms occur. The prognosis is quite variable, with some cases exhibiting aggressive local spread and distant metastases, while others demonstrate very benign behavior for many years.[2]

Carcinoma of the thyroid may occur at any age but is most common during the fifth decade of life. About 60% of children with thyroid carcinoma present with regional lymphadenopathy as the leading symptom. Whole body scanning using I-131 is used to detect local and distant metastases. Only those tumors of the thyroid that are well-differentiated will show accumulation of I-131. In addition to the thyroid gland and metastatic lesions, it should be recognized that there are other regions in the body in which iodine is taken up. These organs include the choroid plexus, nasopharynx, salivary glands, stomach, intestine, and bladder. Complete surgical thyroidectomy is very difficult so that even following total thyroidectomy it is possible to find residual iodine uptake in the thyroid bed (Fig. 12-13). Pulmonary metastases develop in 10–40% of patients with differentiated carcinoma of the thyroid.[46] When searching for metastatic thyroid disease exogenous thyroid medication must be discontinued for at least 2–3 weeks before administering the diagnostic dose of I-131. The endogenous TSH levels in blood must be elevated in order to ensure an adequate metastatic examination. Thyroidectomy is essential for increasing the availability of I-131 to metastatic lesions by increasing TSH secretion. Very rarely, exogenous TSH is used in order to produce a stimulation of metastases when endogenous TSH levels are low. Disadvantages with the administration of exogenous TSH include side effects of the allergic type, ranging from urticaria to anaphylaxis, and the expense.

The treatment for thyroid carcinoma in children is primarily surgical. Subtotal thyroidectomy plus node dissection are frequently performed. Attempts at total thyroidectomy are often unsuccessful and carry a significant risk of permanent hypoparathyroidism. Radical neck dissection is not indicated in children.[9] Ablation of residual normal thyroid tissue or cervical metastases can be accomplished with I-131.[4,15,17,19] This has been shown to reduce the rate of recurrence,[24] though convincing evidence of its increasing longterm survival has not been published and controversy remains regarding the role of I-131 therapy in patients with disease limited to the neck.[7,22,38,43] Patients with distant metastases are candidates for I-131 therapy. The usual dose of I-131 for therapy is 50–150 mCi depending on patient size and extent of disease.[4,9,24,30] Careful dosimetric estimates should be obtained in each case to determine that this modality will be effective, and that the bone marrow dose will be within tolerable limits.[23] Multiple treatments are often necessary to achieve a therapeutic effect. Complications from I-131 therapy are uncommon. Brinckner reported a 1–2% incidence of leukemia in his review of 487 published cases and 194 cases in his own series who were given therapeutic doses of I-131. Fertility and birth histories in a series of 40 patients treated with I-131 prior to 21 years of age were within acceptable norms for the general population.[37] Pulmonary fibrosis following I-131 therapy has been reported, but only in patients with diffuse pulmonary metastases given massive doses.[4] Several precautions are necessary for the handling of patients and their excreta, and these are described in guidelines by the National Council on Radiation Protection and Measurements.[26]

References

1. Barnes JW, Bentley G. Production of iodine-123 in the LASL radiochemistry hot cells. Proc Conf Remote Sy Tech 1980; 27:292–4.

2. Baylin SB, Wells SA. Management of medullary thyroid cancer. in: Greenfield LD, ed. Thyroid cancer. 1979; 151–163. West Palm Beach, FL: CRC Press.
3. Beekhuis H, Piers DA. Radiation risk of thyroid scintigraphy in newborns. Eur J Nucl Med 1983; 8:348–50.
4. Beierwaltes WH. The treatment of thyroid carcinoma with radioactive iodine. Semin Nucl Med 1978; 8:79–94.
5. Bett R, Cuninghame JC. Iodine-123 production and chemical characteristics. Nuklearmedizin 1982; 19(Suppl):289–93.
6. Brinkner H, Hansen HS, Anderson AP. Induction of leukemia by I-131 treatment of thyroid carcinoma. Br J Cancer 1973; 28:232–7.
7. Buckwalter JA, Thomas CG, Freeman JB. Is childhood thyroid cancer a lethal disease? Ann Surg 1975; 181:632–6.
8. Casara D, Zorat PL, Busnardo B, Girelli ME. Pulmonary metastases from thyroid carcinoma detected only by radionuclide imaging. Br J Radiol 1981; 54:362–3.
9. Clayton GW, Kirkland RT. Cancer of the thyroid in children. In: Greenfield LD, ed. Thyroid cancer. 1978; 207–21. West Palm Beach, FL: CRC Press.
10. DeGroot L, Paloyan E. Thyroid carcinoma and radiation: a Chicago endemic. JAMA 1973; 225:487–91.
11. Dorfman SG, Cooperman MT, Nelson RL, Depuy H, Peake RL, Young RL. Painless thyroiditis and transient hyperthyroidism without goiter. Ann Intern Med 1977; 86:24–28.
12. Favus MJ, Schneider AB, Stachura ME, Arnold JE, Ryo UY, Pinsky SM, Colman M, Arnold MG, Fortham LA. Thyroid cancer occurring as a late consequence of head-and-neck irradiation. Evaluation of 1056 patients. N Engl J Med 1976; 294:1019–25.
13. Fisher DA, Dussault JH, Foley TP, La Franchi S, Mitchell ML, Klein AH, Larsen PR, Murphey WH, Walfish PG. Screening for congenital hypothyroidism: results of screening one million North American infants. J Pediatr 1979; 94:700–5.
14. Hamburger JI. Subacute thyroiditis: diagnostic difficulties and simple treatment. J Nucl Med 1974; 15:81–89.
15. Harness JK, Thompson NW, Nishiyama RH. Childhood thyroid carcinoma. Arch Surg 1971; 102:278–84.
16. Heyman S, Crigler JF, Treves S. Congenital hypothyroidism: I-123 thyroidal uptake and scintigraphy. J Pediatr 1982; 101:571–4.
17. Jareb B, Lowhagen T. Carcinoma of the thyroid in children and young adults. Acta Radiol 1972; 11:411–21.
18. Jingerman JM, Lagunas-Solar MC. Cyclotron production of high purity I-123 for medical applications. J Radioanal Chem 1981; 65:31–45.
19. Joppich I, Roher HD, Hecker WC, Knorr D, Daum R. Thyroid carcinoma in childhood. Prog Pediatr Surg 1983; 16:23–28.
20. Kaplan M, Kauli R, Lubin E, Grunebaum M, Laron Z. Ectopic thyroid gland, a clinical study of 30 children and a review. J Pediatr 1978; 92:205.
21. Kaplan MM, Garnick MB, Gelber R. Li FP, Cassady JR, Sallan SE, Fine WE, Osack MJ. Risk factors for thyroid abnormalities after neck irradiation for childhood cancer. Am J Med 1983; 74:272–80.
22. Leeper RD. The effect of I-131 therapy on survival of patients with metastatic papillary or follicular thyroid carcinoma. J Clin Endocrinol Metab 1973; 36:1143–52.
23. Maxon HR, Thomas SR, Hertzberg VS, Keriakes JG, Chen I, Sperling MI, Saenger EL. Relation between effective radiation dose and outcome of radioiodine therapy in thyroid cancer. N Engl J Med 1983; 309:937–41.
24. Mazzaferri EL, Young RL, Oertel JE, Kemmerer WT, Page CP. Papillary thyroid carcinoma: the impact of therapy in 576 patients. Medicine (Baltimore) 1977; 56:171–96.
25. Mochizuki Y, Mowafy R, Pasternack B. Weights of normal thyroids in New York City Health Physics 1963; 9:319–321.
26. NCRP Report No. 37. Precautions in the management of patients who have received therapeutic amounts of radionuclides. 1973; 6–23. NCRP Publications, Washington, DC.
27. New England Congenital Hypothyroidism Collaborative. Effects of neonatal screening for hypothyroidism: prevention of mental retardation by treatment before clinical manifestations. Lancet 1981; ii:1095–8.
28. Ochi H, Sawa H, Fukuda T, Inoue Y, Nakajima H, Masuda Y, Okamura T, Onoyama Y, Sugano S, Ohkita H, Tei Y, Kamino K, Kobayashi Y. Thallium-201 chloride thyroid scintigraphy to evaluate benign and/or malignant nodules. Usefulness of the delayed scan. Cancer 1982; 50:236–40.
29. Perry HA. Solid thyroid nodules. Am Surg 1982; 8:170–4.
30. Pfister-Goedeke L, Stauffer UG. Thyroid carcinoma in childhood. Prog Pediatr Surg 1983; 16:29–37.
31. Pinsky S, Ryo Y. Thyroid imaging: a current status report. In: Freeman L, Weissmann H, eds. Nuclear medicine annual. 1981; 157–94. New York: Raven Press.
32. Reaume CE, Sofie VL. Lingual thyroid. Review of the literature and report of a case. Oral Surg 1978; 45:841–5.

33. Refetoff S, Harrison J, Karanfilski BT, Kaplan EL, DeGrott LJ, Bekerman C. Continuing occurrence of thyroid carcinoma after irradiation to the neck in infancy and childhood. N Engl J Med 1975; 292:171–5.
34. Richards P, Prach T, Srivastava SC, Meinken GE. An iodine-123 generator/iodination kit: a preliminary report. J Radioanal Chem 1981; 65:47–50.
35. Safa AM, Schumacher OP. Follow up of children treated with I-131 (letter to the editor). N Engl J Med 1976; 294:54.
36. Safa AM, Schumacher OP, Rodriguez-Antunez A. Long term follow-up results in children and adolescents treated with radioactive iodine (I-131) for hyperthyroidism. N Engl J Med 1975; 292:167–71.
37. Sarker SD, Beierwaltes WH, Gill SP, Cowley BJ. Fertility and birth histories of patients treated with I-131 for thyroid cancer before 1969 at age of 20 years or less. J Nucl Med 1976; 17:460–4.
38. Varma VM, Beierwaltes WH, Nofal MM, Nishiyama RH, Copp JE. Treatment of thyroid cancer: death rates after surgery and after surgery followed by sodium iodide I-131. JAMA 1970; 214:1437–42.
39. Vincent JS, Dougan AH, Lyster DL, Blue JW. A facility for the production of iodine-123 by spallation of cesium. J Radioanal Chem 1981; 65:17–29.
40. Volpe R. Subacute (de Quervain's) thyroiditis. Clin Endocrinol Metab 1979; 8:81–95.
41. Webster EW, Alpert NM, Brownell GL. Radiation doses in pediatric nuclear medicine and diagnostic x-ray procedures. In: James AE, Wagner HN, Cooke RE, eds. 1974; 34–58. Pediatric nuclear medicine. Philadelphia: WB Saunders.
42. Wellington H, August GP, Randolph JG, Schisgall RM, Chandra R. Solitary thyroid nodules in children and adolescents. J Pediatr Surg 1982; 17:225–9.
43. Wilson SM, Block GE. Carcinoma of the thyroid metastatic to lymph nodes of the neck. Arch Surg 1971; 102:285–91.
44. Winship T, Rosvoll RV. Thyroid carcinoma in childhood: final report on a 20 year study. Clin Proc Child Hosp Natl Med Cent 1970; 26:327–48.
45. Winter J, Eberlein WR, Bongiovanni AM. The relationship of juvenile hypothyroidism to chronic lymphocytic thyroiditis. J Pediatr 1966; 69:709.
46. Worm AM, Holten I, Taaning E. Nuclear imaging of pulmonary metastases in thyroid carcinoma. Acta Radiol Oncol 1980; 19:401–3.

Chapter 13 Brain

S. T. Treves
Roy L. Strand
Robert K. Crone
Annalise Lipp

The introduction of computed tomography, with its high sensitivity and reasonable specificity, has resulted in a decrease in the use of scintigraphy of the brain. Routine use of both radionuclide scintigraphy and computed tomography is not currently justifiable. At Children's Hospital in Boston about 700 scintigraphic studies of the brain were performed in 1972 while only 30 were done during 1983. Another important contribution in the diagnosis of cerebral disorders in newborns that has contributed to the decrease in radionuclide scans of the brain has been the development of cranial ultrasonography. Scintigraphic studies, however, remain useful in some clinical settings. In addition, hospitals that do not have access to computed tomography equipment rely more heavily on radionuclide studies in the evaluation of disorders of the central nervous system.

The radionuclide method is attractive due to the low radiation dose to the patient, the high sensitivity, and the lack of risk.[5,15,21,28]

Indications for radionuclide studies of the brain include the following: symptoms and signs suggesting the presence of an intracranial tumor such as persistent headache, vomiting, seizures, papilledema, focal motor signs, ataxia, or nistagmus; head trauma for the possibility of subdural hematoma, effusion, or hydrocephalus; inflammatory conditions such as meningitis or brain abscess; acute hemiplegia; and vascular abnormalities.

In a previous study in our institution, radionuclide brain scanning had a true-positive rate of 83%, and a true-negative rate of 99%. Patients with symptoms of increased intracranial pressure, focal motor signs, bacterial infection, suspected tumor, trauma, congenital malformations, ataxia, nystagmus, and dizziness have the highest percentage of abnormal radionuclide studies. Brain abscess, subarachnoid bleeding, intracranial tumors, cerebrovascular accidents, and immune complex disease result in a high yield of scintigraphic abnormality. Diseases that have the least likelihood to result in abnormal radionuclide scans include seizure disorder, headache, mental retardation, demyelinating disease, and hydrocephalia.[28]

Cerebral radionuclide angiography permits evaluation of cerebral vascular territories following intravenous injection of a radionuclide.

Static scintigraphy of the brain reflects changes in the permeability of the blood–brain barrier. Increased permeability of the blood–brain barrier to radionuclides is nonspecific. Most lesions in the brain reveal increased radionuclide uptake, while a small number of them are not detectable. Rarely a lesion exhibits lower concentration of tracer than the surrounding brain matter, for example, a cerebral or subarachnoid cyst.

Method

Radiopharmaceuticals

Technetium-99m (Tc-99m) as sodium pertechnetate has been widely used for both cerebral radionuclide angiography and static scintigraphy of the brain. Most technetium-labelled tracers commonly used for scintigraphy are normally excluded from the brain substance. After intranveous injection, Tc-99m sodium pertechnetate is loosely bound to serum albumin and red blood cells. This tracer is lost from the vascular space with a clearance half-time of 30–40 min. It is eliminated by the gastrointestinal tract and the kidneys. Approximately 20% of the administered activity remains in the blood at 2 h. Any abnormality that disturbs the blood–brain barrier permit tracers to penetrate the brain substance. A usual dose of this tracer is 200 μCi/kg of body weight with a total minimal dose of 2 mCi. Patients receiving Tc-99m pertechnetate are premedicated with sodium (intravenous) or potassium (oral) perchlorate in a dose of 3–6 mg/kg of body weight in order to block uptake of the tracer by the choroid plexus. Tc-99m DTPA or Tc-99m glucoheptonate may be used also at the same dose levels as pertechnetate. These tracers have been suggested as alternatives to Tc-99m pertechnetate, offering higher lesion-to-background ratios. Both have more rapid blood disappearance rates than pertechnetate, and they do not concentrate in the choroid plexus; therefore, premedication with perchlorate is not necessary. See Chapter 16 for absorbed dose estimates with pertechnetate, and Chapter 4 for dosimetry of Tc-99m DTPA.

Examination Technique

A computerized gamma camera equipped with high sensitivity, high resolution, converging and pinhole collimators is recommended. The high-sensitivity collimator is useful for cerebral radionuclide angiography; the high-resolution collimator is used for static scintigraphy. The converging collimator may be useful for cerebral radionuclide angiography in small children and the pinhole collimator, with its greater resolution, is useful for spot imaging of the brain and the posterior fossa.

Other than premedication with perchlorate when using pertechnetate no additional patient preparation is necessary. Sedation is indicated with irritable or uncooperative patients.

Cerebral radionuclide angiography is usually performed with the patient in the supine position and the camera viewing the head anteriorly. Other projections may be chosen as appropriate according to the clinical situation. A rapid bolus of radiotracer is given intravenously and recording on the computer is begun immediately at one frame/sec for 60 sec. Simultaneous analog images are recorded on film at a rate of one/2–3 sec for 60 sec.

Approximately 30 min after the cerebral radionuclide angiogram, static images of the brain are recorded on the computer and on analog format. Anterior, laterals, posterior, and vertex views are obtained for 500,000 counts each. Lateral views are obtained for the same time exposure. Additional delayed views at 2–4 h after injection of the tracer are obtained in some cases in order to attempt to localize a lesion not detected on the early views, to enhance the lesion-to-background ratio, and/or to assess better the extent of lesions already detected on early views.

Experience with radionuclide computed tomography in children is limited. Some initial evidence suggests that tomography results in an improvement in the diagnostic capability of radionuclide imaging of the brain (Figure 13-1).[3,13,16,20]

Clinical Applications

Normal Study

A normal anterior cerebral radionuclide angiogram reveals three phases: the arterial phase, the capillary phase, and the venous phase. The arterial phase reveals the bolus of tracer as it circulates in the carotid and vertebral arteries, the area of the circle of Willis, and the territories of the anterior and middle cerebral arteries. These two arterial territories appear on the angiogram as a characteristic symmetric "trident." This appearance will be distorted in the presence of tumors, vascular accidents, hydrocephalus, vasculitis, etc. In cerebral death the intracranial vascular territories are not visualized. The capillary phase shows rather diffuse distribution of the tracer and the venous phase reveals activity within the venous sinuses (Fig. 13-2).

Normal static cerebral scintigraphy reveals lack of radiotracer concentration in the brain matter with some activity in the vascular spaces of the Sylvian fissures, the sagittal and transverse sinuses, and superficial tissues, skull, and skin. The cerebral hemispheres appear symmetric. Activity in prominent superficial veins and/or the temporal muscle may cause confusion in the interpretation of images obtained immediately after the injection. Later images may be helpful in this regard. The choroid plexus is not visualized unless perchlorate is inactive, or has not been absorbed, or in the presence of a choroid plexus papilloma (Fig. 13-3).

Radionuclide images of the brain can be im-

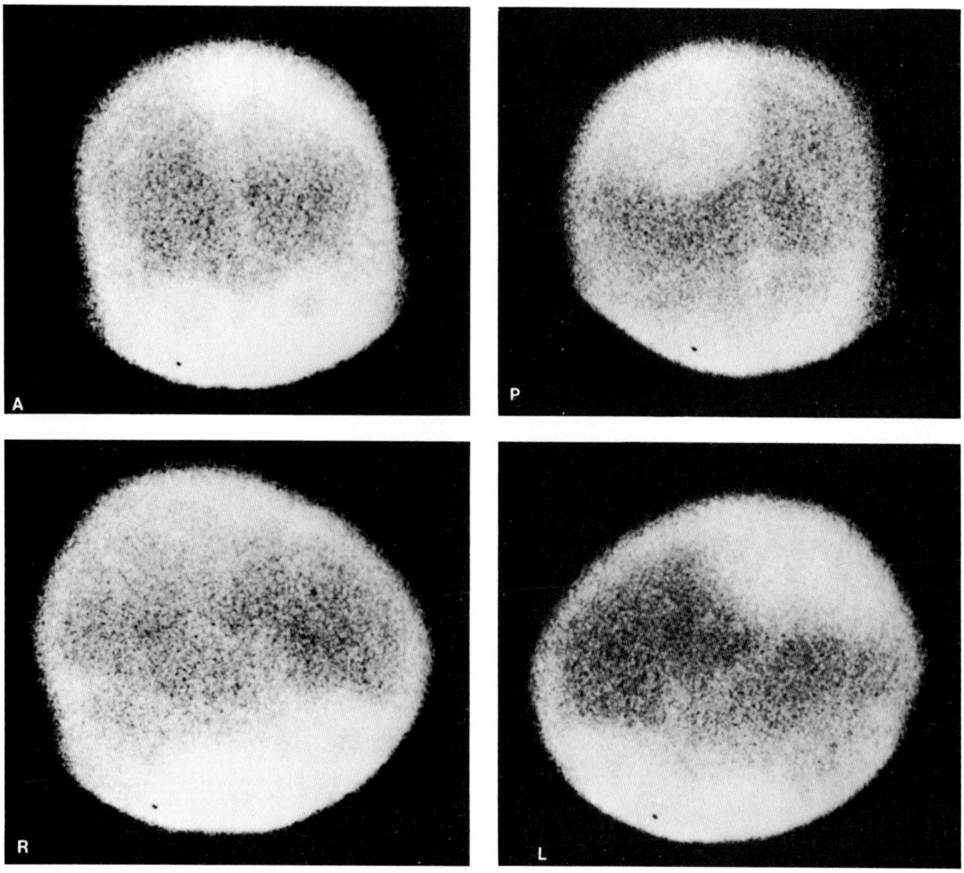

Figure 13-1. A: Radionuclide brain scan from a young patient with a massive meningioma. A, Anterior; P, Posterior; R, Right lateral; L, Left lateral.

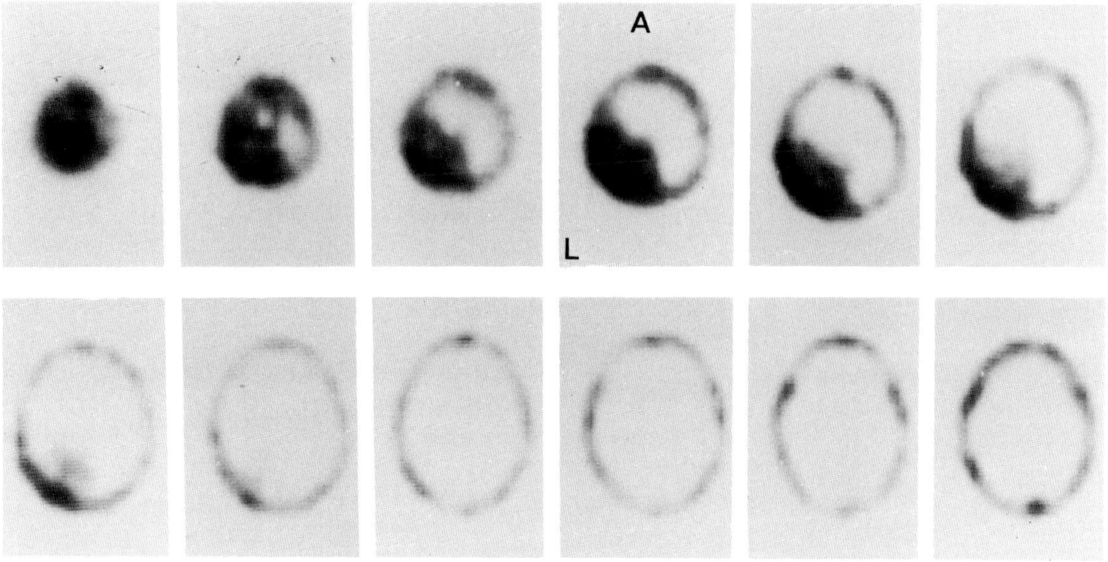

Figure 13-1. B: Single-photon (Tc-99m pertechnetate) tomography on the same patient outlines the extent of the tumor better than the images obtained with the stationary gamma camera.

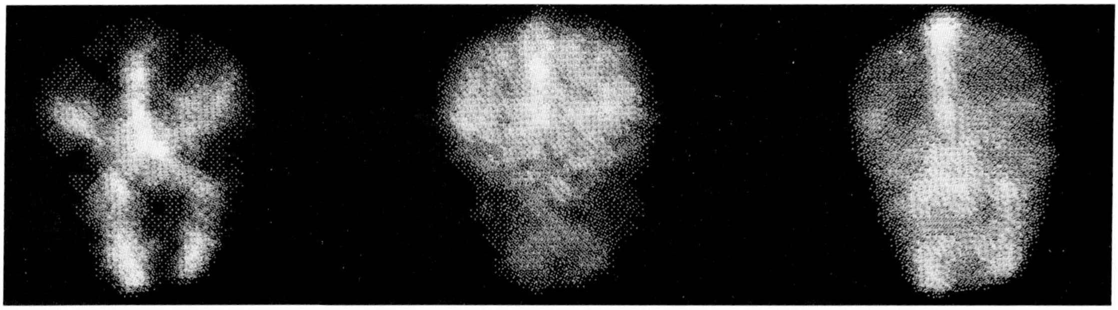

Figure 13-2. Normal Tc-99m NaO_4^- cerebral radionuclide angiogram (CRA). Selected frames; each image represents 2 sec. The arterial, capillary, and venous phases are shown.

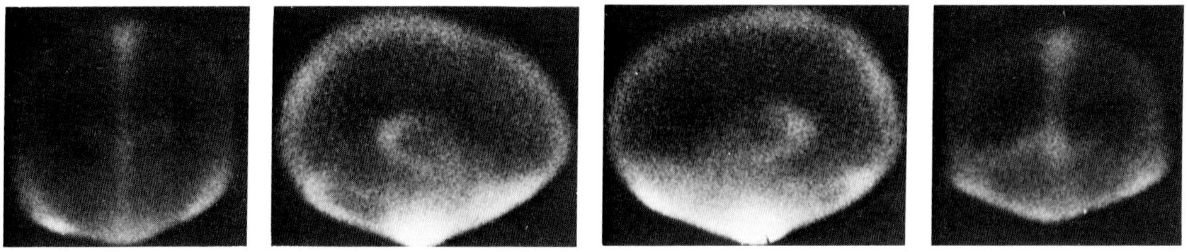

Figure 13-3. Normal Tc-99m NaO_4^- brain scan with visualization of normal choroid plexus activity. This patient had not been premedicated with potassium perchlorate in the investigation of a possible choroid plexus papilloma. (Anterior, right lateral, left lateral, posterior views.)

proved by computer contrast enhancement in order to reduce the effect of high activity from salivary glands and soft tissues, and to augment visualization of intracranial activity (Fig. 13-4).

Tumors

Scintigraphic detection of tumors depends on various factors including location, size, vascularity, intactness of the blood–brain barrier, rate of tumor growth, histology, and technique. Our findings for tumor detectability are similar to those published in the literature (85–90%). Infratentorial tumors are more difficult to detect than supratentorial tumors (Figs. 13-5–13-9). Craniopharyngiomas and optic gliomas can be detected in the majority of instances with multiple projections and magnification scintigraphy. Brain stem glioma is particularly difficult to detect with scintigraphy, due to its deep location and overlying bony structures. Certain benign tumors (usually cystic) do not concentrate radiopertechnetate significantly. In this regard it is important to note that the degree of tracer concentration in tumors does not correlate with histologic type or degree of malignancy of the tumor.

Routine administration of perchlorate has been reported not to interfere with scintigraphic detection of choroid plexus papilloma. In two cases, however, we observed that perchlorate produced either total or partial suppression of pertechnetate uptake by such tumor[17] (Figs. 13-10 and 13-11). Since tumors of the posterior fossa are more common in children than in adults, careful technique with appropriate projections and magnification should be employed. Tc-99m DTPA or Tc-99m glucoheptonate, with their rapid blood disappearance and lack of uptake by the nasooral mucosa and the salivary glands, may be of value in identifying posterior fossa tumors.

Trauma

Acute complications of head trauma include leak of cerebrospinal fluid, fracture of the skull, sub-

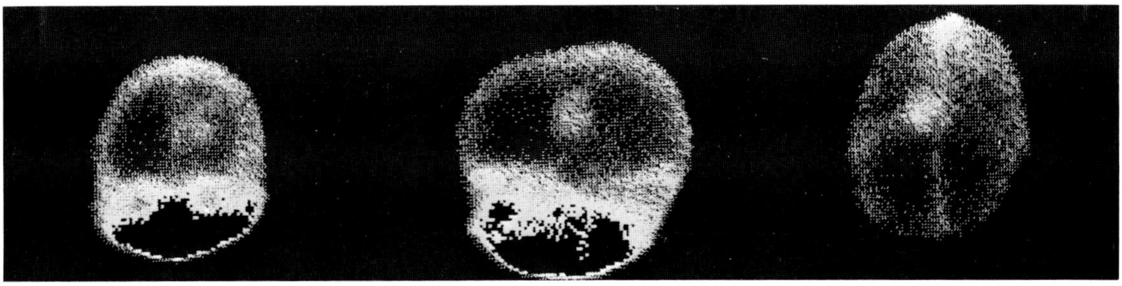

Figure 13-4. Maliganant glioma. Tc-99m NaO_4^- brain scan. Background and activity corresponding to salivary and facial concentration of the tracer was reduced by computer enhancement. (Anterior, left lateral, vertex views.)

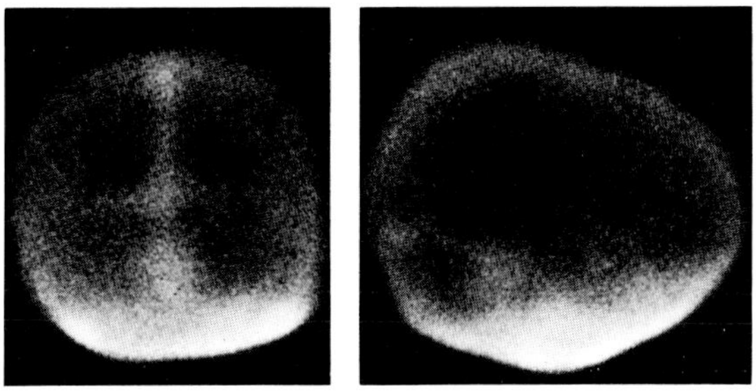

Figure 13-5. Microcystic astrocytoma. Tc-99m NaO_4^- brain scan shows a well-defined area of increased uptake in the posterior fossa at the midline. *Left:* posterior view; *right:* right lateral view.

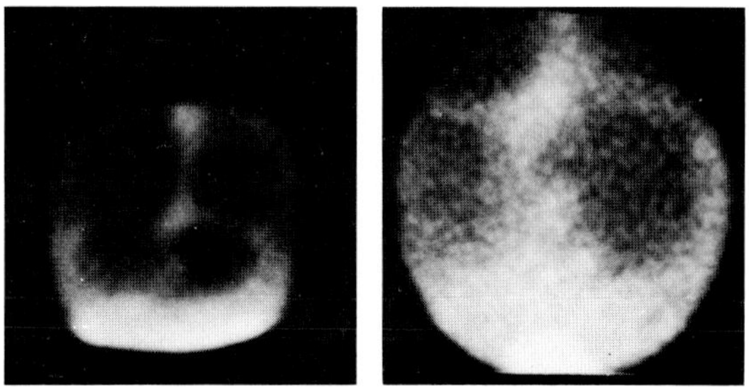

Figure 13-6. Astrocytoma. Tc-99m NaO_4^- brain scan from a 3.5-year-old male with a history of hyperactivity. The posterior view reveals a well-defined area of increased concentration of the tracer in the posterior fossa at the midline *(left)*. The lesion is appreciated better on the image obtained with the pinhole collimator *(right)*.

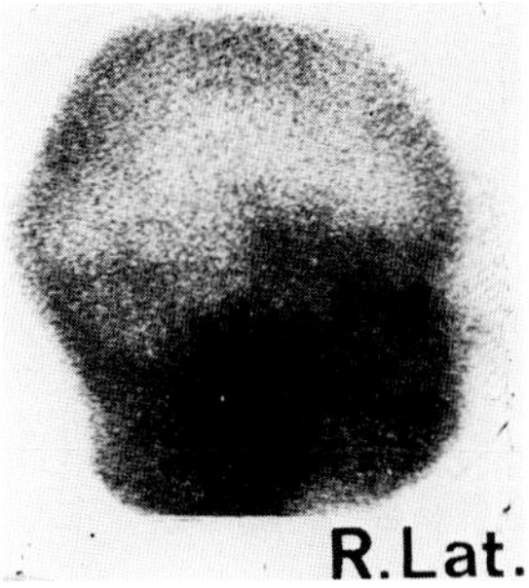

Figure 13-7. Tumor of the hypothalamus and the third ventricle. Tc-99m NaO_4^- brain scan reveals increased uptake projecting on the lateral view over the suprasellar region. R. Lat., right lateral view.

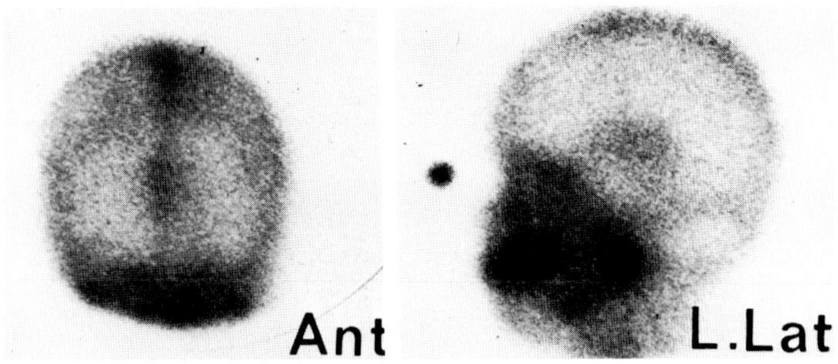

Figure 13-8. Medulloblastoma of the posterior region of the third ventricle. Tc-99m NaO_4^- brain scan shows increased concentration of the tracer in the region of the tumor. Ant., anterior view; L. Lat., left lateral view.

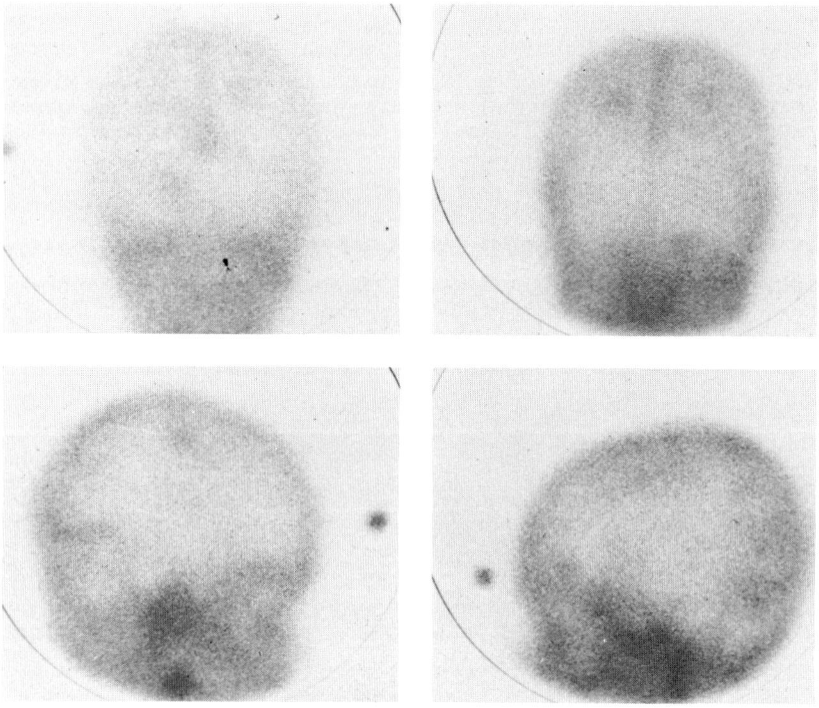

Figure 13-9. Malignant mesothelioma of the myocardium with brain metastases visualized on a Tc-99m NaO_4^- brain scan.

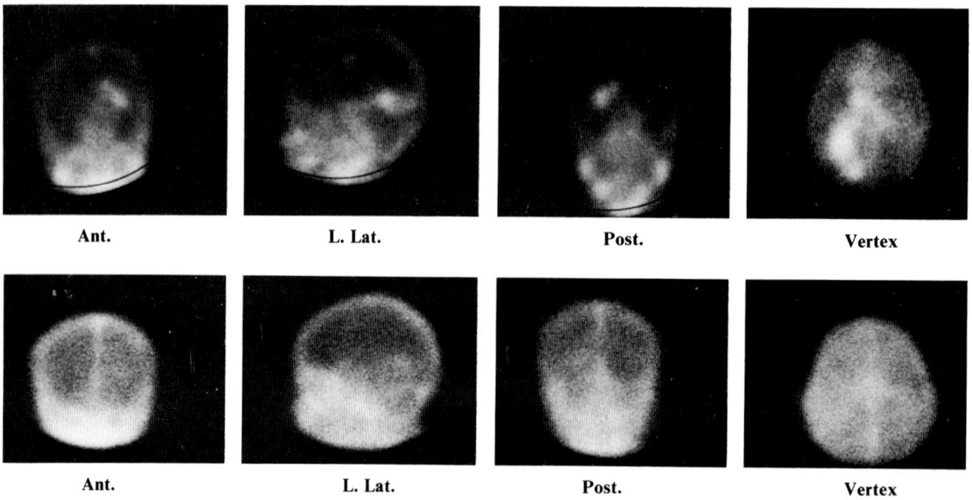

Figure 13-10. Malignant choroid plexus papilloma, Tc-99m NaO_4^- brain scan without *(top)*, and with *(bottom)* premedication with potassium perchlorate. This tumor extends into a large portion of the ventricular system, particularly on the left side. Perchlorate results in a marked reduction of radiotechnetium uptake by the tumor.

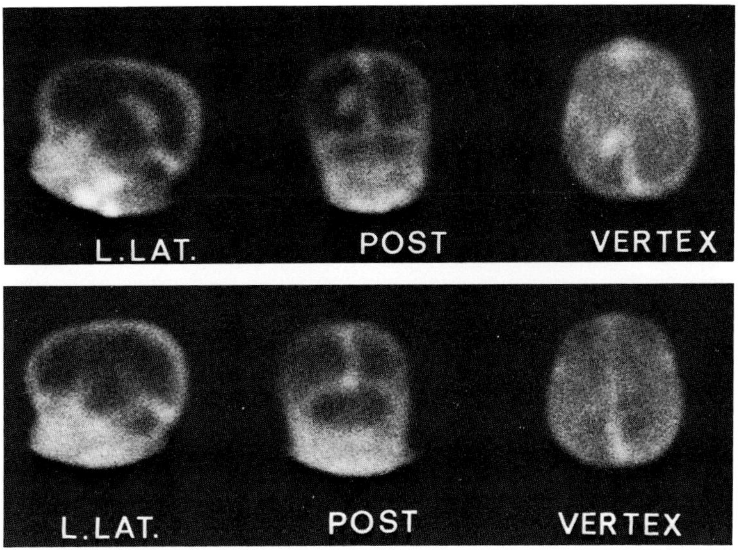

Figure 13-11. Choroid plexus papilloma. Suppression of Tc-99m NaO_4^- uptake by perchlorate. *Top:* Scan without premedication reveals intense uptake of the tracer in the tumor. *Bottom:* Perchlorate blocks uptake of radiotechnetium in the choroid plexus papilloma.

dural hematoma, edema, intracerebral hemorrhage, and intraventricular hemorrhage. Late complications include arteriovenous fistula, brain abscess, CSF leak, subdural hematoma, and atrophy of the brain.

Early in the development of a subdural hematoma or effusion, radionuclide angiography may demonstrate a superficial area of reduced to absent perfusion during the arterial and capillary phases of the study.[14]

Subdural hematomas on static scans appear as superficial areas of increased uptake that extend anteroposteriorly. Detection with scintigraphy will depend on the size of the hematoma and on the timing of the study relative to the acute episode. The likelihood of a positive result is greatest at 5–10 days following injury. Very small effusions may not be detected at all and small bilateral effusions (common in children) may be difficult to recognize, particularly if they are symmetric. The best projections to evaluate for subdural hematomas and effusions are the anterior, vertex, and posterior projections.

The heads of patients with established or suspected head trauma must be inspected for evidence of heamtomas, laceration, infection, or inflammation of the soft tissues, sites of subdural taps, and intravenous infusion in the superficial veins of the head. Any of these may produce increased uptake of tracer and confuse interpretation of cerebral scintigraphs. Skull fracture will also cause focal increase in tracer uptake. Burr holes and surgical flaps also create positive results. Brain scintiscans may remain abnormal for several months to several years following skull trauma, or after surgical intervention in the skull.

Other processes that may reveal a pattern of abnormal uptake similar to that of subdural hematoma include meningitis and superficial tumors.

Brain abscess which may occur following trauma will be detected by scintigraphy in almost all cases.

Cerebral Death

With the advent of organ system support technology, traditional methods of determining that death has occurred have become less well defined. Although irreversible cessation of cardiorespiratory function is still the most common criterion by which death is determined, cardiopulmonary assist devices may prolong these functions even after brain function has ceased. Permanent cessation of brain function is a clinical and legal definition of death.

Several committees have attempted to define criteria by which death can be declared under these circumstances, starting with the Beecher Committee in 1968 and more recently by the report, *Defining Death,* by the President's Commission for the Study of Ethical Problems in Medicine and Biomedical and Behavioral Research. These reports have carefully outlined the criteria for determining brain death in adults. These same reports have consistently suggested that caution be used when applying these criteria to children, presumably due to a lack of experience.

It is generally accepted that the clinical triad of coma, apnea, and absent brain stem reflexes, as evaluated for adults, also applies to children.[1,2,7,24] It is important to emphasize that the clinical examination is considered to be the most important component of the criteria for the determination of brain death. Laboratory studies can be used as adjuncts in determining brain death; however, they are only confirmatory in nature and may not be necessary depending upon the circumstances. Each clinical situation must be considered individually to decide which, if any, of these studies will be helpful.

Determination of Death

Death has occurred whenever an individual has suffered either an irreversible cessation of circulatory and respiratory function, or when he or she has suffered an irreversible cessation of all functions of the entire brain, regardless of cardiopulmonary status.

1. *Determination of cardiopulmonary death.* Clinical examination will disclose at least the absence of responsiveness to external stimulation, heartbeat, and respiratory effort in the absence of hypothermia or circulatory assist devices. Confirmatory laboratory tests may include electroencephalography, or blood pressure measurement by sphygmomanometry or transduced intraarterial pressure. Irreversibility is recognized by persistent cessation of functions during a period of time appropriate for the history and clinical conditions. In situations where death is observed and expected, 5 min may be a reasonable period of observation, whereas in the unobserved or unexpected situation resuscitative measures should be instituted and maintained for a more prolonged period of time. In the hypothermic patient, death cannot be determined until a core temperature of 30°C is reached, unless rigor mortis or putrefaction has occurred.

2. *Determination of brain death.* Brain death has occurred when cerebral and brain stem functions are irreversibly absent. Absent cerebral function is recognized clinically as the lack of responsivity; that is, there is no autonomic or somatic response to any sort of external stimulation, mediated through the brain stem. Absent brain stem function is recognized clinically when pupillary light, corneal, oculocephalic, oculovestibular, oropharyngheal, and respiratory reflexes are irreversibly absent. Procedures for testing for these reflexes are listed below. Particularly in children, peripheral nervous activity including spinal cord reflexes may persist after brain death; however, decorticate or decerebrate posturing is inconsistent with brain death.

Irreversibility is recognized when the cause of coma is established and when the possibility of recovery is excluded by observation for an appropriate period of time. It is important that the cause of coma be established whenever possible. Absence of brain function due to head trauma has different implications than that due to a metabolic abnormality or intoxication. Important reversible causes that may mimic irreversibility are sedation, hypothermia, neuromuscular blockade, and shock. If the cause of coma cannot be established, these reversible conditions must be ruled out by appropriate laboratory studies. These studies include analysis of blood and urine for clinically significant levels of toxic substances that might produce coma, such as sedatives, hypnotics, and anesthetics; measurement of core body temperature, which must be greater than 32°C, and measurement of peripheral neuromuscular function.

The period of time of observation will also vary depending on the circumstances and possible causes. In most cases where the etiology is established and seems appropriate, such as severe inoperable head trauma, a period of 6 h seems reasonable and is commonly recommended, whereas with hypoxic-ischemic encephalopathy, a period of 24 h may be more appropriate.

Confirmatory laboratory finding may be appropriate in determining brain death, and possibly accelerate the determination of irreversibility. However, if etiology and irreversibility are established and the clinical examination is unequivocal, confirmatory tests are unnecessary.

Historically, laboratory studies have been relied on in many instances where not strictly necessary because pediatricians have been reluctant to depend exclusively on their skills for making such an important decision. Also, parents in a state of shock and disbelief at the loss of a previously healthy child frequently need time and objective data before accepting the death as real. Lastly, many cases of brain death in pediatrics involve medicolegal concerns that require substantial documentation.

The Clinical Examination for Brain Death

In order for the neurological examination to be valid, the following preexisting conditions must be met:

1. Normotension
2. Normothermia
3. Absence of clinically significant levels of anesthetic, psychotropic, hypnotic, or analgesic drugs
4. Confirmation of normal peripheral neuromuscular function
5. Absence of mydriatic drugs
6. Absence of clinically significant metabolic abnormalities.

Cerebral unresponsiveness is manifested by deep coma, that is, there must be no spontaneous movement and no response to either auditory or painful somatic stimulation delivered to each extremity and both sides of the face.

Brain stem unresponsiveness is confirmed by the absence of the following reflexes mediated by the brain stem:

1. Absent pupillary light reflex
2. Absent ciliospinal reflex
3. Absent corneal reflex
4. No spontaneous eye movement
5. Absent doll's eye movements
6. Absent oculovestibular reflex. After confirmation of the patency of the external auditory canal, 25–50 ml of saline should be injected against each tympanic membrane, confirming the absence of associated nystagmus.
7. Absent gag response to oropharyngeal stimulation.
8. Absent cough reflex to tracheal and carinal stimulation.
9. Apnea. Absence of respiration is confirmed by administering 100% oxygen through the ventilator for 5 min with a ventilator rate adjusted to produce an arterial P_{CO_2} of 35 torr or greater. With continual flow of 100% oxygen, the ventilator rate is turned to zero for an additional 5 min. Apnea is confirmed if there is no evidence of spontaneous respiration with an associated arterial P_{CO_2} of 60 torr or greater.

Cerebral radionuclide angiography has been used for confirmation of brain death in children and adults. This technique is particularly useful in coma due to drugs. In cerebral death the radionuclide angiogram reveals absence of perfusion to the territories of the anterior and middle cerebral arteries. In addition, there is lack of visualization of the sagittal sinus on the venous phase of the study (Fig. 13-12). There will be evidence of activity in the superficial tissues over the head. The territories of the carotid and vertebral arteries usually are visualized to the level of the circle of Willis.[25]

Cerebral Complications of Congenital Heart Disease

Acute cerebral vascular occlusion and brain abscess are relatively frequent complications in patients with cyanotic congenital heart disease. Overwhelmingly, the former occurs in patients under 2 years of age and the latter in patients over 2 years of age. Cerebral radionuclide angiography in conjunction with static brain scintigraphy is useful in the evaluation of patients with acute cerebrovascular compromise. Cerebral radionuclide angiography is capable of demonstrating a reduction in cerebral blood flow almost immediately after the accident (Fig. 13-13). Cerebral infarction is usually not detected on the static images until 3–6 days following the onset of symptoms. In children, however, we have seen positive brain scans within a few hours to 1 day after infarction (Fig. 13-14).

Scintigraphy is a very sensitive and reliable method for the detection of brain abscesss and can delineate the lesion quite precisely (Figs. 13-15 and 13-16). We have never encountered a patient with a brain abscess and a normal radionuclide brain scan. External detection with the aid of small radioactive markers is useful in localizing the abscess in relation to superficial structures and thus facilitates surgical drainage. Several brain abscesses have been surgically drained successfully after localization by brain scintigraphy alone.

Delayed images at 3–6 h after the injection of

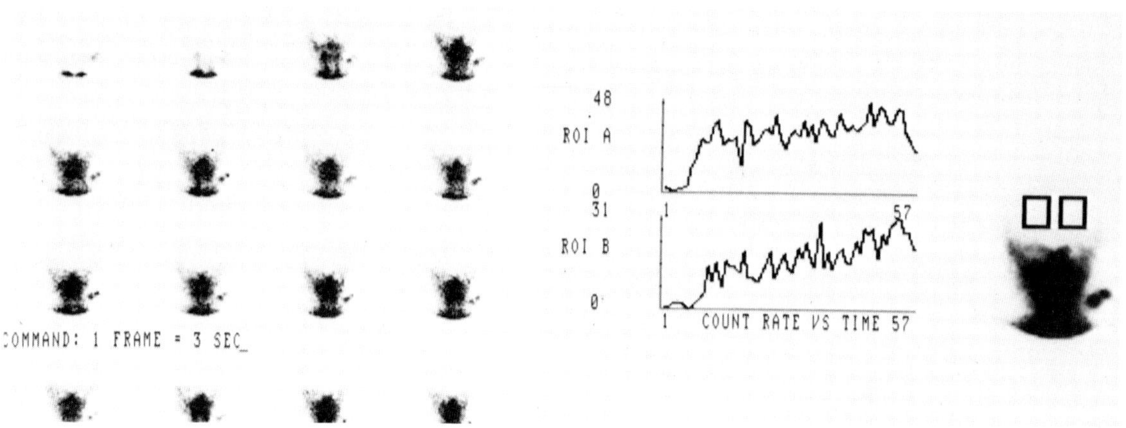

Figure 13-12. A: Cerebral death. *Left:* CRA (one fame/3 sec) with Tc-99m NaO_4^-. The injection of the tracer was made into a catheter placed into the superior vena cava. The territories of the carotid and the vertebral arteries are visualized on the second and third frames. There is no evidence of perfusion in the anterior and the middle cerebral artery territories. Only slowly circulating activity in the tissues of the surface of the head is visualized. In addition there is no visualization of the sagittal sinus during the venous phase. *Right:* Time-activity curves of the cerebral hemispheres reveal low amplitude and lack the normal arterial peak.

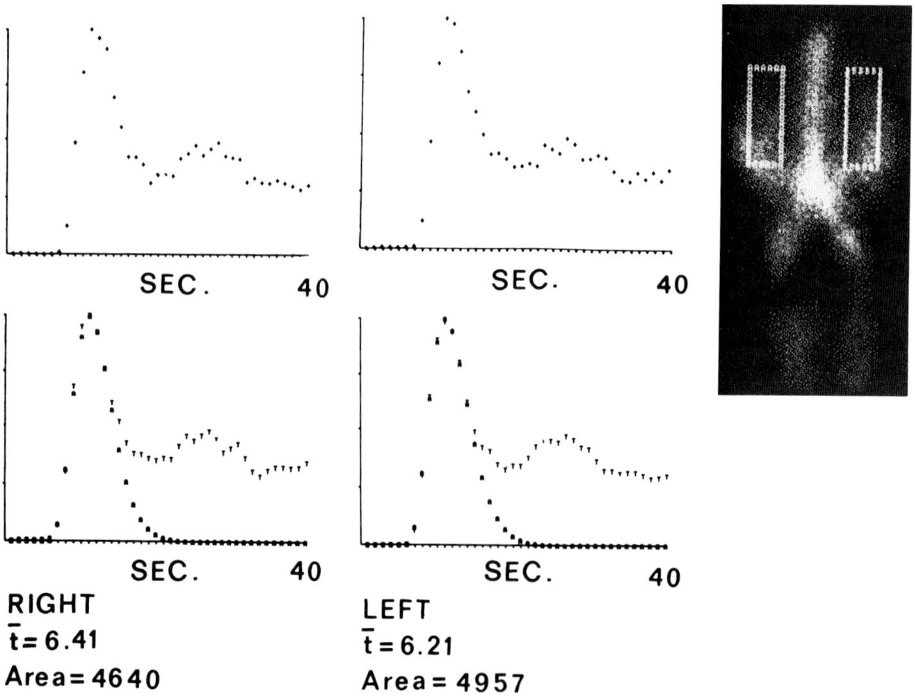

Figure 13-12. B: Normal time-activity curves from a CRA.

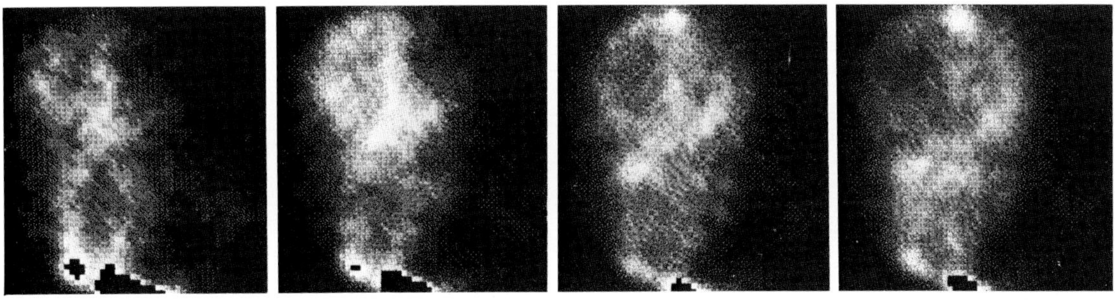

7 sec. 9 sec. 12 sec. 16 sec.

Figure 13-13. Cerebrovascular accident. Patient with congenital heart disease. Tc-99m NaO_4^- CRA shows lack of blood flow to the territory irrigated by the left middle cerebral artery (7–9 sec). There is delayed arrival of the tracer to the right side. Anterior view.

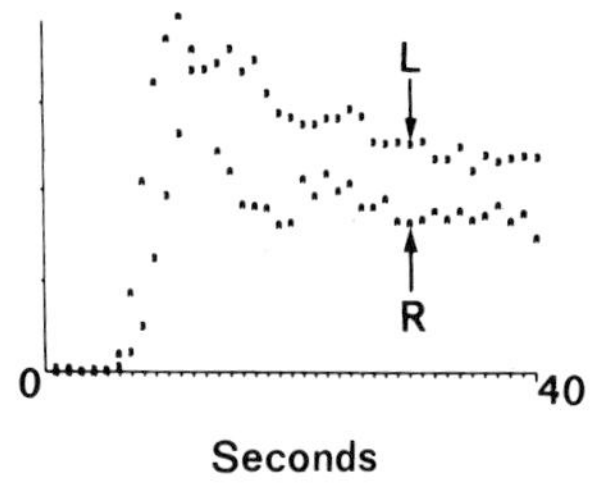

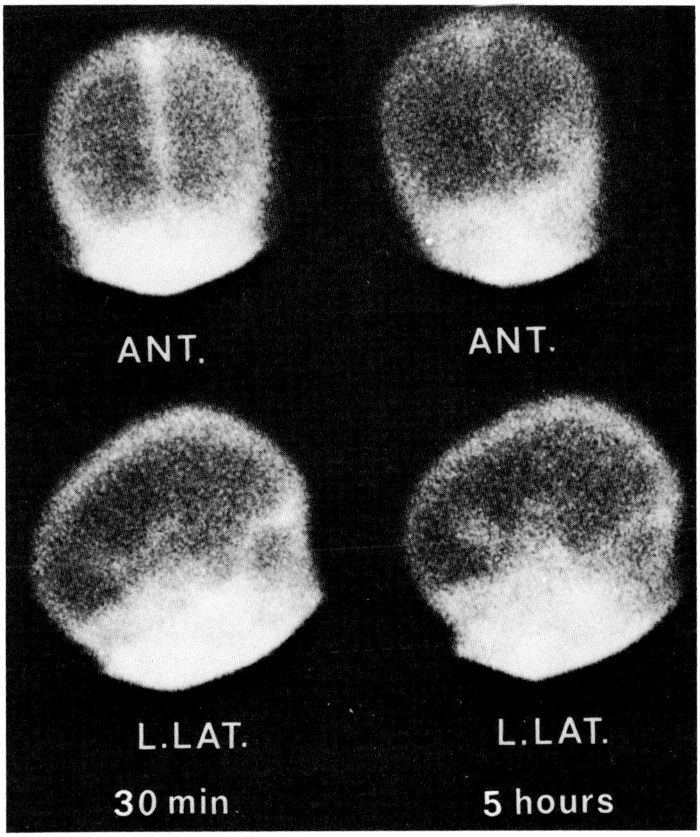

Figure 13-14. Cerebral infarct. Tc-99m NaO_4^- brain scan 1 day after an infarct. There is increased uptake of the tracer in the left frontoparietal region, which is more evident on images obtained 5 h after the injection of the tracer.

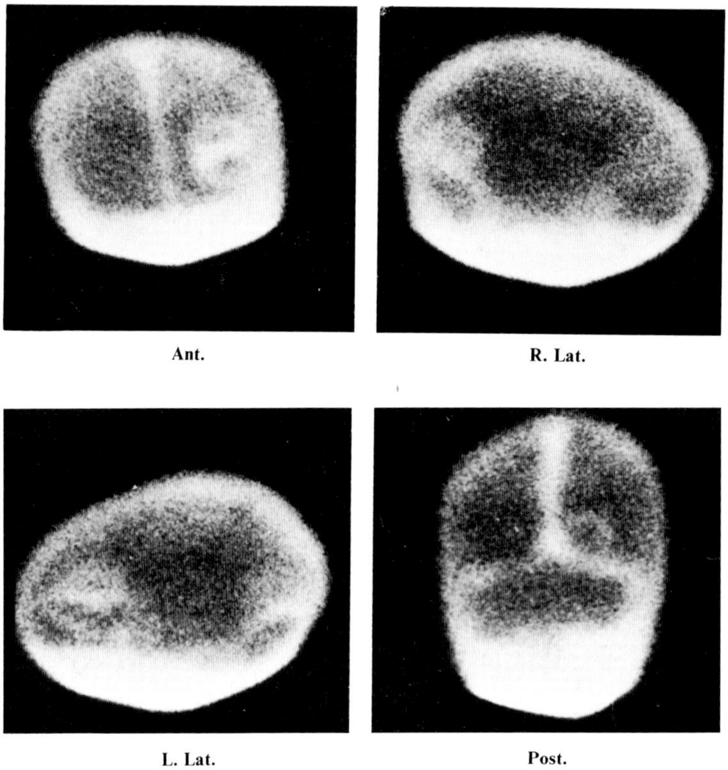

Figure 13-15. Multiple cerebral abscesses in a patient with cyanotic congenital heart disease (left frontal and right occipital regions). Tc-99m NaO_4^- brain scans. Ant. anterior view; R. Lat., right lateral view; L. Lat., left lateral view; Post., posterior view.

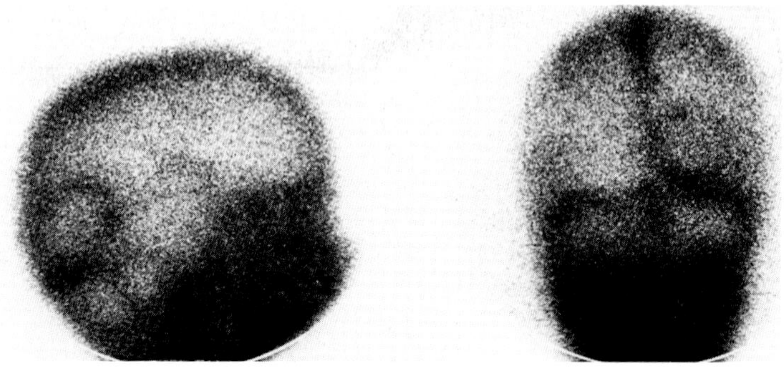

Figure 13-16. Brain abscess in a patient with cyanotic congenital heart diesase. The TC-99m NaO_4^- brain scan reveals a rounded area of increased tracer uptake to the right of the sagittal sinus and just above the right transverse sinus.

radiotracer should be employed, as they are useful for the detection and/or better localization of brain infarct (Fig. 13-14) and brain abscess, particularly in the presence of an initially normal or suspicious radionuclide brain scintigraph.[6,26]

Diseases of the Subdural Space

Subdural collections are frequently bilateral and in children they may occur higher over the convexity than in adults.[29] Subdural collections are bilateral in about two-thirds of pediatric cases and in only about 15% of adult cases.[6] Although they are usually more severe on one side, the contrast between normal and abnormal sides may be low, and this can make scintigraphic diagnosis of subdural collection difficult. On radionuclide scans, subdural collections appear as areas of superficial increased uptake of the tracer (Fig. 13-17).

Infectious Diseases

As discussed before, radionuclide imaging is a sensitive and efficacious technique for the detection and localization of brain abscess. Scintigraphy is almost always abnormal even before there is central liquefaction during the phase of cerebritis (Fig. 13-18).

Radionuclide brain scanning may be more sensitive than computerized axial tomography in the demonstration of intracranial infectious diseases.[23]

Meningitis usually reveals superficial, localized, and/or generalized increased uptake of radiotracer. In meningitis due to *Haemophilus influenzae* unilateral concentration of radiotracer over one hemisphere has been found simulating the scintigraphic appearance of subdural hematoma. This pattern of activity may be found in meningitis with or without the presence of subdural fluid. About 50% of cases of *Haemophilus influenzae* meningitis have an effusion. This may be subclinical, but can be demonstrated by subdural tap or by computed tomography. This type of meningitis is the most common cause of subdural effusion in infants. Alternately, multiple areas of increased uptake may be seen that probably represent infection or cortical vein thombosisss.[6]

In meningoencephalitis radionuclide scanning demonstrates an increase in concentration of the tracer peripherally over the brain. Focal encephalitis can be detected as well on radionuclide images of the brain. Diffuse encephalitis usually demonstrates a nonspecific and diffuse pattern of increased radionuclide uptake on brain scanning. Ventriculitis causes a focal or diffuse increase in tracer uptake in the region of the ventricles.

Herpes encephalitis is visualized on radionuclide brain scanning as foci of increased uptake in one or both temporal lobes. Less frequently, the frontal or parietal lobes are affected. Cerebral radionuclide angiography may demonstrate hyperperfusion of the affected region of the brain early in the disease. Later in the course of the disease, when a region of necrosis develops, the angiogram may show decreased cerebral perfusion. Abnormalities on radionuclide studies are present as early as 3–5 days after the onset of symptoms.

Radionuclide brain scans in pyogenic meningitis may be initially normal, but most frequently they reveal increased peripheral uptake (Fig. 13-19).

Deep foci of increased radionuclide uptake may be found in subacute sclerosing panencephalitis. This is an uncommon, progressive, and frequently fatal disease. This disease of the brain affects children and young adults. There is widespread destruction of myelin in the cerebral hemispheres and focal lesions in the brain stem. This disorder, which evolves over months, is believed to be caused by a measles type of virus.

Seizure Disorders

Seizures are common in pediatric patients. The majority are benign and self-limited convulsions associated with fever. The majority of pediatric patients with seizure disorders do not demonstrate abnormality on the cerebral radionuclide angiogram or on the static radionuclide brain scan. In children with whom the initial problem is generalized seizure with a normal neurlogic examination and normal or nonspecific electroencephalogram the likelihood that a brain scan will reveal focal abnormality is very low. Only about 0.5% of patients with seizure disorder will have an abnormal radionuclide brain scan.[28] Scintigraphy may well be abnormal in patients with seizures due to arteriovenous malformation or tumor. Patients with seizure disorders and findings suggestive of focal or expanding intracranial lesion will be more likely to reveal focal abnormality on the radionuclide brain scan.[10,28] Tumor is an important but uncommon cause of seizure in children. Cerebral radionuclide

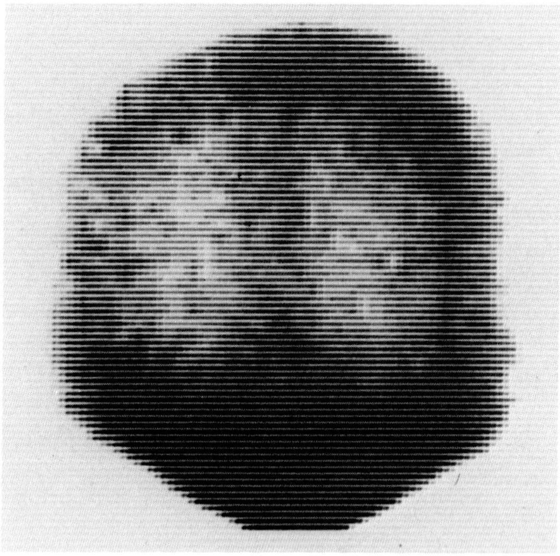

Figure 13-17. Left subdural effusion. Tc-99m brain scan shows increased tracer uptake along the left convexity. Anterior view.

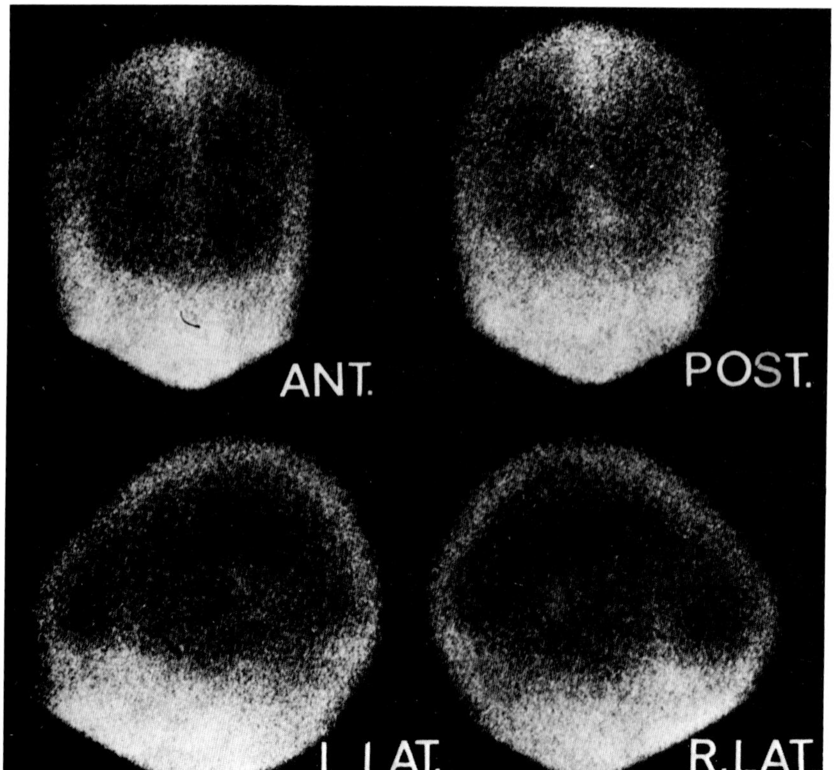

Figure 13-18. Cerebritis. Small, not well-defined area of increased uptake of Tc-99m NaO_4^- in the right posterior parietal region.

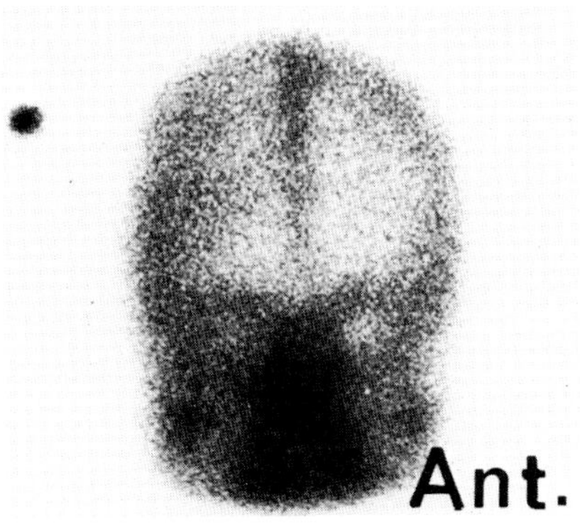

Figure 13-19. Pneumococcal meningitis in a 7-month-old male. Tc-99m NaO_4^- brain scan shows increased uptake of the tracer over the right convexity.

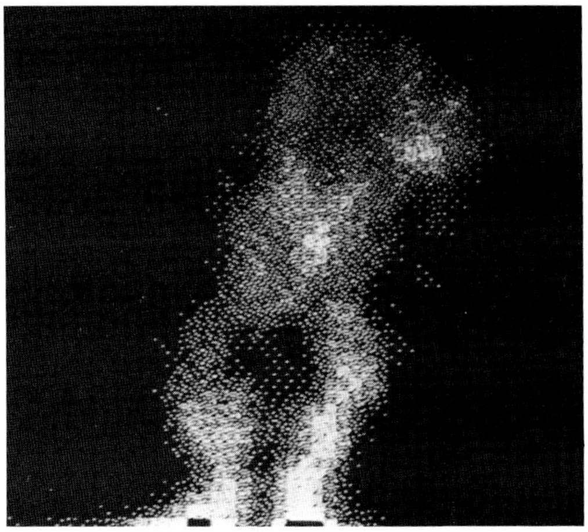

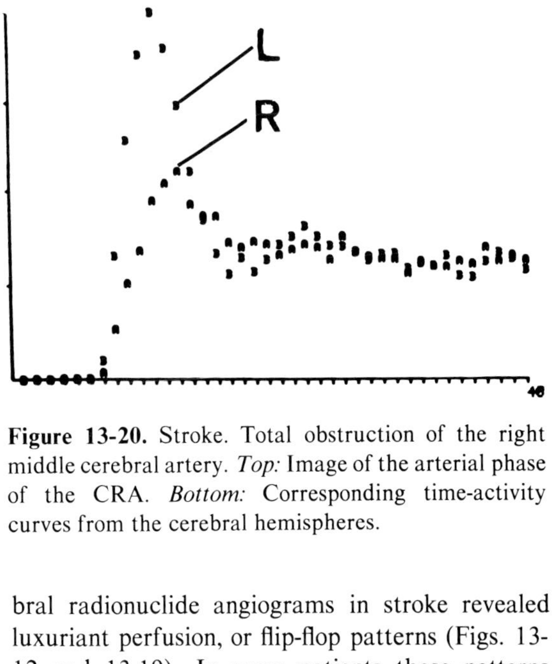

Figure 13-20. Stroke. Total obstruction of the right middle cerebral artery. *Top:* Image of the arterial phase of the CRA. *Bottom:* Corresponding time-activity curves from the cerebral hemispheres.

angiography, if performed soon after a seizure, may reveal increased perfusion to the affected hemisphere. Similarly, static scintigraphy may demonstrate transient increase in radiotechnetium uptake, on images obtained soon after an ictal episode.

Headache—Mental Retardation

Headache alone as the presenting symptom has one of the lowest probabilities of resulting in abnormal brain scans. Equally low is the possibility of finding abnormal brain scans in patients with mental retardation.

Stroke

Vascular disorders may be caused by vascular occlusion or cerebral hemorrhage. Vascular obstruction may be caused by emboli, thrombosisss, or abnormality of the walls of vessels. Cerebral hemorrhage may be present with aneurysm, arteriovenous malformation, arterial or venous occlusion, trauma, and infection.

Cerebral radionuclide angiography is a sensitive method for the detection of stroke during the first week of the episode in children. Gates et al. in examining 33 children found that the accuracy of cerebral radionuclide angiography for detection of stroke during the first week of clinical symptoms was 94%, while computed tomography was 60% accurate and static scintigraphy only 11% accurate. During the second week the accuracy of computed tomography rose to 100%; however, static radionuclide scintigraphy improved only to 50%. Cerebral radionuclide angiograms in stroke revealed luxuriant perfusion, or flip-flop patterns (Figs. 13-12 and 13-19). In some patients these patterns changed to that of cerebral hemispheric ischemia.[9] Initially, in cerebrovascular accidents the static brain scan is normal while the cerebral radionuclide angiogram shows decreased to absent perfusion to an arterial territory. This is followed by a persistent abnormality in the cerebral radionuclide angiogram, and a focal area of increased uptake on the static brain scan that follows a vascular territory (Fig. 13-20).[28]

Arteriovenous Malformation

Arteriovenous malformation is recognized on cerebral radionuclide angiography as an area of rapid and abundant perfusion of radiotracer on the ar-

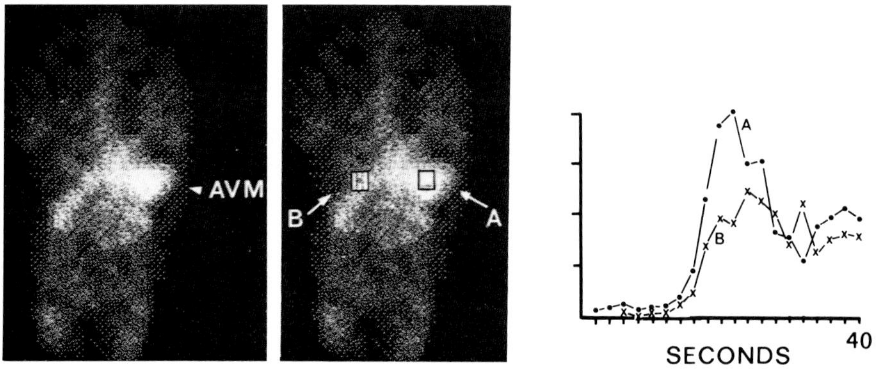

Figure 13-21. Arteriovenous malformation. Anterior CRA. Images are a composite of the arterial and capillary phases demonstrating an area of hyperperfusion over the left sides. Time-activity curves from the AVM on the left and a symmetric area on the right side are shown. The time course of activity is more rapid and the amplitude of the peak greater over the AVM. Static scintigraphy (not shown) revealed a normal pattern of distribution of the tracer.

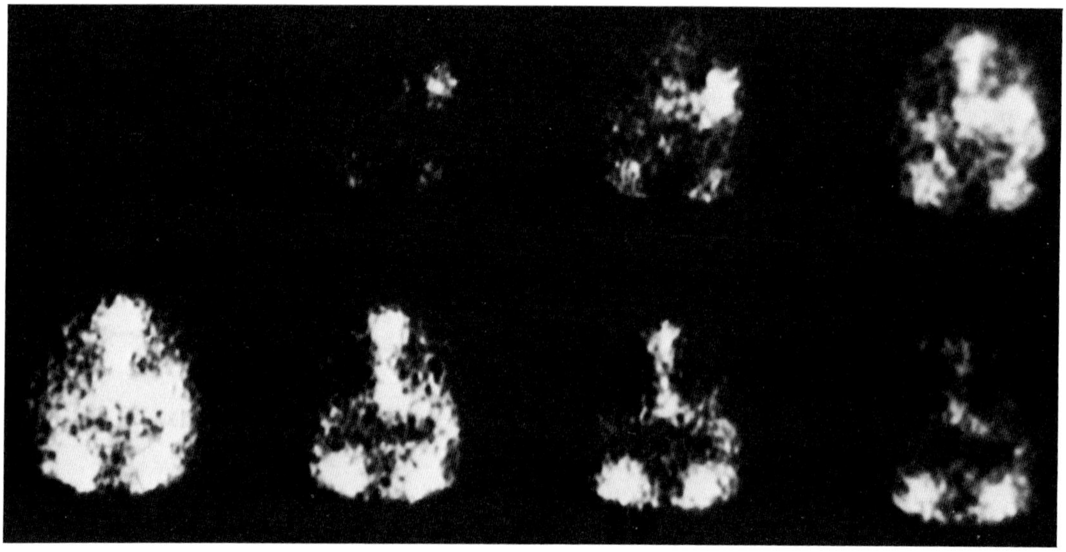

Figure 13-22. Arteriovenous malformation in the right occipital region. Posterior Tc-99m NaO_4^- CRA reveals an area of arterial "blush" in the right occipital region. The tracer disappears rapidly from this lesion and static scintigraphy obtained later revealed no focal abnormality. 1 frame = 2 seconds.

terial and capillary phases, and sometimes extending into the venous phase of the study. Compared with the normal side, time-activity curves over the arteriovenous malformation reveal a greater amplitude and more rapid transit of the tracer (Figs. 13-21 and 13-22).

A set of static scintigraphs should be obtained immediately following the radionuclide angiogram for more optimal localization of the lesion. As the intravascular concentration of radiotechnetium decreases with time it is not uncommon to observe a normal distribution of tracer on delayed static views.

Degenerative Neurologic Diseases

Abnormal radionuclide brain scans have been reported in a number of degenerative diseases of the

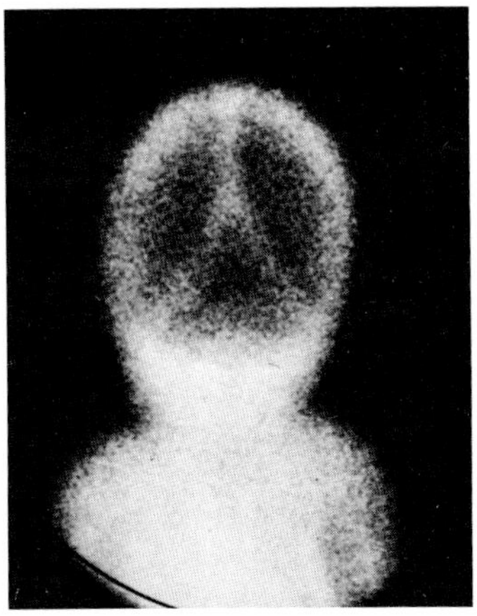

Figure 13-23. Dandy-Walker malformation. Posterior Tc-99m NaO_4^- brain scan shows an inverted Y appearance of the venous sinus.

central nervous system including demyelinating diseases, progressive multifocal leucoencephalopathy, adrenal leukodystrophy, Schilder's disease, and multiple sclerosis.[4,8,12,19,22,27] The value of radionuclide imaging of the brain in the diagnosis of these disorders is questionable, since generally degenerative diseases of the brain are diagnosed clinically and with other laboratory investigations.

Congenital Malformations and Abnormal Head Size and Shape

Asymetry of the skull and abnormal position of the venous sinuses and their confluence can be produced by unilateral cortical atrophy, large congenital cysts, chronic subdural collection, premature closure of one or more sutures, and congenital tumor. If an intracranial cyst is large it may appear as an area of decreased tracer uptake.

Dandy-Walker malformation, or enlargement of the posterior fossa due to congenital arachnoid cyst, will reveal an inverted Y appearance of the venous sinuses (Fig. 13-22). The inferior angle of the transverse sinus in this malformation is more acute (about 110°) than normal. Congenital aqueductal stenosis of the Arnold-Chiari malformation type II may result in an inferior displacement of the torcula herophili. Radionuclide studies in evaluation of congenital hydrocephalus are of limited if any value at present.

Diseases of the Skull

Many lesions of the skull result in scintigraphic abnormality. These include fibrous dysplasia, histiocytosis, metastatic neuroblastoma, hemangioma, bony metastases, and fibrosarcoma of the calvarium.[18]

References

1. A Report of the Ad Hoc Committee of the Harvard Medical School to examine the definition of brain death. A definition of irreversible coma. JAMA 1968; 205:85–88.
2. An Appraisal of the Criteria of Cerebral Death. A Summary Statement. A Collaborative Study. JAMA 1977; 237:982–6.
3. Carril JM, MacDonald AF, Dendy PP, Keyes WI, Undrill PE, Mallard JR. Cranial scintigraphy: value of adding computed tomographic section to conventional pertechnetate images (512 cases). J Nucl Med 1979; 20:1117–23.
4. Chatterton BE. Progressive abnormalities in the brain scan in adrenal leukodystrophy. AJR 1977; 129:939–40.
5. Conway JJ. Radionuclide imaging of the central nervous system in children. Radiol Clin North Am 1972; 10:291–312.
6. Conway JJ, Vollert J. The accuracy of radionuclide imaging in detecting pediatric dural fluid collections. Radiology 1972; 105:77–83.
7. Crone RK. Brain death (Editorial). Am J Dis Child 1983; 137:545–6.
8. Furuse M, Obayasi T, Tsuji S, Miyatake T. Adrenoleukodystrophy. Radiology 1978; 126:707–10.
9. Gates GF, Fishman LS, Segall HD. Assessment of cerebral perfusion in childhood strokes. Clin Nucl Med 1982; 7:502–11.
10. Golden GS, Erenberg G. Radionuclide brain scans in convulsive disorders. Pediatrics 1972; 49:787.
11. Report of the Medical Consultants on the Diagnosis of Death to the President's Commission for the Study of Ethical Problems in Medicine and Biochemical and Behavioral Research. Guidelines for the determination of death. JAMA 1981; 10:62–64.
12. Higgins CB, Taketa RM, Halpern SE. Abnormal brain scans in adrenal leukodystrophy. Radiology 1975; 114:667–9.
13. Hill TC, Costello P, Gramm HF, Lovett R, McNeil BJ, Treves S. Early clinical experience with a radionuclide emission computed tomographic brain imaging system. Radiology 1978; 128:803–6.
14. Hopkins GB, Kristensen KAB. Rapid sequential

scintiphotography in the radionuclide detection of subdural hematomas. J Nucl Med 1973; 14:288–90.

15. Hurley PJ, Wagner HN. Diagnostic value of brain scanning in children. JAMA 1972; 221:877–81.
16. Jarrit PH, Ell PJ, Myers MJ, Brown JG, Deacon JM. A new transverse-section brain imager for single-gamma emitters. J Nucl Med 1979; 20:319–27.
17. Kaplan W, McComb G. Strand R, Treves S. Suppression of technetium-99m pertechnetate uptake in a choroid plexus papilloma. Radiology 1973; 109:395–6.
18. Kieffer SA, Loken MK. Positive brain scans in fibrous dysplasia and other lesions of the skull. Am J Roentgenol 1969; 106:731–8.
19. Kirsh J, Rosenthall L, Finlayson MH, Wee R. Progressive multifocal leukoencephalopathy. Radiology 1976; 119:399–400.
20. Kuhl DE, Edwards RQ, Ricci AR, Yacob RJ, Mich TL, Alavi A. The Mark IV system for radionuclide computed tomography of the brain. Radiology 1976; 121:405–13.
21. Mishkin F. Brain scanning in children. Semin Nucl Med 1972; 2:328–42.
22. Moses DC, Davis LE, Wagner H. Brain scanning with Tc-99m O_4 in multiple sclerosis. J Nucl Med 1972; 13:847–8.
23. Pinsky S, Yum HY, Patel D, Beckerman C, Ryo UY. Comparison of radionuclide brain and computerized tomography for the detection of intracranial infections. Clin Nucl Med 1981; 6:12–18.
24. Rowland TW, Donnelly JH, Jackson AH, Jamioz SB. Brain death in the pediatric intensive care unit. A clinical definition. Am J Dis Child 1983; 137:547–50.
25. Schwartz JA, Baxter J, Brill D, Burns JR. Radionuclide cerebral imaging confirming brain death. JAMA 1983; 14:246–7.
26. Treves S, Yalaz RD, Yalaz K. Radionuclide investigation of the central nervous system in children. Prog Pediatr Radiol 1976; 5:86–111.
27. Weisbaum SD, Garnett ES. Brain scan in Schilder's disease. J Nucl Med 1973; 14:291–2.
28. Yalaz K. Treves S. Brain scanning and cerebral radioisotope angiography (CRA) in children. Pediatrics 1974; 54:696–703.
29. Zingesser LH. Scanning in disease of the subdural space. Semin Nucl Med 1971; 1:41–47.

Chapter 14 Cerebrospinal Fluid

S. T. Treves
Keasley Welch
Alvin Kuruc

RADIONUCLIDE CISTERNOGRAPHY

As in the case of radionuclide studies in the evaluation of disorders of the brain, the introduction of computed tomography has resulted in a major reduction in the use of radionuclide cisternography. This method has been used in conjunction with clinical examination and other neurological procedures in children to aid in the evaluation of hydrocephalus. Radionuclide cisternography permits the observation of the mixing and absorption of the cerebrospinal fluid (CSF). Normally after the introduction of a tracer into the lumbar subarachnoid space, the material progresses rapidly upward so that at about 6 h the basal cisterns and Sylvian fissures are outlined and at 24 h the material is over the cerebral hemispheres or in the parasagittal region[10,11] (Fig. 14-1). The CSF is a secretion. Two processes, however, occur in series. There is filtration from the capillary lumen to the interstitial spaces of the choroid plexus, and that filtrate is the fluid from which the secretion is elaborated by the lining epithelium.[41] The concept that CSF actually circulates in the spinal region with downward and upward currents of fluid may not be necessary, probable, or in any case the only mechanism that explains the movement of this fluid. It has been shown that with each pulse, about 0.75 ml of fluid from the cranium moves down into the spinal canal during systole and returns to the head in diastole. During this to-and-fro movement, mixing would occur and the kinetics of distribution of the tracer would be of the diffusional type and with a very high coefficient of diffusion.[12,41]

The production rate of CSF in children is about 0.30 ml/min, but lower in infancy. This represents 0.5% of the total volume of CSF/min.[25] Other workers measured CSF flows of 0.35–0.37 ml/min in patients.[5,6,37] CSF produced in the lateral ventricles flows through the foramina of Monro to join the CSF that is formed in the third ventricle. The movement of CSF continues through the aqueduct of Sylvius to the fourth ventricle, where the contribution of the rhombencephalic plexus is added, and through the foramen of Magendie mainly and to some extent the foramina of Luschka into the lateral and great cisterns. From the basal cisterns, the CSF moves up through the chiasmatic cisterns, Sylvian fissures, the pericallosal cisterns, and then laterally over the cerebral hemispheres, posteriorly around the cerebellum by way of the quadrigeminal cistern, and the posterior callosal cistern. A small quantity proceeds caudally around the spinal subarachnoid space. The major points of CSF reabsorption are the arachnoid villi.[8,9] Arachnoid granulations are not present at birth but progressively develop by 18 months of age. Both the arachnoid granulations and villi protrude through the dura into the superior sagittal sinus. The cranial villi are capable of absorbing three to five times the normal production of CSF. Communication with the granulations from the CSF is to vascular channels through which CSF passes preferentially in an outward direction.[42]

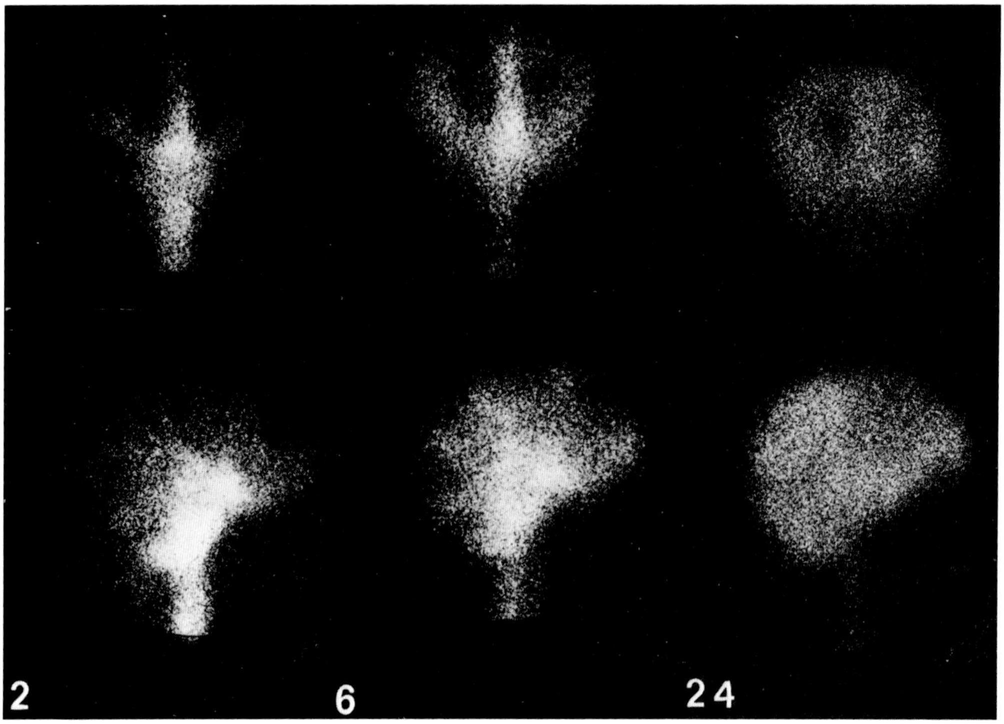

Figure 14-1. Normal In-111 DTPA cisternography. Anterior (Ant) and right lateral (R. Lat) views obtained 2, 6, and 24 h after the injection of the tracer into the lumbar subarachnoid space.

Method

Radiopharmaceuticals

Tracers used for radionuclide cisternography are confined to the CSF space and are quickly eliminated through the arachnoid without being metabolized. Either indium-111 (In-111) diethylenetriamine pentaacetic acid (DTPA) or technetium-99m (Tc-99m) DTPA is given in the subarachnoid space. Usual administered doses for Tc-99m DTPA are 0.3–1.0 mCi and for In-111 DTPA 50–200 μCi. For routine cisternography in children we prefer Tc-99m DTPA for its higher photon flux and lower radiation dose. The relatively short physical half-life of Tc-99m is not an obstacle to the evaluation of CSF in children because it is distributed more quickly. In older children and adults, In-111 DTPA is preferable. The radiation dose to the spinal cord and the surface of the brain with Tc-99m DTPA is about 1.0 rad/mCi administered. The radiation absorbed dose with In-111 DTPA is approximately 2.5 rad/mCi. Iodine-131 (I-131) albumin, which is not recommended for the evaluation of children, results in an absorbed radiation dose of about 7 rad with the usual administered dose of 0.1 mCi.

Method of Examination

The tracer is usually administered into the lumbar subarachnoid space. Other sites of injection include the cisterna magna or a lateral ventricle. Careful technique is essential. Following the subarachnoid administration of the tracer an image of the injection site is obtained in order to establish the adequacy of the injection. Epidural injections may produce a typical "Christmas tree" or a "railroad" appearance on the scintigraph and will result in an unsatisfactory examination. Routinely, series of images with the gamma camera are obtained on the anterior, posterior, and lateral projections at 2, 6, and 24 h after the administration of the tracer. Since the turnover of CSF in children is more rapid than in adults more frequent imaging is necessary. A high-resolution, low-energy collimator is used.

In the evaluation of CSF leaks more frequent images are obtained soon after the administration of the tracer. This is important in order to increase the chances of localizing the leakage. It is important that the patient be studied while there is active CSF leak in the position at which the leak is most profuse; otherwise visualization of the leak by this method may not be possible. For this purpose the patient is maintained in the position in which he may be known to leak more profusely, and images are obtained every half hour in the appropriate projection in an attempt to localize any extracranial activity. If extracranial activity due to a CSF leak is detected the patient is imaged on other projections in order to allow for a localization in two dimensions. The timing of the lateral and the anterior views is critical, as the CSF leak may be transient.

Small leaks may not be detectable by scintigraphy. In some instances it may be useful to place cotton pledgets in the nasal orifices which should be changed and carefully labeled every 2–4 h and counted for activity. In some instances it may be necessary to place small cotton pledgets in selected locations deeper inside the nasal cavity, for example, over the orifices of drainage of the nasal sinuses, in order to determine the site of leak. However, a CSF leak can be stopped with cotton plegets.

Placement and maintenance of nasal cotton pledgets in children is difficult and in many cases impossible and we regard this technique as unreliable. An additional problem with pledgets is that tracers used in cisternography diffuse in the blood and may appear in nasal secretions. The pledgets should be weighed and counted, and the activity in the plasma measured. This helps to account for normal nasal activity and to facilitate recognition of differences in absorption. Activity ratios of the nose/serum of less than 1.5 should not be considered indicative of CSF leak.[30] In some instances children had cotton pledgets placed and maintained under general anesthesia in an attempt to localize a CSF leak. We do not recommend general anesthesia because it tends to decrease or stop leakage of CSF.

Clinical Applications

Normal Radionuclide Cisternogram

On images at 2 and 6 h the tracer can be seen as it migrates upward into the interhemispheric fissure and the Sylvian fissures. By 24 h the tracer can be seen over the convexity (Fig. 14-1).

Hydrocephalus

Hydrocephalus is caused by a relative obstruction of CSF absorption, and rarely, by overproduction. The most common cause of hydrocephalus in the neonate is congenital malformation. In infants and older children, hydrocephalus is caused by trauma, inflammation, bleeding, or intracranial tumor. In most cases, computed tomography of the brain distinguishes extraventricular from intraventricular obstructive hydrocephalus. Difficult cases may be solved by radionuclide cisternography.

In hydrocephalus there is an active and progressive increase in the size of the spaces containing CSF. In infants, open sutures allow for an increase in the volume of the ventricles initially without much increase in intracranial pressure. A persistent increase in intracranial pressure ultimately results in atrophy of the brain. This is due to a reduction in the cerebral blood flow which results in cerebral hypoxia.

In communicating hydrocephalus (extraventricular obstructive hydrocephalus) the radiotracer circulates into the ventricular system and does not appear in the cerebral fissures and on the convexity. Persistence of the tracer within ventricles for more than 24 h was thought to indicate a progressive form of hydrocephalus that eventually needed shunting. In other instances of communicating hydrocephalus a mixed pattern is seen, some tracer appears in the ventricular system, and some in the fissures and over the convexity (Fig. 14-2).[2,3,16,28,33,34] This pattern may indicate a partially compensated form of hydrocephalus and these patients probably do not need CSF shunting immediately, but must be followed carefully in order to detect any worsening. Radionuclide cisternography, however, has not been found to be a reliable test for determining the need for shunting in adults, and there is not enough experience with it in children.[17,35,39,40] It was recently proposed that the pattern of turnover of tracer in CSF is a reflection of ventricular size and the increased volume of distribution of the CSF.[32] This idea is in keeping with the poor correlations found by earlier investigators.

Obstructive hydrocephalus is equated to intraventricular obstructive hydrocephalus. If intraventricular obstructive hydrocephalus is considered, the tracer is injected into a lateral ventricle.

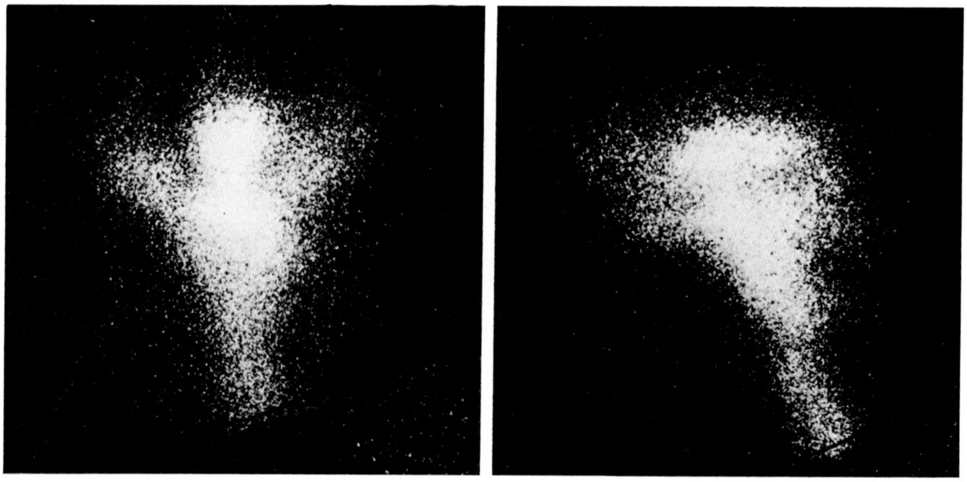

Figure 14-2. Communicating hydrocephalus with both intra- and extraventricular diffusion of the tracer. In-111 DTPA cisternography. Image 2 h following injection. *Left:* anterior view; *right:* right lateral view.

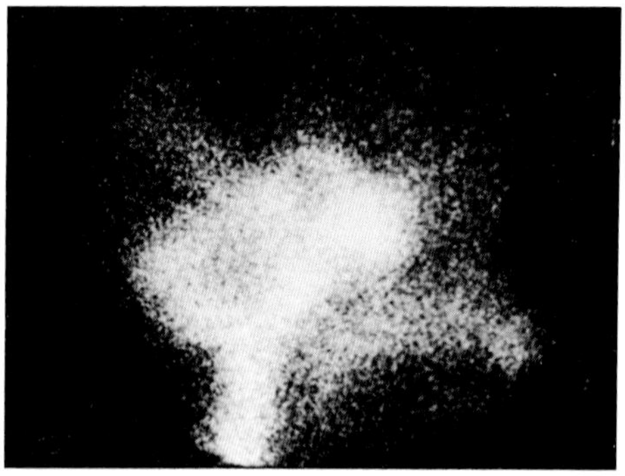

Figure 14-3. CSF leak. Tc-99m DTPA cisternography. Right lateral view 4 h after injection of the tracer into the lumbar subarachnoid space. This is one of multiple images obtained every 15 min. Activity in the oropharynx due to a CSF leak is obvious. This was a posttraumatic leak through the fossa of Rosenmuller.[20]

Hydrocephalus due to oversecretion of CSF is in most cases caused by a papilloma of the choroid plexus.[13,22,26,27,36] CSF production rates of 0.75–1.45 ml/min in patients with papilloma of the choroid plexus have been measured.[13,21]

CSF Liquorrhea

Cerebrospinal fluid liquorrhea is generally manifested by dripping from the nose or ear. Profuse leakage suggests communication with a large cistern. If rhinorrhea is invariably unilateral an opening into the nose or a paranasal sinus is suggested. If the side that drips alternates with position, a nasopharyngeal site, either directly or from the ear, is suggested. In leaks of CSF, radionuclide cisternography reveals extracranial activity due to leak of the tracer outside the cranial cavity. CSF leak complicates up to one-third of fractures of the base of the skull. The majority of these leaks cease spontaneously within a week. Meningitis can occur in about one-fourth of the patients if they are not treated with antibiotics.[29] Both rhinorrhea and otorrhea are amenable to investigation with radionuclide cisternography (Figs. 14-3 and 14-4).[1,4,7,19,20,24]

Loculations of CSF

It is possible to have loculations of CSF in free communication with the subarachnoid pathways without loss of fluid to the external environment. Loculations of CSF appear on radionuclide cysternography as areas of accumulation and retention of the tracer over a relatively long period of time, for example, a nasal encephalocele or a subconjunctival loculation of CSF (Figs. 14-5 and 14-6).[31]

Porencephalic Cyst

Porencephalic cysts are caused by infection, trauma, or vascular problems that cause localized atrophy of the brain. These cysts have a pia-arachnoid lining and communicate with a ventricle. These abnormalities lead to stasis of tracer on radionuclide cisternography, suggesting a one-way valve mechanism for the movement of CSF.[14,15]

Figure 14-4. Otorrhea. In-111 DTPA cisternography. Anterior view 4 h after injection of the tracer in the lumbar subarachnoid space. Extracranial activity in the region of the right ear is visualized (arrow).

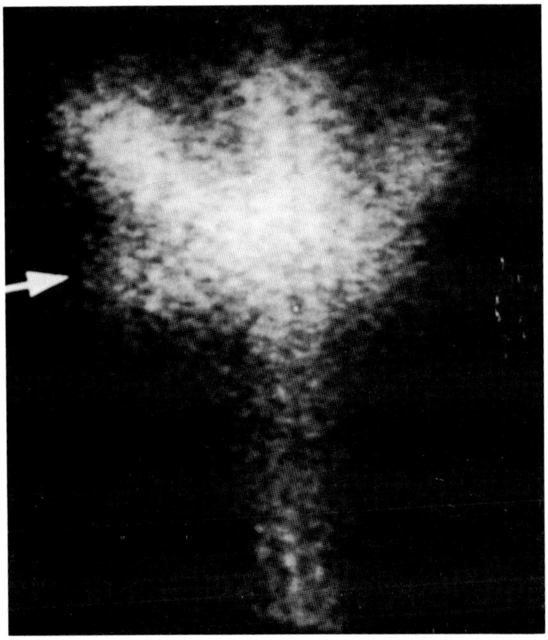

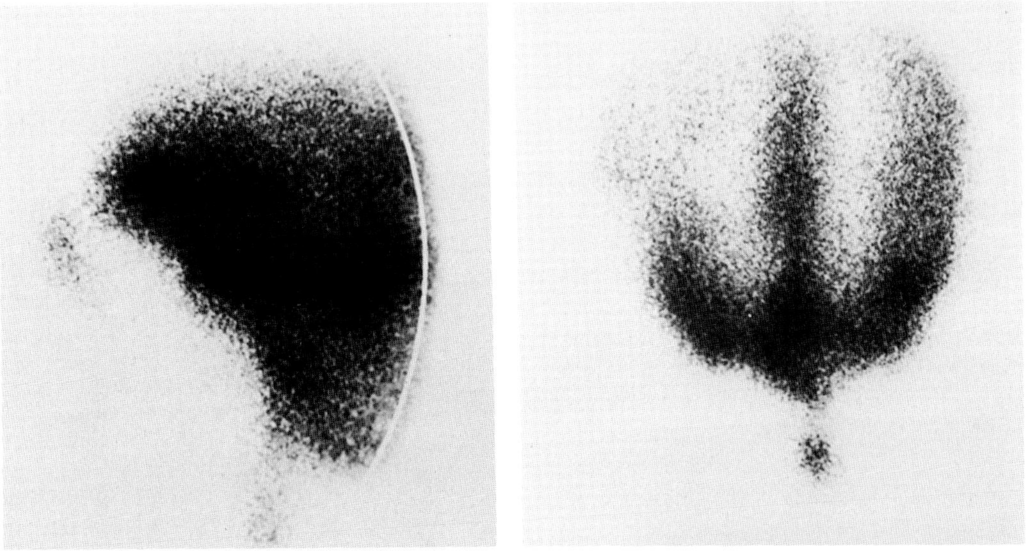

Figure 14-5. Nasal encephalocele. Tc-99m DTPA cisternography, left lateral and anterior views 4 h after injection of the tracer in the lumbar subarachnoid space. A pool of extracranial activity is visualized anteriorly, corresponding to a nasal encephalocele.

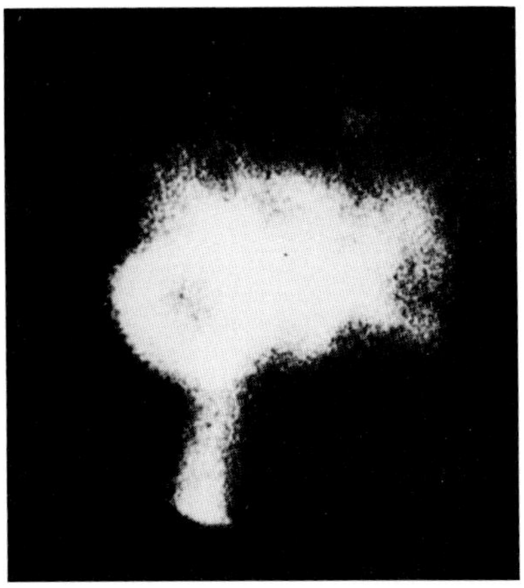

Figure 14-6. Subconjuctival CSF loculation. Right lateral view of an In-111 DTPA cisternogram. There is focal extracranial activity corresponding to a massive subconjuctival CSF loculation.[31]

Block of Spinal CSF Flow

Tumors or other lesions in the spine may cause blockage of CSF flow. These are seen on radionuclide cysternography as filling defects in which the radiotracer does not circulate or accumulate (Fig. 14-7).

CSF SHUNTS

Assessment of patency and quantitation of flow of CSF shunts can be made with radionuclide techniques in a rapid, safe, and accurate way.

Method

Radiopharmaceutical

Tc-99m as sodium pertechnetate in a dose of 250–500 μCi in a volume of 0.01–0.02 ml is used.

Examination Technique

The patient should rest in a horizontal position for 30–60 min before the study in order to be able to measure shunt flow at baseline CSF pressures. The patient is positioned under the gamma camera equipped with a collimator of high sensitivity, and for low energies. The patient must remain immobile for the duration of the study.

The radiotracer is injected in a retrograde direction into the valve of the shunt and its disappearance is monitored with the gamma camera and the computer at a rate of one frame/5 sec for 5 min. At the end of this time a series of images are obtained along the course of the shunt in order to detect any interruption of the flow of CSF. The series of images obtained are evaluated visually (Fig. 14-8).

A time-activity curve is calculated from a region over the valve of the shunt. By knowing the volume of the valve (volume of distribution) and the disappearance rate of the tracer, the CSF shunt flow can be calculated (Fig. 14-9).[18,38]

Alternately the radionuclide can be injected into the ventricle in order to follow its flow into the shunt. This method only allows for qualitative estimation of shunt flow.

The half-disappearance time in normally functioning shunts is 0.5–6.0 min. The Holter valve measures 0.2 ml. As mentioned before the volume injected must be small in order to minimize fluid

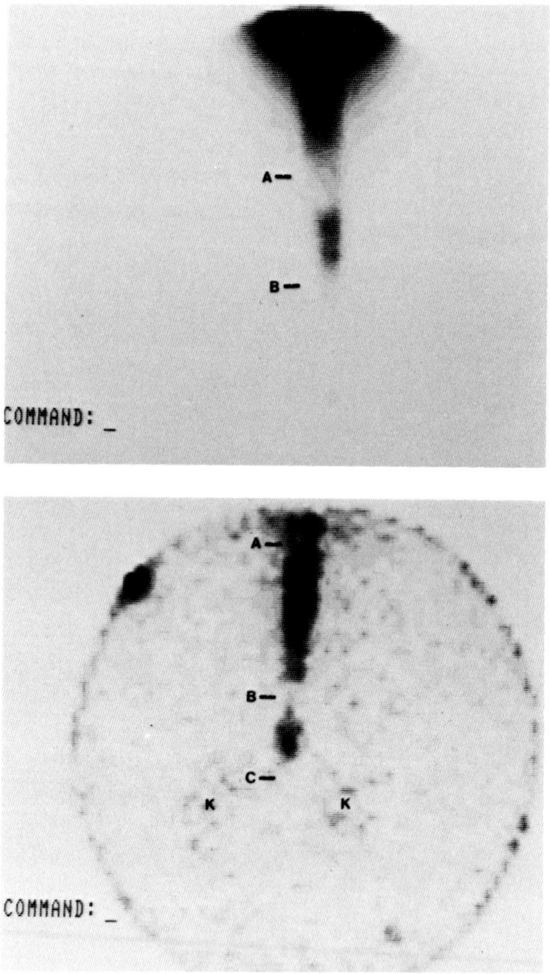

Figure 14-7. Block of CSF diffusion due to metastatic medulloblastoma in the spine. Tc-99m DTPA was injected into a lateral ventricle. *Top:* Posterior view of the cervical and thoracic spine 1 h after injection of the tracer. There are two "filling defects" corresponding to tumor mass (A and B). *Bottom:* View of the lower thoracic and lumbar spine reveals another block of tracer movement in the CSF (C). Renal activity is visualized bilaterally (K).

displacement due to the injection. Optimal results are obtained with a uniform injection technique.[23] If the volume of the valve into which the tracer is injected is unknown, quantitation of CSF shunt flow is not possible.

The exponential method models the valve as a single, well-mixed compartment. The term well-mixed means that the tracer becomes equilibrated with the entire volume of the compartment immediately after its introduction and remains so throughout the period of observation, independent

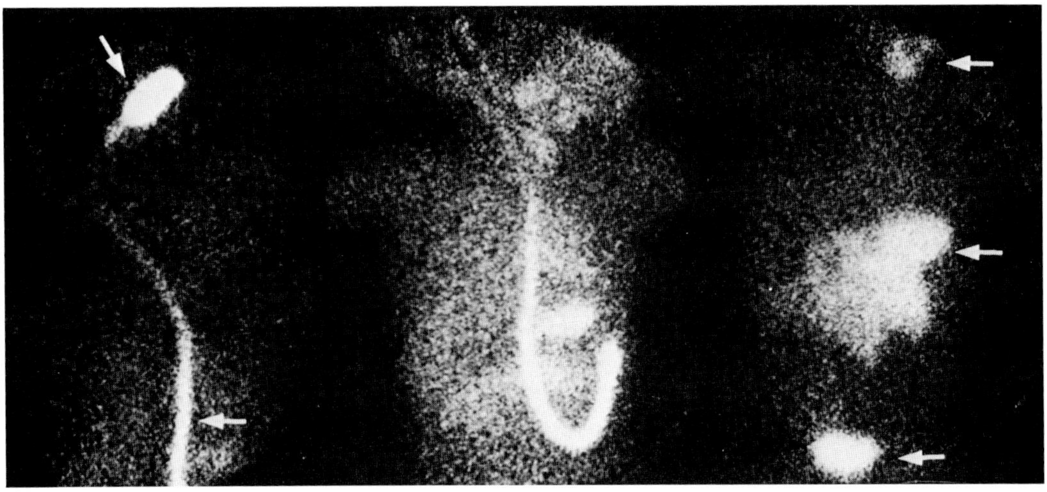

Figure 14-8. Patent ventriculo-peritoneal CSF shunt. *Left:* Image obtained almost immediately after administration of 300 μCi of Tc-99m NaO_4^- in a volume of 0.1 ml in the valve. Activity in the valve and in the tubing is visualized *(arrows)*. *Center:* Image 5 min later shows the trajectory of the tube, activity in the stomach, thyroid, salivary glands, and soft tissues indicating rapid absorption of the tracer. *Right:* Two and a half hours later most of the activity is concentrated in the bladder, the gastrointestinal tract, and the thyroid *(arrows)*.

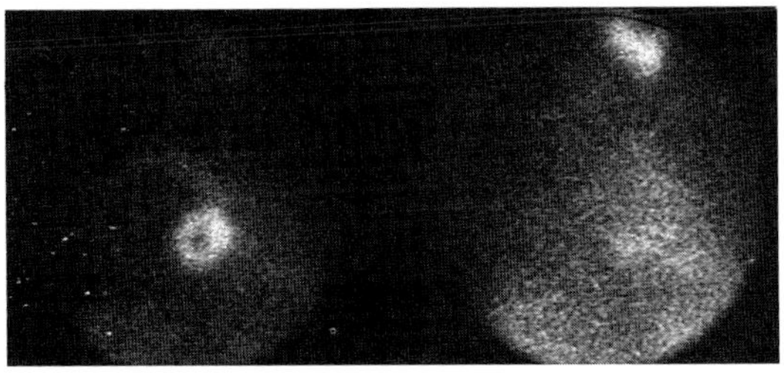

$$\text{Flow rate} = \frac{\text{Vol}\ (\ln A_1 - \ln A_2)}{T_{A1} - T_{A2}}$$

Flow rate = 0.21 cc/min.

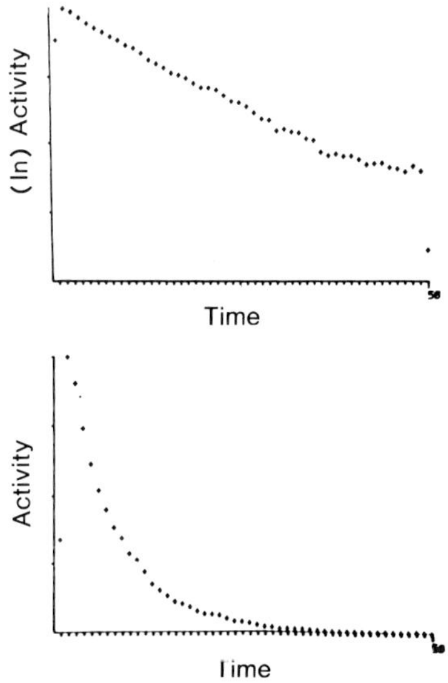

Figure 14-9. Patent ventriculo-peritoneal shunt. *Upper left:* Anterior views of the chest and abdomen 10 min after injection of Tc-99m NaO_4^- into the valve of the shunt. Both images show widespread distribution of the tracer in the body indicating patency of the shunt. *Right:* logarithmic *(top)* and linear *(bottom)* time-activity curves from the valve obtained from images at one frame/5 sec. Calculation of CSF shunt flow are shown.

of the site of introduction of the tracer. In such a system, the disappearance curve is of the form

$$A(t) = A(0)\ e^{-t/k} \qquad [1]$$

where t is time and k is the time constant of the system. The time constant is equal to the mean time the radionuclide remains in the compartment or the mean transit time (*MTT*). Flow is calculated using the formula

$$F = V/k \qquad [2]$$

where V is the volume of distribution.

Two observations cast some doubt on the well-mixed compartment model. One is that the apparent volumes of distribution, calculated using Eq. [2], are in general significantly different from the physical volumes of the valve. The other is that the observed disappearance curve differs significantly from the exponential curve predicted by the model. We therefore developed an alternative approach to estimating flow. If a radiotracer is instantaneously introduced so that the tracer is uniformly distributed across the fluid entering the compartment one may estimate flow by calculating the *MTT* using the formula

$$MTT = A/H \qquad [3]$$

where A is the total area under the disappearance curve and H is the initial height of the disappearance curve. Flow is calculated using the formula

$$F = V/(A/H) \qquad [4]$$

This is illustrated in Fig. 14-10.

This method, which is based on the area-over-height ratio (A/H), was found to result in greater precision than the exponential method.

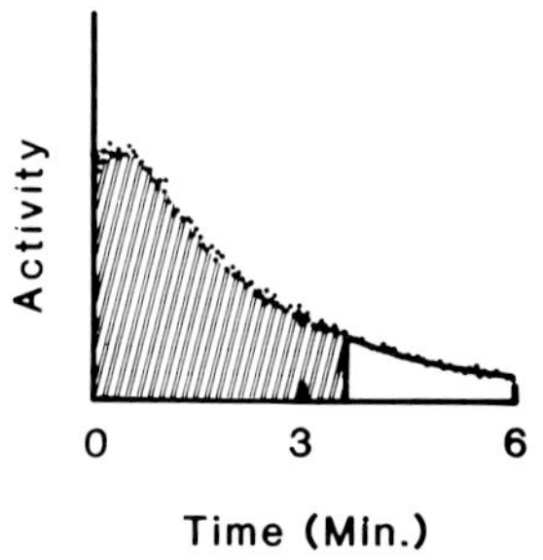

Figure 14-10. CSF flow may be estimated from the area under the valve disappearance curve using Eq. [3]. Since the curve may not have reached zero before the end of the recording period, the curve is extrapolated by fitting an exponential function to its final portion. The fit starts when the activity is <25% of the maximum activity or when 75% of the recording period has expired, whichever comes first. The total area is computed by numerically integrating the initial portion and adding the area under the exponential fit.

Clinical Applications

Ventriculo-peritoneal and ventriculo-atrial shunts are used in hydrocephalic patients to divert CSF into a body space so it can be absorbed. Mechanical failure, occlusion, or the development of loculated spaces around the ventricular or the distal end of the shunt are causes of malfunction of a shunt. Such malfunction can usually be determined on clinical grounds, but in doubtful cases, special measures may be indicated. Radionuclide studies can measure the shunt flow, determine the presence of an obstruction, and diagnose loculation of CSF at the distal end of the shunt.

References

1. Ashburn WL, Harbert JC, Briner WH. Cerebrospinal fluid rhinorrhea studied with the gamma scintilliation camera. J Nucl Med 1968; 9:523.
2. Bannister R, Gilford E, Kocen R. Isotope encephalography in the diagnosis of dementia due to communicating hydrocephalus. Lancet 1967; 2:1014–7.
3. Benson DF, Lemay M, Patten DH, Rubens AB. Diagnosis of normal pressure hydrocephalus. N Engl J Med 1970; 283:609–15.
4. Caldicott WGH, Northe JB, Simpson DA. Traumatic cerebrospinal fluid fistulas in children. J Neurosurg 1973; 38:1–9.
5. Cutler RWP, Page L, Galicich J, Watters GV. Formation and absorption of cerebrospinal fluid in man. Brain 1968; 91:707–20.
6. Cutler RWP, Murray JE, Moody RA. Overproduction of cerebrospinal fluid in communicating hydrocephalus. Neurology (Minneap) 1973; 23:1–5.
7. Cowan RJ, Maynard CD. Trauma to the brain and extracranial structures. Semin Nucl Med 1974; 4:319–38.
8. Davson H, Segal MB. Secretions and drainage of the cerebrospinal fluid. Acta Neurol Lat Am 1971; 17(Suppl):99.
9. Davson H, Hollingsworth G, Seagal MB. The mechanism of drainage of the cerebrospinal fluid. Brain 1970; 93:665.
10. DiChiro G. Movement of the cerebrospinal fluid in human beings. Nature 1964; 204:290–1.

11. DiChiro GD, Hammock MK, Bleyer WA. Spinal descent of cerebrospinal fluid in man. Neurology (Minneap) 1976; 26:1–8.
12. duBoulay G, Shah SH, Currie JC, Logue V. The mechanism of hydromyelia in Chiari type I malformations. Br J Radiol 1974; 47:579–87.
13. Eisenberg HM, McComb JG, Lorenzo AV. Cerebrospinal fluid overproduction and hydrocephalus associated with a choroid plexus papilloma. J Neurosurg 1974; 40:381–5.
14. Ferreira S, Jhingram SG, Johnson PC. Radionuclide cisternography for the study of arachnoid cysts: a case report. Neuroradiology 1980; 19:167–9.
15. Front D, Minderhoud JM, Beks JW, Penning L. Leptomeningeal cysts diagnosed by isotope cisternography. J Neurol Neurosurg Psychiatry 1973; 36:1018–23.
16. Glasaue FE, Alker GJ, Leslie EV, Nicol CF. Isotope cisternography in hydrocephalus with normal pressure. Case report and technical note. J Neurosurg 1968; 29:555–61.
17. Greitz T, Grepe A. Encephalography in the diagnosis of convexity block hydrocephalus. Acta Radiol [Diag] (Stockholm) 1971; 11:232–42.
18. Harbert J. Haddad D, McCullough D. Quantitation of cerebrospinal fluid shunt flow. Radiology 1974; 112:379–87.
19. Harwood-Nash DC. Fractures of the petrous and tympanic parts of the temporal bone in children: a tomographic study of 35 cases. Am J Roentgenol 1970; 110;598–607.
20. Jaffe B, Welch K, Strand R, Treves S. Cerebrospinal fluid rhinorrhea via the fossa of Rosenmuller. Laryngoscope 1976; 86:903–7.
21. Johnson RT. Clinicopathological aspects of the cerebrospinal fluid circulation. In: Wolsetenholme GEW, O'Connor CM, eds. CIBA Foundation symposium on production, circulation, and absorption of the cerebrospinal fluid. 1958; 265–78. Boston: Little Brown & Co.
22. Khan EA, Luros JT. Hydrocephalus from overproduction of cerebrospinal fluid. J Neurosurg 1952; 9:59–67.
23. Kuruc A, Treves S, Welch K, Merlino D. Radionuclide estimation of cerebral spinal fluid shunt flow: Evidence supporting an alternative theoretical model. J Neurosurg 1984; 60:361–364.
24. Lantz EJ, Forbes GS, Brown ML, Laws ER. Radiology of cerebrospinal fluid rhinorrhea. AJR 1980; 135:1023–30.
25. Lorenzo AV, Page LK, Watters GV. Relationships between cerebrospinal fluid formation, absorption, and pressure in human hydrocephalus. Brain 1970; 93:679.
26. Matson DD. Hydrocephalus in a premature infant caused by papilloma of the choroid plexus: with report of surgical treatment. J Neurosurg 1953; 10:416–20.
27. Matson DD, Crofton FDL. Papilloma of the choroid plexus in childhood, J Neurosurg 1960; 17:1002–27.
28. McCullough DC, Harbert JC, Di Chiro G, Ommaya AK. Prognostic criteria for cerebrospinal fluid shunting from isotope cisternography in communicating hydrocephalus. Neurology (Minneap) 1970; 20:594–8.
29. McKusic KA. The diagnosis of traumatic cerebrospinal rhinorrhea. J Nucl Med 1977; 18:1234–5.
30. McKusic KA, Malmud LS, Kordela PA, Wagner HN. Radionuclide cisternography: normal values for nasal secretion of intrathecally injected In-111 DTPA. J Nucl Med 1973; 14:933–4.
31. McLennan JE, Mickle JP, Treves S. Radionuclide cisternographic evaluation and follow-up of posttraumatic subconjunctival CSF loculation. J Neurosurg 1976; 44:496–9.
32. O'Brien MD, Haggith GW, Appleton D. Cerebrospinal fluid dynamics in dementia. Exp Brain Res 1982; 5(suppl):196–200.
33. Patten DH, Benson DF, Diagnosis of normal-pressure hydrocephalus by RISA cisternography. J Nucl Med 1968; 9:457–61.
34. Philippon J, Ancri D, Pertuiset B. Hydrocephalie a pression normale. Rev Neurol (Paris) 1971; 125:374–85.
35. Rau H, Flas A, Horst W, Baumgartner G. Clinical observations on communicating hydrocephalus of unknown etiology. J Neurol 1974; 207:279–87.
36. Ray BS, Peck FC. Papilloma of the choroid plexus of the lateral ventricles causing hydrocephalus in an infant. J Neurosurg 1956; 13:405–10.
37. Rubin RC, Henderson ES, Ommaya AK, Walker MD, Rall DP. The production of cerebrospinal fluid in man and its modification by acetazolamine. J Neurosurg 1966; 25:430–6.
38. Rudd TG, Shurtleff DB, Loeser JD, Nelp WB. Radionuclide assessment of cerebrospinal fluid shunt function in children. J Nucl Med 1973; 14:683–6.
39. Shenkin HA, Crowley JN. Hydrocephalus complicating pituitary adenoma. J Neurol Neurosurg Psychiatry 1973; 36:1063–8.
40. Tator CH, Murray S. A clinical pneumoencephalographic and radioisotopic study of normal pressure communicating hydrocephalus. Can Med Assoc J 1971; 105:573–9.
41. Welch K. Selected topics relating to hydrocephalus. Exp Eye Res 1977; 25:(Suppl) 345–75.
42. Welch K, Friedman J. The cerebrospinal valve. Brain 1960; 83:454.

Chapter 15 Dacryoscintigraphy

Sydney Heyman
James A. Katowitz

An adequate flow of tears is important for the normal function of the eye. The tears serve several purposes, such as providing an optically uniform field, a lubricating and antibacterial function, as well as nourishing the cornea. The lacrimal gland, accessory lacrimal gland tissue, and secretions of the meibomian and mucous glands of the conjunctiva contribute to the formation of tears.

Tearing occurs when the tear production is excessive or there is an abnormality of drainage. Tearing (epiphora) is the most frequent symptom of lacrimal drainage dysfunction. The diagnosis and treatment of tearing disorders present some of the most common challenges facing the clinician.

The commonest anomaly of the lacrimal apparatus is a congenital obstruction of the nasolacrimal duct. Whereas 30% of newborns have a physiologic obstruction that clears completely in the first few weeks of life, a treatable nasolacrimal block persists in 1–6% of neonates.[15] Bilateral abnormalities are found in up to 33% of these patients.[9] Less frequent defects include an anomalous location of a punctum and canaliculus, atresia, or absence of the puncta or multiple puncta. Supernumerary puncta (anlage ducts) may occur on a familial basis.[11] These may open into a normal canaliculus or into a separate duct that in turn empties into the nasolacrimal sac. Atresia and total absence of the puncta may be inherited as an autosomal dominant trait with variable penetrance.[12]

While obstruction in infants is usually congenital in origin, in older children it may be secondary to infection, mechanical obstruction (polyps, foreign bodies), or following traumatic or surgical fractures of the facial or nasal bones. Congenital abnormalities of the lacrimal pump mechanism may also occur despite patent nasolacrimal passages.[7]

Epiphora usually begins in the second or third week of life after tear production is normally established. In both children and adults 88% of those with epiphora have obstruction to flow.[10] The resulting stasis leads to conjunctivitis and if both openings to the lacrimal sac close off, then dacryocystitis can occur. Acute dacryocystitis may lead to an abscess within the sac and possible fistula formation, while cellulitis of the overlying skin occurs frequently. With chronic duct obstruction, but a patent common canaliculus, a mucocele of the lacrimal sac may form, presenting as a painless swelling, in contrast with the tense and painful swelling of acute dacryocystitis.

While children with major facial anomalies should always be suspected of having abnormalities of the nasolacrimal apparatus, it appears that involvement is actually less than might be expected. However, in a series of 75 patients with clefts of the palate and prepalate, there was a 10% incidence of duct obstruction and 12% incidence of associated lacrimal abnormalities.[16]

Children with tumors in the region of the orbit requiring radiation therapy are theoretically at risk for the development of obstructive lesions. Although the nasolacrimal drainage system appears to be resistant to the low doses of radiation currently used, it is still recommended that the status of the system be evaluated prior to radiation therapy or surgery when the inner canthus is involved, or when epiphora exists or is a potential complication.[1]

Anatomy and Physiology

The nasolacrimal apparatus consists of the lacrimal lake, puncta, canaliculi, nasolacrimal sac, and the nasolacrimal duct (Fig. 15-1). The puncta carry tears from the lacrimal lake into the ampulla and both upper and lower canaliculi. Usually the canaliculi join to form a common canaliculus opening into the lacrimal sac at the internal common punctum. The walls of the canaliculi contain elastin and collagen, maintaining an open lumen. Thus fluid can flow from the punctum into the sac by capillary action. The lacrimal sac lies on the anteromedial wall of the bony orbit, in a fossa partly within the orbital cavity. The nasolacrimal duct arises from the sac and opens just below the anterior end of the inferior nasal turbinate.

In the resting state the lateral and medial walls of the duct are in contact, and separate only with the flow of fluid. In addition to the effects of gravity and capillary action, a lacrimal pump system appears to be important in the transport of tears from the puncta to the nose. Blinking is important in moving tears to the puncta. Closure of the lids causes the punctum to move nasally, decreasing the volume of the canaliculi. At the same time contraction of the orbicularis oculi muscles is associated with a dilatation of the sac creating a negative pressure. Thus tears are forced into the nasolacrimal sac. Opening of the lids reverses the process. As the canaliculi reexpand, tears are drawn into the system from the punctum. With the relaxation of the orbicularis the sac collapses, forcing the accumulated tears down into the nasolacrimal duct, since the valve of Rosenmuller blocks retrograde flow back into the common internal punctum.

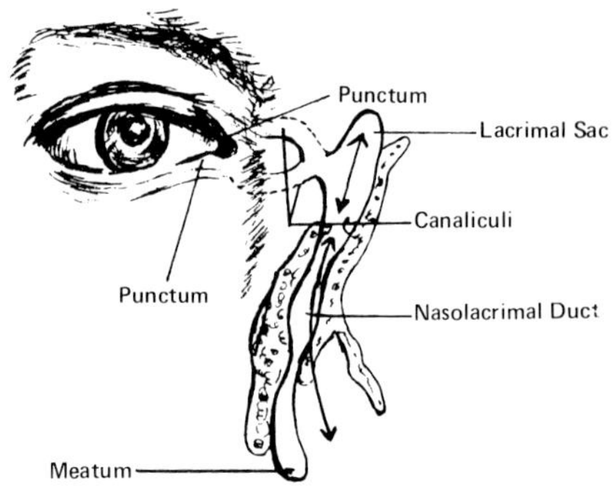

Figure 15-1. Anatomy of the nasolacrimal apparatus.

Assessment of Lacrimal Drainage

Children presenting with epiphora, or unexplained chronic conjunctivitis, may be evaluated by one or more of several techniques (Table 15-1). Observation may indicate an increase in the height of the tear meniscus between the lower lid and the cornea. Notice should be made of any lid margin abnormalities. Ectropion of the lid or punctum may lead to epiphora due to reflex tearing from exposure, and lashes of an entropic lid may also stimulate reflex tearing by direct surface irritation. While observing the patient, abnormalities of the lacrimal pump mechanism may become evident. Pressure on the lacrimal sac, producing reflux of its contents from the puncta, may provide additional information indicating a mucocele.

In addition to observation of the tear meniscus, the Schirmer I test with a local anesthetic is useful. Unfortunately it is of almost no value in the pediatric age group. A strip of No. 41 Whatman filter paper is folded at one end and inserted into the lower conjunctival sac, at the junction of the middle and temporal third of the lower lid. Less than 10 mm of wetting of the filter paper over a 5-min period suggests a problem with baseline tear production. This test helps to rule out false-positive problems caused by decreased baseline flow producing a reflex outflow of tears from the lacrimal gland.

The Jones dye tests are likewise of limited value in the pediatric population. The test requires recovery of 2% fluorescein dye from the nose after instillation into the conjunctival cul de sac. Although helpful in adult epiphora, the response of a conscious child to attempts at collecting the dye make

Table 15-1. Studies to Assess Lacrimal Drainage in Children

Tear meniscus level
Dye disappearance test
Irrigation and probing
Dacryocystography
Dacryoscintigraphy

it too difficult to attempt safely. The results may also be difficult to interpret meaningfully due to questions of dilution secondary to crying.[8] Taste tests that are completely subjective have little value in assessing pediatric nasolacrimal function.

In the dye disappearance test a single drop of 2% fluorescein is instilled into the anesthetized conjunctival cul-de-sac of each eye. Excess fluid or overflow is wiped away, and the tear meniscus observed over a 5-min period. In a negative test (normal) the tear meniscus will become relatively unstained within 5 min. When positive (obstruction) the meniscus will either increase or be diluted only slightly. The test is simple but subjective. The results are not entirely reliable and are often difficult to evaluate with certainty. Further, if a blockage is present, the level at which it occurs is not evident. In children the dye disappearance test may be facilitated by using the blue cobalt filter of the biomicroscopic slit lamp opened wide at a distance of 2–3 feet. The patients are then more easily observed at a less threatening distance while seated on a parent's lap.

Irrigation and probing require a general anesthetic, except in infants under 6 months, who may be probed without an anesthetic. Without the controlled environment provided by general anesthesia, irrigation in newborns or very young infants should be avoided. It is more difficult to perform and there is the risk of iatrogenic trauma to the canaliculus and internal punctum. Hydrostatic pressure may open mild obstruction and should be employed prior to probing when doing this under general anesthesia. Extreme care is needed to avoid the creation of false passages.

Dacryocystography is a useful test in adults but in the child also requires a general anesthetic, and is mostly indicated for special problems in diagnosis where functional blocks, mucoceles, or neoplasms (which are rare) are in question. A radioopaque dye is injected into each lower canaliculus. After obtaining a baseline anterior-posterior and lateral views of the orbits, anterior-posterior and oblique films are taken and repeated at 15 and 30 min. It is possible to delineate fistulae, diverticulae, mucoceles, neoplasms, nonopaque foreign bodies, and casts of the sac. Further, slow clearance of the dye by 30 min is suggestive of a functional block. However, the use of a relative supine position and general anesthesia renders the study less physiologic, and reduces its value somewhat as a functional study in children. The radiation dose to the patient has been estimated to be 3 rads, compared with 370 mrads from an anterior-posterior x-ray of the skull.

Dacryoscintigraphy is another method of evaluating lacrimal flow, and has been found to be a useful adjunctive study for evaluating epiphora in children. It is noninvasive and physiologic, and provides quantitative data.[3,4] In comparison with dacryocystography the absorbed dose to the lens of the eye is only between 4 and 14 mrads/100 μCi Tc-99m pertechnetate under normal physiologic conditions, although with blockage of the lacrimal drainage apparatus the lens dose could increase to 40 mrads.[1,13,14]

Dacryoscintigraphy, or the use of a radioactive tracer to evaluate nasolacrimal drainage, was first described by Rossomondo in 1972.[14] Since that time attention has been drawn to the quantitative aspects of the study[3,5,6] and the clinical utility of the study has been reviewed.[2] While the early studies have virtually all been in adult patients, reference to the efficacy of dacryoscintigraphy in children has been infrequent. More recently we have reported on our experience using this technique in the pediatric age group.[4]

Method

Patients are premedicated with potassium perchlorate, 6 mg/kg given orally to block thyroidal uptake. They are seated in front of a gamma camera fitted with a pinhole collimator. A 1-mm insert is preferred to increase the resolution of the study. The distance from the collimator is such that the outer canthi of both eyes and the tip of the nose are in the field of view. Tilting the head back, 100 μCi Tc-99m pertechnetate in 10 μl is rapidly instilled into each lower temporal marginal tear strip. The use of a micropipette greatly facilitates the administration of the 10 μl drop. A drop size of 10 μl was chosen since this could be comfortably accommodated by all patients without overflow. Following administration of the drops, the head is immediately repositioned. Utilizing a chin support (Fig. 15-2) aids in the immobilization of the head. Sequential analogue images are obtained every minute for the next 20 min, with simultaneous computer acquisition at four frames/min.

Interpretation is by visual inspection of the images and computer playback. By placing regions of interest (ROIs) around each orbit, the rate of

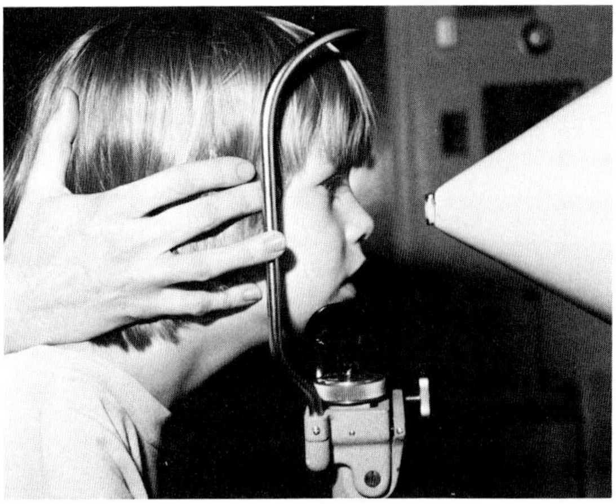

Figure 15-2. Positioning of the patient in front of the pinhole collimator.

washout may be quantitated. When clearance is delayed, older patients are asked to either blink forcefully, inspire deeply and rapidly through the nose, or both. Forceful blinking increases the pressure in the nasolacrimal sac, while forceful sniffing creates a low pressure within the nose due to a venturi effect. The placement of a further three or four drops of normal saline in the canthal region to encourage progression of the previously administered radioactive drops has also been suggested.[3] Maneuvers such as these may distinguish an anatomic block from a functional delay.

In normal patients activity is usually evident within the sac by 1 min, with evidence of flow into the duct by 2–3 min. Progression down the nasolacrimal duct to the distal end is more variable. Quantitative analysis in normal adults in the erect position has shown that significant amounts of tracer can be expected in the sac by 12 sec,[3] while the time to reach maximum activity may range between 1 and 15 min (mean 5.2).[5,6]

Infants and small children, who may not be cooperative, have been studied under sedation. This is usually accomplished with oral chloral hydrate (in a dose of 40 mg/kg). Because blinking is not spontaneous while the patient is under sedation, passive movement of the lids has been resorted to in four patients. Care must be taken not to massage over the sac. While the validity of performing the study in this manner needs to be documented, useful information was obtained in two of these studies.

Clinical Application

Dacryoscintigraphy has been found to be useful both in the initial workup of a patient presenting with tearing, as well as in the postoperative assessment. This is illustrated by the following examples.

Case 1

A 15-year-old girl complaining of right-sided epiphora was found to have an increased tear meniscus on the same side. As she was too apprehensive to allow investigative irrigation and probing without a general anesthetic a dacryoscintigram was performed. The scintigraphic study was normal (Fig. 15-3), and no surgical procedures were required, since she has shown gradual symptomatic improvement with prolonged followup.

Case 2

In another 15-year-old girl with a similar complaint, the dacryoscintigram confirmed an obstruction on the right at the level of the common canaliculus (Fig. 15-4). She underwent a dacryocystorhinostomy with the insertion of silastic tubing with a good result.

In the postoperative period the study may confirm the recurrence of an obstructive lesion in a symptomatic patient, or indicate the possibility of an impending problem.

Case 3

Following a probing and irrigation under general anesthesia for bilateral obstruction, this 5-year-old boy was asymptomatic. However, although the drainage on the left side was normal, the flow into the right nasolacrimal sac was significantly delayed, indicating the probable need for further intervention (Fig. 15-5). Further examples of abnormal nasolacrimal drainage after surgery are shown in Figs. 15-6–15-10. These demonstrate the utility of the study when planning further management.

The value of performing the study with sedation may be questioned. Since blinking has been shown to be important for promoting normal drainage, it is not surprising that a marked delay is noted in sedated infants and children. In uncooperative patients sedation with chloral hydrate has allowed the placement of drops into each eye while the patient

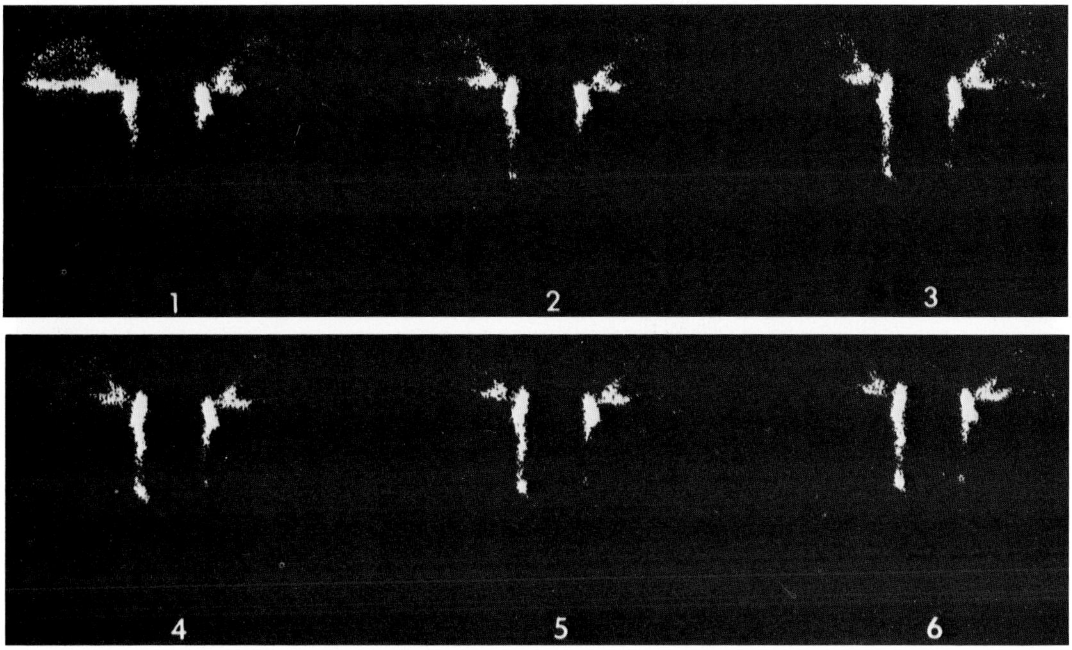

Figure 15-3. A normal study in a 15-year-old girl complaining of right-side epiphora.

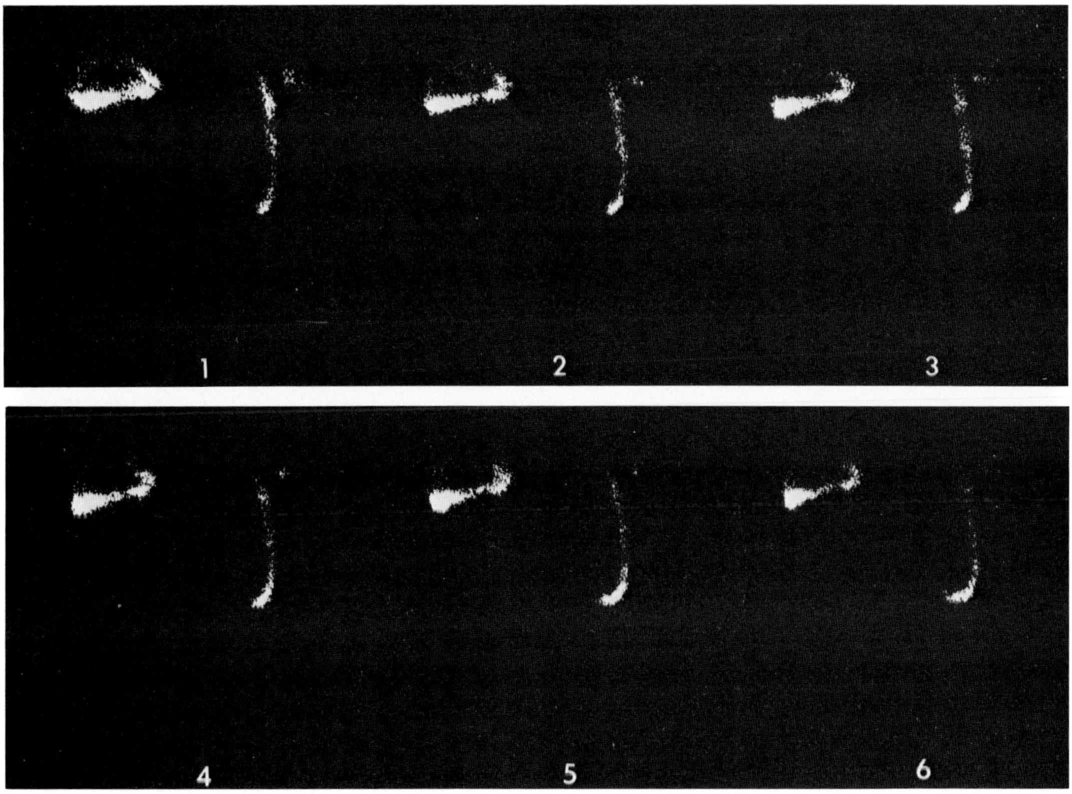

Figure 15-4. The scintigram in this 15-year-old girl revealed normal flow on the left, but an obstruction at the level of the common canaliculus on the right. Her complaint was of right-sided tearing. The numbers below each image indicate the time in min.

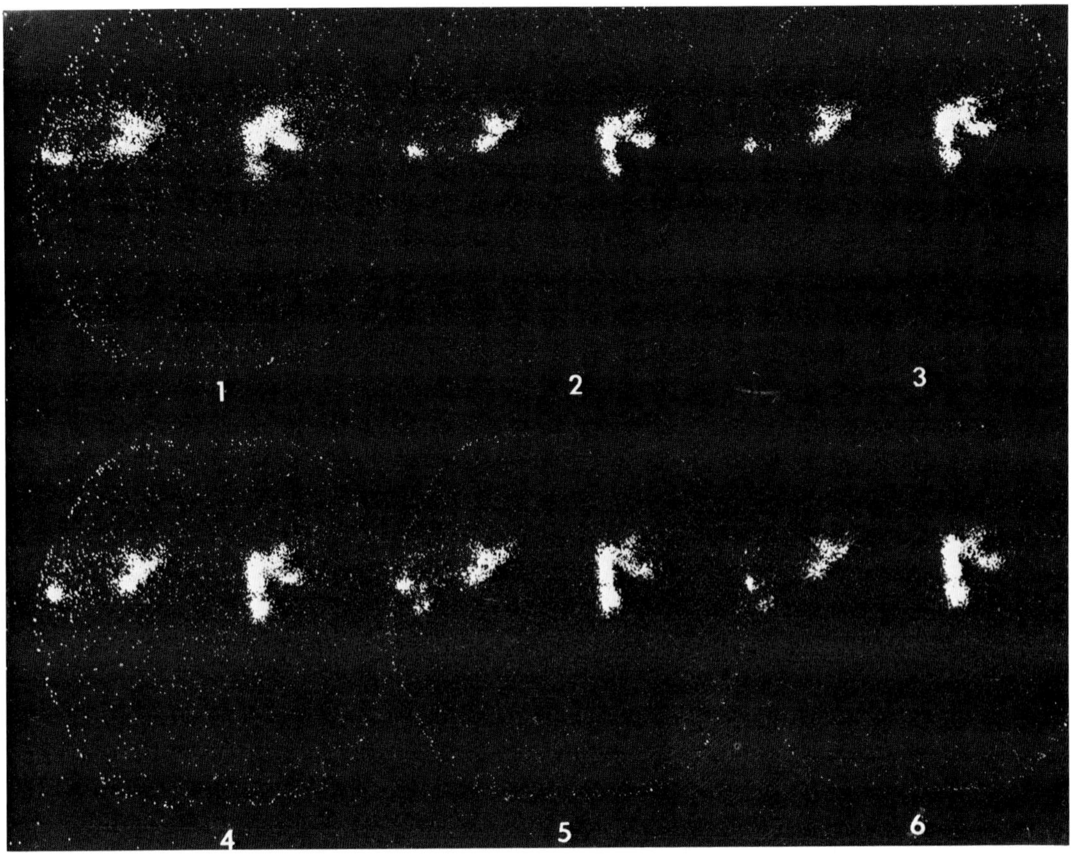

Figure 15-5

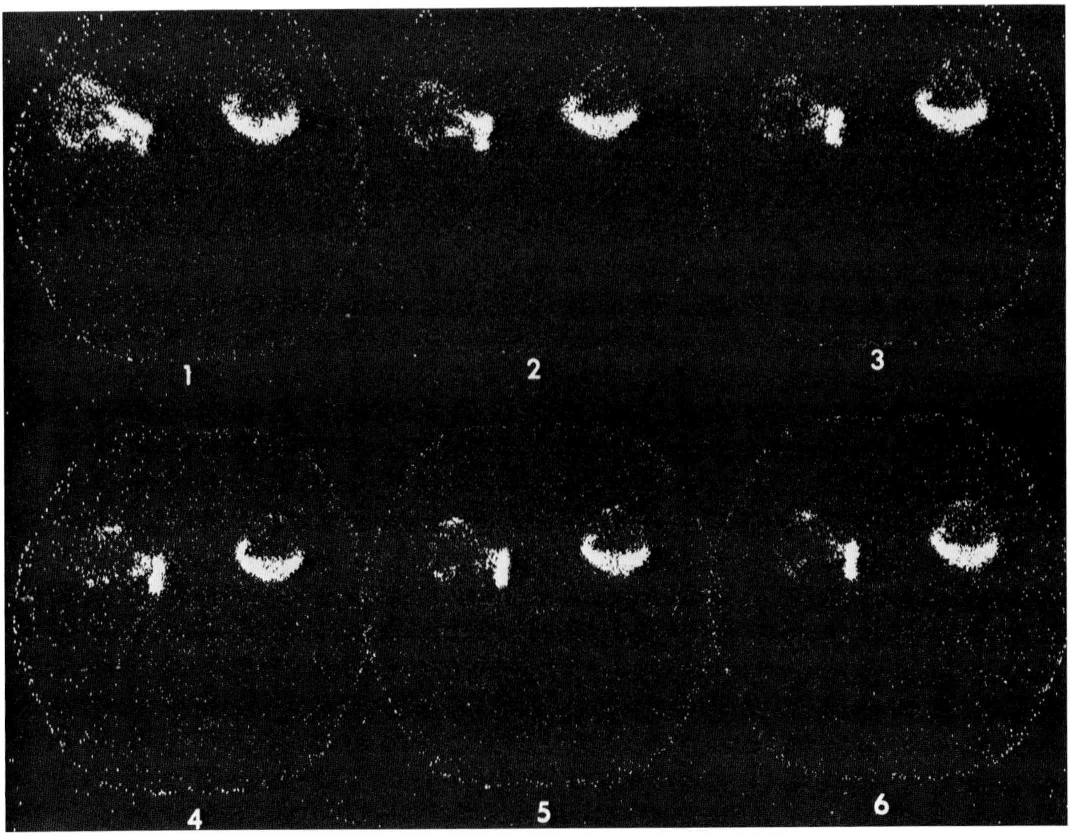

Figure 15-6

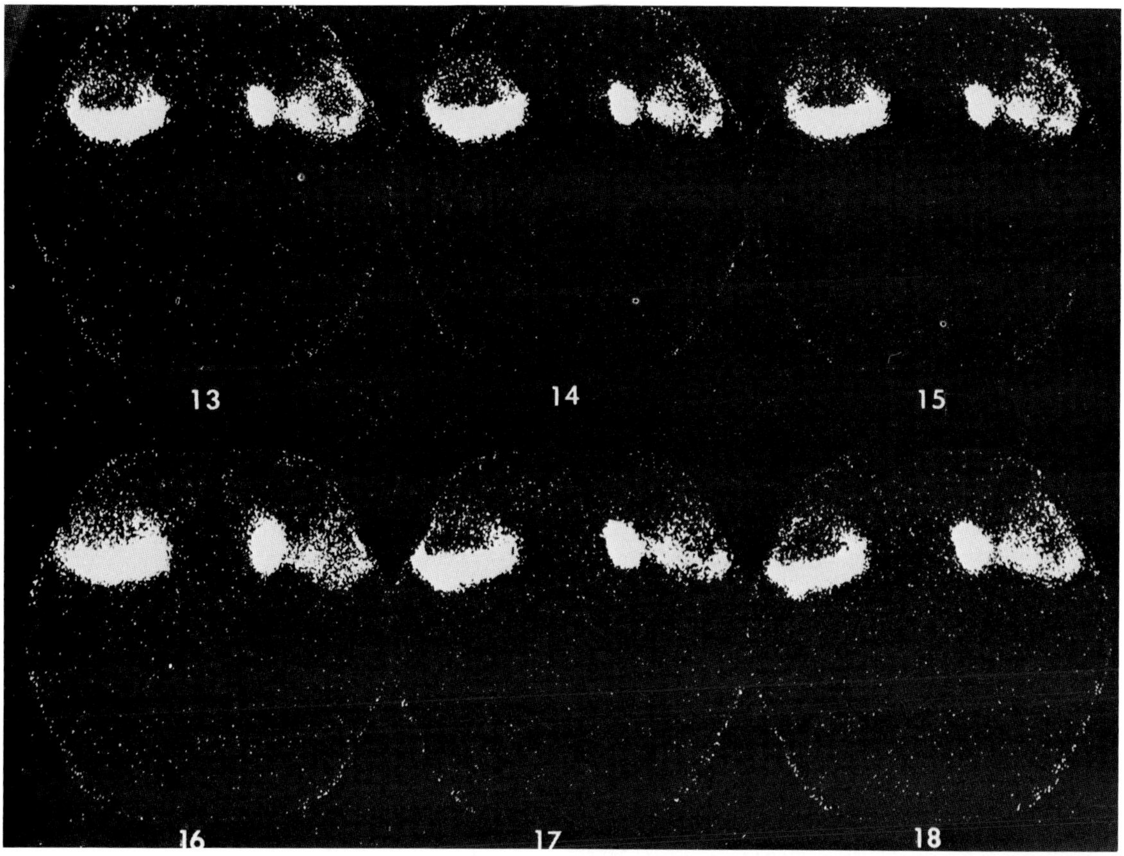

Figure 15-7

Figure 15-5. This study was performed after surgery for bilateral obstruction in a 5-year-old boy. The flow into the right nasolacrimal sac is delayed. The need for further surgical intervention is suggested, and will be determined by further followup.

Figure 15-6. This 18-year-old boy had a left-sided orbital hemangioma, necessitating a dacryocystorhinostomy because of obstruction to flow. Postoperatively he complained of left-sided epiphora. The dacryoscintigram confirms the absence of flow into the left nasolacrimal sac.

Figure 15-7 Silastic tubes were placed bilaterally because of tearing in this 10-year-old girl with a craniofacial disorder. When these failed, bilateral dacryocystorhinostomies were performed with a good result. However, at followup the scintigraphic study shows pooling in the right nasolacrimal lake with no progression, while on the left side there was no flow distal to the nasolacrimal sac.

Figure 15-8. There is evidence of a blockage to flow through the common canaliculus on the right, and delayed flow distal to the sac on the left, in this 12-year-old boy. He complained of right-sided tearing. The tear meniscus level was increased on this side. Following rapid nasal inspiration there was normal flow down the nasolacrimal duct on the left, but no change on the right. He underwent a right-sided dacryocystorhinostomy and has remained asymptomatic.

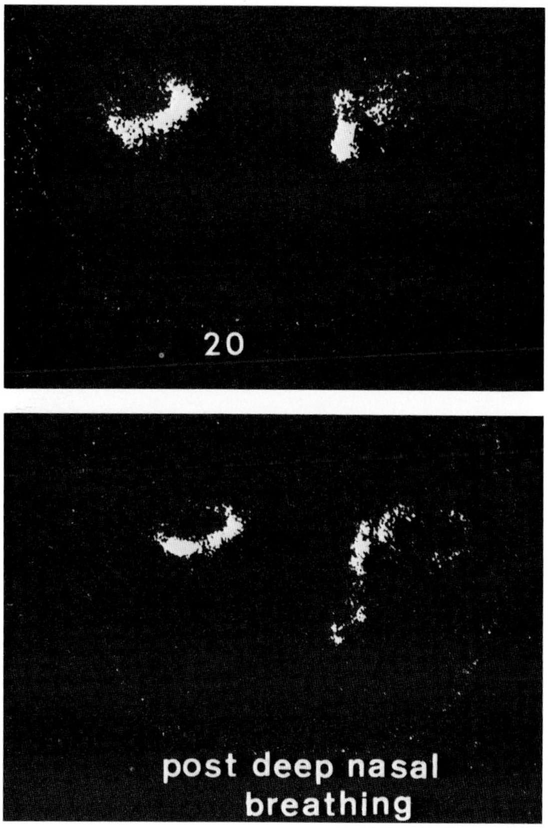

Figure 15-8

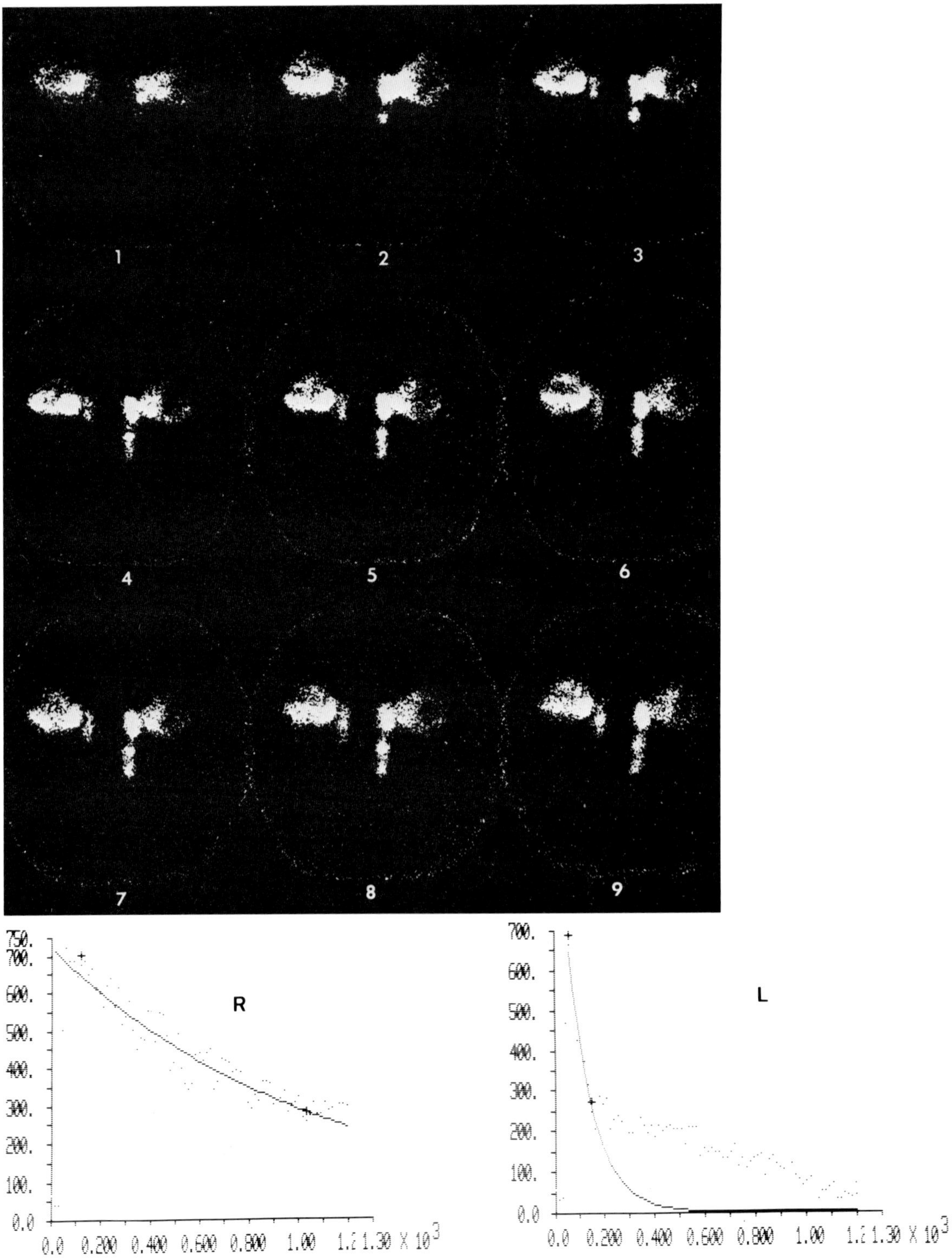

Figure 15-9. This 12-year-old boy complained of persistent right sided tearing after surgery. Both the tear meniscus level and the dye disappearance test were abnormal on this side. The dacryoscintigram showed normal flow on the left, but no flow beyond the nasolacrimal sac on the right. He was known to have medial canthal dystopia. The time activity curves derived from regions of interest around the orbits show normal clearance on the left, but a significant delay on the right.

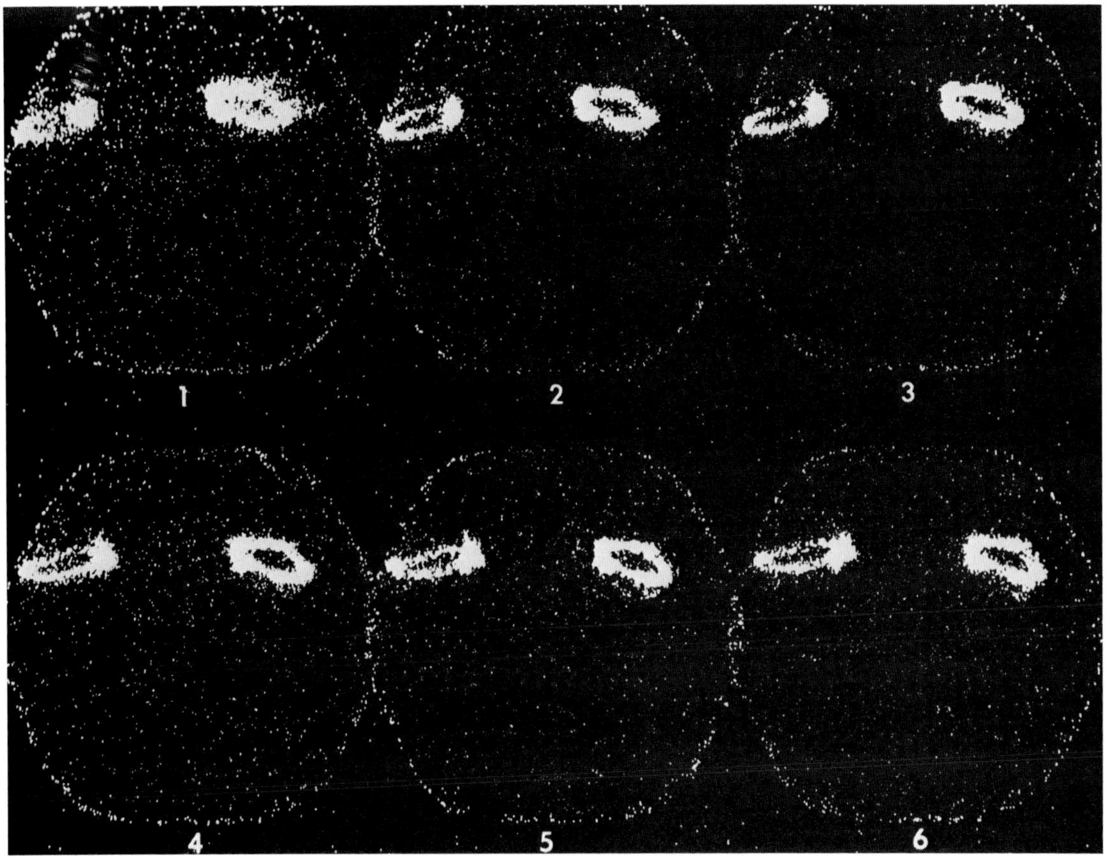

Figure 15-10. The postoperative study in this 12-year-old girl shows a persistent bilateral block at the level of the common canaliculi. Symptomically there was only minimal improvement, and this study indicated the need for further treatment.

is supported in a slightly inclined sitting position. We have used either an infant seat for this purpose, or the child may be held in a parent's arms.

Case 4

The patient, a 21-month-old boy, was sedated with chloral hydrate. There was no clearance of activity from the conjunctival sacs, until the lids were passively opened and closed in a rhythmic fashion (Fig. 15-11). Care must be taken not to massage the nasolacrimal sacs. This produced flow into both nasolacrimal sacs and ducts. Although he had bilateral tearing at this time, with increased tear meniscus levels, he was treated conservatively based on the scintigraphic findings. At followup his symptoms continued to improve considerably.

Dacryoscintigraphy has proved to be a useful noninvasive study in children presenting with epiphora. Our own experience in 34 patients (74 eyes studied) showed agreement with either the clinical findings or the results of other tests in 63 cases, 34 being abnormal and 29 normal (Table 15-2). There was discordance in 11 studies. In nine of these the scans altered the clinical management, either because the systems were functionally normal, or an abnormality was revealed suggesting further appropriate therapy (Table 15-3). The findings were misleading in two patients. One 4-year-old boy with a craniofacial disorder had left-sided epiphora. The scan showed a bilateral abnormality but the patient improved spontaneously without specific therapy. In another 11-year-old boy the scan showed delayed clearance on the right, but suggested an obstruction on the left. His only complaint was right-sided epiphora. Clinically he had an absent punctum on the right.

In our experience children over the age of 5

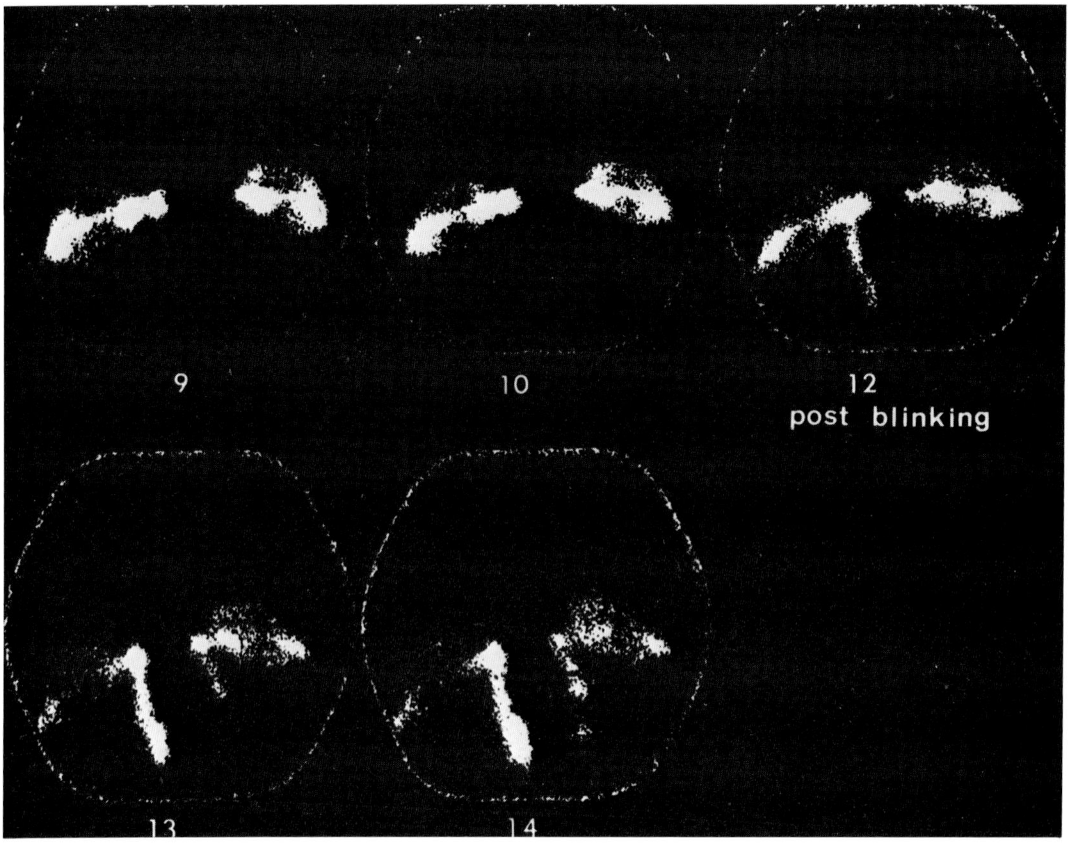

Figure 15-11. The dacryoscintigram in this 21-month-old boy was performed while sedated with chloral hydrate. There was no clearance from the conjunctival sacs until both lids were actively opened and closed in a rhythmic manner. Flow was noted into both ducts prompting further conservative management though he had significant bilateral tearing. At follow up his symptoms had improved considerably.

Table 15-2. Dacryoscintigraphy Compared with Other Tests

		Scan		Other	
Clinical	Patients	N	A	C	D
Epiphora	12	12	14	19	7
Postsurgery	18	17	23	36	4
Trauma	4	6	2	8	—

N, Normal; A, abnormal; C, concordance; D, discordance.

Table 15-3. Scintigraphy Altering Management

Name	Age	Sex	Comment
JS	5	M	Further surgery
SH[a]	1	F	Cancelled surgery
JA	14	F	Unilateral surgery only
RD	7	m	Unilateral punctectomy
EB	2	F	Delayed probing-improved
LF	7	F	Conservative-improved
JP[a]	2	M	Conservative-improved
MG	15	F	Conservative-improved
SK	17	F	Postsurgery-improved

[a]Sedated

years are in general cooperative. Smaller children may be apprehensive, and of course the study cannot be performed in a crying patient. It is in the latter group that sedation may be useful. In two of four patients studied in this way the information obtained altered the further management (Table 15-3).

Dacryoscintigraphy is potentially a valuable tool for evaluating epiphora in children. Attention to some of the noninvasive interventional procedures referred to may further decrease the small number of misleading studies.

References

1. Brizel HE, Sheils WC, Brown M. The effects of radiation therapy on the nasolacrimal system as evaluated by dacryoscintigraphy. Radiology 1972; 16:373.
2. Brown M, El Gammal TAM, Lukenberg MN, Eabig C. The value, limitations, and applications of nuclear dacryocystography. Semin Nucl Med 1981; XI:250.
3. Chavis RM, Welham RAN, Maisey MN. Quantitative lacrimal scintillography. Arch Ophthalmal 1978; 96:2066.
4. Heyman S, Katowitz JA, Smoger B. Dacryoscintigraphy in children. (in press).
5. Hurwitz JJ, Maisey MN, Welham RAN. Quantitative lacrimal scintillography. I. Method and physiological application. 1975; Br J Ophthalmol 59:308.
6. Hurwitz JJ, Maisey MN, Welham RAN. Quantitative lacrimal scintillography. II. Lacrimal pathology. Br J Ophthalmol 1975; 59:313.
7. Jones LT. Anatomy of the tear system. Int Ophthalmol Clin. 1973; 13:3.
8. Jones LT, Wobig JL. Newer concepts of tear duct and eyelid anatomy and treatment. Trans Am Acad Ophthalmol Otolaryngol 1977; 82:603.
9. Mahindra S, Dalgit R, Jamwal N, Mathew M. Lateral nasal proboscis. J Laryngol Otol 1973; 87:177.
10. Malik SRK, Gupta AK, Chaterjee S, Bhardwaj OP, Saha M. Dacryoscystography of normal and pathological lacrimal passages. Br J Ophthalmol 1969; 53:174.
11. Pico G. Congenital anomalies of the lacrimal system. In: Veirs ER, (ed.) The lacrimal system: Proceedings of the First International Symposium. 1970; 3–9. St. Louis: CV Mosby.
12. Putterman A: Treatment of epiphora with absent lacrimal puncta. Arch Opthalmol 1973; 89:125.
13. Robertson JS, Brown ML, Coloard DM. Radiation absorbed dose to the lens in dacryoscintigraphy with $^{99m}TcO_4$. Radiology 1979; 133:747.
14. Rossomondo RM, Carlton WH, Trueblood JH, Thoma PR. A new method of evaluating lacrimal drainage. Arch Ophthalmol 1972; 88:523.
15. Veirs ER. Disorders of the nasolacrimal apparatus in infants and children. J Pediatr Ophthalmol 1966; 3:32.
16. Whitaker LA, Katowitz JA. Facial anomalies involving the nasolacrimal apparatus. In: Tessier P et al. (eds.) Symposium on plastic surgery in the orbital region. 1976; 159–66. St. Louis: CV Mosby.

Chapter 16 Heart

S. T. Treves
Roger Hurwitz
Alvin Kuruc
H. W. Strauss

Application of radionuclides to the study of the cardiovascular system was first investigated by Blumgart and Yens[11] and by Blumgart and Weiss[12] in 1927 when they used radium-C and a primitive radiation detector in studies on the velocity of blood flow. In 1948, Prinzmetal et al.[95,96] described radiocardiograms of three patients with congenital heart disease using iodine-131 (I-131) sodium iodide and a Geiger-Mueller counter.

Over the past three decades, improvements in cardiovascular surgery permitted first palliation and then total correction of many congenital cardiac abnormalities. These advances, combined with the advent of short-lived radionuclides and computerized gamma cameras, have provided much of the impetus for development of nuclear medical methods for evaluation of the cardiovascular system.

Radionuclide applications in pediatric cardiology include first-pass radionuclide angiography, gated blood-pool scintigraphy, and myocardial perfusion scintigraphy. Frequent indications for radionuclide studies in pediatric cardiology are listed in Table 16-1.

FIRST-PASS RADIONUCLIDE ANGIOGRAPHY

First-pass radionuclide angiography in pediatric cardiology is used primarily for detection, localization, and quantitation of cardiovascular shunts.* The technique relies principally on the indicator-dilution theory, which has also been the subject of much review.† Other quantitative applications of this method include calculations of right and left ventricular ejection fractions, cardiac output, pulmonary transit time, stroke volume, diastolic volume, circulation time, and pulmonary blood volume. With this technique it is also possible to image normal and abnormal circulatory patterns within the heart, lungs, and great vessels.

First-pass radionuclide angiography has the advantage of being only minimally invasive, requiring a small intravenous injection. It carries no known risk, produces no significant hemodynamic disturbance, and delivers a low dose of radiation to the patient. Therefore, this examination can be used repeatedly in the same patient without much discomfort or hazard. Limitations of first-pass radionuclide angiography include its relatively low anatomic resolution and the lack of direct measurement of intracardiac pressures and oxygen saturation. Coupled with a careful history, with a physical examination, and often with complementary diagnostic methods, radionuclide angiography provides the physician with a useful noninvasive approach to the diagnosis and followup of certain cardiovascular disorders in children.

*References 1, 4, 5, 13, 15, 17, 20, 32, 38, 39, 45, 52, 57, 62, 66, 75, 78, 91, 112, 113, 115, 121, 127a, 131.
†References 22, 26, 35, 42, 82, 84, 89, 117, 134, 138.

Table 16-1. Application of Radionuclides in Pediatric Cardiology

Differentiation between pulmonary and cardiac causes for cyanosis in the newborn
Evaluation of the premature infant with patent ductus arteriosus (PDA)
Differentiation of small atrial septal defect (ASD) from mild pulmonic stenosis (PS)
Evaluation of patients in whom criteria of operability are equivocal
Confirmation of the closing of intracardiac shunts
Detection and quantitation of residual shunts and other postoperative complications
Evaluation of cardiac function in patients with congenital or organic heart disease (cardiac output, ejection fraction, end-diastolic volume, stroke volume, etc)
Assessment of myocardial perfusion: ischemia, infarction, cardiomyopathies
Diagnosis of right ventricular hypertrophy
Determination of regurgitant fraction

Method

Equipment

A gamma scintillation camera connected to a digital computer is used for first-pass radionuclide angiography. The most commonly used collimator is one with parallel holes and high sensitivity, designed for low gamma energies. Converging collimators of high sensitivity are useful in the evaluation of premature infants and newborns because they provide magnification and increased sensitivity. Conventional pinhole collimators provide even greater magnification but unfortunately are relatively insensitive, requiring a higher dose of radiotracer to be administered.

The anterior projection is adequate for detection and quantitation of shunts and for determination of cardiac output. Better separation of the atria from the ventricles is achieved with the parallel slant-hole collimator (30°) caudally tilted and positioned over the patient in the left anterior oblique projection. For determination of right and left ventricular ejection fractions, a right anterior oblique projection is taken with the face of the slant-hole collimator in contact with the patient's anterior chest. The slant-hole collimator in the left anterior oblique projection with the holes oriented caudally is helpful in the localization of shunts. The computer system associated with the camera should have convenient recording, storage, playback, interaction, and analysis capabilities.

Radiopharmaceuticals

Technetium-99m Radiopharmaceuticals

The most commonly used radiopharmaceutical for first-pass radionuclide angiography is technetium-99m (Tc-99m) as sodium pertechnetate (half-life, 6 h; energy, 140 keV). A usual dose schedule is 200 μCi/kg of body weight with a minimal total dose of 2–3 mCi. The volume injected should be small (0.2–0.5 ml) in order to obtain a compact bolus and facilitate temporal resolution. The solution of tracer must therefore have a high specific activity. Prior to administration of Tc-99m pertechnetate, patients are premedicated with sodium or potassium perchlorate. Perchlorate blocks uptake of technetium pertechnetate by the choroid plexus, thyroid, salivary glands, and stomach and promotes its urinary elimination. Tc-99m can be used in almost any chemical form as long as the activity level is appropriate because it is assumed that during the first pass most radiotracers remain largely intravascular. No perchlorate is necessary when other technetium radiopharmaceuticals are used. Tc-99m human serum albumin or Tc-99m red blood cells are used if a cardiac output determination is desired. Similarly, one of these two agents is used for the first-pass angiogram if a gated blood-pool scan is to follow this study.

Iridium-191m

Iridium-191m (Ir-191m), with a physical half-life of only 4.96 sec, is advantageous for radionuclide angiography. It emits photons at energies of 65 keV and 129 keV, which are in 58% and 30% abundance, respectively.[126] Both energy peaks can be imaged with modern gamma scintillation cameras. Because of its short physical half-life, relatively large amounts of Ir-191m activity can be administered to a patient with much lower absorbed radiation dose than with smaller amounts of Tc-99m. The high photon flux available with Ir-191m permits rapid imaging with high information density.

With Ir-191, the heart and great vessels can be evaluated in a variety of physiologic conditions such as rest, exercise, or under the effect of cardioactive drugs.

Ir-191m is the product of beta decay of osmium-191m (Os-191m), which has a physical half-life of 15.4 days. An Os-191 → Ir-191m generator system, which can deliver multiple doses of Ir-191m for rapid intravenous injection, has been developed in our laboratory and used in humans.[23,47,124,126,136,137] If Ir-191m is used, the time-activity curve from the angiogram should be corrected for radioactive decay and count losses due to gamma camera dead time before analysis.

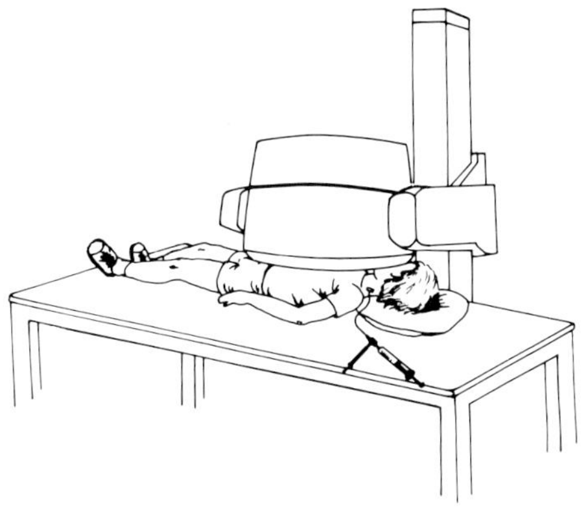

Figure 16-1. First-pass radionuclide angiogram. The patient is supine on the examination table with the gamma camera viewing his chest. An external jugular vein has been entered. The syringes containing the radiotracer and saline flush are connected to the butterfly set and ready for injection.

Patient Preparation

In our experience, most patients do not require sedation. An aide or two are necessary for restraining patients who cannot cooperate. Sedation may be given in certain cases. The sedation should be chosen on the basis of the patient's problem and in consultation with the referring physician. We find, however, that most sedatives used in pediatric practice are not effective, especially during introduction of the needle, and that manual restraint of the patient is necessary in most cases. In many instances sedatives will cause children to be more irritable.

Injection and Imaging

Qualitative and quantitative analyses of first-pass radionuclide angiography are best done if the radiotracer is delivered to the cardiopulmonary system as a rapid, compact injection.

Meticulous injection technique is necessary in order to obtain accurate quantitative results. This cannot be emphasized enough. With the patient in the supine position on the examining table, a vein is entered using a 21-, 23-, or 25-gauge needle in a butterfly set. The preferred site for injection is one of the external jugular veins. Once the vein has been entered, the needle is secured to the skin with adhesive tape. In our laboratory, almost all studies are performed with injection in one of the external jugular veins. In our experience, injection in the external jugular veins ensures success in > 95% of studies, while injection in the antecubital veins results in a fragmented bolus in about 30% of the cases.

In adult patients (and particularly obese ones) with inaccessible jugular veins, a small intravenous catheter placed as close to the superior vena cava as possible is helpful. In premature and small infants whose intrathoracic resistance is low and for whom the intravenous volume to be displaced is small, an adequate bolus can be injected via antecubital veins or even scalp veins. Scalp veins should be used as a last resort because of a high incidence of fragmented bolus in this case.

Once the vein has been entered, the patient's chest is centered in the field-of-view of the gamma camera (Fig. 16-1). We have developed a disposable injector (Paramedical Disposables, Inc., Watertown, MA, U.S.A.) for rapid and simultaneous injection of the radionuclide and saline flush (Fig. 16-2). The volume of saline flush ranges from 0.5 ml in a premature infant to 10 ml in an adult. Before the radionuclide is injected, a trial injection with saline alone should be made to ensure against accidental extravasation of the radionuclide solution. If there is no frank and free flow into the vein or if there are doubts about the adequancy of the venipuncture, the tracer must not be injected and the needle should be withdrawn. The injection should be made when the patient is not crying or breathing irregularly because rapid changes in intrathoracic pressure will most likely cause fragmentation of the bolus and render the study inadequate. Injecting the tracer and the saline simultaneously allows for uniform delivery of the tracer followed by uniform and uninterrupted

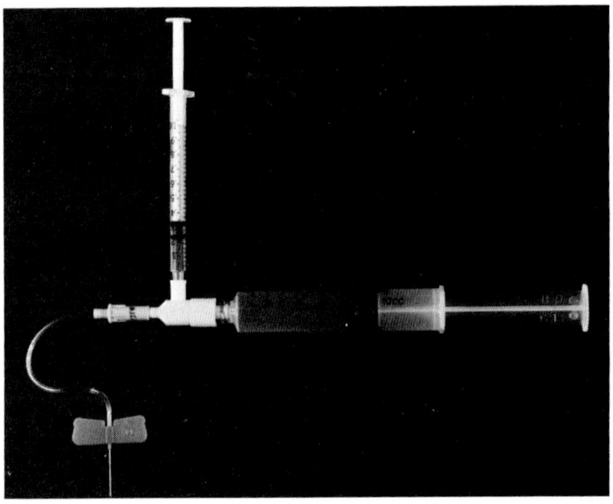

Figure 16-2. Injection assembly. A small disposable injector facilitates rapid intravenous injection of small volumes of radiotracer with simultaneous saline flush. The injector has a one-way valve, which prevents reflux of the radiotracer into the syringe containing the saline. The small syringe (usually a tuberculin syringe) contains the radiotracer; the 10-ml syringe contains the saline. The whole assembly is connected to the butterfly needle set already in place.

flushing. The injection should be given in one continuous motion without interruption.

Computer recording is started simultaneously with the injection. Once recording is completed, the quality of the tracer bolus is determined by inspection of a time-activity curve generated from a small area over the superior vena cava. We consider a bolus acceptable if the spike of the curve is about 3 sec in duration and if it is not followed by a secondary peak (Fig. 16-3). This evaluation is done while the patient is still under the gamma camera with the needle in place and supervised by an aide.

If the first injection is unsatisfactory due to poor injection technique or to a Valsalva maneuver, a second injection may be given with a dose of Tc-99m about 50% greater than the first dose. Data recording for the second angiogram is begun a few seconds before the injection to allow for background correction (Fig. 16-4). If both injections fail, the study should be repeated on another day.

Deconvolution analysis of the pulmonary curve can correct for some inadequate injections and avoid the necessity of repeating a study.[3,8,68] The

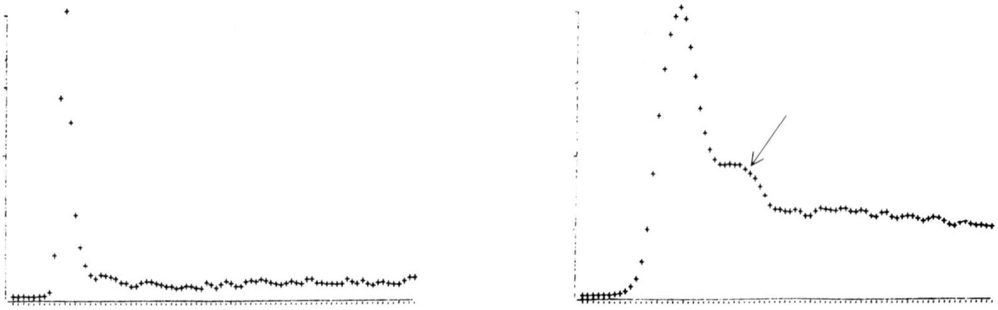

Figure 16-3. Time-activity curves at two frames/sec (2 fps). **A:** Time-activity histograms of the superior vena cava *(left)* and the right lung *(right)*. The bolus of radiotracer is adequate because it produced a single peak. The lung curve is that of a left-to-right shunt showing premature recirculation of the tracer.

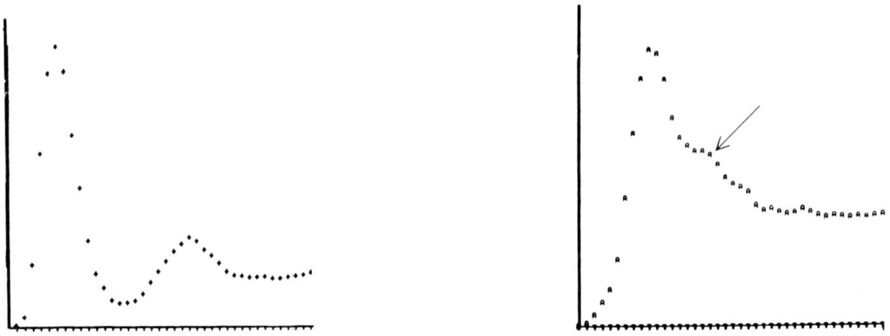

Figure 16-3. B: Pulmonary time-activity curves. Normal *(left)*. Left-to-right shunt *(right)*.

use of ultrashort-lived radionuclides such as Ir-191m is advantageous because it permits repeat angiograms within a short period of time without interference from background radiation (Fig. 16-5).

Data Recording

Angiography is recorded on a computer using either a matrix (frame) mode or list mode. For detection, localization, and quantitation of shunts, a rate of two to four frames/sec is adequate. For measurement of ejection fraction, a rate of at least 25 frames/sec should be used. Cardiac output determinations can be obtained at a slower frame rate, such as one frame/s. Multiple measurements may be made from one angiogram. If many of these measurements need to be made, a rapid frame rate should be used and the study compressed in time when necessary.

Data Display

For anatomic evaluation of the study, a series of images of 0.5, 1, 2, or 4 sec (depending on the patient's circulation time) are displayed on the computer monitor. The images may be interpolated into a finer matrix with or without contrast enhancement to facilitate recognition of anatomic features. Also, it may be desirable to add and subtract images corresponding to various phases of the angiogram to facilitate selection of regions of interest (ROIs) and avoid overlap with adjacent cardiovascular structures. As an example, the images corresponding to the cardiac blood pool and the great vessels may be subtracted from the pulmonary phase of the angiogram in order to aid selection of ROIs over the lungs to be used for quantitation of left-to-right shunts. A cine-like display that can be replayed in an endless loop at varied speeds is often useful in evaluating the angiogram initially.

Clinical Applications

Normal First-Pass Angiogram

A normal anterior radionuclide angiogram shows the bolus of radiotracer circulating within the superior (or inferior) vena cava and consecutively in the right atrium, the right ventricle, the lungs, the left atrium, the left ventricle, and the aorta. The left atrium is normally difficult to see on the ante-

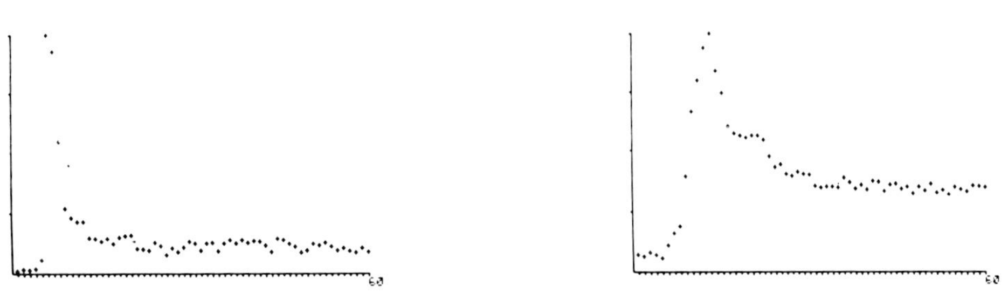

Figure 16-4. Two injection of Tc-99m pertechnetate in the same patient. On the *top* are shown two time-activity curves. One represents a fragmented and prolonged bolus of tracer in the superior vena cava (SVC, *top left*). Note the three consecutive peaks on that curve. The pulmonary curve wrongly indicates a very large left-to-right shunt with a pulmonary-to-systemic flow ratio (Q_p:Q_s) > 3 *(top right)*. On the *bottom panels*, curves from a second injection are shown. The curve of the SVC reflects a good bolus *(bottom left)*, and the pulmonary curve shows a left-to-right shunt with a Q_p:Q_s of 1.8 *(bottom right)*. Each point represents 0.5 sec.

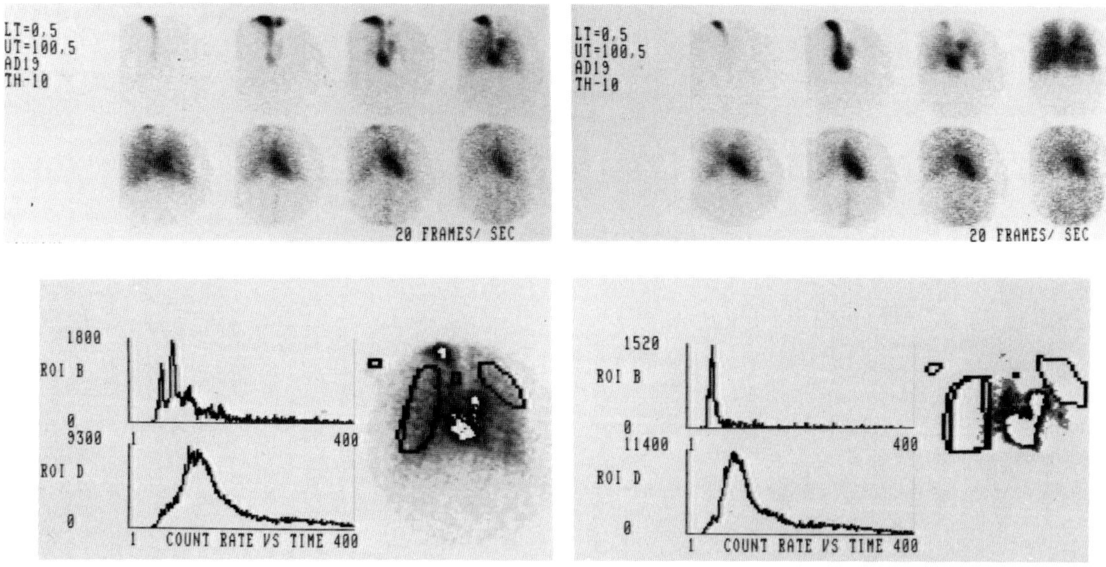

Figure 16-5. Two consecutive Ir-191m radionuclide angiograms performed on the same patient. The first study *(top left)* shows the effect of crying on the integrity of the bolus of radiotracer. Transit of Ir-191m through the right subclavian vein is delayed and there is reflux into the left subclavian vein. Each frame represents 1 sec. The time-activity curve of the superior vena cava (ROI B, *bottom left*) reveals multiple peaks, which indicate fragmentation of the bolus. The pulmonary curve (ROI D) analysis reveals a Q_p:Q_s of 1.6. After a second injection of Ir-191m through the same right jugular vein, the angiogram reveals good passage of the tracer through the superior vena cava *(top right)*. Time-activity curves of the second study *(bottom right)* show adequacy of the bolus (ROI B) and the corresponding pulmonary curve (ROI D). The estimated Q_p:Q_s from this curve was 1.2.

rior projection. The left side of the heart and the aorta are clearly visible with the lungs almost totally devoid of any activity. The normal relative sizes of the cardiac chambers and of the great vessels can be appreciated.

A pulmonary time-activity curve of a normal radionuclide angiogram is characteristic. It shows a small segment where there is almost no activity, corresponding to the circulation time from the injection site to the pulmonary vasculature. This is followed by a relatively rapidly ascending slope of increasing activity that culminates on a peak as the center of the bolus reaches the lungs. The curve then descends at a slower rate to almost reach the baseline as the tail of the bolus leaves the lungs. Following this valley another peak of lower amplitude becomes visible. This second peak represents a fraction of the initial amount of tracer returning to the lungs following systemic circulation. Also, this second peak is wider than the first one due to dilution of the bolus in the circulation. A normal Tc-99m first-pass radionuclide angiogram is shown in Fig. 16-6.

Left-to-Right Shunting

In left-to-right shunting, the radionuclide angiogram shows persistently high levels of activity in the lungs and in the right side of the heart due to early recirculation of the radioindicator (Figs. 16-7–16-10). In large atrial septal defects, it is possible to detect dilution of the radiotracer as it reaches the level of the shunt (Fig. 16-8). In addition, there is poor visualization of the left side of the heart and aorta. This dilution effect is accentuated with increasing shunt flow. Persistent pulmonary activity and poor visualization of the left side of the heart on a radionuclide angiogram are diagnostic features of left-to-right shunting.

The pulmonary time-activity curve in a left-to-right shunt is characteristic. Radiotracer prematurely reentering the pulmonary vascular bed through the shunt produces an early second peak that interrupts the decrease in counts after the first peak. This curve can be used to quantitate the shunt by calculating the pulmonary-to-systemic flow ratio (Q_p:Q_s) (Fig. 16-11).

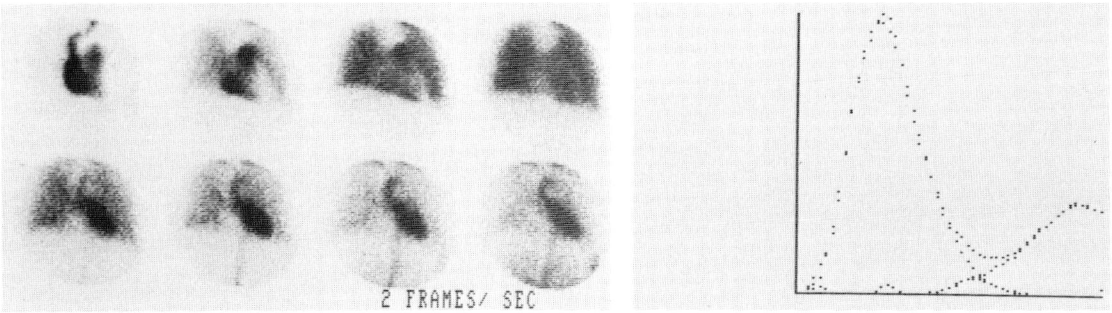

Figure 16-6. Normal anterior radionuclide angiogram with Tc-99m sodium pertechnetate. The tracer was injected into a left external jugular vein. Each image represents 1.5 sec. The radiotracer successively circulates through the superior vena cava, right atrium, right ventricle, pulmonary artery, lungs, left atrium, left ventricle, and aorta. The pulmonary artery appears dilated and probably accounts for the patient's systolic murmur. The estimated pulmonary-to-systemic flow ratio (Q_p:Q_s) from the right lung curve is 1.0. Therefore, this patient has no evidence of left-to-right shunt.

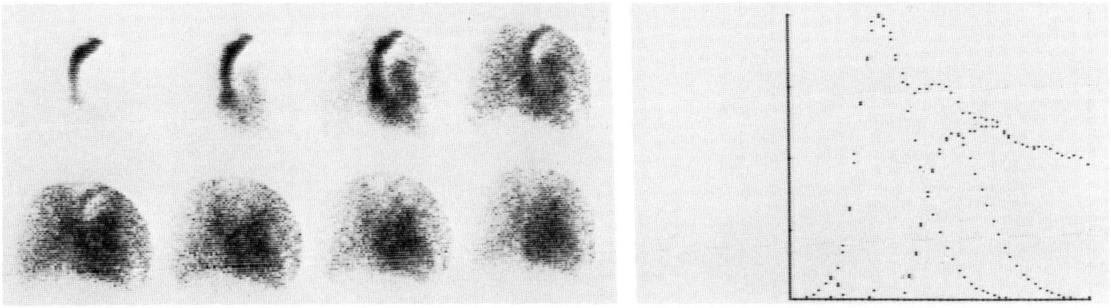

Figure 16-7. Left-to-right shunt in a 10-year-old boy with a clinical question of atrial septal defect. He had a fixed, split-second sound and a I/IV systolic murmur at the left upper sternal border. His chest radiograph showed increased pulmonary markings, and the electrocardiogram showed a right bundle branch block. The echocardiogram revealed paradoxical motion of the interventricular septum and right ventricular enlargement consistent with right ventricular volume overload. No septal defect was identified on the echocardiogram, however. The cardiologist's clinical impression was a small left-to-right shunt through an atrial septal defect. The radionuclide angiogram is typical of a moderate left-to-right shunt with dilution of the tracer by nonradiolabelled blood at the atrial level, poor visualization of the left side of the heart and aorta, and persistent activity in the lungs due to shunt recirculation. Each image represents 1 sec. The estimated Q_p:Q_s was 2.7.

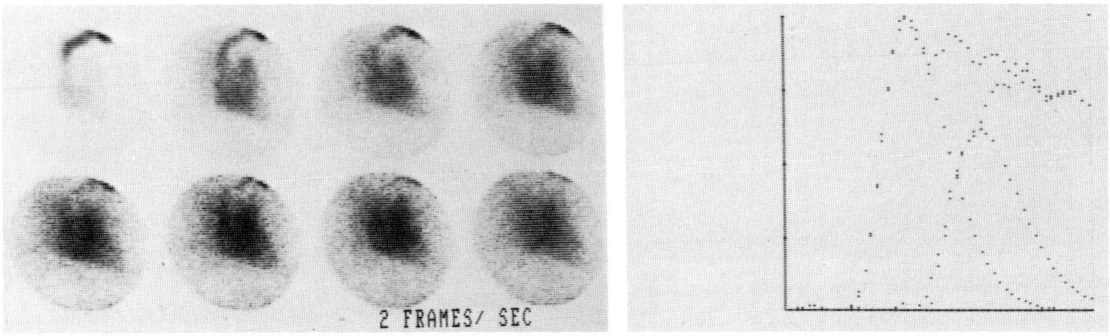

Figure 16-8. Large left-to-right shunt in a 14-year-old girl with a question of partial anomalous venous return. Echocardiography demonstrated right ventricular dilatation and no evidence of an atrial septal defect. Auscultation revealed a split-second sound. The chest roentgenogram showed mildly increased pulmonary markings and probable right ventricular enlargement. The radionuclide angiogram *(left)* shows poor definition of the left side of the heart and the aorta with significant early pulmonary recirculation. The estimated Q_p:Q_s is >3 *(right)*.

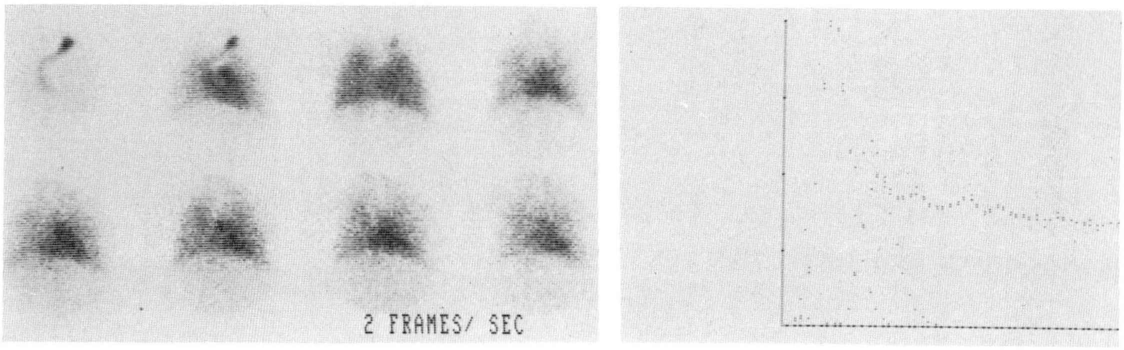

Figure 16-9. Left-to-right shunting in a 3-year-old boy. He had a fixed second sound with a III/VI systolic murmur. His chest radiograph revealed a large pulmonary artery. The electrocardiogram revealed an incomplete right bundle branch block. Echocardiography revealed a large right ventricle and a large right atrium without evidence of an atrial septal defect. The clinical impression was a left-to-right shunt through an atrial septal defect. The radionuclide angiogram is diagnostic of a left-to-right shunt. The Q_p:Q_s is 2.2.

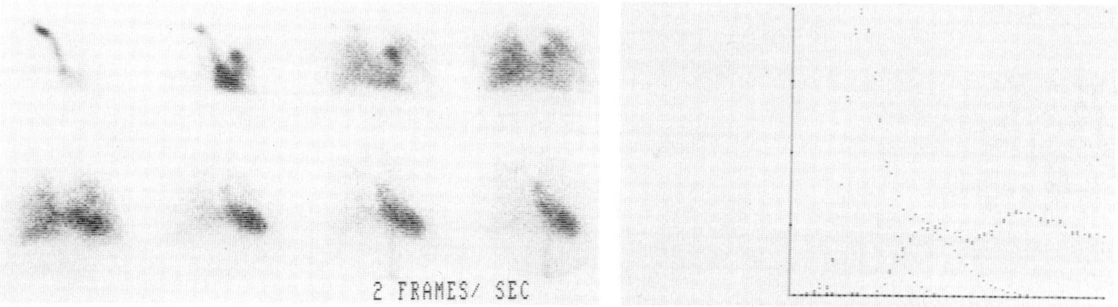

Figure 16-10. Left-to-right shunting in an 11-year-old male with a grade IV/VII shrill and a blowing systolic murmur heard best at midprecordium. The clinical impression was a ventricular septal defect. The radionuclide angiogram reveals some early pulmonary recirculation due to left-to-right shunting. Each frame represents 1 sec. The estimated Q_p:Q_s was 1.7.

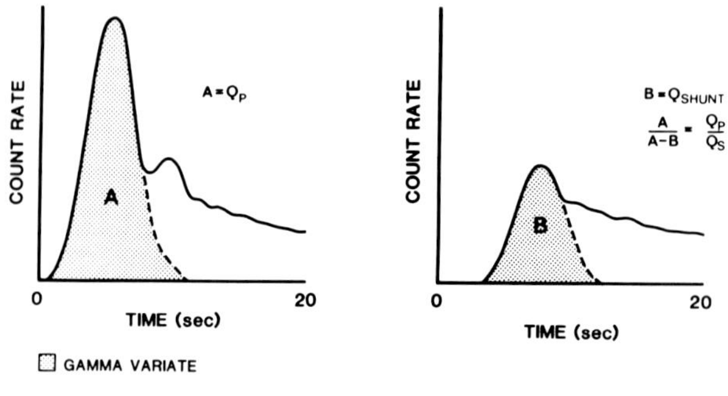

Figure 16-11. Calculation of pulmonary-to-systemic flow ratio (Q_p:Q_s) using pulmonary time-activity curves and the gamma variate model. *A,* Area under the first pass of tracer through the lungs as defined by a gamma variate extrapolation. Q_p, pulmonary flow. *B,* area under the portion of the curve corresponding to radiolabelled blood returning prematurely to the lung by the left-to-right shunt. *Q* shunt, shunt flow. $A - B = Q_s$ = systemic flow.[80]

It is often possible to determine the level of a left-to-right shunt by visually analyzing time-activity curves generated from the superior vena cava, right atrium, right ventricle, and lungs, thus defining the site of recirculation. A left anterior oblique projection with a 30° caudal tilt is useful for this purpose. For example, in partial anomalous pulmonary venous return to the superior vena cava, there is early recirculation in the superior vena cava, right atrium, right ventricle, and lungs. In atrial septal defect, there is early recirculation in the right atrium, right ventricle, and lungs. In ventricular septal defect there is premature recirculation in the right ventricle and lungs. In patent ductus arteriosus, there is early recirculation only in the lungs. If more than one shunt is present, it is possible to localize only the most proximal one.[121] Detecting shunt recirculation in the superior vena cava may be difficult due to overlap of the right pulmonary artery.

Analytic Model

The pulmonary time-activity curve recorded from a normal subject is composed of several sequential components. The first component, appearing at time t_p, is due to detection of radiotracer passing through the pulmonary vascular bed before ever entering the systemic vascular bed. We term this component $P(t)$. The second component, appearing at time t_{r1}, is due to detection of radiotracer passing through the pulmonary vascular bed after one circuit through the systemic vascular bed. We term this component $R1(t)$. The third and later components are due to detection of radiotracer passing through the pulmonary vascular bed after more than one circuit of the systemic vascular bed. The observed normal pulmonary curve, $O(t)$, may therefore be described by the formula:

$$O(t) = P(t) + R1(t) + \cdots.$$

In the case of a patient with a left-to-right shunt, a fraction (K) of radiotracer leaving the pulmonary vascular bed may bypass the systemic vascular bed by traveling through the shunt (Fig. 16-12). The remaining fraction ($1 - K$) of radiotracer will pass through the systemic vascular bed. Assuming the radiotracer is well mixed with blood in the pulmonary bed, these fractions are equal to the relative blood flows through the shunt and systemic vascular beds. The pulmonary-to-systemic flow ratio ($Q_p{:}Q_s$) is therefore equal to $1/(1 - K)$.

As in the normal patients, the first component of the observed pulmonary curve, $P(t)$, is the radiotracer detected as it passes through the pulmonary vascular bed the first time: that is, before it passes through the shunt or the systemic vascular bed. The minimum transit time for passing through the shunt and back to the pulmonary system is generally less than that for passing through the systemic vascular bed to the pulmonary system. Therefore, the second component of $O(t)$, appearing at time t_{S1}, represents radiotracer that is passing through the pulmonary vascular bed after one circuit of the shunt. We term this component $S1(t)$. The area under $S1(t)$ is equal to K times the area under $P(t)$. The next two components of $O(t)$, appearing at times t_{R1} and t_{S2}, are due to detection of radiotracer passing through the pulmonary vascular bed after one circuit of the systemic vascular bed and two circuits of the shunt, respectively. We term these components $R1(t)$ and $S2(t)$. The remaining components of $O(t)$ are due to radiotracer passing

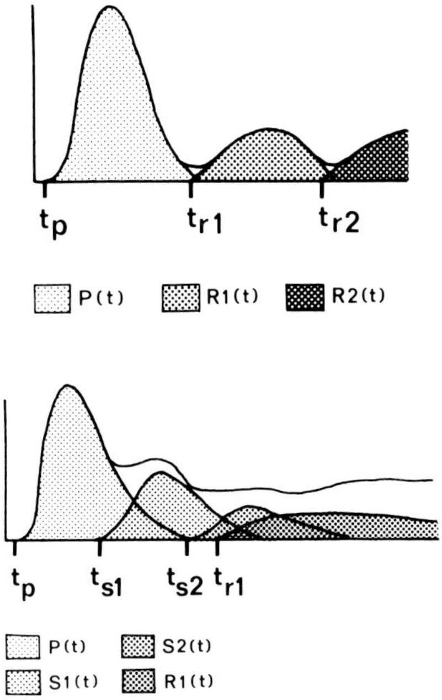

Figure 16-12. Sequential components of the pulmonary time-activity curves in a normal patient *(top)* and in a patient with a left-to-right shunt *(bottom)*. See text for an explanation of the abbreviation.

through the pulmonary vascular bed following multiple circuits of the shunt and systemic vascular bed. The observed pulmonary curve is equal to:

$$O(t) = P(t) + R1(t) + S2(t) + R1(t) + \cdots.$$

This curve is illustrated in Fig. 16-12. Shunt quantitation is the problem of determining K. K may be quantitated as a ratio of blood flow by dividing the area under $S1(t)$ by the area under $P(t)$. Thus by recovering $P(t)$ and $S1(t)$ from $O(t)$ we can obtain an estimate of K.

Gamma Variate Analysis

A method of recovering $P(t)$ and $S1(t)$ from the observed pulmonary curve, $O(t)$, is the gamma variate method. Consider the $O(t)$ obtained from a normal patient. The portion of $O(t)$ for $t_p \leq t \leq t_{r1}$ is due solely to the component $P(t)$. At time t_{r1}, the component $R1(t)$ appears. In most cases, almost the entire area of $P(t)$ is to the left of t_{R1}. It is therefore possible to almost completely recover $P(t)$.

It has been found experimentally that the $P(t)$ obtained after a compact bolus injection of radiotracer can be closely approximated by a gamma variate function of the form:

$$P(t) = C(t - t_0)A\, e^{-(t-t_0)/B}$$

in which t_0 is the time at which activity first appears and C, A, and B are variable parameters. The gamma variate function can be fitted to a portion of an observed data curve by a weighted least squares technique.[109] Thus, it is possible to estimate $P(t)$ by fitting the gamma variate function to $O(t)$ for $t_p \leq t \leq t_{R1}$ and extrapolating.

Consider the $O(t)$ obtained from a patient with a left-to-right shunt. The initial portion of the curve is again solely due to the component $P(t)$. At time t_{s1}, the component $S1(t)$ begins to appear. In this case, t_{s1} is smaller than t_{r1} and a substantial portion of area under $P(t)$ occurs after t_{s1}. However, it is possible to approximately recover $P(t)$ by fitting a gamma variate to $O(t)$ for $t_p \leq t \leq t_{s1}$ and extrapolating. We denote the area under $P(t)$ as $A1$. In practice, it is necessary to infer the limits of the gamma variate fit from $O(t)$. This can be done by visually interpreting the curve and manually choosing the points or by using a computer algorithm that automatically chooses the points.

We now need to recover the component $S1(t)$. Subtracting the gamma variate fit for $P(t)$ from $O(t)$ yields the recirculation curve:

$$RC(t) = S1(t) + R1(t) + S2(t) + \cdots$$

which is equal to $S1(t)$ for $t_{s1} \leq t \leq \min(t_{S2}, t_{R1})$. We denote $\min(t_{s2}, t_{r1})$ as t_{rC}. A gamma variate function is fit to this portion of the recirculation curve and extrapolated to recover $S1(t)$. We denote the area under $S1(t)$ as $A2$. Again, in practice it is necessary to manually or automatically infer the limits of the fit from $RC(t)$.

K is equal to the ratio $A2/A1$. The pulmonary-to-systemic flow ratio ($Q_p{:}Q_s$) is equal to $1/(1 - K)$. Substituting for K, we obtain the formula:

$$Q_p{:}Q_s = A1/(A1 - A2).$$

This method provides accurate determinations of $Q_p{:}Q_s$ within a range of 1.2 to 3.0. Values of 1.0–1.2 will be obtained in patients with no shunt or a very small left-to-right shunt.[1,2,6,80,121,122] When the flow ratio is < 1.6, the shunt may not be recognized by visual inspection of the angiogram.

A number of alternative methods to estimate $Q_p{:}Q_s$ from pulmonary time-activity curves have been suggested.[89] Some promising results have been reported for a proposed method based on a linear time invariant model of the circulation similar to that described here. This method uses a signal processing technique known as homomorphic deconvolution to recover $P(t)$ and $S1(t)$.[87]

Correction for Radiotracer Delivery

Shunt quantitation by the gamma variate method assumes that $P(t)$ and $S1(t)$ can be described by gamma variate functions. In addition, the method assumes that sufficiently large portions of $P(t)$ and $S1(t)$ occur before t_{s1} and t_{rC}, respectively, to allow accurate extrapolation. The validity of both of these assumptions is dependent upon the time course of delivery of the radiotracer to the cardiopulmonary system. This delivery can be monitored using a ROI over the superior vena cava.

Ideally, one would like to deliver the radiotracer to the cardiopulmonary system as an instantaneous pulse because this facilitates shunt quantitation by the gamma variate method. In practice, it is impossible to attain this goal by intravenous injection. It is possible, however, to estimate the pulmonary curve that would be produced from an instantaneous pulse of radiotracer from the observed superior vena caval and pulmonary curves by using a mathematical technique known as deconvolution.[8,35,69]

Studies on dogs and humans have shown that deconvolution may improve the accuracy of shunt quantitation by radionuclide angiocardiography.[3,41,68] Figure 16-13 shows the effect of deconvolution on Ir-191m radionuclide angiocardiography performed on a dog with a left-to-right shunt. The pulmonary curve obtained after a fragmented injection is distorted relative to the pulmonary curve obtained after a compact injection in the same animal. After deconvolution, both lung curves are nearly identical.

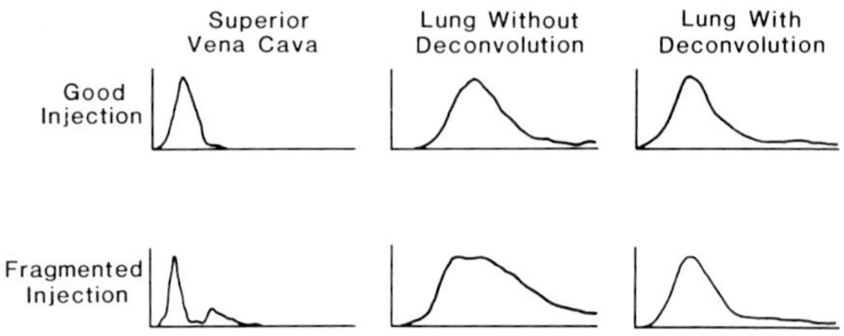

Figure 16-13. Effect of deconvolution on time-activity curves after an adequate injection and after a fragmented injection. Ir-191m angiocardiography.

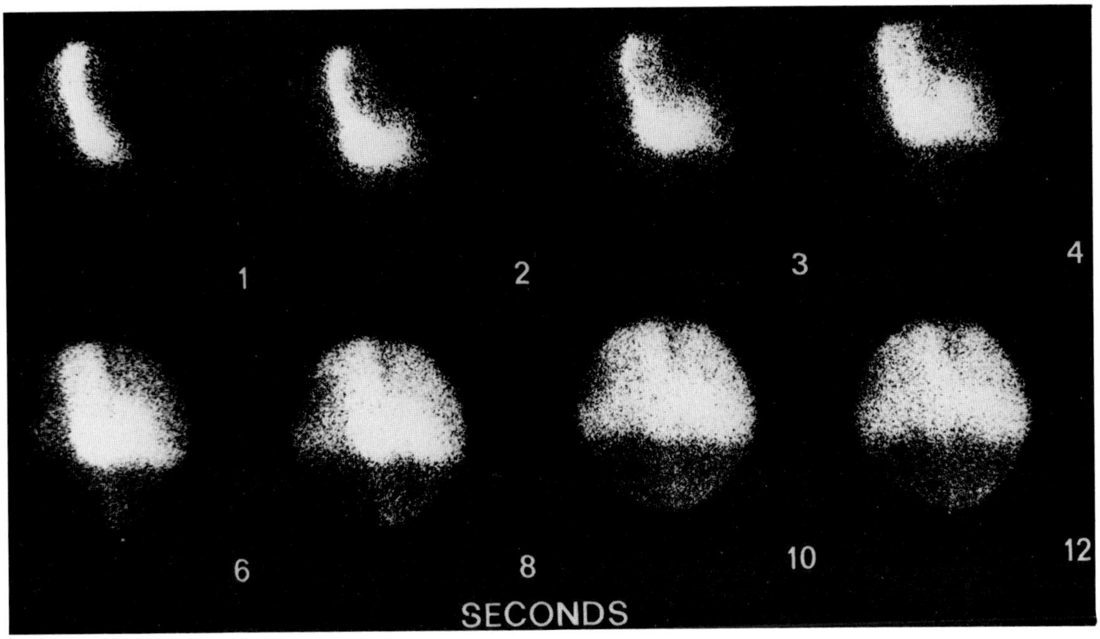

Figure 16-14. Right-to-left shunting in tetralogy of Fallot. The tracer is seen in the superior vena cava (1–3 sec), in the right side of the heart (2–3 sec), and rapidly within the left side of the heart (2–6 sec). The pulmonary activity begins at 6 sec when the abdominal aorta also becomes active.

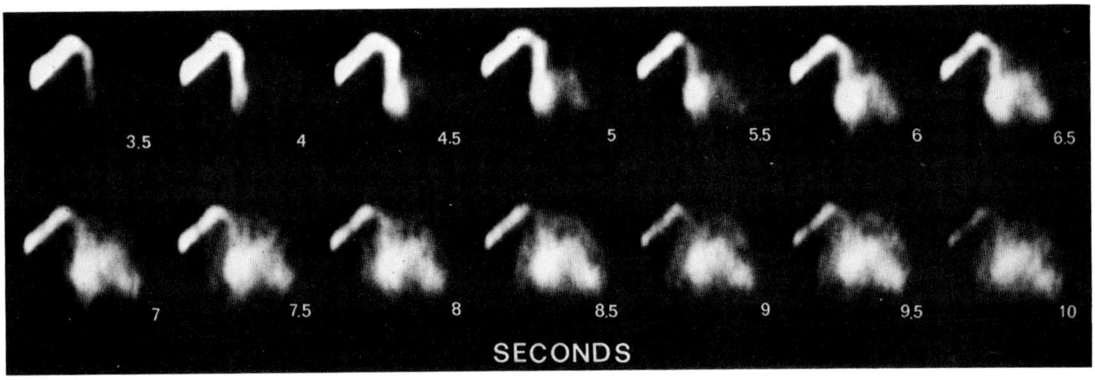

Figure 16-15. Tricuspid atresia. Right-to-left shunting at the atrial level is apparent on frames at 4.5–6.5 sec. The left atrium and left ventricles can be seen at 5–7 sec. The right ventricle is very small and essentially acts as an outflow tract to the right atrium. On the angiogram the area normally occupied by the right ventricle appears as a filling defect, and an area of no activity.

Right-to-Left Shunting

In right-to-left shunting the first-pass radionuclide angiogram reveals passage of the radiotracer within the superior (or inferior) vena cava, the right atrium, and the right ventricle. There is, depending on the level of the shunt, rapid appearance of the tracer within the left atrium and/or the left ventricle and the aorta which on the angiogram appears to occur at the same time or before the tracer reaches the lungs (Fig. 16-14). Characteristically, in tricuspid atresia, the tracer is seen to circulate from the right atrium into the left ventricle, presenting a rather unique angiographic pattern (Fig. 16-15).

Two approaches to detection and quantitation of

right-to-left shunts have been taken. The angiocardiographic technique is the same as described for left-to-right shunting except that the patient should be imaged in the left anterior oblique projection to obtain maximum separation between the right and left ventricles. ROIs are marked over the superior vena cava, right ventricle, left ventricle, and lungs. The time-activity curve from a curve from a small ROI over the left ventricle is analyzed. Care must be taken to avoid contamination of counts from the right side of the heart in the ROI selected. A first peak of activity due to blood shunted from the right to the left heart is followed by a second peak of activity due to the radioactive blood that has circulated through the lungs. Using an exponential extrapolation of the downslope following these peaks, shunt flow can be estimated as the ratio of the area under the first peak to the whole area under both peaks (Fig. 16-16).[51,103,120,132]

Another technique uses radioactive particles (Tc-99m macroaggregated albumin). A major assumption in this method is that the particles are completely extracted from the circulation in one pass through either the pulmonary or the systemic capillary beds. This condition is largely met for particles > 10 μm in diameter. It is also assumed that the particles are mixed uniformly in the blood, that the particles themselves do not affect the blood flow, and that the particles traverse the system in the same manner as the blood. After intravenous administration of radioactive particles to a patient with a right-to-left shunt, the ratio of particles that enter the pulmonary and systemic circulations will equal the ratio of pulmonary blood flow to shunt flow.

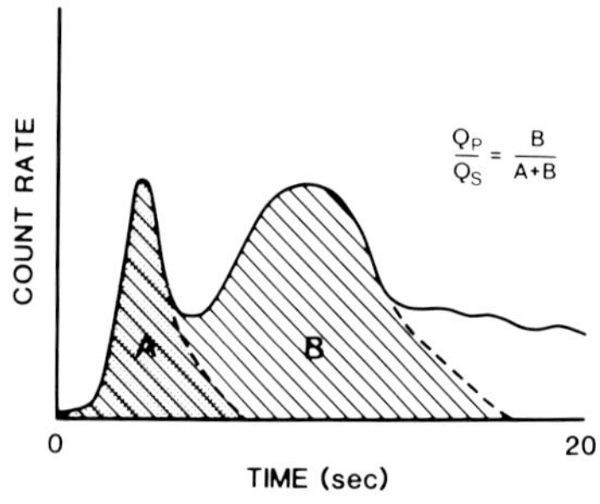

Figure 16-16. Right-to-left shunt. Left ventricular time-activity curve showing two peaks. The first peak corresponds to tracer being shunted from right-to-left. The second peak corresponds to tracer reaching the left ventricle after having circulated through the pulmonary circuit. Q_p, Pulmonary flow; Q_s, systemic flow; *A*, area under the right-to-left shunt curve; *B*, area under the two peaks.

The activity in the whole body is measured and compared with that in the lungs. Gates et al.,[36] using posterior scintiphotos, and Lin,[74] using a whole-body profile device, employed this method. The theoretical difficulty is that the pulmonary and systemic circulations may be detected with different sensitivities due to counting geometry and self-absorption. Complete separation of pulmonary and systemic activities may pose a minor difficulty, but good clinical results have been reported with this method (Fig. 16-17). Although no adverse reactions have been reported from the intravenous administration of particles in patients with right-to-left shunting, one should be reminded that these particles produce microembolization of systemic territories including the brain and the kidneys. When it is necessary to perform this study, we empirically employ a small number of particles (< 10,000) in order to reduce systemic embolization.

Right-to-left shunting can also be detected by angiocardiography with an inert gas. An inert gas is almost completely removed from the blood in one transit through the lungs. Appearance of systemic activity after intravenous injection of an inert gas (dissolved in saline) indicates a right-to-left shunt. Some investigators feel that use of both an inert gas and a nondiffusible indicator helps to define the nature of the cardiac defect, especially in more complicated patients.[13,16,76,77,90]

Cardiac Output

Cardiac output can be calculated by analysis of time-activity curves generated from a ROI over the heart. A bolus of Tc-99m human serum albumin (HSA) or Tc-99m red blood cells is given intravenously and the computer recording is set at one or two frames/sec for 5 min. Two initial peaks appear on the precordial curve: the first peak corresponds to the radioactivity circulating within the right side of the heart, and the second peak corresponds to the activity as it passes within the left side of the heart. After a few minutes the curve reaches a steady amplitude as equilibrium of the indicator in the blood pool occurs. Tc-99m HSA preparations tend to break down slightly in vivo, however, and usually there is indeed a minimal downslope on the portion of the precordial curve corresponding to equilibrium.

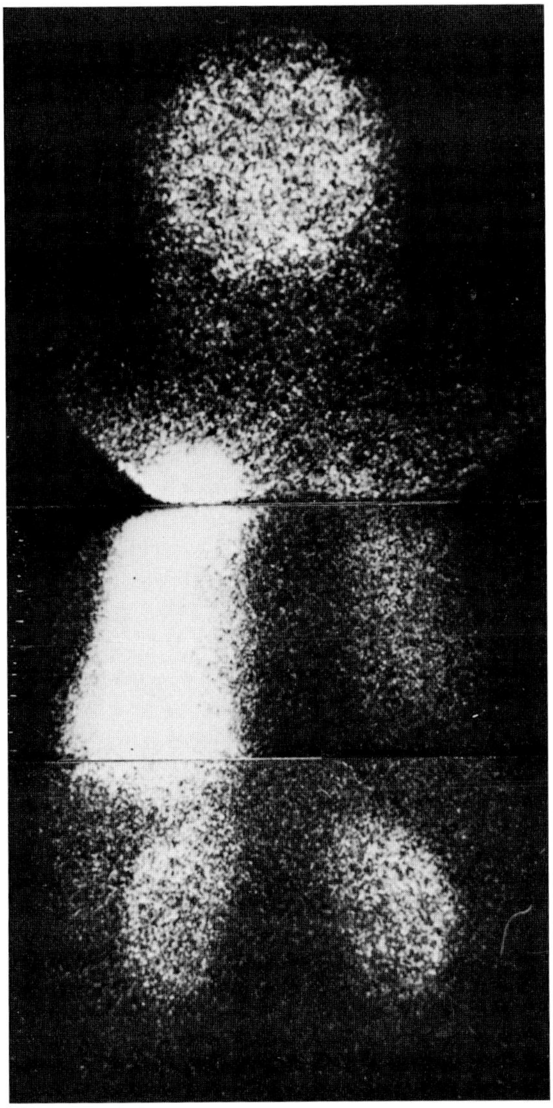

Figure 16-17. Right-to-left shunting in a 12-year-old male with tetralogy of Fallot and a Glenn shunt. Tc-99m macroaggregated albumin was injected intravenously in a vein of one of his feet. There is a significant systemic penetration of the tracer (including brain and kidneys), and the left lung receives most of the pulmonary artery flow from the right side of the heart. The right pulmonary artery receives blood from the superior vena cava by way of the Glenn shunt.

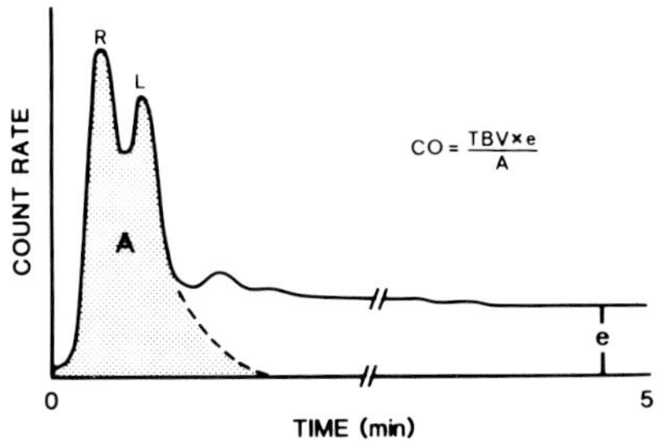

Figure 16-18. Precordial curve for calculation of cardiac output. *CO*, Cardiac output; *TBV*, total blood volume; *A*, area under the curve of the first-pass of tracer in the heart; *R*, right heart peak; *L*, left heart peak; *e*, equilibrium of the tracer in the cardiac blood pool.

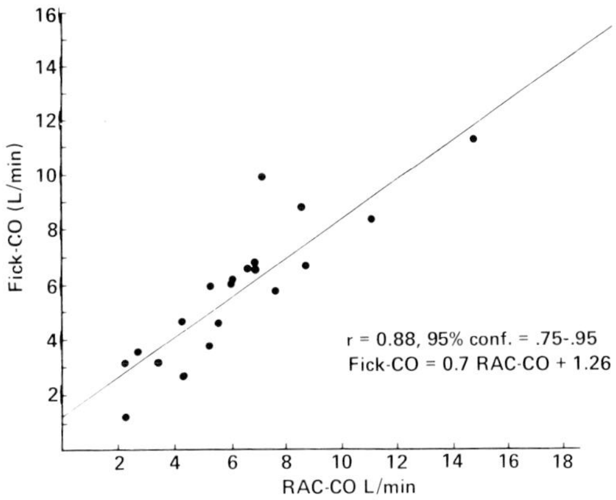

Figure 16-19. Cardiac output in children calculated using radionuclide angiography and the Fick method at cardiac catheterization.

An exponential extrapolation of the downslope of the second peak determines an area of the first pass of radioindicator through the heart (A) (Fig. 16-18). An equilibrium value (e) is determined on the stable portion of the curve, and the total blood volume (TBV) is determined independently. With these parameters, cardiac output (CO) is calculated:

$$CO = \frac{TBV \times e}{A} \text{ ml/min.}$$

While the first two peaks represent intracardiac activity at equilibrium, a portion of the activity during equilibrium arises outside of the heart chambers (e.g., in the chest wall). Empirically, it has been found that the value obtained from this calculation should be multiplied by 0.83 to correct for such extracardiac activity.[19,28,29,132] We have studied 17 pediatric patients with simultaneous determinations of cardiac output by radionuclide angiocardiography and oxygen consumption and found a good agreement by the two techniques ($r = 0.88$) (Fig. 16-19).[97]

Ejection Fraction

Estimation of right and left ventricular ejection fractions requires a recording frame rate of at least 25 frames/sec (or list mode recording) for 25 sec. We use a right anterior projection with a 30° slanted parallel-hole collimator on contact with the patient's chest. The patient can be studied in the supine, sitting, or standing position. After recording, the study is played back and ROIs are marked over the right and left ventricles. Time-activity curves from these regions are calculated and plotted in order to identify the frames in the study corresponding to end-diastole and end-systole. These curves are corrected for radioactive decay if Ir-191m is used. In addition, an adaptive low-pass filter is used to eliminate high-frequenty noise.

Consecutive frames of end-diastole and end-systole are selected over several cycles during the first pass of radionuclide through the right and left ventricles. Composite images of end-diastole and end-systole for each ventricle are formed by adding the previously selected frames at the corresponding times (Figs. 16-20–16-22). Subtracting the end-systolic image from the end-diastolic image produces a so-called stroke-volume image, which is used to help mark the atrioventricular valve planes. ROIs for the right end-diastolic and right end-systolic, left end-diastolic, and left end-systolic ventricular outlines are marked. Ejection fraction can then be calculated by the following formula:

$$\text{Ejection fraction } (RV \text{ or } LV) = \frac{\text{End diastolic counts} - \text{End systolic counts}}{\text{End diastolic counts}}.$$

In this method background subtraction is not used. Limitations with this method include relatively low temporal resolution within a cardiac cycle, some difficulty in detecting the edges of the ventricular blood pools, and the need for careful injection technique. This method is accurate, however, and ideally suited for children because a long period of immobilization is not needed. Further, no assumptions need to be made about shape of the ventricles because the estimation of ejection fraction is based on count rate in the ventricles, which is directly proportional to chamber volume(s).

We have employed this method in children and compared it with biplane angiography performed almost simultaneously. Evaluation of a small number of patients yielded a correlation coefficient of 0.91.[67] In our laboratory, we measured right and left ventricular ejection fractions in 74 children who were referred for skeletal scintigraphy and had normal cardiovascular systems.[55] Values for normal ejection fractions in these children are listed in Table 16-2.

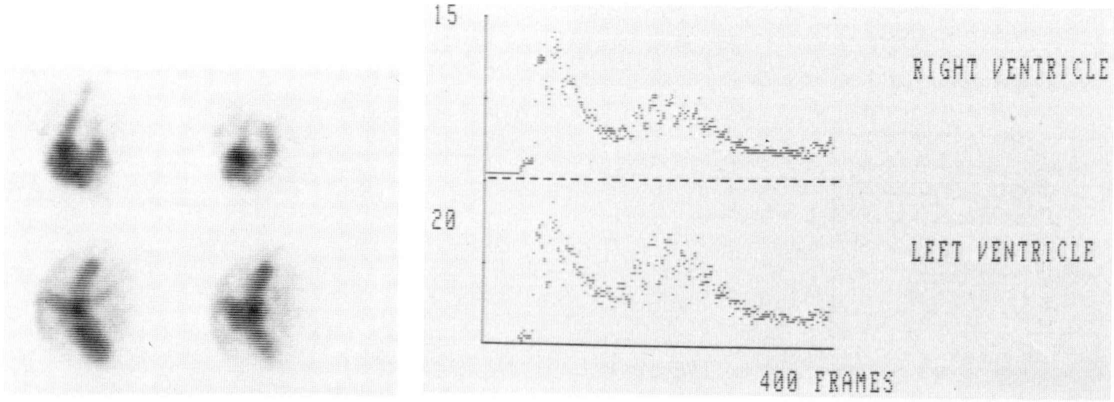

Figure 16-20. Right and left ventricular ejection fractions calculated from first-pass radionuclide angiography in a normal patient. *Left:* Selected frames representing right ventricular end-diastole *(top left)*, right ventricular end-systole *(top right)*, left ventricular end-diastole *(bottom left)*, and left ventricular end-systole *(bottom right)*. *Right:* Time-activity curves from ROIs over the right and left ventricles. Because the study was recorded in the right anterior oblique projection, the ventricular ROIs contain information from both ventricles.

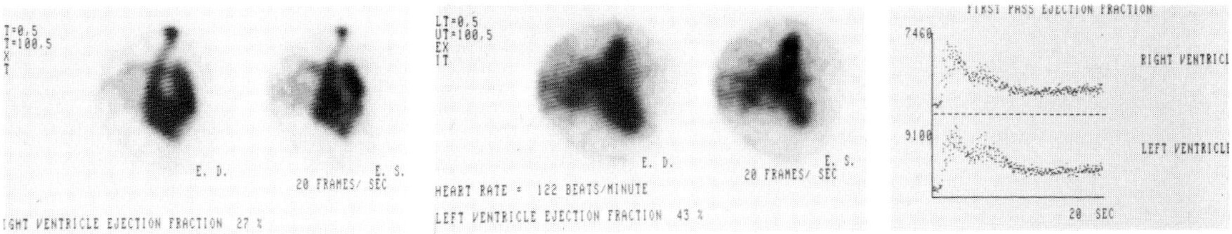

Figure 16-21. Ventricular ejection fractions from Tc-99m first-pass radionuclide angiography. This study was obtained on a 20-year-old patient with cystic fibrosis. *Left:* Right ventricular end-diastole and end-systole. The right ventricular ejection fraction is 27%. *Center:* Left ventricular end-diastole and end-systole. The left ventricular ejection fraction is 43%. *Right:* Corresponding right and left time-activity curves of right and left ventricles.

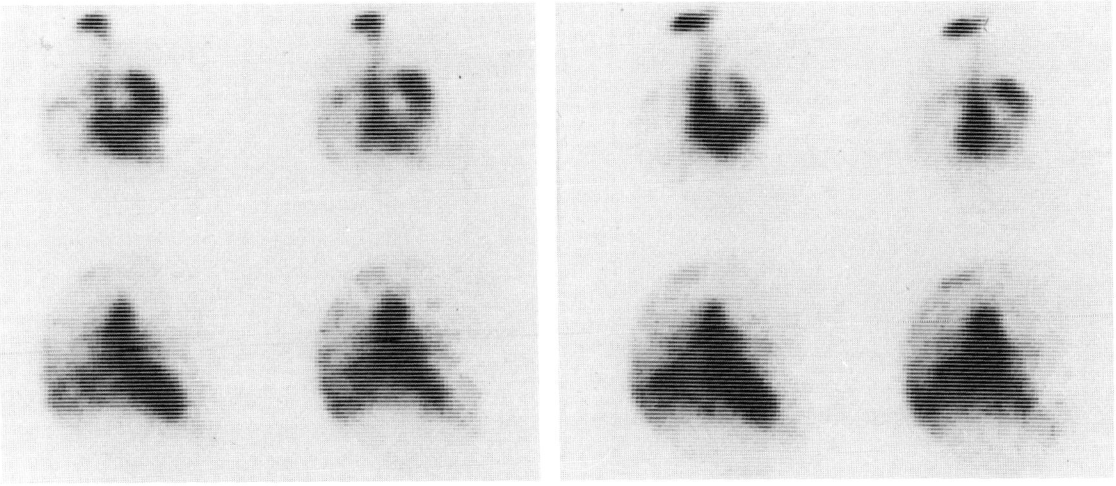

Figure 16-22. Right and left ventricular ejection fractions in a 22-year-old patient with cystic fibrosis. Tc-99m first-pass angiogram. *Left:* Study at rest with right end-diastole and right end-systole represented *above* and the corresponding left ventricular phases *below*. *Right:* Study performed with the patient breathing a rich oxygen mixture. The right ventricular ejection fraction went from 42% to 48% and the left ventricular ejection fraction from 42% to 56%.

Table 16-2. Right and Left Ventricular Ejection Fractions in Children

Age (years)	Patients	RVEF	Patients	LVEF
< 1	5	0.54 ± 0.09	5	0.68 ± 0.13
1–5	12	0.53 ± 0.07	11	0.62 ± 0.09
6–10	16	0.52 ± 0.05	15	0.69 ± 0.08
11–15	19	0.54 ± 0.03	18	0.65 ± 0.09
16–20	22	0.53 ± 0.06	23	0.70 ± 0.08
Totals/Means	74	0.53 ± 0.06	72	0.68 ± 0.09

RVEF, Right ventricular ejection fraction; LVEF, left ventricular ejection fraction

Data from Hurwitz RA et al. Am Heart J, 1983.

Forward Stroke Volume

The forward stroke volume (FSV) is calculated by dividing the cardiac output (CO) by the heart rate.

$$FSV = \frac{CO}{\text{Heart rate}}$$

End-Diastolic Volume of Left Ventricle

The end-diastolic volume of the left ventricle ($EDVLV$) is calculated by dividing the forward stroke volume (FSV) by the left ventricular ejection fraction ($LVEF$).

$$EDVLV = \frac{FSV}{LVEF}$$

This calculation assumes that there is no shunting or regurgitation.

End-Diastolic Volume of Right Heart

The end-diastolic volume of the right heart ($EDVRH$) is equal to the cardiac output (CO) times the mean transit time of the right heart ($MTTRH$.)

$$EDVRH = CO \times MTTRH$$

The mean transit time of the right heart ($MTTRH$) is:

$$MTTRH = \frac{\int_0^\infty tc(t)\, dt}{\int_0^\infty c(t)\, dt}$$

in which $c(t)$ is the right ventricular time-activity curve extrapolated to the baseline.

Pulmonary Blood Volume

Pulmonary blood volume (PBV) is equal to the mean pulmonary transit time ($MPTT$) times the cardiac output (CO).

$$PBV = MPTT \times CO$$

The $MPTT$ is calculated as the mean transit time between the right heart and left atrium.[33,58]

Evaluation of Premature and Newborn Infants

The most important applications of radionuclide angiography in this age group are the differentiation of cardiac from pulmonary causes of cyanosis and the measurement of left-to-right shunting.

In infants with pulmonary disorders, the radionuclide angiogram is usally normal. In patients with increased pulmonary vascular resistance, however, the angiogram may reveal right-to-left shunting through a patent foramen ovale, a patent ductus arteriosus, or both.

The coexistence of prematurity, respiratory distress syndrome, and congestive heart failure due to patent ductus arteriosus is a frequent and complex problem in neonatal care units. Despite intensive research in the pharmacologic, diagnostic, surgical, and epidemiologic aspects of respiratory and ductal physiology, there are still high morbidity and high mortality rates associated with that triad of disorders. The diagnosis of patent ductus arteriosus may be made with reasonable certainty by clinical, radiologic, or echocardiographic examination.

Premature infants with respiratory distress syndrome and congestive heart failure due to patent ductus arteriosus are treated medically or surgically, based on the clinical judgment, experience, and philosophy of the neonatologist and cardiologist. There are no definitive criteria for surgical ligation of the ductus arteriosus. Cardiac catheterization, which until recently was the only method available for measurement of shunt flow, is usually avoided because of the risk to the infant. Radionuclide angiography in this clinical setting provides an objective estimate of the pulmonary-to-systemic flow ratio ($Q_p:Q_s$). This has become possible with the use of small, gamma scintillation camera-computer systems that can be transported to neonatal care units and used to evaluate the patient at the bedside. Even patients on ventilatory assistance and those with severe pulmonary disease can be studied in this way.

We have studied several premature infants with respiratory distress syndrome and patent ductus arteriosus. In this population, radionuclide angiography has been helpful in demonstrating and quantitating left-to-right shunting, deciding when to operate, and assessing spontaneous closure of the ductus arteriosus. In a very small number of these patients who had undergone surgical ligation of a patent ductus arteriosus, postoperative radionuclide angiography estimated a $Q_p:Q_s$ of 1.4–1.5. A likely explanation for this finding is that the left atrial enlargement in patients with a large patent ductus arteriosus may have resulted in a stretched foramen ovale and left-to-right shunting at the atrial level. Other explanations include the existence of intracardiac malformations (ventricular septal defect or atrial septal defect). Rarely, postoperative detection of a large residual left-to-right shunt through the ductus arteriosus is due to surgical failure such as accidental ligation of the main left pulmonary artery.[127]

Quantitation of left-to-right shunting in children with patent ductus arteriosus may provide the information required to establish definite criteria for medical treatment or surgical ligation of the ductus. Indomethacin appears to induce closure of patent ductus arteriosus in some infants. Radionuclide angiography can be used to document decreasing shunt flow, complete closure, or the presence of additional defects such as a patent foramen ovale. Sometimes closure of patent ductus arteriosus by indomethacin is not complete. In other instances reduction of left-to-right shunting is transient and shunt flow subsequently increases (Fig. 16-23).

In children with a patent ductus arteriosus, it is possible to observe evidence of greater shunt recirculation in the left lung as compared with the right (Fig. 16-24). Due to cardiomegaly, however, it is often not possible to draw a ROI over the left lung. The net left-to-right shunt in patent ductus arteriosus is the average value of the $Q_p:Q_s$ of both lungs. Another angiographic characteristic of patent ductus arteriosus is the relatively clear definition of the left side of the heart in spite of left-to-right shunting (Fig. 16-25).

In 15 premature infants with patent ductus arteriosus, we evaluated left-to-right shunting by simultaneous echocardiography and radionuclide angiography.[123] The echocardiographic results were expressed as ratios between the left atrial dimension and the aortic dimension (LA/Ao) Radionuclide angiography provided pulmonary-to-systemic flow ratios ($Q_p:Q_s$) directly. Most of these patients were studied in the neonatal care unit. In general, there was good agreement with these two modalities, but there were some significant discrepancies. In three patients (two of them postoperative patients with large ducts), echocardiography suggested small left-to-right shunts while the radionuclide study demonstrated a shunt ratio of 1.8 in one patient and ratios > 3 in the two postoperative patients. In another patient, echocardiography suggested a large left-to-right shunt, but the radionuclide angiogram revealed a left-to-right shunt with a pulmonary-to-systemic flow ratio of only 1.5. This patient did well without surgery. Radionuclide angiographic estimation of left-to-right shunting is more reliable than echocardiography. Therefore, newborns with left-to-right shunts of questionable magnitude should be studied by radionuclide angiography.[123]

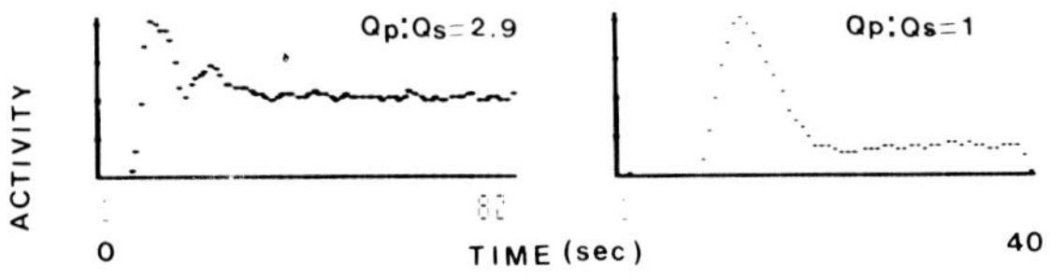

Figure 16-23. Patent ductus arteriosus treated with indomethacin. An initial radionuclide angiogram *(left)* in a premature infant with a patent ductus arteriosus reveals a $Q_p:Q_s$ of 2.9. Twenty-four hours after treatment with indomethacin *(right)*, there is no evidence of left-to-right shunting. One day later, however, a left-to-right shunt was present again.

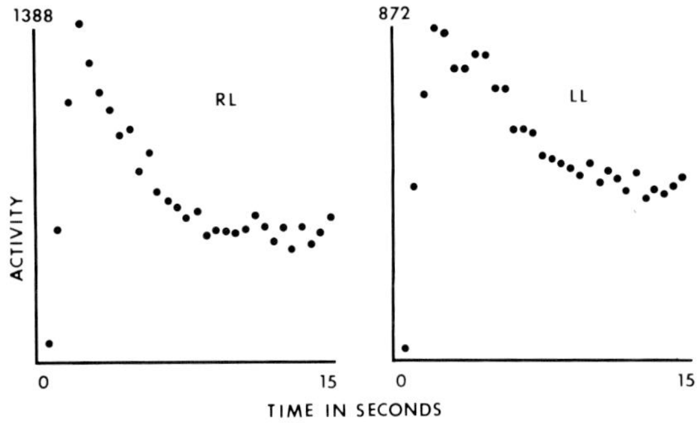

Figure 16-24. Patent ductus arteriosus. Pulmonary time-activity curves from a 2-month-old boy. There is a greater amount of shunt recirculation in the left lung (LL) as compared with the right lung (RL).

In another study, we used Ir-191m angiography in 34 premature and newborn infants. Nine of these patients had simultaneous measurement of pulmonary-to-systemic flow ratios by oxymetry during cardiac catheterization. We found a correlation coefficient of 0.90 with these two methods.[128]

The degree of pulmonary vascular resistance has an important effect on the appearance of radionuclide angiograms and on the amount of left-to-right

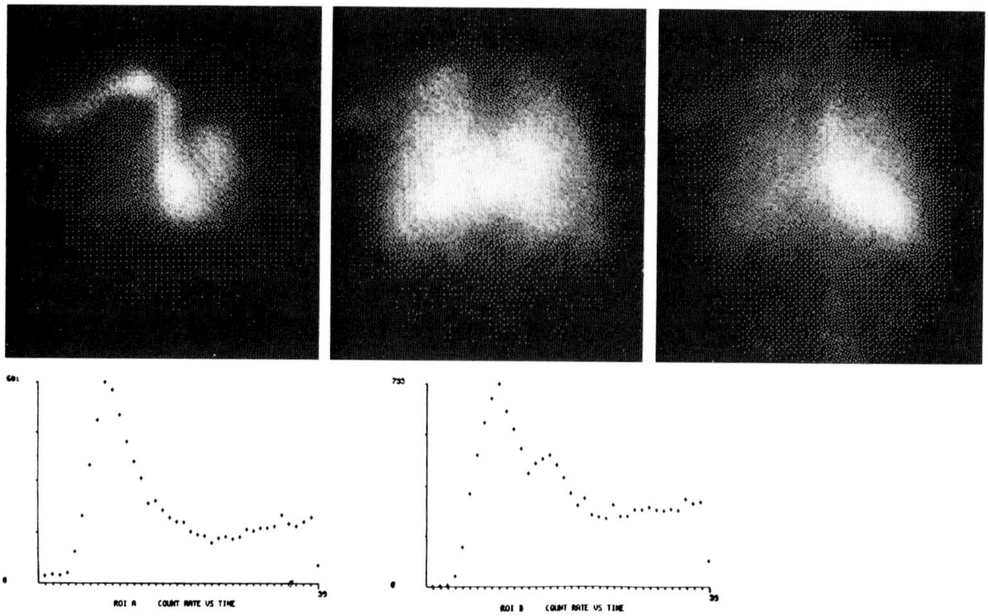

Figure 16-25. Patent ductus arteriosus. Selected frames of a radionuclide angiogram reveal clear visualization of the left side of the heart. There is a definite difference in the time-activity curves of the right and left lungs. The estimated Q_p:Q_s from the left lung curve is significantly greater than that estimated from the right lung curve.

shunting. During the first days of life, pulmonary resistance is high and the net amount of left-to-right shunting through a ventricular septal defect may be low or imperceptible on the radionuclide angiogram. Later, when the pulmonary vascular resistance decreases, the left-to-right shunting increases and the defect can be appreciated on the radionuclide study (Fig. 16-26).

Even in the presence of improving surgical techniques, repair of a ventricular septal defect in infants is not without risk. McNicholas et al.[83] found a 17% operative mortality in the repair of 24 patients with isolated ventricular septal defect in infancy. In that circumstance, if a patient is not in intractable heart failure, it would seem prudent to postpone surgical intervention beyond infancy if the clinician can be assured that obstructive pulmonary vascular disease is not developing.

In newborn infants with cyanosis due to cardiac disease (for example, transposition of the great arteries or a large right-to-left shunt with severe pulmonary stenosis), radionuclide angiocardiography will demonstrate early appearance of the radionuclide in the aorta at the same time or before it appears in the lungs (Fig. 16-27). Precise anatomic diagnoses of these complex congenital abnormalities require catheterization and angiography.

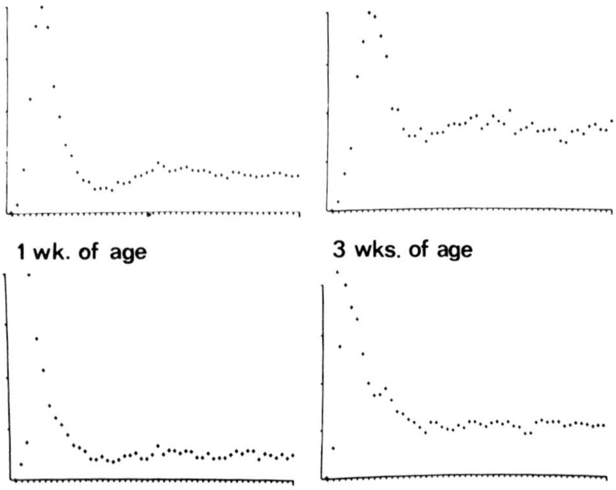

Figure 16-26. Ventricular septal defect. Pulmonary time-activity curve obtained from a radionuclide angiogram on a 1-week-old boy with a murmur *(top left)*. There is no evidence of left-to-right shunting. Another study obtained when the patient was 3 weeks of age reveals evidence of left-to-right shunting *(top right)*. A time-activity curve over the right atrium does not show evidence of shunting at that level *(bottom left)*. The right ventricular curve shows evidence of premature recirculation due to a ventricular septal defect *(bottom right)*.

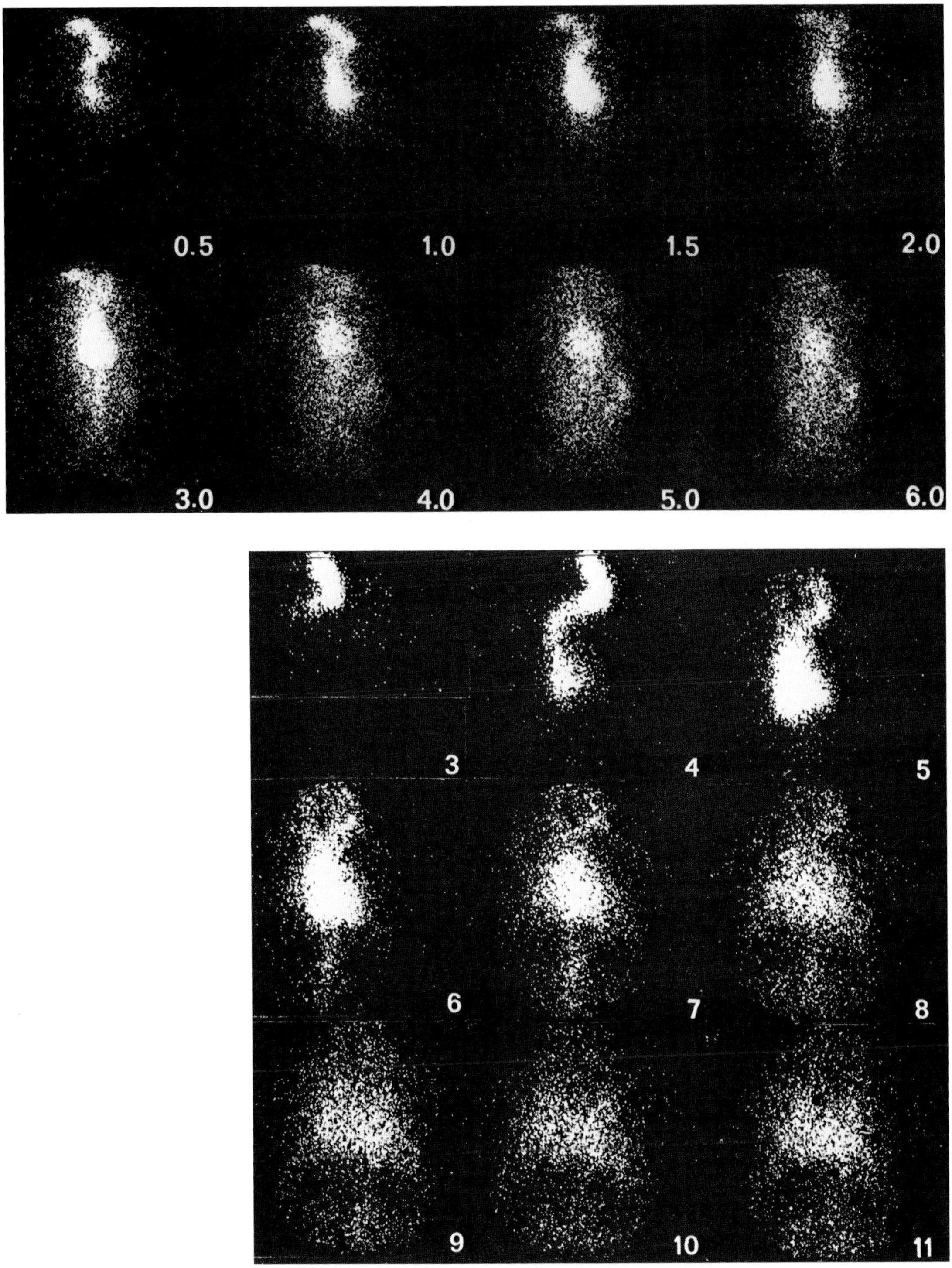

Figure 16-27. Transposition of the great arteries. *top:* Four-day-old boy. The Tc-99m radionuclide angiogram shows early appearance of the tracer in the aorta (2.0–3.0 sec) and no evidence of much pulmonary activity. This appearance suggests very poor mixing of blood within the heart. *Bottom:* Seven-day-old boy. This radionuclide angiogram was obtained after balloon atrial septostomy. Here also there is early appearance of the tracer in the aorta (5.0–6.0 sec) but there is more pulmonary activity, suggestive of a degree of intracardiac mixing.

Atrial Septal Defect and Pulmonic Stenosis

In some instances, the origin of a cardiac murmur may be difficult to determine clinically. A systolic ejection murmur with wide splitting of the second heart sound may be encountered in both pulmonic stenosis and atrial septal defect. In addition, in both instances there may be enlargement of the pulmonary artery segment on the chest radiograph and signs of right ventricular overload on the electrocardiogram. At this point, radionuclide angiography can be helpful because it can firmly establish the diagnosis and cardiac catheterization may be obviated. A decision for surgical closure can be made then or the patient may be either followed clinically (if the shunt is small) or discharged with the diagnosis of mild pulmonic stenosis if there is no shunting (Fig. 16-6). We have documented in a small number of patients natural closure of atrial septal defects diagnosed previously by cardiac catheterization.

Although it is well recognized that echocardiographic abnormalities are found in most patients with atrial septal defect (Figs. 16-8 and 16-9), the hemodynamic significance of these defects can be difficult to quantitate.[10,133] The utility of radionuclide angiocardiography in assessing the magnitude of left-to-right shunting has been evaluated in 27 patients with suspected secundum atrial septal defects (ASD) by comparing the radionuclide findings with shunt size determined at cardiac catheterization and during surgical closure.[53] These authors demonstrated close correlation (r = 0.90) between $Q_p:Q_s$ estimates by radionuclide angiography and cardiac catheterization in the 27 patients. Direct surgical appraisal revealed a "moderate-large" defect in all 22 patients with $Q_p:Q_s$ estimated by radionuclide angiography as > 1.5.

In our own study conducted during 1979–1980, radionuclide assessment of 74 patients suspected of having atrial septal defect had the following clinical impact: cancellation of surgery in three, cancellation of cardiac catheterization in one, surgery scheduled or performed (without catheterization) in 12, and discharge from further cardiac care (exclusion of atrial septal defects) in 13 patients.[54]

Ventricular Septal Defect

In ventricular septal defect, the character of the murmur, the electrocardiogram, and the chest radiograph may permit approximation of the size of the shunt. Radionuclide angiography provides precise estimation of the shunt flow and can contribute significantly to clinical management of patients. In left-to-right shunting through a small ventricular septal defect but without increase of pulmonary arterial pressure, radionuclide angiography can document decreasing shunt flow and complete closure. In patients with large ventricular or atrial septal defects, preoperative cardiac catheterization is necessary to diagnose the location and number of defects and to assess pulmonary arterial pressures.

Pulmonary Vascular Hypertension with Shunts

Certain children with a large, relatively unrestrictive ventricular or atrial septal defect and pulmonary hypertension develop with time a fixed elevation of pulmonary vascular resistance with severe structural changes in the peripheral pulmonary arteries.[27,48,49,56,107] When such changes have occurred, the patient's heart defect should no longer be corrected by surgery. With the availability of surgical repair in infancy, development of fixed pulmonary hypertension may be avoided.[21,83,105,108]

In patients with a high pulmonary vascular resistance and a reactive pulmonary vascular bed, the pulmonary resistance will drop when the patient breathes 100% oxygen. This in turn will cause the left-to-right shunt to increase. The assumption is made that these patients do not have severe structural changes in their pulmonary arteries and therefore are candidates for surgical correction of their defect.

Fujii et al.[34] in our laboratory used radionuclide angiography to assess pulmonary vascular reactivity in eight patients (nine studies) with a large intracardiac defect and pulmonary hypertension. Radionuclide angiocardiograms were performed first with the patient breathing room air and then after 10 min of breathing a mixture containing 90% or more of oxygen (Fig. 16-28). The pulmonary-to-systemic flow ratios obtained by radionuclide angiography were compared with those calculated with the Fick principle during cardiac catheterization. There was a good correlation with these two methods both in studies conducted on room air (r = 0.88) and in those obtained with oxygen (r = 94). All six studies in five patients with a reactive pulmonary vasculature (judged by a pulmonary vascular resistance at cardiac catheterization of less than 6 units/m^2 with oxygen or after tolazoline) had a radionuclide pulmonary-to-systemic flow ratio of 3.0 or greater with oxygen. The three

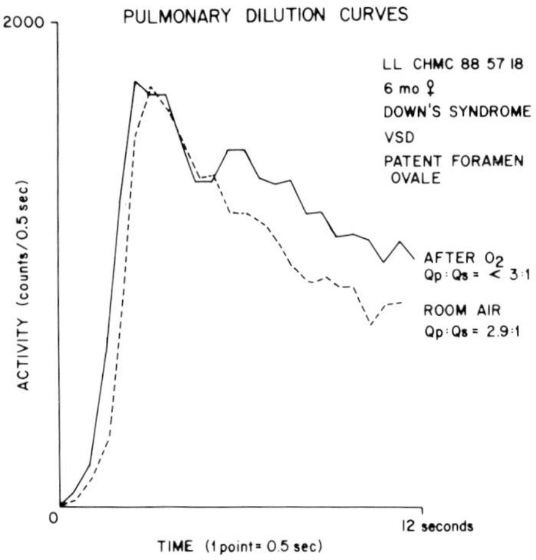

Figure 16-28. Effect of rebreathing a mixture rich in oxygen on the magnitude of left-to-right shunting. The dotted pulmonary curve was obtained with the patient breathing room air. The $Q_p{:}Q_s$ was 2.0. After breathing oxygen the secondary peak due to the left-to-right shunt has a higher amplitude reflecting an increase in shunt flow. The $Q_p{:}Q_s$ was >3.0.

patients with a nonreactive pulmonary vasculature had a radionuclide pulmonary-to-systemic flow ratio of 2.3 or less with oxygen, a value that was unchanged from the room air value. These data suggest that radionuclide angiocardiography may be a useful, relatively noninvasive method of assessing pulmonary vascular reactivity in patients with a large, relatively nonrestrictive intracardiac defect. The use of ultrashort-lived radionuclides is advantageous in this setting because multiple studies can be performed without background interference.

Increase of the pulmonary artery pressure produces an increase in the right myocardial mass and flow. This results in increased uptake of thallium-201 (Tl-201) in the right ventricle. The magnitude of this increase in the right ventricular uptake of Tl-201 seems to relate to the magnitude of pulmonary artery pressure.[25,98,100] Thus it is possible to make gross estimates of peak right ventricular pressure by observation of thallium scintigrams taken at rest.

Postoperative Assessment

After cardiovascular surgery, the appearance of new murmurs, persistent murmurs, or congestive heart failure may suggest patch detachment, surgical failure, valvular abnormalities, or residual defects. During the early postoperative period, cardiac catheterization may be too hazardous. Radionuclide angiography using mobile gamma camera computer systems can be carried out in the intensive care unit at the bedside without disruption of monitoring and other special care that these severely ill patients need. This technique can rapidly, safely, and accurately detect and quantify residual or new shunts in these instances. Immediate results are available, and reoperation can be carried out

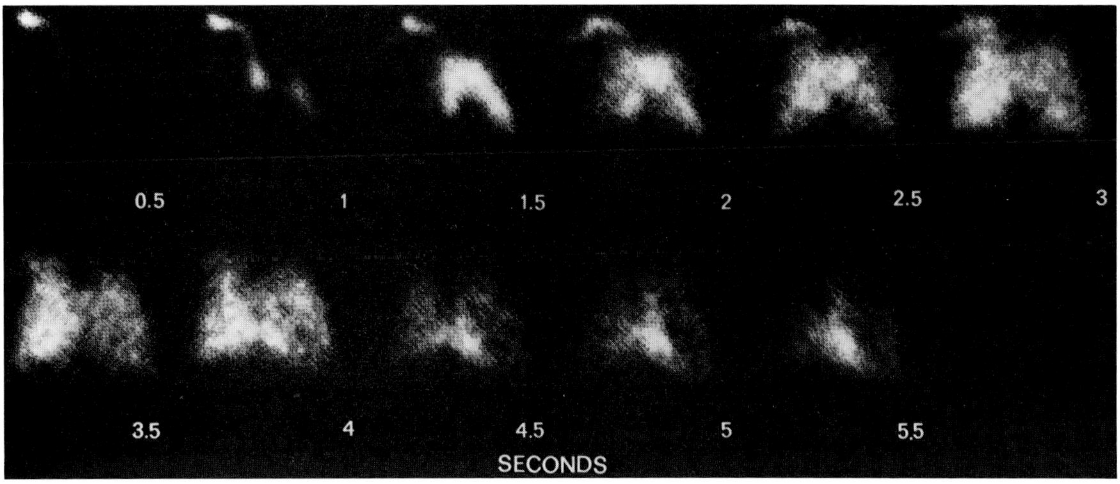

Figure 16-29. Successful Mustard operation. Anterior Tc-99m radionuclide angiogram. The tracer is shown as it circulates through the superior vena cava, the neoatrium, the left ventricle (1.0–1.5 sec), the pulmonary artery, the lungs (2.0–2.5 sec), the right side of the heart, and the aorta (4.0–5.5 sec). There is no evidence of a shunt.

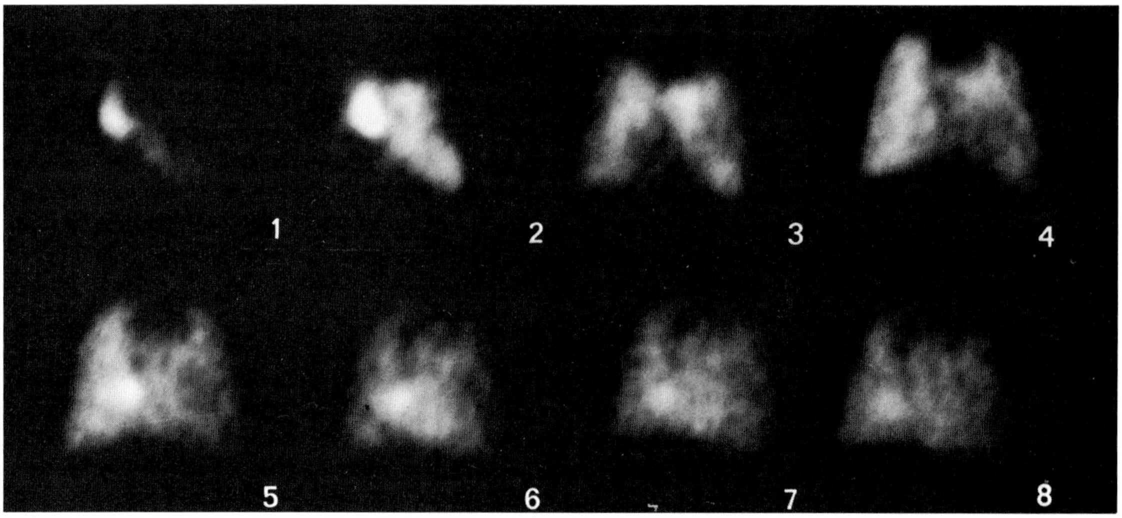

Figure 16-30. Large left-to-right shunt following a Mustard operation. The tracer is shown in the neoatrium (1 sec), left ventricle (2–3 sec), and the lungs (3–5 sec). The anatomic right side of the heart and the aorta are barely visible due to residual hemodynamic left-to-right shunting (5–8 sec).

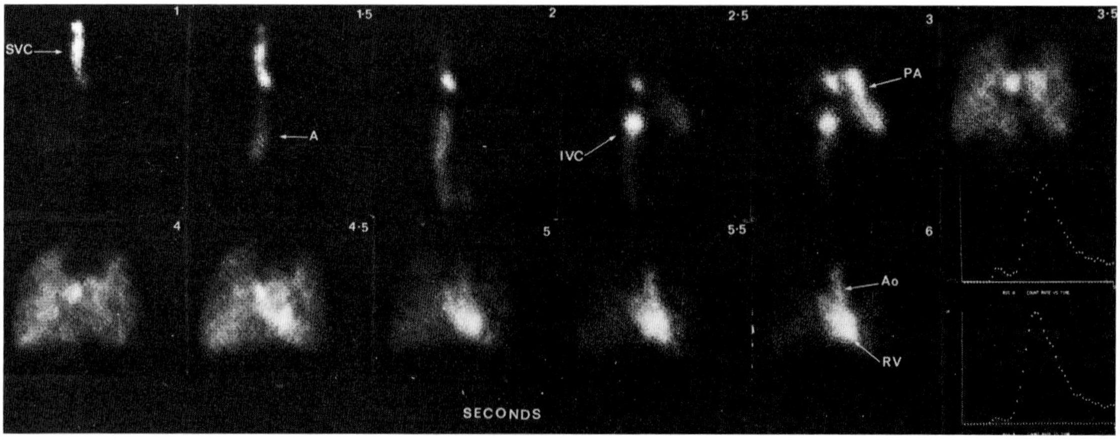

Figure 16-31. Superior vena caval obstruction after Mustard operation. The tracer appears in the superior vena cava (SVC, 1 sec), the azygos vein (A, 1.5 sec), the inferior vena cava (IVC), the neoatrium, the left ventricle, and the pulmonary artery (PA, 3 sec), then the lung, the right side of the heart, and the aorta (RV, Ao, 4.5–6 sec).

promptly if necessary and, in certain instances, without cardiac catheterization.

Similarly, during the late postoperative period, radionuclide angiography can document the success of surgery and detect complications or residual defects. For example, residual shunting or obstruction of the superior or inferior vena cava following the Mustard operation for transposition of the great arteries is detectable with this technique (Figs. 16-29–16-31). Serial evaluations will document spontaneous closure of a small residual shunt.

Hurwitz et al.[53] used first-pass radionuclide angiography to detect and quantitate residual intracardiac shunts and systemic venous obstruction after repair of transposition of the great arteries in 29 children. Information from the radionuclide angiograms was compared with data obtained during cardiac catheterization. In the group as a whole,

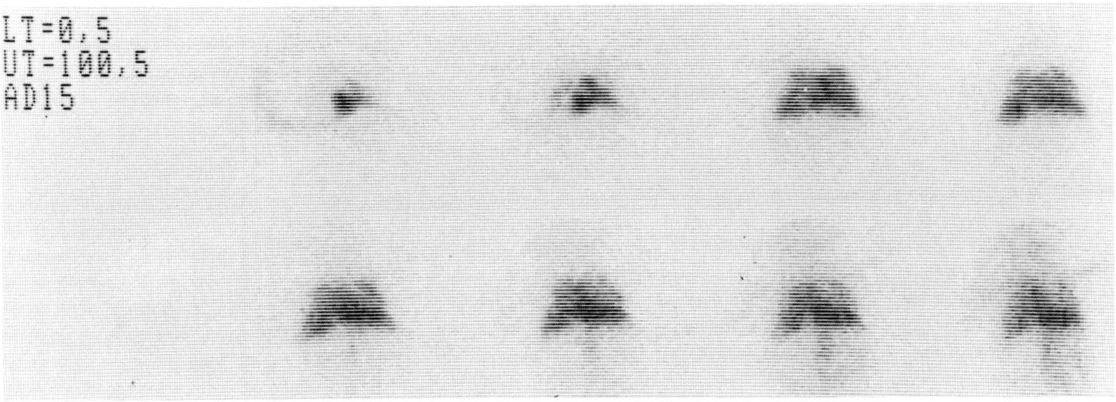

Figure 16-32. Arterial switch operation in transposition of the great arteries in a 1-month-old infant. An almost normal circulatory pattern is shown on the angiogram.

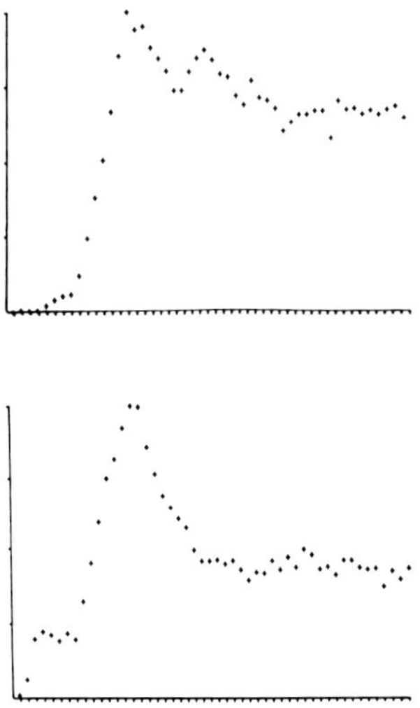

Figure 16-33. Pulmonary time-activity curves after surgical anastomosis. **A:** Right Blalock-Taussig anastomosis. Pulmonary curves reveal greater early pulmonary recirculation in the right lung, which signifies that the anastomosis is patent.

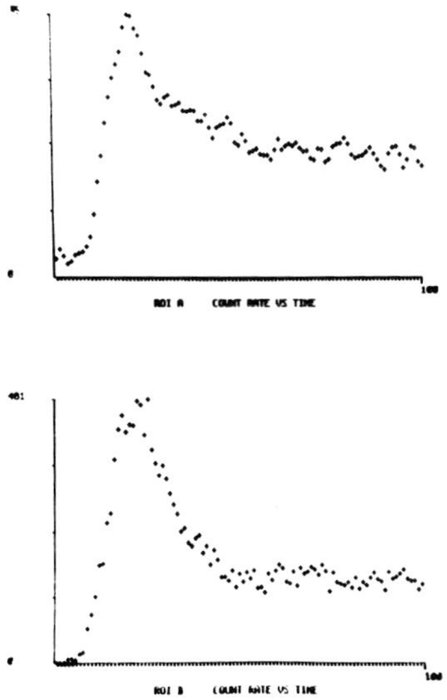

Figure 16-33. B: Patent Waterston anastomosis. There is greater early pulmonary recirculation in the right lung. (In a patent Potts anastomosis there will be greater recirculation in the left lung.)

information obtained with radionuclide angiography correlated well with cardiac catheterization data in evaluation of residual shunts and obstruction to systemic venous return.[53,79,81,86,104] Radionuclide angiography also permits assessment of circulating integrity in the switch procedure in transposition of the great arteries (Fig. 16-32).

Radionuclide angiography can be used to determine whether a palliative shunt is patent. For example, after Blalock-Taussig, Potts, and Waterston anastomoses, the pulmonary time versus activity curve of the lung on the side of the anastomosis will reveal a greater amount of early recirculation compared with the opposite lung if the shunt is patent (Fig. 16-33). After the Glenn operation, transit of radioindicator in the superior vena cava, pulmonary artery, lung, and left side of the heart is characteristic (Fig. 16-34). Peripheral vascular surgical procedures could also be evaluated with this technique.

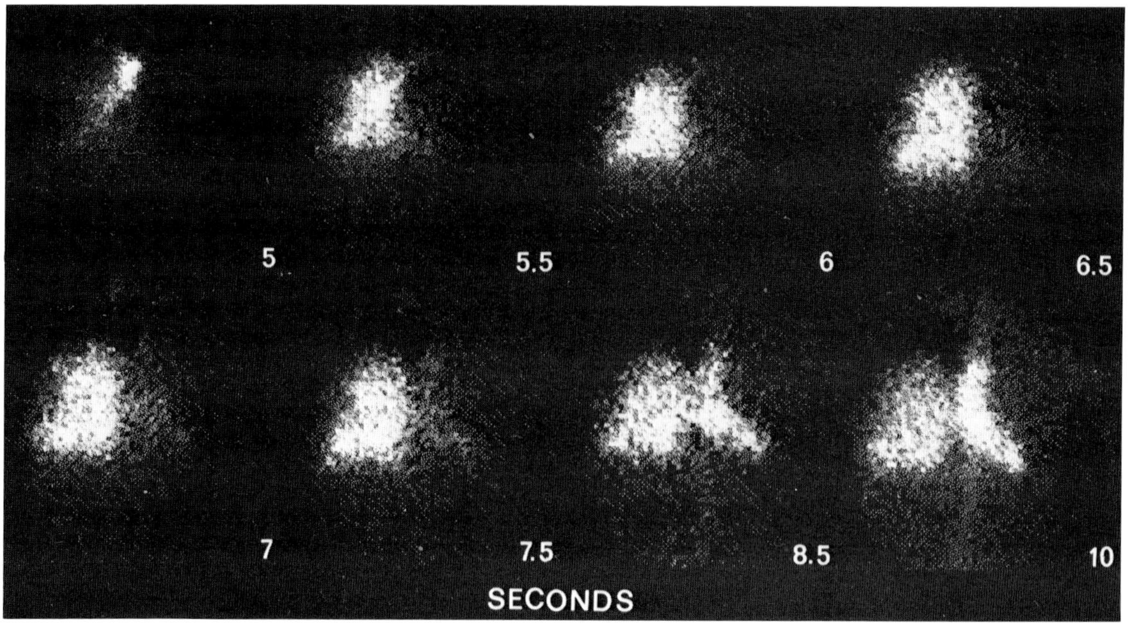

Figure 16-34. Glenn operation. Tc-99m pertechnetate first-pass radionuclide angiogram. The tracer was injected in an external jugular vein and is shown as it circulates into the superior vena cava (5 sec), right lung (5.5–7 sec), left side of the heart, and aorta (8.5–10 sec).

GATED BLOOD POOL ANGIOGRAPHY

Gated blood-pool angiography is the most frequently performed cardiovascular radionuclide study in adult patients, and results of these investigations have been very extensively published. The method has been less widely employed in children.

The gated blood-pool scan is a means of imaging the blood-pool of the heart by synchronizing the recording of scintillation data with an indicator of cardiac contraction such as the electrocardiogram, pulse wave tracing, or heart sounds[9,114] (Figs. 16-35 and 16-36). This technique permits repetitive sampling of a specific phase of the cardiac cycle from each of many cycles until an image of reasonable count density is recorded. Certain conditions must be met in order for the gated scan to be performed adequately: constant cardiac function during the study, no patient motion, minimal diaphragmatic motion, largely intravascular location of the tracer, and sufficient count density.

The gated blood pool scan permits an evaluation of both global and regional ventricular function. Generally, no patient preparation is needed for this study, but some young patients may require sedation in order to keep them still for the 20–30 min required to record.

Method

Radiopharmaceuticals

A good blood-pool label is critical for an adequate study. Tc-99m red blood cells or Tc-99m human serum albumin have been used.[43,92,114,119] Images with Tc-99m HSA usually have a lower blood pool-to-lung ratio compared with Tc-99m red cells. Both in vivo and in vitro methods have been proposed for red cell labelling, and there appears to be little clinical difference with these two methods.[46] Some workers administer a solution of stannous pyrophosphate intravenously followed in 15–30 min by a bolus of Tc-99m as sodium pertechnetate. With this technique, the Tc-99m activity appears to bind almost instantly to the globin portion of the hemoglobin, giving in most instances a high labelling efficiency.[92] In our institution we employ Tc-99m red blood cells in a dose of 300 μCi/kg with a minimum dose of 2–3 mCi. We use a modification of the Brookhaven National Laboratory kit for labelling the red cells.

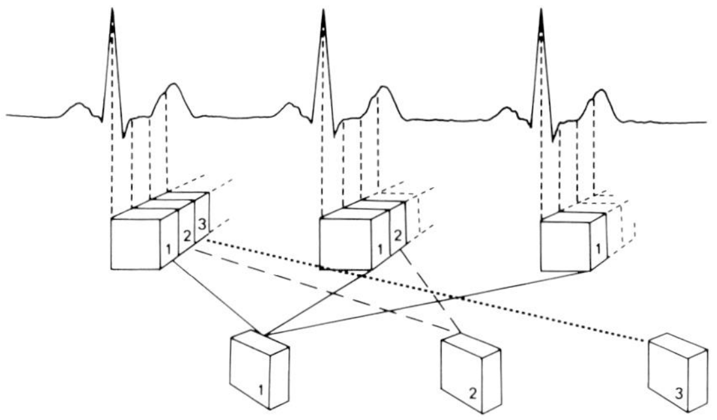

Figure 16-35. Technique for gated blood pool scintigraphy.

Instrumentation

A computerized gamma camera is necessary for performing gated blood-pool scintigraphy. A collimator frequently employed is a parallel-hole collimator because it has no significant spatial distortion with depth and thus is useful for estimating size of the cardiac chambers. A collimator with shorter holes will provide a higher count rate than one with larger holes and will allow for shorter recording times, but this is accompanied by some loss in spatial resolution. If one is interested in global cardiac function and not as much in abnormalities of regional wall motion as in most children, a high-sensitivity collimator will be adequate.

In our laboratory, we employ a parallel hole collimator with holes slanted 30°. This collimator is placed flat in contact with the patient's chest in a left anterior oblique projection with the holes pointing caudally. The degree of obliquity is dictated by the ability to clearly distinguish the interventricular septum. Even with some spatial distortion, it is possible to estimate ventricular volumes with this collimator. For gated blood-pool scans in newborns and infants, we employ a converging or pinhole collimator even though both of these cause spatial and count/depth distortion and accurate estimation of volumes may not be made.

Data Recording

At least 20 frames in each cardiac cycle are required to attain reasonable temporal resolution,[44] and usually 20–30 min are necessary to record a study.

Data recording programs usually allow an opportunity to tailor the study to each patient. One of the most common frame rates required for an adequate study is 40 msec/frame; however, this may be lengthened or shortened depending on the patient's heart rate. Some correction for arrhythmias is usually available to specify the maximum acceptable range in R-R interval. Usually, the maximum acceptable change in R-R interval is 100 msec. This arrhythmia rejection method helps to prevent distortion of data that occurs with aberrant beats.

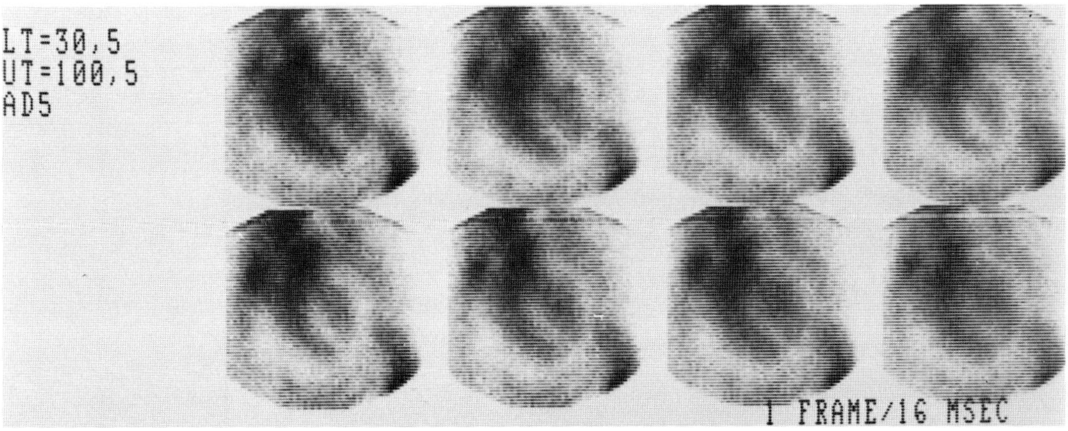

Figure 16-36. Gated blood pool scan obtained on a 15-year-old male after surgical repair of an atrial septal defect. The first frame was taken during during end-diastole; end-systole is shown on the fourth frame *(above right)*. The area surrounding the cardiac blood pool represents a large pericardial effusion. This patient's right and left global ejection fractions were depressed.

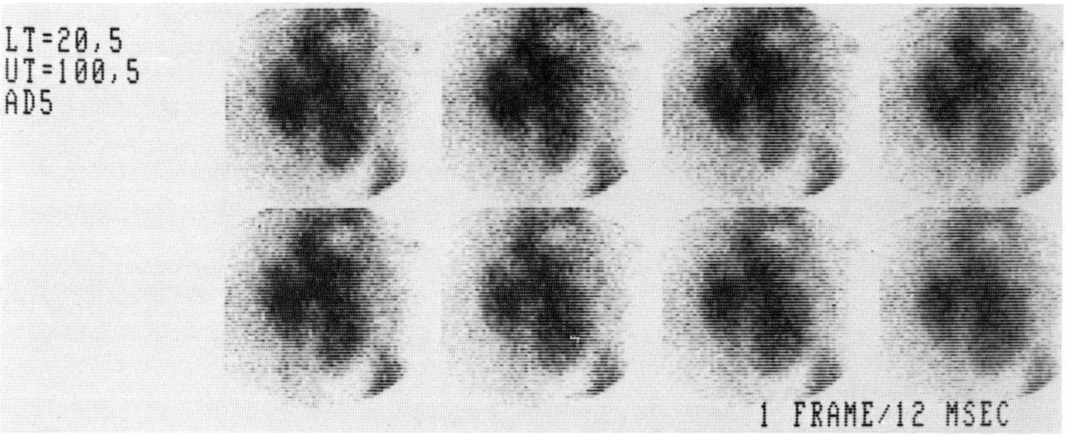

Figure 16-37. Gated blood pool study on a patient with cardiomyopathy. Both ventricles contact poorly.

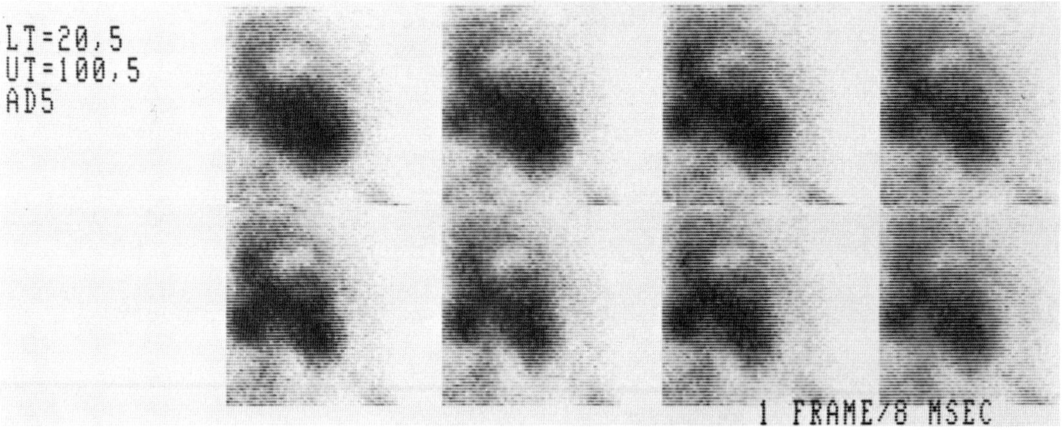

Figure 16-38. Tricuspid atresia. Three-year-old male. A poorly contracting, large left ventricle is visible.

If aberrant beats occur frequently (more than 10% of the beats) or if other arrhythmias are present (atrial fibrillation), this method of recording cannot be used. Alternatively, it is possible to record all scintigraphic events and the electrocardiogram on list mode and then evaluate various R-R intervals after the study is recorded. The end of the study can be determined by a preset number of cardiac cycles or a preset amount of time. We usually record 5–10 million counts in each study.

Quality Control

Before analyzing the gated blood-pool scan, it is important to assess the technical adequacy of the study. The following items should be evaluated: adequate tracer labelling, patient motion, positioning, sharpness of the image, and adequate gating.

Analysis

There are two parts to the analysis of gated blood-pool scans: visual evaluation of the study on a series of images (Figs. 16-37–16-39) or on cine-like display (continuous loop) of the heart cycle and measurement of function and volumes. Because the detected count rate is proportional to blood volume in the heart chambers, ventricular volume changes can be quantitated by analyzing time-activity curves from ROIs over the ventricles. The time-ac-

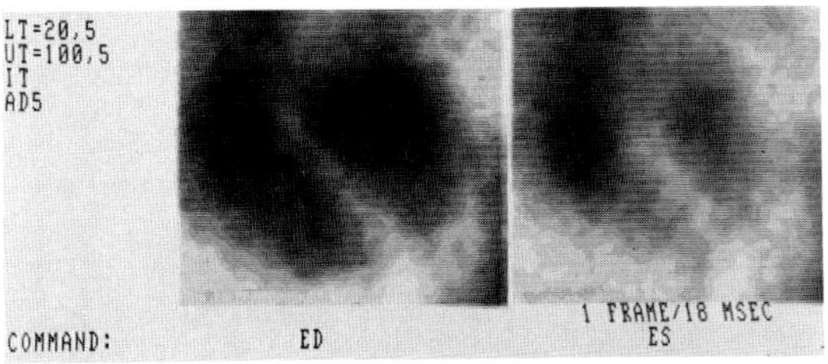

Figure 16-39. End-diastolic *(left)* and end-systolic *(right)* frames of a gated blood pool study performed after surgical repair of a tetralogy of Fallot.

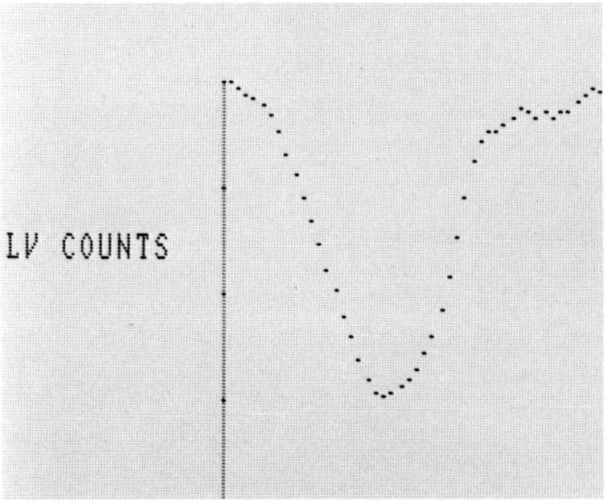

Figure 16-40. Time-activity curve of the left ventricular blood pool from a patient with normal ejection fraction. One average heart cycle is represented.

tivity curve (background corrected) of a ROI over the left ventricle is very similar to the ventricular volume curve that can be generated at angiography. From this time-activity curve, global ventricular ejection fraction, ejection rate, and filling rate can be calculated (Figs. 16-40 and 16-41). Left ventricular volume can be estimated using geometric measurements.

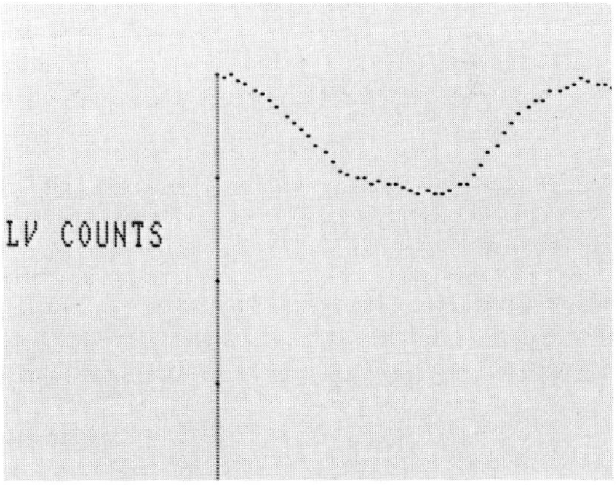

Figure 16-41. Time-activity curve of the left ventricular blood pool from a patient with tetralogy of Fallot and low ventricular function (35%).

Clinical Applications

Several potential applications of gated blood-pool scanning in children have been proposed. These include: determination of regurgitant fraction; measurement of cardiac output, left and right ventricular ejection fractions, stroke volume, and end-diastolic volume; and evaluation of ventricular wall motion. Note that several of these determinations can also be made with first-pass radionuclide angiography. Similarities and differences with these two methods are listed in Table 16-3.

Myocardial Wall Motion Abnormalities

Focal myocardial wall motion abnormalities are more unusual in children than in adults and are as readily evident on blood-pool angiograms. In anomalous left coronary artery departing from the pulmonary artery, the segment of myocardial wall involved is usually quite large, and its abnormal motion can, therefore, be detected by both the gated blood-pool scan and the first-pass radionuclide angiogram (Fig. 16-42). Focal abnormalities in wall motion in children can also be seen in myocardial involvement in the mucocutaneous lymph node syndrome, in certain patients with cardiomyopathy such as thalassemia, and in tumors of the heart.

Blood-pool angiography also may be useful for assessment of global ventricular function in patients with cystic fibrosis (Fig. 16-43), cardiomyopathy,[93] or congenital heart diseases. Liberthson et al.[73] found that in patients with an atrial septal defect, sequential gated blood-pool studies done be-

Table 16-3. Comparison of ECG-Gated Blood-Pool Scan and First-Pass Radionuclide Angiography

	Gated blood pool scan	First-pass angiogram
ECG computer interface	Yes	No
Injection technique importance	No	Yes
Counting statistics and spatial resolution	Good	Fair
Shunt quantitation	No	Yes
Temporal separation of structures	No	Yes
Background	High (60–80%)	Low ($\leq$ 20%)
Recording time	20–30 Min	$<$ 30 Sec
Multiple studies within a short time	Yes	Yes
Quantitation of valvular insufficiency	Yes	Maybe
Transit times	No	Yes

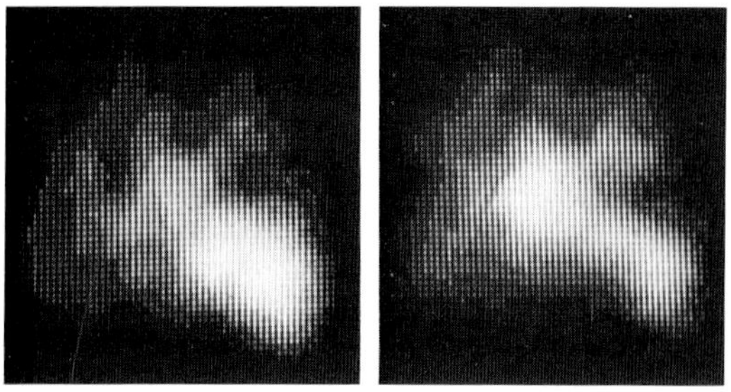

Figure 16-42. Anomalous left coronary artery in an infant. Selected left ventricular end-diastolic *(left)* and end-systolic *(right)* frames of a Tc-99m first-pass radionuclide angiogram show poor contraction of the left ventricle with bulging of the anterolateral wall at end-systole.

fore and after operation demonstrated right ventricular hypokinesis that persisted after operation.

Measurement of Valvular Regurgitation

A ratio of the change in count rates in the left ventricle between end-diastole and end-systole divided by the change in count rates in the right ventricle between end-systole and end-diastole (regurgitant volume index, stroke volume ratio) provides a unique way to quantitate valvular regurgitation.[3,14,70,102,106,129] Rigo et al.[102] developed the method based on cardiac blood-pool scanning. In the left anterior oblique projection, this study permits simultaneous assessment of the left and right ventricles. Measurement of the change in counts between end-diastole and end-systole over the right and left ventricles reflects the respective total stroke volume variations. The mean left ventricular to right ventricular stroke ratio (LV:RV) in normal patients is 1.19. In patients with aortic and/or mitral regurtitation, this ratio is elevated. These authors found good agreement between the LV:RV stroke ratio and angiographic grading of valvular regurgitation. The technique is simple and does not require elaborate data processing (Fig. 16-44).

Hurwitz et al.[54] in our laboratory evaluated the capacity of this method to quantitate aortic and/or mitral regurgitation in children and young adults at rest and during isometric exercise. There was good correlation with cineangiographic results in 47 of 48 patients. The stroke-volume ratio was used to classify severity: the group with equivocal regurgitation differed from the group with mild regurgitation ($p < 0.02$); patients with mild regurgitation differed from those with moderate regurgitation ($p < 0.001$); and those with moderate regurgitation differed from those with severe regurgitation ($p < 0.01$). The stroke volume ratio was responsive to isometric exercise, remaining constant or increasing in 16 of 18 patients. After corrective surgery the stroke volume ratio significantly decreased from preoperative measurements in all seven patients evaluated. The stroke volume in normals varied between 1.0 and 1.3.

This study suggests that a stroke volume ratio $>$ 2.0 is compatible with moderately severe regurgitation and that a ratio $>$ 3.0 indicates severe regurgitation. This technique should be useful for quantitating aortic and/or mitral regurgitation and

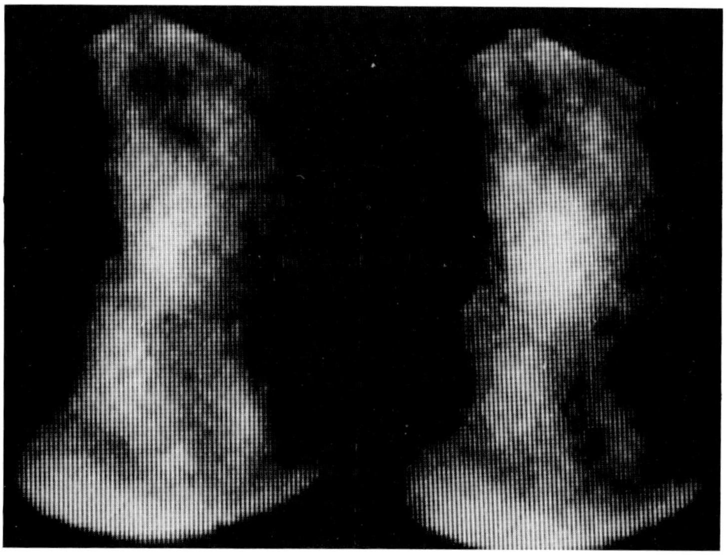

Figure 16-43. Gated blood pool scan on a 14-year-old male with cystic fibrosis. A left anterior oblique view demonstrates that the left ventricle contracts adequately while the enlarged right ventricle contracts poorly. *Left:* End diastole; *right:* end systole.

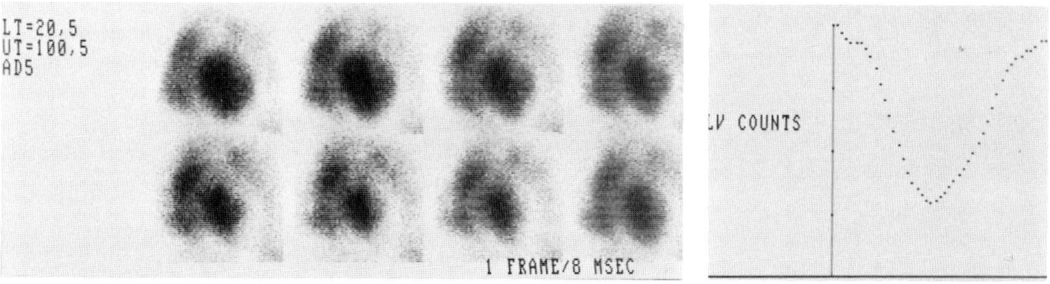

Figure 16-44. Gated blood pool study obtained on a 7-year-old male with a ventricular septal defect and aortic regurgitation. The ratio of left ventricular over right ventricular stroke volume (LV/RV stroke volume) was 5:1.

helping to follow the course of young patients with left-sided valvular regurgitation.

MYOCARDIAL PERFUSION SCINTIGRAPHY

Method

Radiopharmaceuticals

At present, myocardial scintigraphy in children is carried out using Tl-201. Thallium is produced in a cyclotron; it has a physical half-life of 73 h and decays by electron capture. In its decay, it produces mercury K x-rays of 69–83 keV (98% abundance) and gamma rays of 135 and 167 keV (10% abundance).[71] A minimum dose of 0.150 mCi and a maximum dose of 2.0 mCi are appropriate guidelines. See Table 16-4 for a more detailed dose schedule and absorbed dose estimates.

Tl-201 is considered a potassium analog, and as such it appears to be transported via the cell membrane bound as Na^+, K^+-ATPase.[60,71] Clearance of potassium from the myocardium is faster than that of thallium, however.[37,116] After intravenous injection, the blood disappearance half-time of thallium is less than 1 min. The peak myocardial uptake,

Table 16-4. Tl-201 Absorbed Dose in rads

Age (years)	Newborn	1	5	10	15	Adult
Administered dose mCi	0.15	0.300	0.600	1.0	1.6	2.0
Absorbed dose (rad)						
Heart	0.76	0.69	0.84	1.00	0.46	0.50
Liver	0.76	0.66	0.90	0.81	0.98	0.86
Kidneys	1.53	1.32	1.50	1.80	2.20	2.40
Lung	0.05	0.08	0.06	0.06	0.08	0.10
Testes	0.78	0.60	0.78	1.00	0.75	0.82
Ovaries	0.87	0.60	0.78	0.90	0.96	1.00
Whole body	0.48	0.31	0.37	0.43	0.45	0.36

about 3–4% of the injected dose, occurs at approximately 10 min. At this time, the distribution of radiothallium in the heart appears to correlate with myocardial perfusion.[116]

Imaging Technique

In some instances, such as in congestive heart failure, early imaging reveals poor myocardium/background ratio so that imaging at a later time (4–6 h) is necessary for better assessment of regional myocardial perfusion (Fig. 16-45). Early imaging is useful in detecting myocardial ischemia especially if the test is done after exercise. Viable myocardium will show uptake on later views due to redistribution of thallium. Infarcted areas, on the other hand, will retain less radiotracer than the rest of the myocardium even on late images.

A high-resolution, parallel-hole collimator designed for low energies is used on most patients, but for small children, the converging collimator is advantageous. In prematures and infants, the pinhole collimator is indispensable. Anterior, 30°, 45°, and/or 60° left anterior oblique and 45° right anterior oblique projections are obtained. Images are obtained at 150,000–500,000 counts and recorded on film and on the computer. Computer image enhancement is useful for evaluation of Tl-201 myocardial scintiscans (background subtraction, smoothing, interpolation into finer matrices, and elimination of high activity present in the liver).

In certain complex congenital heart malformations, a radionuclide angiogram and in the same projection help to indentify the structures that may not be obvious on the radiothallium image. Ultrashort-lived radionuclides such as Ir-191m serve very well for this purpose.

Clinical Applications

Anomalous Coronary Artery

Tl-201 is used to assess distribution of myocardial perfusion in patients with anomalous departure of the left coronary artery from the pulmonary artery.[31,40,99,101] In anomalous coronary artery of the infantile type, there are inadequate intercoronary anastomoses so that the patient presents early in infancy with severe congestive heart failure and electrocardiographic evidence of ischemia or infarction (Figs. 15-45 and 16-46). The timing of operative intervention in this group is a subject of controversy.[24,30,88,94] Recent reports indicate that surgery can be performed in early infancy even with evidence of infarction, but the outcome in this group is grim and the longterm prognosis unknown.[130]

In the adult type of defect, there are abundant intercoronary anastomoses so the patient is rarely symptomatic. The lesion is brought to the attention of the cardiologist usually in the patient's later childhood for evaluation of an unusual heart murmur.[85] Controversy exists also in this group as to whether it is necessary to create a two-coronary system by means of a bypass graft (Fig. 16-47).

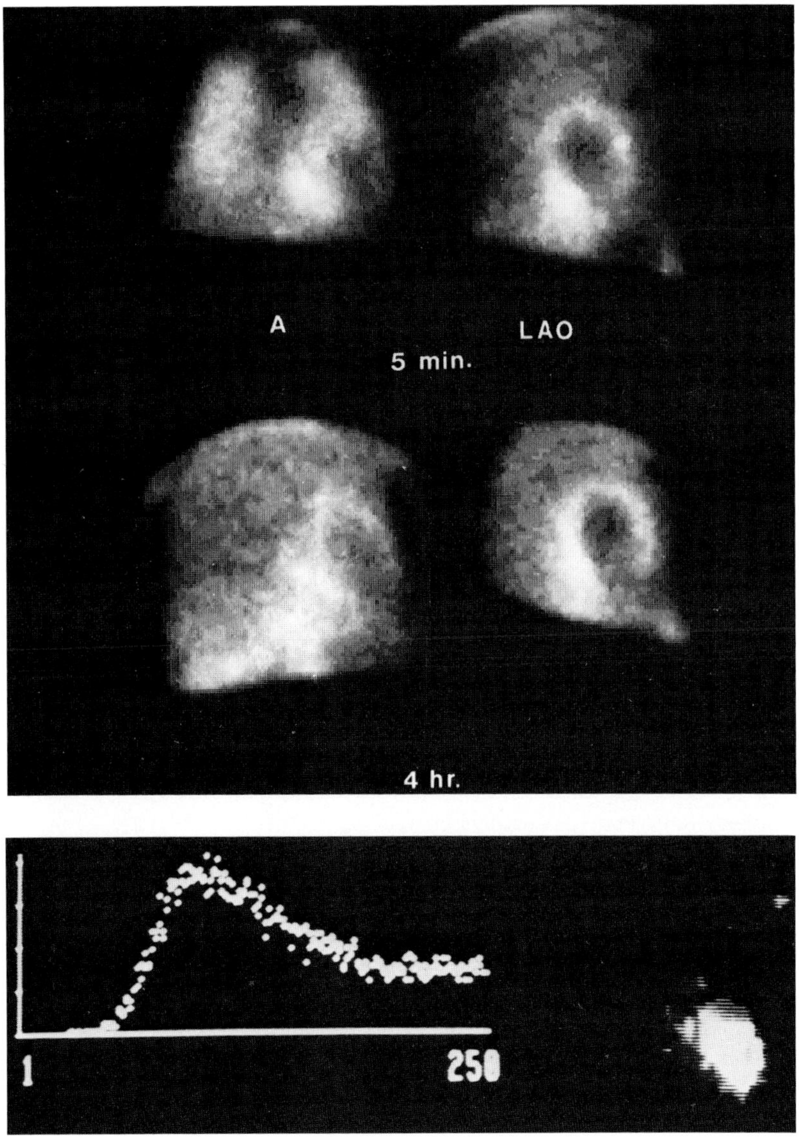

Figure 16-45. Anomalous origin of left coronary artery from pulmonary artery in a 3.5-month-old baby girl who presented with respiratory distress. She had signs of left ventricular hypertrophy and ischemic STP wave changes on the electrocardiogram. The chest radiograph revealed cardiomegaly and left lower lobe atelectasis. At cardiac catheterization an anomalous left coronary artery arising from the main pulmonary artery was found. The patient developed congestive heart failure and severe ventricular dysfunction. Tl-201 myocardial scintigrams *(left)* obtained 5 min after injection of the tracer reveal relatively high pulmonary Tl-201 activity, probably due to congestive heart failure. Repeat images obtained 4 h later reveal much lower Tl-201 activity in the lungs, permitting clearer evaluation of myocardial perfusion. The large perfusion defect in the anterolateral and inferior walls of the left ventricle represents a myocardial infarct. Note also the dilatation of the left ventricular cavity and the relatively thin myocardial wall. A Tc-99m first-pass angiogram revealed very poor contractility of the left myocardium *(right)*. At autopsy there was fibroelastosis and infarction in the same areas where the Tl-201 activity was abnormal.

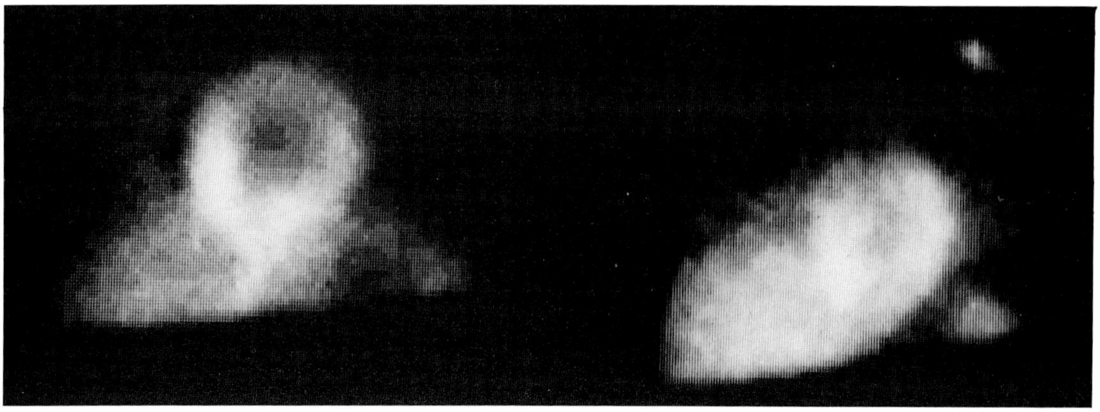

Figure 16-46. Anomalous left coronary artery in a 13-year-old boy. This patient's chest radiograph revealed cardiomegaly. The electrocardiogram suggested left ventricular and left atrial enlargement. Cardiac catheterization revealed anomalous origin of the left coronary artery from the main pulmonary artery. The left-to-right shunt had a $Q_p{:}Q_s$ of 2.0. There was a massive collateral network arising from the right coronary artery and filling the left coronary system. The preoperative Tl-201 scintigrams reveal uniform myocardial perfusion, an enlarged left ventricular chamber, and slight activity in the right ventricle on the study performed at rest *(left)*. The postoperative Tl-201 scans show again normal myocardial perfusion but the left ventricular chamber is normal in size *(right)*.

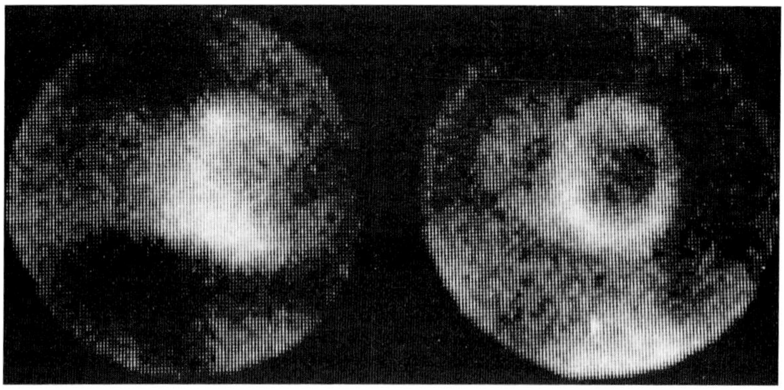

Figure 16-47. Anomalous left coronary artery in a 15-year-old male. A Tl-201 study performed after exercise reveals a large perfusion defect in the apex of the left ventricle (*left,* anterior view; *right,* left anterior oblique). The right ventricular free wall can be seen as expected on an exercise study. In addition, a first-pass radionuclide angiogram *(not shown)* revealed a left-to-right shunt caused by the anomalous coronary artery with a $Q_p{:}Q_s$ of 2.0.

Right Ventricular Hypertrophy and Hypertension

In normal individuals, the right ventricular myocardium is not visible on radiothallium scintiscans taken at rest, even with computer enhancement. The right ventricular wall can be seen in the normal individual if the injection of radiothallium is made during or just after exercise. Increased Tl-201 uptake in the right myocardium has been reported in patients with right ventricular hypertrophy.[63–65,110]

We have studied the effect of right ventricular hypertrophy on the myocardial distribution of Tl-201 in rats.[98] A small group of rats were maintained in a hypobaric chamber (air at 380 mm Hg) for 2 weeks to cause pulmonary arterial hypertension. Another group of rats maintained in room air served as controls. At the end of this period, the rats were injected with Tl-201 intravenously and sacrificed at 10 min after injection. The right ventricle was surgically separated from the intact left ventricle (including septum), weighed, and counted for activity. The hypoxic rats showed significant right ventricular hypertrophy, and the ratio between the masses of the left ventricle (LV) and right ventricle (RV) decreased from 4.2 $\pm$ 0.2 in controls to 2.4 $\pm$ 0.1 SD in hypoxic animals. The LV/RV activity ratios in both the hypoxic and control rats were almost identical to the respective mass ratios ($r = 0.97$). Radiographic and microscopic studies confirmed the changes of pulmonary arterial hypertension in the lungs of hypoxic rats. The right ventricle hypertrophied in response to this increased pressure load while the left ventricle remained the same in weight-adjusted comparisons of the two groups.[98]

In another study, Tl-201 myocardial scintigraphy was performed in patients with congenital heart defects to determine whether, by quantification of right ventricular uptake, it would be possible to assess the degree of right ventricular hypertrophy and so predict the level of right ventricular pressure.[100] Prior to injection, the syringe with the radiothallium was counted at the center of the collimator. The same was done for the syringe after the injection. Subtracting the counts after injection from the counts before injection gave an estimate of the injected counts. After the myocardial scintiscans were obtained, ROIs were outlined in the left anterior oblique projection to include the left myocardium, the right myocardium, and an area of the lung for background correction. The percentage of injected counts in the myocardium, corrected for background and normalized for pixel size, was computed. No attempt was made to correct for tissue absorption (muscle, blood, ribs). In addition the relative uptake between the right and left myocardial muscle was computed.

A total of 24 patients ranging in age from 7 months to 30 years were studied; 18 were studied before corrective surgery and 6 after operation. All but three had congenital heart defects that had resulted in pressure and/or volume overload of the right ventricle. During routine cardiac catheterization, Tl-201 was injected through the venous catheter, and myocardial images were recorded in anterior and left anterior oblique projections. These were subsequently analyzed quantitatively and qualitatively.

Insignificant right ventricular Tl-201 counts judged as being $< 1\%$ of the injected dose or $< 0.3\%$ of the left ventricular counts were present in six patients, all with a right ventricular peak systolic pressure of < 30 mm Hg. In the remaining 18 patients, there was a good correlation between the right ventricular/left ventricular peak systolic pressure ratio and the right ventricular/left ventricular Tl-201 counts ratio. All patients with right ventricular/left ventricular peak systolic pressure < 0.5 mm Hg had a ratio of right ventricular to left ventricular Tl-201 counts of < 0.4. Qualitative evaluation of right ventricular uptake proved helpful mainly in distinguishing the patients with right ventricular pressures at or above systemic levels. Figure 16-48 shows five left anterior oblique Tl-201 scintigrams obtained on patients with increasing right ventricular pressures.

Although these results are preliminary, it appears that external quantitation of Tl-201 myocardial uptake could be used as an index of right ventricular mass and its increase secondary to increased pressure in the right ventricle.[25,100,111] Such information would be useful in pulmonic stenosis, in septal defects altering the pulmonary vasculature, and in primary pulmonary disorders such as cystic fibrosis. Further, an estimate of left ventricular mass with radiothallium would be possible. Such estimates over time could be used to document an increase in left ventricular mass in patients with aortic stenosis.[7,18]

One should keep in mind, however, that these es-

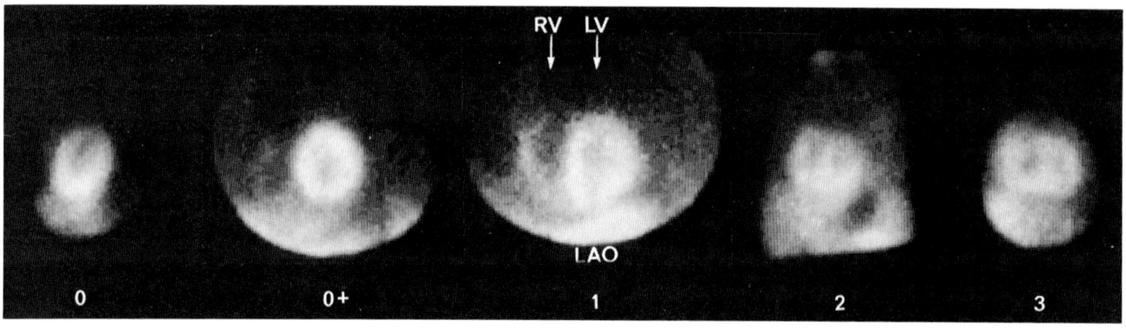

Figure 16-48. Tl-201 scintigrams on the left anterior oblique projection in patients with increasing right ventricular pressure. The tracer was injected with the patients at rest. The image on the left is from a patient with normal pulmonary pressure. The greater the pressure in the pulmonary artery, the more intense the visualization of the right ventricle. The image on the right corresponds to a 2-year-old patient with critical pulmonic stenosis and a pulmonary pressure close to the systemic pressure.

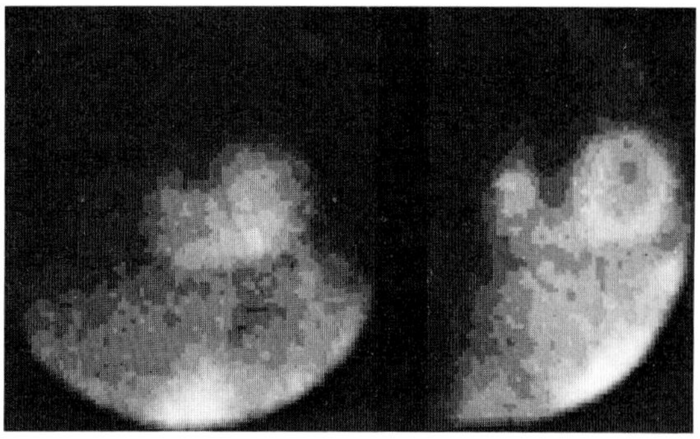

Figure 16-49. Tetralogy of Fallot. Anterior *(left)* and left anterior oblique *(right)* Tl-201 scintigram on a patient with tetralogy of Fallot. The images obtained with the patient at rest reveal concentration of the tracer in a thickened right ventricular free wall.

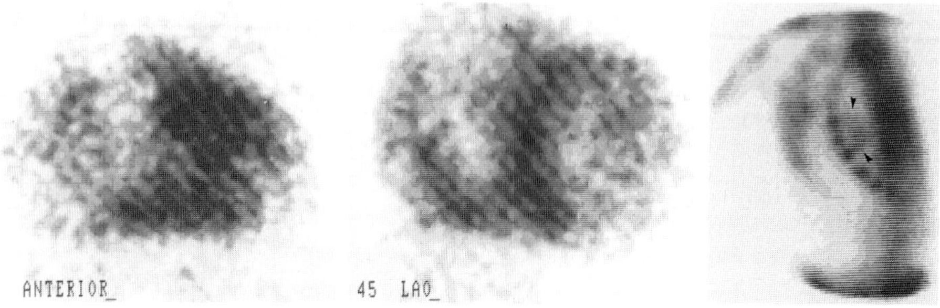

Figure 16-50. Transposition of the great vessels. *Left and center:* Anterior and left anterior oblique (LAO) projections of a Tl-201 study. This scan is from a 2-month-old infant following an arterial switch operation for transposition of the great arteries. There is significant hypoperfusion of a large portion of the left ventricle as evidenced by very low Tl-201 uptake within its wall. *Right*: A Tc-99m methylene diphosphonate image obtained on the left anterior oblique projection reveals extensive accumulation of the tracer in the left ventricle *(arrowheads)*, suggesting extensive left myocardial infarction.

timates of myocardial uptake were obtained in patients with a normal coronary circulation. Should there be an abnormal coronary circulation (i.e., anomalous coronary artery), then the distribution of Tl-201 uptake in the myocardium might be altered independently of the changes related to increased ventricular load. Visualization of the right ventricle on Tl-201 studies is also present in lesions including tetralogy of Fallot (Fig. 16-49) and transposition of the great arteries (Fig. 16-50).

Cardiomyopathies

A number of cardiomyopathies could be studied with radiothallium to determine the absolute uptake as a function of total myocardial mass or to define areas within the myocardium that become dysfunctional, are replaced by fibrosis, or may be necrotic. Glycogen storage disease, thalassemia, adriamycin therapy, and other disorders may also produce cardiomyopathy and are suitable for evaluation of regional myocardium perfusion with Tl-201. A complete discussion of cardiomyopathies has been published in an article by Hudson.[50]

An example of cardiomyopathy is the patient shown in Fig. 16-51, a 7-year-old male with thalassemia. This patient was in high-output failure, and the scintiscans reveal an area of decreased uptake of radiothallium. Pathogenesis of the heart failure and the nature of the cardiac disturbance are obscure, but the former has been attributed to extensive deposition of hemosiderin and myocardial degeneration. Occasionally there is destruction of muscle and replacement fibrosis in such patients.[118] There may also be intracellular biochemical disturbances of the myocardium caused by the hemosiderin deposits with resulting impairment in enzyme systems required for the glycolytic cycle in myocardial metabolism.[72]

Mucocutaneous Lymph Node Syndrome

Mucocutaneous lymph node syndrome (Kawasaki disease) is an acute, febrile, mucocutaneous condition accompanied by swelling of cervical lymph nodes.[61] One or two percent of the patients initially reported by Kawasaki died suddenly of cardiac failure. At autopsy, these patients had arteritis similar to infantile periarteritis nodosa accompanied by coronary thrombosis and aneurysm. About 65% of the children affected with this disease have various degrees of cardiac involvement. An excellent review of Kawasaki disease has been written by Yanagihara and Todd.[135] Tl-201 scintigraphy can aid in the diagnosis of coronary involvement in this disease (Fig. 16-52).

Kato et al.[59] found that 15% of 290 patients with mucocutaneous lymph node syndrome who underwent coronary angiography had coronary aneurysms. During followup studies up to 8 years, these authors found that in 50% of the patients no observable lesions were seen. These patients had no symptoms referred to the cardiovascular system and normal electrocardiography, exercise stress testing, and thallium scintigraphy. In 24% of these patients, the aneurysms shrank in size; in about 17% the aneurysms had disappeared but the coronary arteries were completely obstructed or markedly stenosed. In four (10%) of 42 patients irregularities of the coronary arterial wall without stenosis were seen.

Of 34 patients who underwent Tl-201 scintigraphy, all 15 with regression of the coronary aneurysms had normal findings. For six of the 19 patients with abnormal followup, coronary angiography showed perfusion defects with Tl-201. In followup angiography, all six patients had obstruction or marked stenosis of the coronary arteries. Tl-201 scintigraphy seemed as effective as electrocardiography in the detection of coronary abnormalities.[59]

Diagnosis of myocardial ischemia or infarction in some cases, however, cannot be made by planar Tl-201 imaging (Fig. 16-52). Single-photon emission tomography seems to increase the detectability of myocardial lesions in these patients.[125]

Other Disorders

Tl-201 scintigraphy could be used in children as in adults to detect myocardial ischemia and infarction. Arteriosclerotic heart disease, stress diseases, asymmetric septal hypertrophy (Fig. 16-53), and tumors of the heart (Fig. 16-54) are other disorders in which Tl-201 scintigraphy may be useful in pediatrics. Strauss et al. have demonstrated the value of Tl-201 cardiac scintigraphy for anatomic definition of certain congenital heart lesions, such as single ventricle, in children.[116]

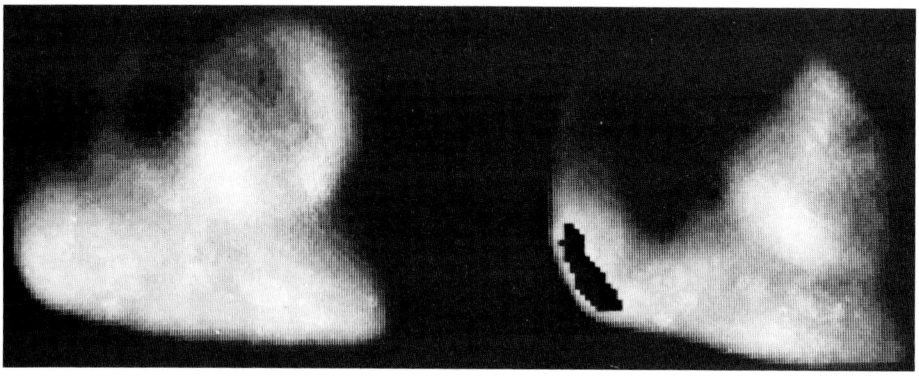

Figure 16-51. Cardiomyopathy and global cardiac failure in thalassemia. Images obtained with Tl-201 reveal focal deficits of perfusion in the left myocardium. Cardiologic assessment suggested a high-output low-resistance type of failure. The left ventricular ejection fraction estimated by first-pass radionuclide angiography was 18%. The focal decrease in radiothallium uptake is probably due to fibrosis secondary to hemosiderosis.

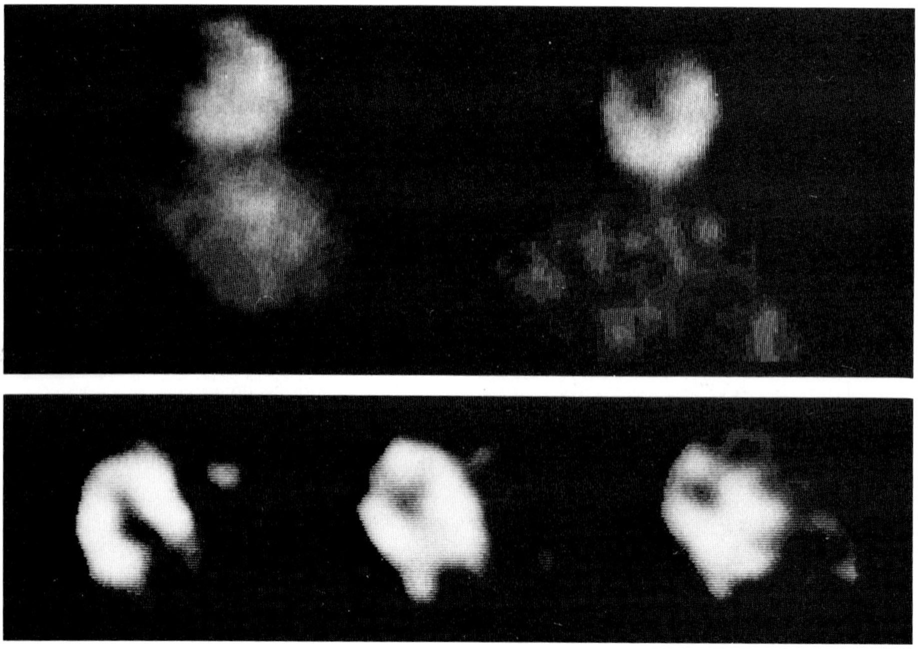

Figure 16-52. Mucocutaneous lymph node syndrome (Kawasaki disease) in a 3.5-month-old male. *Top:* Anterior *(left)* and left anterior oblique *(right)* projections of a Tl-201 study reveal essentially normal distribution of the tracer in the myocardium. *Bottom:* Single-photon emission computed tomograms in a transverse reconstruction show a perfusion deficit in the apex (L, left; A, anterior). Postmortem examination confirmed the presence of acute myocardial infarction in the apex and anterior wall corresponding to the area of decreased Tl-201 uptake.[125]

L R

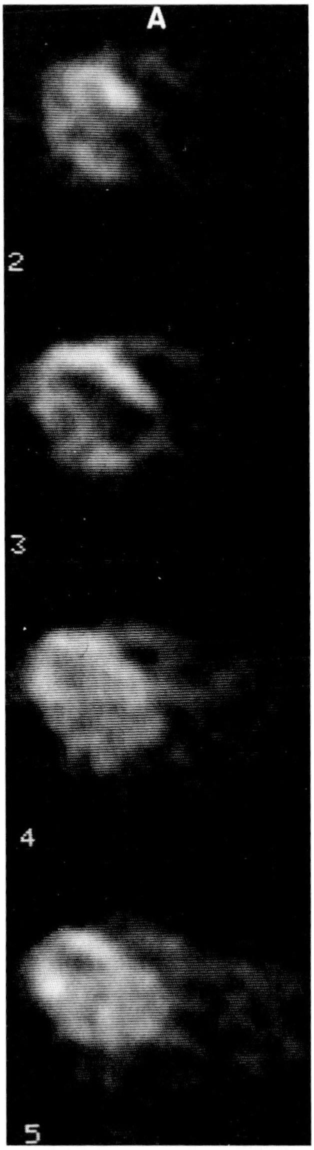

A

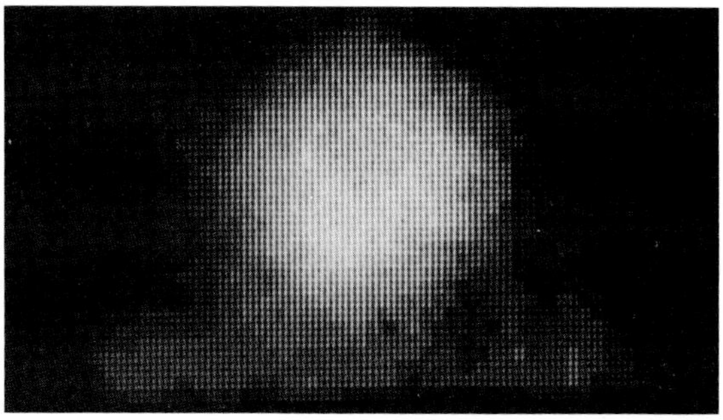

Figure 16-53. Idiopathic hypertrophic subaortic stenosis (IHSS) in a 14-month-old male. The Tl-201 scintiscan on the left anterior oblique projection shows a thickened left myocardial wall and a relatively small ventricular chamber.

Figure 16-54. Myocardial tumor. The Tl-201 images reveal a thickened myocardial wall but no perfusion abnormalities *(left)*. The single-photon emission tomogram shows a normal septum and apex. The left ventricular free wall is thickened and distribution of tracer within the tumor is irregular *(right)*. This 10-year-old male had been well until 7 years of age when he suffered three episodes of chest pain over the course of a year. At 8 years of age a systolic murmur was heard at the apex. His chest radiograph and fluoroscopy were normal. At 10 years of age an echocardiogram revealed a thick left ventricular wall, which was suspected of harboring a myocardial tumor. Angiocardiography showed marked thickening of the left myocardial free wall and the anterolateral papillary muscle. The diagnostic impression was a rhabdomyoma, a fibroma, or localized hypertrophy.[125] **A:** *Left,* anterior; *center,* left anterior oblique; *right,* left lateral; **B:** L, left; R, right; A, anterior.

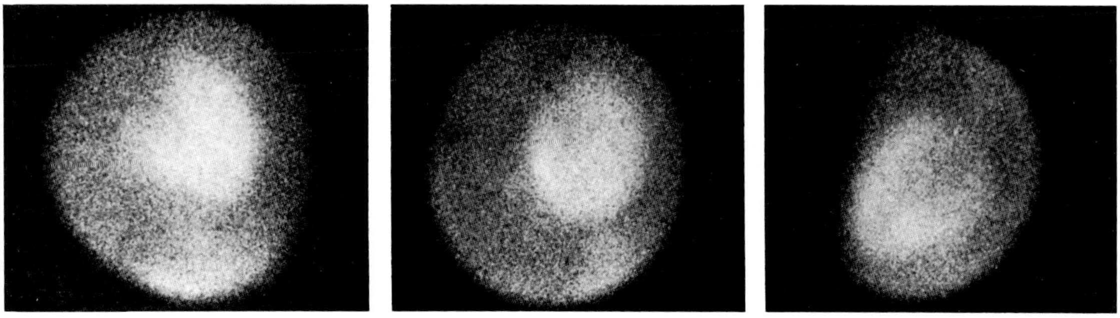

B

References

1. Alderson PO, Jost RG, Strauss AW, Boonvisut S, Markham J. Detection and quantitation of left-to-right cardiac shunts in children: a clinical comparison of count ratio and area ratio techniques (abstract). J Nucl Med 1975; 16:511.
2. Alderson PO, Gaudiani VA, Watson DC. Quantitation radionuclide angiocardiography in animals with experimental atrial septal defects. J Nucl Med 1978; 19:364–9.
3. Alderson PO, Douglass KH, Mendenhall KG, Guadiani VA, Watson DC, Links JM, Wagner HN Jr. Deconvolution analysis in radionuclide quantitation of left to right cardiac shunts. J Nucl Med 1979; 20:502–6.
4. Ashburn WL, Alazraki NP. Cardiovasular shunt quantitation. In: Handmaker H, Lowenstein JM, eds. Nuclear medicine in clinical pediatrics. New York: Society of Nuclear Medicine, 1975.
5. Ashburn W, Braunwald E. Diagnosis of congenital heart disease. In: Blahd WH, ed. Nuclear medicine, 2nd ed. New York: McGraw-Hill, 1971.
6. Askenasi J, Ahnberg DS, Korngold E, LaFarge CG, Maltz DL, Treves S. Quantitative radionuclide angiocardiograph: detection and quantitation of left-to-right shunts. Am J Cardiol 1976; 37:382–7.
7. Bailey IK, Come PC, Kelly DT, Burow RD, Griffith LSC, Strauss HW, Pitt B. Thallium-201 myocardial perfusion imaging in aortic valve stenosis. Am J Cardiol 1977; 40:889–99.
8. Bassingthwaihte JB. Circulatory transport and the convolution integral. Mayo Clin Proc 1967; 42:137–54.
9. Berman DS, Salel AF, De Nardo GL, Bogren HG, Mason DT. Clinical assessment of left ventricular regional contraction patterns and ejection fraction by high resolution gated scintigraphy. J Nucl Med 1975; 16:865–74.
10. Bierman FZ, Williams RG. Subxiphoid two-dimensional imaging of the interatrial septum in infants and neonates with congenital heart disease. Circulation 1979; 60:80–90.
11. Blumgart HL, Yens OC. Studies on the velocity of blood flow. I. The method utilized. J Clin Invest 1927; 4:1–13.
12. Blumgart HL, Weiss S. Studies on the velocity of blood flow. VII. The pulmonary circulation time in normal resting individuals. J Clin Invest 1927; 4:399–425.
13. Bosnjakovic VB, Bennet LR. Dynamic isotope studies in cardiology. AEC Symposium Series 1972; 27:562.
14. Bough EW, Gandsman EJ, North DL, Shulman RS. Gated radionuclide angiographic evaluation of valve regurgitation. Am J Cardiol 1980; 46:423–8.
15. Braunwald E, Morrow AG. Newer diagnostic technics in congenital heart disease. Adv Intern Med 1960; 10:41–80.
16. Braunwald E, Long RTL, Morrow AG. Injections of radioactive krypton (Kr^{85}) solutions in the detection of cardiac shunts. J Clin Invest 1959; 38:990.
17. Braunwald E, Morrow AG, Folse R. The use of radioisotopes in clinical studies of the central circulation. Prog Cardiovasc Dis 1962; 4:543–64.
18. Bulkley BH, Rouleau J, Strauss HW, Pitt B. Idiopathic hypertrophic subaortic stenosis: detection by thallium-201 myocardial perfusion imaging. N Engl J Med 1975; 293:1113–6.
19. Burke G, Halko A, Goldberg D. Dynamic clinical studies with radioisotopes and the scintillation camera: ^{99m}Tc-sodium pertechnetate cardiac blood-flow studies. J Nucl Med 1969; 19:270–80.
20. Case RB, Hurley HW, Keating P. Detection and measurement of circulatory shunts by use of a radioactive gas. Prog Cardiovasc Dis 1959; 2:186–95.
21. Castaneda AR, Rosenthal A. Persistent abnormalities after repair of congenital heart defects. Ventricular septal defects. Ventricular septal defect and tetralogy of Fallot. Adv Cardiol 1977; 20:110–6.
22. Castellana FS, Bassingthwaighte JB. Mathematical modeling of the central circulation. In: Pierson RN, Kriss JP, Jones RH, eds. Quantitative nuclear cardiography. New York: Wiley, 1975.
23. Cheng C, Treves S, Samuel A, Davis MA. A new osmium-191 → iridium-191m generator. J Nucl Med 1980; 21:1169–76.
24. Chiariello L, Meyer J, Reul GJ, Hallman GL, Cooley DA. Surgical treatment for anomalous origin of left coronary artery from pulmonary artery and cardiovascular surgery. Ann Thorac Surg 1975; 19:443–50.
25. Cohen HA, Baird MG, Rouleau JR, Fuhrmann CF, Bailey IK, Summer WR, Strauss HW, Pitt B. Thallium 201 myocardial imaging in patients with pulmonary hypertension. Circulation 1976; 54: 790–5.
26. Conn HL Jr. Use of indicator-dilution curves in the evaluation of acquired heart disease. Prog Cardiovas Dis 1959; 2:166–85.
27. Dammann JF, Ferencz C. The significance of the pulmonary vascular bed in congenital heart disease. III. Defects between the ventricles or great vessels in which both increased pressure and blood

flow may act upon the lungs and in which there is a common ejectile force. Am Heart J 1956; 52:210–31.
28. Donato L. Basic concepts of radiocardiography. Semin Nucl Med 1973; 3:111–30.
29. Donato L, Giuntini C, Lewis ML, Durand J, Rochester DF, Harvey RM, Cournand A. Quantitative radiocardiography. I. Theoretical considerations. Circulation 1962; 26:174–82.
30. El-Said GM, Ruzyllo W, Williams RL, Mullins CE, Hallman GL, Cooley DA, McNamara DG. Early and late results of saphenous vein graft for anomalous origin of left coronary artery from pulmonary artery. Circulation 1973; 3 (Suppl):2–6.
31. Finley JP, Howman-Giles R, Gilday DL, Olley PM, Rowe RD. Thallium-201 myocardial imaging in anomalous left coronary artery arising from the pulmonary artery. Applications before and after medical and surgical treatment. Am J Cardiol 1978; 42:675–80.
32. Freedman GS. Radionuclide angiocardiography in the adult. In: Strauss HW, Pitt B, James AE, eds. Cardiovascular nuclear medicine. St. Louis: CV Mosby, 1974.
33. Freedman GS, Dwyer A, Walberg J. Radionuclide determination of cardiac chamber flow/volume characteristics. J Nucl Med 1976; 17:84–87.
34. Fujii AM, Rabinovitch M, Keane JF, Fyler DC, Treves S. Radionuclide angiocardiographic assessment of pulmonary vascular reactivity in patients with left-to-right shunt and pulmonary hypertension. Am J Cardiol 1982; 49:356–61.
35. Gamel J, Rousseau WF, Katholi CR, Mesel E. Pitfalls in digital computation of the impulse response of vascular beds from indicator-dilution curves. Circ Res 1973; 32:516–23.
36. Gates GF, Orme HW, Dore EK. Measurement of cardiac shunting with technetium labeled albumin aggregates. J Nucl Med 1971; 12:746–9.
37. Gehring PJ, Hammond PB. The interrelationship between thallium and potassium in animals. J Pharmacol Exp Ther 1967; 155:187–201.
38. Greenfield LD, Bennett LR. Detection of intracardiac shunts with radionuclide imaging. Semin Nucl Med 1973; 3:139–52.
39. Greenfield LD, Vincent WR, Graham LS, Bennett LR. Evaluation of intracardiac shunts. CRC Crit Rev Clin Radiol Nucl Med 1975; 6:217–51.
40. Gutgessell HP, Pinsky WW, Depuey EG. Thallium-201 myocardial perfusion imaging in infants and children. Value in distinguishing anomalous left coronary artery from congestive cardiomyopathy. Circulation 1980; 61:596–9.
41. Ham HR, Dobbeleir A, Viart P, Piepz A, Lenaers A. Radionuclide quantitation of left-to-right cardiac shunts using deconvolution analysis: concise communication. J Nucl Med 1981; 22:688–92.
42. Hamilton WF. Measurement of cardiac output. In: Hamilton WF, Dow P, eds. Handbook of physiology, section 2, circulation. Washington: American Physiological Society, 1962.
43. Hamilton RG, Alderson PO. A comparative evaluation of techniques for rapid and efficient in vivo labelling of red cells with Tc-99m pertechnetate. J Nucl Med 1977; 18:1010–13.
44. Hamilton GN, Williams DL, Gould KL. Selection of appropriate frame rates for radionuclide angiography (abstract). J Nucl Med 1976; 17:556–7.
45. Hayden WG, Kriss JP. Scintiphotographic studies of acquired cardiovascular disease. Semin Nucl Med 1973; 177–90.
46. Hegge FN, Hamilton GW, Larson SM, Ritchie JL, Richards P. Cardiac chamber imaging: a comparison of red blood cells labeled with Tc-99m in vitro and in vivo. J Nucl Med 1978; 19:129–34.
47. Hnatowich DJ, Kulprathipanja S, Treves S. An improved ^{191}Os-^{191m}Ir generator for radionuclide angicardiography. Radiology 1977; 123:189–94.
48. Hoffman JIE, Rudoph AM. The natural history of ventricular septal defects in infancy. Am J Cardiol 1965; 16:634–53.
49. Hoffman JIE, Rudolph AM. Increasing pulmonary vascular resistance during infancy in association with ventricular septal defect. Pediatrics 1966; 38:220–30.
50. Hudson REB. The cardiomyopathies: order from chaos. Am J Cardiol 1970; 25:70–77.
51. Hurley PJ, Poulose KP, Wagner HN Jr. Radionuclide angiocardiography for detecting right-to-left intracardiac shunts (abstract). J Nucl Med 1969; 10:344.
52. Hurley PJ, Wesselhoeft H, James AE. Use of nuclear imaging in the evaluation of pediatric cardiac disease. Semin Nucl Med 1972; 2:353–72.
53. Hurwitz RA, Papanicolaou N, Treves S, Keane JF, Castaneda A. Radionuclide angiocardiography in evaluation of patients after surgical repair of transposition of the great arteries. Am J Cardiol 1982; 49:761–5.
54. Hurwitz RA, Treves S, Keane JF, Girod DA, Caldwell RL. Current value of radionuclide angiocardiography for shunt quantification and management in patients with secundum atrial septal defect. Am Heart J 1982; 103:421–5.
55. Hurwitz RA, Treves S, Freed M, Girod DA, Caldwell RL. Quantitation of aortic and mitral regurgitation in the pediatric population: evaluation of radionuclide angiocardiography. Am J Cardiol 1983; 51:252–5.

55a. Hurwitz RA, Treves S, Kuruc S. Right ventricular and left ventricular ejection fraction in pediatric patients with normal hearts: first pass radionuclide angiocardiography. Am Heart J 1983.
56. Iverson RE, Linde LM, Kegel S. The diagnosis of progressive pulmonary vascular disease in children with ventricular septal defects. J Pediatr 1966; 68:594–600.
57. Jones RH, Anderson PAW. Congenital heart disease: imaging and analytic methods. In: Pierson RN, Kriss JP, Jones RH, eds. Quantitative nuclear cardiography. New York: Wiley, 1975.
58. Jones RH, Sabiston DC Jr, Bates BB, Morris JJ, Anderson PAW, Goodrich JK. Quantitative radionuclide angiocardiography for determination of chamber-to-chamber cardiac transit times. Am J Cardiol 1972; 30:855–64.
59. Kato H, Ichinose E, Yoohioka F, Takechi T, Matsunaga S, Suzuki K, Rikitake N. Fate of coronary aneurysms in Kawasaki disease: serial coronary angiography and long-term follow-up study. Am J Cardiol 1982; 49:1758–66.
60. Kawana N, Krizeh H, Porter J, Lathrop KA, Charleston D, Harper PV. Use of Tl-201 as a potassium analog in scanning (abstract). J Nucl Med 1970; 11:333.
61. Kawasaki T, Kosaki F, Okawa S, Shigematsu I, Yanagawa H. A new infantile acute febrile mucocutaneous lymph node syndrome (MLNS) prevailing in Japan. Pediatrics 1974; 54:271–6.
62. Keane JF, Williams R, Treves S, Rosenthal A. Assessment of the postoperative patient by noninvasive techniques. Prog Cardiovasc Dis 1975; 18:57–74.
63. Khaja F, Alam M, Goldstein S, Anbe DT, Marks DS. Diagnostic value of visualization of the right ventricle using thallium-201 myocardial imaging. Circulation 1979; 59:182–8.
64. Kondo M. Thallium-201 myocardial imaging in patients with various heart diseases. Nippon Igaku Hoshasen Gakkai Zasshi 1979; 39:942–54.
65. Kondo M, Kubo A, Yamazaki H, Ohsuzu F, Handa S, Tsugu T, Masaki H, Kinoshita F, Hoshimoto S. Thallium-201 myocardial imaging for evaluation of right ventricular overloading. J Nucl Med 1978; 19:1197–1203.
66. Kriss JP. Cardiovascular radiosotopic angiocardiography. In: Handmaker H, Lowenstein JM, eds. Nuclear medicine in clinical pediatrics. New York: Society of Nuclear Medicine, 1975.
67. Kurtz D. Ahnberg DS, Freed M, LaFarge CG, Treves S. Quantitative radionuclide angiography: determination of left ventricular ejection fraction in children. Br Heart J 1976; 38:966–73.
68. Kuruc A, Treves S, Parker JA, Cheng C, Zimmerman RE, Sawan A. An improved deconvolution technique for radionuclide angiocardio graphic quantitation of left-to-right shunting: experimental results in dogs with and without atrial septal defects (abstract). J Nucl Med 1982; 23:69–70.
69. Kuruc A, Treves S, Parker JA. Accuracy of deconvolution algorithm assessed by simulation studies: concise communication. J Nucl Med 1983; 24:258–63.
70. Lam W, Pavel D, Byron E, Sheikh A, Best D, Rosen K. Radionuclide regurgitant index: value and limitations. Am J Cardiol 1981; 47:292–8.
71. Lebowitz E, Green MW, Fairchild R, Bradley-Moore PR, Atkins HL, Ansari AN, Richards P, Belgrave E. Thallium-201 for medical use I. J Nucl Med 1975; 16:151–5.
72. Lewis HP. Cardiac involvement in hemochromatosis. Am J Med Sci 1954; 227:544–8.
73. Liberthson RR, Pohost GM, Dinsmore RE. Atrial septal defect: pre- and postoperative evaluation by gated cardiac scanning (abstract). J Nucl Med 1979; 19:750.
74. Lin CY. Lung scan in cardiopulmonary disease. I: Tetralogy of Fallot. J Thorac Cardiovasc Surg 1971; 61:370–9.
75. Long RTL, Cornell WP. Experimental detection of left-to-right circulatory shunts with injections of krypton[85]. Proc Soc Exp Biol Med 1959; 101:836–8.
76. Long RTL, Waldhausen JA, Cornell WP, Sanders RJ. Detection of right-to-left circulatory shunts: a new method utilizing injections of krypton.[85] Proc Soc Exp Biol Med 1959; 102:456–8.
77. Long RTL, Braunwald E, Morrow AG. Intracardiac injection of radioactive krypton. Clinical applications of new methods for characterization of circulatory shunts. Circulation 1960; 21:1126–33.
78. MacIntyre WJ, Kriss JP. The normal heart. In: Pierson RN, Kriss JP, Jones RH, eds. Quantitative nuclear cardiography. New York: Wiley, 1975.
79. Mair DD, Ritter DG, Danielson GK, Wallace RB, McGoon DC. The palliative Mustard operation: rationale and results. Am J Cardiol 1976; 37:762–8.
80. Maltz DL, Treves S. Quantitative radionuclide angiocardiography: determination of Q_p:Q_s in children. Circulation 1973; 47:1049–56.
81. Marcelletti C, Mair DD, McGoon DC, Wallace RB, Danielson GK. The Rastelli operation for transposition of the great arteries: early and late results. J Thorac Cardiovasc Surg 1976; 76:427–34.

82. Marshall HW, Helmholz HF, Wood EH. Physiologic consequences of congenital heart disease. In: Hamilton WF, Dow P, eds. Handbook of physiology, section 2 circulation. Washington: American Physiological Society, 1962.
83. McNicholas KW, Bowman FO, Ellis K, Hayes C, Malm JR. Repair of ventricular septal defect in infants. NY State J Med 1977; 77:232–3.
84. Meier P, Zierler KL. On the theory of the indicator-dilution method for measurement of blood flow and volume. J Appl Physiol 1954; 6:731–44.
85. Moodie DS, Cook SA, Gill CC, Napoli CA. Thallium-201 myocardial imaging in young adults with anomalous left coronary artery arising from the pulmonary artery. J Nucl Med 1980; 21:1076–9.
86. Mustard WT, Keith JD, Trusler GA, Fowler R, Kidd L. The surgical management of transposition of the great vessles. J Thorac Cardiovasc Surg 1964; 48:953–8.
87. Nakamura M, Suzuki Y, Nagasawa T, Sugehara M, Takahashi T. Detection and quantitation of left-to-right shunts from radionuclide angiocardiography using the homomorphic deconvolution technique. IEEE Trans Biomed Eng 1982; BME-29:192–201.
88. Neches WH, Mathews RA, Park SG, Lenox CC, Zuberbuhler JR, Siewers RD, Bahnson HT. Anomalous origin of the left coronary artery from the pulmonary artery. A new method of surgical repair. Circulation 1974; 50:582–7.
89. Parker JA, Treves S. Radionuclide detection localization and quantitation of intracardiac shunts and shunts between the great arteries. Progr Cardiovasc Dis 1977; 20:121–50.
90. Parker JA, Secker-Walker R, Hill R, Siegel BA, Potchen EJ. A new technique for the calculation of left ventricular ejection fraction. J Nucl Med 1972; 13:649–51.
91. Parker H, Weber PM, Van Dyke DC, Davies H, Steele P, Sullivan R. Evaluation of central circulatory dynamics with the radionuclide angiocardiogram. In: Strauss HW, Pitt B, James AE Jr, eds. Cardiovascular nuclear medicine. St. Louis: CV Mosby, 1974.
92. Pavel DG, Zimmer AM, Patterson VN. In vivo labelling of red cells with Tc-99m: a new approach to blood pool visualization. J Nucl Med 1977; 18:305–8.
93. Pohost GM, Fallon JT, Strauss HW. Radionuclide techniques in cardiomyopathy. In: Strauss HW, Pitt B, eds. Cardiovascular nuclear medicine, 2nd ed. St. Louis: CV Mosby, 1979.
94. Primo G, Wellens F, Crickx A, Deuvaert F, Le Clerc JL. Anomalous origin of the left coronary artery from the pulmonary artery. Successful correction by direct implantation in the aorta. Acta Paediatr Belg 1981; 34:171–3.
95. Prinzmetal M, Corday E, Bergman HC, Schwartz L, Spritzler RJ. Radiocardiography: a new method for studying the blood flow through the chambers of the heart in human beings. Science 1948; 108:340–1.
96. Prinzmetal M, Corday E, Spritzler RJ, Flieg W. Radiocardiography and its clinical applications. JAMA 1949; 149:617–22.
97. Rabinovitch M, Rosenthal A, Ahnberg DS, Nadas AS, Treves S. Cardiac output determination by radionuclide angiography in patient with congenital heart disease (abstract). Am J Cardiol 1977; 39:309.
98. Rabinovitch M, Fischer KC, Gamble W, Reid L, Treves S. Thallium-201: quantitation of right ventricular hypertrophy in chronically hypoxic rats. Radiology 1979; 130:223–5.
99. Rabinovitch M, Rowland TW, Castaneda AR, Treves S. Thallium-201 scintigraphy in patients with anomalous origin of the left coronary artery from the pulmonary artery. J Pediatr 1979; 94:244–7.
100. Rabinovitch M, Fischer KC, Treves S. Quantitative thallium-201 myocardial imaging in assessment of right ventricular pressure in patients with congenital heart defects. Br Heart J 1981; 45:198–205.
101. Rajfer SI, Oetgen WS, Weeks KD Jr, Kaminski RJ, Rocchini AP. Thallium-201 scintigraphy after surgical repair of hemodynamically significant primary coronary artery anomalies. Chest 1982; 81:687–92.
102. Rigo P, Alderson PO, Robertson RM, Becker LC, Wagner HN. Measurement of aortic and mitral regurgitation by gated cardiac pool scans. Circulation 1979; 60:306–12.
103. Riihimaki E, Heiskanen A, Tahti E. Theory of quantitative determination of intracardiac shunts by external detection. Ann Clin Res 1974; 6:45–49.
104. Senning A. Surgical correction of transposition of the great vessels. Surgery 1959; 45:966–80.
105. Sigmann JM, Perry BL, Behrendt DM, Stern AM, Kirsh MM, Sloan HE. Ventricular septal defect: results after repair in infancy. Am J Cardiol 1977; 39:66–71.
106. Sorensen SG, O'Rourke RA, Chaudhuri TK. Noninvasive quantitation of valvar regurgitation by gated equilibrium radionuclide angiography. Circulation 1980; 62:1089–98.
107. Stanton RE, Fyler DC. The natural history of pulmonary hypertension in children with ventricular

septal defects assessed by serial right-heart catheterization. Pediatrics 1961; 27:621–26.
108. Stark J, Hoffman JIE. Debate on congenital heart disease. Adv Cardiol 1976; 17:51–72.
109. Starmer CF, Clark DO. Computer computation of cardiac output using the gamma function. J Appl Physiol 1970; 28:219–20.
110. Stevens RM, Baird MG, Fuhrmann CF, Rouleau J, Summer WR, Strauss HW, Pitt B. Detection of right ventricular hypertrophy by thallium 201 myocardial perfusion imaging (abstract). Circulation 1975; 51/52 (Suppl II):243.
111. Strauer BE, Burger S, Bull U. Multifactorial determination of thallium-201 uptake of the heart: an experimental study concerning the influence of ventricular mass, perfusion and oxygen consumption. Basic Res Cardiol 1978; 73:298–306.
112. Strauss HW. Detection and quantification of intracardiac shunts. In: Strauss HW, Pitt B, James AE, eds. Cardiovascular nuclear medicine. St. Louis: CV Mosby, 1974.
113. Strauss HW, Pitt B. Nuclear cardiology. In: Weissler AM, ed. Noninvasive cardiology. New York: Grune & Stratton, 1974.
114. Strauss HW, Zaret BL, Hurley PH, Natarajan TK, Pitt B. A scintiphotographic method for measuring left ventricular ejection fraction in man without cardiac catheterization. Am J Cardiol 1971; 28:575–80.
115. Strauss HW, Wagner HN Jr, Wesselhoeft H, Hurley PJ. Radionuclide angiocardiography in pediatrics. In: James AE, Wagner HN Jr, Cooke RE, eds. Pediatric nuclear medicine. Philadelphia: WB Saunders, 1974.
116. Strauss HW, Harrison K, Tanjan JK, Lebowitz E, Pitt B. Thallium-201 for myocardial imaging. Circulation 1975; 51:641–5.
117. Swan HJC. Indicator-dilution methods in the diagnosis of congenital heart disease. Prog Cardiovasc Dis 1959; 2:143–65.
118. Swan WGA, Dewar HA. The heart in haemochromatosis. Br Heart J 1952; 14:117–24.
119. Thrall JH, Freitas JE, Swanson D, Rogers WL, Clare JM, Brown ML, Pitt B. Clinical comparison of cardiac blood pool visualization with technetium-99m red blood cells labeled in vivo and with technetium-99m human serum albumin. J Nucl Med 1978; 19:796–803.
129. Treves S. Detection and quantitation of cardiovascular shunts with commonly available radionuclides. Semin Nucl Med 1980; 10:16–26.
121. Treves S, Maltz DL. Radionuclide angiocardiography. Postgrad Med 1974; 56:99–197.
122. Treves S, Maltz DL, Adelstein SJ. Intracardiac shunts. In: James AE, Wagner HN Jr, Cooke RE, eds. Pediatric nuclear medicine. Philadelphia: WB Saunders, 1974.
123. Treves S, Collins-Nakai R, Ahnberg D, Lang P. Quantitative radionuclide angiocardiography (RAC) in premature infants with patent ductus arteriosus (PDA) and respiratory distress syndrome (RDS)(abstract). J Nucl Med 1976; 17:554.
124. Treves S, Kulprathipanja S, Hnatowich DJ. Angiocardiography with iridium-191m. An ultrashort-lived radionuclide (T1/2 4.9 sec). Circulation 1976; 54:275–9.
125. Treves S, Hill TC, VanPraagh R, Homan BL. Computed tomography of the heart using thallium-201 in children. Radiology 1979; 132:707–10.
126. Treves S, Cheng C, Samuel A, Lambrecht R, Babchyck B, Zimmerman R, Norwood W. Iridium-191m angiocardiography for the detection and quantitation of left-to-right shunting. J Nucl Med 1980; 21:1151–7.
127. Treves S, Fogle R, Lang P. Radionuclide angiography in congenital heart disease. Am J Cardiol 1980; 46:1246–55.
127a. Treves S, Royal H. Babchyck B. Pediatric nuclear cardiology. In: Engle ME, ed. Pediatric cardiovascular disease. Philadelphia: FA Davis, 1980.
128. Treves S, Fyler D, Fujii A, Kuruc A. Low radiation iridium-191m radionuclide angiography: detection and quantitation of left-to-right shunts in infants. J Pediatr 1982; 101:210–5.
129. Urquhart J, Patterson RE, Pacer M, Goldsmith SJ, Horowitz SF, Litwack R, Gorlin R. Quantitation of valve regurgitation by radionuclide angiography before and after valve replacement. Am J Cardiol 1981; 47:287–91.
130. Venugopal P, Subramanian S. Anomalous origin of the left coronary artery from the pulmonary artery. Definitive surgical treatment by saphenous vein interposition in a 17 month old child. Ann Thorac Surg 1975; 19:451–6.
131. Wagner HN, Rhodes BA. Radioactive tracers in diagnosis of cardiovascular disease. Prog Cardiovasc Dis 1972; 15:1–24.
132. Weber PM, Dos Remedios LV, Jasko IA. Quantitative radioisotopic angiocardiography. J Nucl Med 1972; 13:815–22.
133. Weyman AE, Wann LS, Caldwell RL, Hurwitz RA, Dillon JC, Feigenbaum H. Negative contrast echocardiography: a new method for detecting left-to-right shunts. Circulation 1979; 59:498–505.
134. Wood EH, ed. Symposium on use of indicator-dilution technics in the study of the circulation. Circ Res 1962; 10:377–581.

135. Yanagihara R, Todd J. Acute febrile mucocutaneous lymph node syndrome. Am J Dis Child 1980; 139:603–14.
136. Yano Y. Radionuclide generators: current and future applications in nuclear medicine. In: Subramanian G, Rhodes BA, Copper JF, Sodd VJ, eds. Radiopharmaceuticals. New York: Society of Nuclear Medicine, 1975.
137. Yano Y, Anger HO. Ultrashort-lived radioisotopes for visualizing blood vessels and organs. J Nucl Med 1968; 9:1–6.
138. Zierler KL. Circulation times and theory of indicator-dilution methods for determining blood flow and volume. In: Hamilton WF, Dow P, eds. Handbook of physiology, section 2 circulation. Washington: American Physiological Society, 1962.

Chapter 17 Lung

S. T. Treves
G. B. C. Harris

Scintigraphy of the lungs is a unique method that provides quantitative regional information on pulmonary blood flow, ventilation, volume, and gas diffusion. Radiography of the chest provides anatomic information but is not as specific and quantitative for ventilation and perfusion. Pulmonary function tests are quantitative of global pulmonary function but do not give regional information.

Regional pulmonary ventilation can be assessed using either xenon-133 (Xe-133) or krypton-81m (Kr-81m). In either case, the radioactive gas is administered by inhalation while the gamma camera images the lungs. Kr-81m has a half-life of 13 sec and delivers very little radiation to the patients so that it is ideal for use in pediatrics.

Regional pulmonary perfusion is assessed by intravenous Xe-133 dissolved in saline, Kr-81m, or technetium-99m (Tc-99m) macroaggregated albumin. Xe-133 and Kr-81m can be used in all patients including those with pulmonary vascular hypertension, severe pulmonary insufficiency, and right-to-left shunting. Studies with macroaggregated albumin permit multiple projections but do not provide the information about gas exchange or washout that can be obtained with Xe-133. Combination of perfusion and ventilation evaluations with the patient in the same position are helpful in order to map the regional relationship between these two pulmonary functions. The principal use of pulmonary scintigraphy in children is for the assessment of regional lung function. Indications for pulmonary scintigraphy in children include disorders such as pulmonary artery agenesis, pulmonary emboli, pulmonary valve stenosis, pulmonary sequestration, other anomalies including those that are the result of cardiovascular surgery, pectus excavatum; bronchial disorders such as congenital lobar emphysema, acute or chronic bronchial occlusion; allergic and metabolic disorders such as cystic fibrosis, asthma (mucus, trappings, infection); infectious diseases such as pneumonia.

In all instances a recent radiograph of the chest is needed to aid in the interpretation of results.

Methods

Radiopharmaceuticals

Tc-99m MAA

After intravenous injection, particles of macroaggregated albumin (MAA) tagged with Tc-99m embolize arterioles in the lungs in a distribution proportional to regional pulmonary blood flow. Interrupted or decreased blood flow in a portion of the lung is reflected on scanning as a region of absent or reduced concentration of tracer.

The number of arterioles occluded with one typical intravenous injection of Tc-99m MAA is relatively small, and under normal conditions these small obstructions are physiologically insignificant. Most (90%) of these particles of albumin range in size from 10 to 40 μm in diameter. Approximately 280,000,000 pulmonary arterioles are small enough to trap the macroaggregates in adults, and commonly only about 200,000–500,000 particles

Table 17-1. Radiation Dose from Tc-99m MAA (rad)

Age (years)	Newborn	1	5	10	15	Adult
Body weight (Kg)	3.5	12.1	20.3	33.5	55.0	70.0
Administered dose (mCi)	0.2	0.5	1.0	1.5	2.5	3.0
Range of particles administered (x100)	10–50	50–150	200–300	200–300	200–700	200–700
Total body	0.024	0.028	0.031	0.042	0.0375	0.036
Lungs	0.740	0.550	0.580	0.765	0.7	0.6
Liver	0.054	0.055	0.062	0.1035	0.1075	0.096
Bladder wall	0.084(1)	0.125(1)	0.310(2)	0.345(2)	0.375(2)	0.36(2)
Ovaries	0.0152	0.0165	0.019	0.039	0.0375	0.03
Testes	0.0124	0.0105	0.019	0.018	0.0325	0.0192

(1) 2 hour voiding interval
(2) 4.8 hour voiding interval

Calculations by the Radiopharmaceutical Internal Dosimetry Information Center, Oak Ridge, TN.

are administered for a lung scan. Further, the vascular blockade is only temporary because MAA is degraded in the lung into smaller particles and eliminated from the pulmonary vasculature with a biologic half-time of about 6–8 h. The breakdown polypeptides are taken up by cells in the liver and subsequently eliminated by the biliary system.

The minimum toxic dose for albumin is 20 mg/kg, which exceeds the usual imaging dose of less than 10 μg of albumin by a factor of 1000.[130]

Another albumin preparation used for perfusion lung scanning is Tc-99m microspheres, which have a more uniform particle size (20–40 μm) and a longer biologic half-life than macroaggregates. Because allergic reactions have been reported with microspheres, however, we prefer to use macroaggreates.[53]

In newborns and young children whose pulmonary vasculature is immature, a small number of particles should be used. In the human infant, the number of alveoli increases rapidly during the first year of life and then more gradually, reaching adult levels at about 8 years of age.[30,131] While the precise age at which alveolar multiplication ceases is not known with certainty, one study shows a rapid increase from about one-tenth to one-third of adult values during the first year of life and to one-half the adult number by 3 years of age.[38]

Heyman suggests that if 500,000 particles are regarded as safe in the adult, their number should not exceed 50,000 in the newborn or 165,000 at 1 year of age.[65] We suggest that a small number of MAA particles (< 10,000) be used in neonates or patients with severe pulmonary disease. For quantitation of right-to-left shunting a small number of particles is also sufficient because one is not interested in evaluating regional pulmonary flow in detail. In order to attain images with apparent uniform distribution of activity in the lungs, at least 60,000 particles should be injected if the lungs are mature. Table 17-1 lists suggested number of injected particles for patients at various ages, usual administered activity, and absorbed radiation dose.

Tc-99m MAA is usually injected with the patient in the supine position. If possible, the patient should be instructed to take a few deep breaths while the radiotracer is injected slowly (5–10 sec). In the supine position, the distribution of MAA reflects the ventral-to-dorsal gradient of perfusion so that relatively more particles are concentrated in the dependent portions of the lung. The vertical gradient (apex to base) of perfusion in the lung is not as prominent on scans obtained after injection of MAA in the supine as it is in the upright position.

Commercial kits for the preparation of Tc-99m MAA contain macroaggregated albumin with stannous chloride that require only adding an appropriate amount of Tc-99m as sodium pertechnetate followed by brief agitation of the vial. It is extremely important never to allow blood to mix with the MAA in the syringe because clotting of this blood may be accelerated. Injection of any clotted blood must be avoided. We prefer to enter a vein using a butterfly type needle set that has been previously filled with normal saline. A few milliliters of saline are injected to ensure good venous access; the MAA are then injected and the tubing is flushed with saline. A similar technique is used when injecting Tc-99m MAA through any other intravenous tubing. Imaging can begin immediately after injection.

Xe-133

Xe-133 is the most widely used radioactive gas for evaluation of regional lung function.[83] Xenon is an inert gas with low solubility in the body fluids. The solubility of Xe-133 in fat is considerably higher than in blood. The partition coefficients are 8 for fat/blood, about 1 for brain/blood, and lower for other tissues. Xe-133 has a physical half-life of 5.2 days, and its principal photon energy is 80 keV (37% abundance) and decays to stable cesium. A 346-keV beta emission accompanies radioactive decay of this tracer and is responsible for a substantial proportion of the radiation exposure to patients. These beta particles are absorbed by < 1 mm of tissue. The nucleus formed by beta decay reaches the stable state by either emitting gamma rays of 80 keV or by the process of internal conversion, which is accompanied by emission of 30-keV x-rays.

Using the suggested administered doses, for a 1-year-old patient, the estimated radiation absorbed dose to the lungs is 600–800 mrad and the gonadal dose is 5–15 mrad. For a 15-year-old patient, the estimated radiation absorbed dose is 100–300 mrad to the lungs and 4–8 mrad to the gonads.[84] Higher radiation exposure will occur in patients with delayed washout due to airway obstruction or in patients with right-to-left shunting.

Xe-133 can be administered either by inhalation or by intravenous injection. When Xe-133 gas is mixed with air or with an air-oxygen mixture and inhaled in a single breath, its distribution within the lungs reflects regional ventilation. When a patient without airway obstruction breathes an oxygen-air Xe-133 mixture from a closed system over several respiratory cycles (and the volume of the reservoir is maintained at a constant level by absorption of carbon dioxide and replenishment of oxygen), concentration of Xe-133 in the lungs comes to equilibrium with that in the reservoir. Xe-133 distribution in the lungs after rebreathing is more uniform than distribution after a single inhalation of the tracer. This uniform concentration allows calculation of the distribution of aerated lung volume (expressed as volume or equilibrium).

If the patient then breathes room air, the concentration of Xe-133 within the lungs normally will decrease rapidly with a half-time of 5–30 sec, depending on the age of the patient. The younger the patient is, the shorter the washout time will be. The rate of removal of Xe-133 from the lungs depends primarily on alveolar ventilation. Estimates of regional ventilation obtained in this manner permit assessment of aerated lung only.

Xe-133 is poorly soluble, but under appropriate partial pressure, it will diffuse in various fluids including saline. When Xe-133 in saline is exposed to room air, the tracer comes out of solution very rapidly. If a small (0.5–1.5 ml) bolus of Xe-133 in saline is rapidly given intravenously, arrival of the tracer in capillaries of the lungs (peak activity) is directly proportional to regional pulmonary blood flow. As Xe-133 in blood reaches the alveolar-capillary membrane, it comes off solution instantaneously and enters the alveolar air. Removal of Xe-133 from the lungs is then dependent on alveolar ventilation. Therefore, following an intravenous injection of Xe-133 in saline, it is possible to assess regional pulmonary perfusion and ventilation. Estimates of regional ventilation obtained in this way reflect primarily ventilation of perfused lung tissue.

When assessing the distribution of pulmonary perfusion with Xe-133, the effect of intrapulmonary diffusion and rebreathing of this gas within the lung must be kept in mind. Because passage of intravenously injected Xe-133 into the alveolar air is instantaneous, delivery of a small, compact, single bolus of Xe-133 is essential in order to obtain a faithful assessment of regional pulmonary blood flow. If the injection of Xe-133 is prolonged or the volume of solution injected is large, poor temporal resolution will prevent separation of perfusion from ventilation on the resulting images.

Miorner estimated regional lung perfusion with intravenous Xe-133 in saline in humans during breathholding and during normal breathing. The random error was slightly greater when estimating perfusion during normal breathing as compared with breathholding, but the differences were small. Therefore, estimates of regional lung perfusion using Xe-133 in saline during normal breathing are judged acceptable for routine clinical work.[100]

Kr-81m

Kr-81m has a physical half-life of 13 sec and emits a 190-keV gamma ray during decay. This radiotracer is obtained from a rubidium-81 → Kr-81m radionuclide generator. The parent radionuclide, Rb-81, has a 4.7-h half-life and is produced in a cyclotron.[8,42–44,58,120,151]

Advantages of Kr-81m over Xe-133 in the evaluation of regional lung function in children include: favorable physical characteristics for imaging, improved spatial resolution, and the ease in obtaining multiple views, which permit better detection and localization of abnormalities. In addition, studies with Kr-81m result in a lower radiation absorbed dose to the patient. Also sequential studies to evaluate the effect of exercise and/or pharmacologic interventions are conveniently obtainable with Kr-81m. Disadvantages of Kr-81m are that it is not conveniently available on a regular basis and that it may not be as effective as Xe-133 in the assessment of air trapping.

Kr-81m gas is eluted through the generator with humidified O_2 at a rate of about 1 liter/min. Absorbed radiation doses from Kr-81 are lower than those from Xe-133. For a 1-year-old, the estimated radiation absorbed dose to the lungs is about 75 mrad for each Kr-81m view and the gonadal dose is about 4 mrad. For a 15-year-old, the estimated radiation dose to the lungs is 15 mrad and the gonadal dose about 0.78 mrad. The estimated whole-body doses are 0.96 mrad and 0.91 mrad for a 1- and 15-year-old, respectively, for each Kr-81m view.[90]

Examination Technique

Tc-99m MAA Perfusion Studies

After intravenous administration of Tc-99m MAA, anterior, posterior, anterior and posterior obliques, and lateral views are obtained. Delineation of the posterior and lateral basal segments of the lower lobes is achieved best on the oblique projections.[22,140] A gamma camera with a large field-of-view and a high-resolution collimator should be used. Each view is recorded for 300,000–500,000 counts.

Xe-133 Ventilation-Perfusion Studies

Two methods of Xe-133 ventilation-perfusion assessment have been used in children. The one that requires patient cooperation is Xe-133 camera radiospirometry. This method cannot be used in young patients who are unable to hold their breath or to perform the various respiratory maneuvers necessary in the study.[81] The other method, although less rigorous from the pulmonary physiology standpoint, can be used to evaluate ventilation and perfusion in children of all ages including premature infants. Either procedure requires adequate facilities for safe handling and disposal of Xe-133.

Xe-133 Examination of Small Children and Uncooperative Patients

A method for assessing regional lung function in infants and children of all ages was developed in our laboratory[133] (Figs. 17-1 and 17-2). The procedure is explained to the parents and when possi-

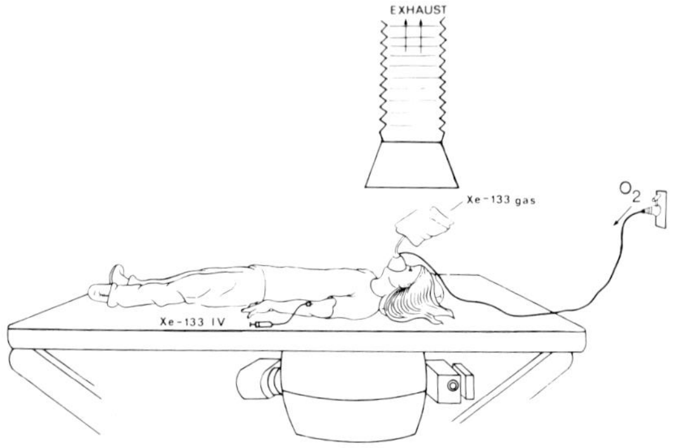

Figure 17-1. Method for examination of ventilation and perfusion in children and uncooperative patients using xenon-133. The patient is supine and the gamma camera is underneath the examining table to view the posterior aspect of the chest. Xe-133 is introduced into a plastic bag (shielding not shown) connected to a pediatric anesthesia mask. External oxygen is added into the mask if needed. The mask is withdrawn and xenon is allowed to wash out of the lungs into the exhaust system. Next, a rapid intravenous bolus of Xe-133 in saline is given to assess regional perfusion and washout. During the time of examination the patient breathes normally.

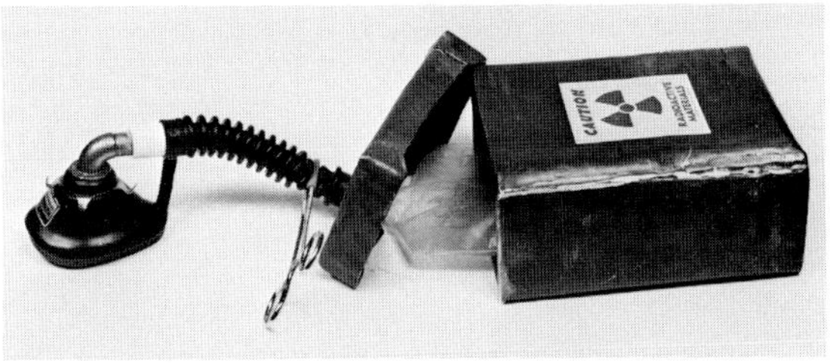

Figure 17-2. Detail of the arrangement for the ventilation part of the Xe-133 study. A pediatric anesthesia mask is connected to a plastic bag of about 800 ml capacity filled with Xe-133 and oxygen. The bag is shielded within a lead box and is closed by means of a clamp. The clamp is released just as the patient begins to breathe from the mask.

ble to the patient. The patient is taken into the examining room and is shown the equipment and the mask. Placement of the mask alone on the patient's face is practiced. A pediatric scalp vein set inserted in a superficial vein is connected to a disposable injector with a one-way valve, which facilitates delivery of a small volume of xenon in saline (Paramedical Instruments Inc., Waltham, MA). The patient is examined in the supine or sitting position. Some children need restraining during the study. Sedation is not used. The study consists of a ventilation phase and a perfusion phase.

Xe-133 as gas or in saline is injected into aplastic bag of about 800 ml capacity. This bag has been previously filled with oxygen almost to capacity, closed with a surgical clamp, and placed in a lead box. When Xe-133 in saline is injected into the bag, the gas diffuses out of solution and a gauze (which was previously inserted in the bag) absorbs the saline, preventing its accidental swallowing. The final concentration of xenon gas in the bag is about 20 μCi/ml.

For the ventilation study, the xenon bag is attached to a pediatric anesthesia mask. The face mask is placed gently but firmly over the nose and mouth of the patient. The clamp closing the bag is released immediately and the patient is allowed to breathe gas from the bag (washin) until similar concentrations of activity are achieved throughout the lungs (equilibrium, volume). The mask is then withdrawn, and the patient breathes room air. Xenon washes out of the patient's lungs into the room air (washout).

For the perfusion phase of the study, Xe-133 in saline is rapidly injected intravenously as a bolus. A usual dose is 300 μCi/kg of body weight (minimum dose, 2 mCi). Specific activity of the solution should be 10–40 mCi/ml. The bolus must be delivered within $<$ 3 sec in order to permit accurate assessment of perfusion. The study is recorded in a computer at one frame/sec. In children, the entire study usually takes 2.0–3.0 min. In patients with obstructive airway disease, xenon in the lungs never reaches equilibrium because its distribution is governed by various and irregular regional air flow rates.

A series of 5-sec images are obtained over the entire study, and these are evaluated visually for distribution of ventilation and perfusion and washout. In most routine clinical settings, this visual assessment provides sufficient information (Fig. 17-3).

The study can also be analyzed quantitatively. For quantitative analysis, an image of lung activity during the equilibrium phase is displayed on the monitor of the computer. A region of interest (ROI) is marked over the lung away from the superior vena cava and the heart in order to calculate a reference time-activity curve. By means of an interactive computer program, various points on the time reference curve are selected by the operator, including equilibrium, start of washout after equilibrium, background activity prior to perfusion, perfusion peak, and perfusion washout. Identical points in time are automatically marked by the computer on time-activity curves corresponding to other lung regions. These curves are then analyzed to determine regional distribution of activity representing ventilation, perfusion, and volume.

Regional distribution of equilibrium and perfusion are calculated with this formula:

$$D_i \text{ (percent)} = \frac{A_i \times 100}{\sum_{i-1}^{N} A_i}$$

in which D_i is the regional distribution expressed as a percentage of total equilibrium and perfusion, A_i is the regional activity measured at peak perfusion, and N is the number of regions (exclusive of the region of reference).

Regional distribution of ventilation is calculated from washout of equilibrated Xe-133 in lung and washout of perfused lung according to an extension of the mean clearance rate formula.[139]

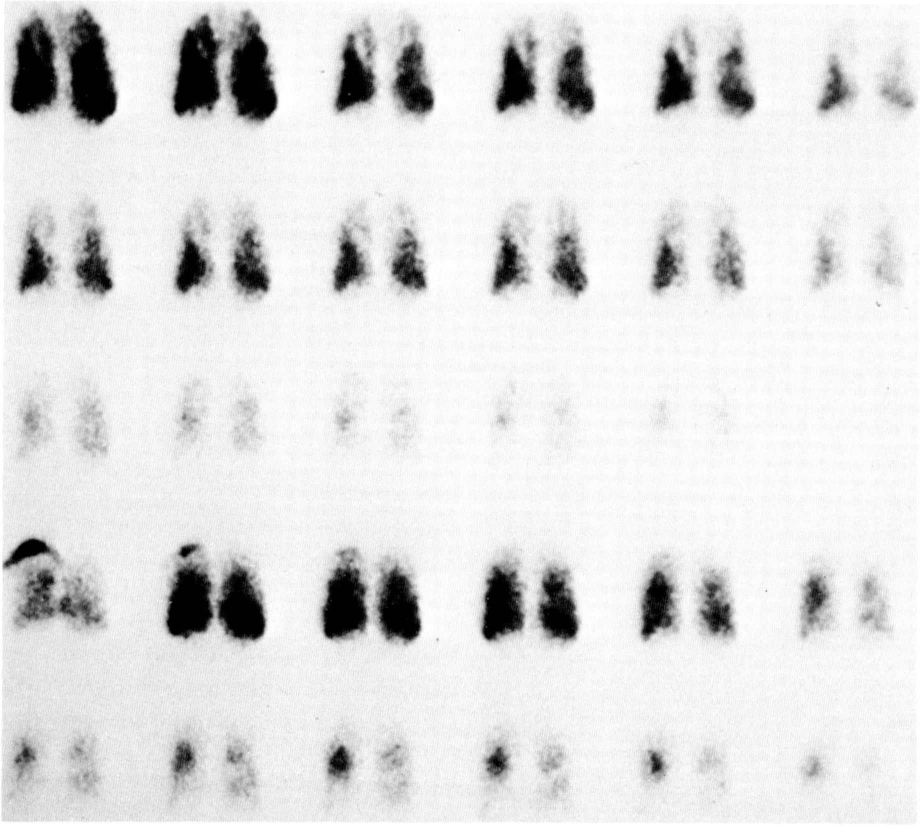

Figure 17-3. Cystic fibrosis. Xe-133 ventilation-perfusion study. Each frame represents 5 sec. Beginning on the left upper corner are the images obtained during rebreathing of the gas. Ventilation is irregular throughout the lung fields and is particularly poor in the upper lung zones. Washout is markedly delayed throughout the lungs. The perfusion phase begins on the third row. Perfusion is irregular throughout both lung fields and is severely reduced in the upper lung fields. The distribution of pulmonary blood flow, although abnormal, appears more uniform than that of ventilation. There is also delayed and irregular washout after intravenous Xe-133.

$$D_i \text{ (percent)} = \frac{\dfrac{\overline{A}_i}{T_{1/2}} \times 100}{\displaystyle\sum_{i-1}^{N} \frac{\overline{A}_i}{T_{1/2}}}$$

in which D_i is the regional distribution, $\overline{A}_i$ is a mean regional activity during the equilibration plateau or perfusion, $T_{1/2}$ is the half-time washout in that region, and N is the number of regions exclusive of the representative region. Distribution ratios of ventilation over equilibrium, ventilation over perfusion, and perfusion over equilibrium are calculated.

Xe-133 Camera Radiospirometry

Technique. The overall procedure is carefully explained to the patient, and the breathing maneuvers are practiced several times with special attention to the need for the patient not to move during the entire examination. Because cooperation is essential for a successful examination, children under about 7 years of age are not suitable candidates for this technique.

A gamma camera with a large field of view equipped with a collimator for low energies is used.[100,132] A 21–23-gauge butterfly type needle is inserted intravenously and flushed with saline. The patient is studied in the sitting position with his back to the detector, breathing through a mouthpiece. The mouthpiece is connected to a magnetic valve, which permits breathing of room air or gas from the closed-system spirometer.

While the patient breathes normally into the closed system, the vital capacity is measured. The continuous external oxygen inflow is adjusted to compensate for the patient's oxygen consumption so that a constant volume is maintained in the system.

Xenon (300 μCi/kg) is injected intravenously as a small, rapid bolus while the patient holds his breath at or near total lung capacity (*TLC*); the corresponding plateau of activity is proportional to regional perfusion ($\dot{Q}$). The patient then breathes into the closed system until equilibrium is reached between the xenon concentration in the spirometer and in the patient's lungs. This is determined by observing stabilization of the count rate from the lungs. When equilibrium is reached (typically 2–5 min of rebreathing), the patient is instructed to hold his breath at or near total capacity for 10–15 sec. This regional Xe-133 activity is proportional to regional aerated lung volume (V). The valve is then opened so that xenon washes out of the lungs and into the exhaust as the patient returns to normal breathing. Xenon (3–5 mCi) is added to the spirometer in order to increase its concentration in preparation for the next maneuver. When background activity in the lungs is approached, the patient is again asked to inhale Xe-133 from the spirometer and then hold his breath at or near *TLC*. After a few seconds of breathholding, the circuit is again opened to the exhaust until pulmonary activity returns to background. The activity in the lungs during breathholding is proportional to regional ventilation ($\dot{V}$).

Analysis. The images of the study are viewed on the monitor of the computer. For visual assessment, series of images (5–10 sec) are obtained during $\dot{Q}$, $\dot{V}$, V, and washout. The image of each lung is usually divided into three zones (upper, middle, and lower) of equal vertical height, and ROIs are marked over these areas. The plateaus corresponding to $\dot{Q}$, $\dot{V}$, and V are identified on time-activity curves by their characteristic appearance as a sequence of relatively stable values. The counts are summed over all ROIs to calculate regional percentages of activity for $\dot{V}$, Q, and V, respectively. Distribution indices ($\dot{V}/V$; $\dot{Q}/V$; $\dot{V}/\dot{Q}$) are calculated for each region.

Normal Distribution. The right and left lung each contribute approximately one-half of the Xe-133 activity during the phases of the study when volume, ventilation, and perfusion are estimated. Anatomically, the right lung makes up about 55% and the left lung 45% of total lung volume. This difference is attenuated when pulmonary Xe-133 is monitored with the gamma camera in the posterior projection. Pulmonary activity during the equilibrium phase of the study reflect the distribution of air volume and the shape of the lungs. The volume of the lung is greatest at the base and gradually diminishes toward the apex.

In the supine position, equal volumes of lung receive nearly equal shares of ventilation and blood flow. The percentages of ventilation and perfusion in each zone are equal, and the mean indices of ventilation and perfusion do not differ significantly from unity. The distribution of function is even. In the erect position, distribution of Xe-133 after a single breath or intravenous Xe-133 (peak activity) reflects the vertical gradients of function whereby the apex of the lung receives less ventilation and blood flow than the base.[9]

The ventilation gradient is caused by differences in the mechanical behavior of lung regions from apex to base. At the apex, the weight of the lung and the elasticity of the chest wall act to overcome lung recoil. Apical pleural pressure is strongly negative, apical alveoli are well expanded, and apical compliance is low. At the base, the weight of the lung acts in synergy with lung recoil. Basal alveoli are poorly expanded and their compliance is high. During slow-breathing maneuvers in radiospirometry, compliance alone normally determines regional distribution of ventilation. Accordingly, when pleural pressure falls with inspiration by the same amount in all parts of the lungs, a greater volume gain occurs at the base than at the apex.[98]

The perfusion gradient is due to hydrostatic pressures affecting the regional pressure in branches of the pulmonary artery and transmural pressure in pulmonary capillaries and veins. Regional perfusion depends on relationships among pulmonary arterial, alveolar, and venous pressures. Studies of isolated perfused lungs have identified four distribution zones from apex to base: zone I, where there is little or no blood flow for lack of perfusing pressure; zone II, where perfusion increases rapidly with an increasing pressure head on the arterial side; zone III, where the perfusion gradient reflects changes in transmural pressure in the whole vascular bed; and zone IV, where blood flow falls because of increased interstitial pressure.[69,142,143]

Changes in lung volume affect the distribution of function in normal lungs. The distribution of ventilation depends mainly on the lung volume from which inhalation of xenon is started because the lung volume determines the regional distribution of alveolar size and compliance. Administration of xenon by a single breath may be started from residual volume to maximize the regional differences in ventilation or the difference from functional residual capacity (*FRC*) to minimize the need for the patient's cooperation. The latter is preferable for sick patients and for all children. With a single breath bringing lung volume from *FRC* to near total lung capacity, regional ventilation normally increases linearly from the apex to the base of the lung. When three vertical lung regions are considered, ventilation to the lower zones of the lung is 1.5–2 times greater than that to the upper zones.

The effect of lung volume on distribution of blood flow results from differences in regional hemodynamic resistance, which offset the action of gravity on perfusing pressures. Near residual volume the dependent regions of the lung are poorly expanded and exhibit high regional vascular resistance, which shifts pulmonary blood flow to the upper lung regions with a consequent loss of vertical gradient. The perfusion gradient increases when lung volume is raised from residual volume to two-thirds of total lung capacity. For lung volumes in the upper third of total lung capacity, the distribution of function becomes independent of lung volume[70] and regional perfusion normally increases by a factor of 2–2.5 from the upper to the lower third of the lung.

Regional Volume. Good measurements of regional volume are essential for strict interpretation of distribution data. These measurements depend largely on adequate equalization of regional xenon concentrations as produced by rebreathing in a closed-system spirometer. Technical requirements applicable to this part of the radiospirometric examination include: airtight spirometer with a mixing fan, zero pressure at the mouthpiece, effective CO_2 absorption, continuous and stable O_2 input, and sufficient time for equilibration to take place. Time is the major factor. Two to 4 min of rebreathing results in complete mixing between lungs and spirometer only in normal persons. Inadequate mixing is common in patients with lung disease, and this worsens as airway obstruction increases in severity.[45]

Patients with airway obstruction can be identified by radiologic examination and global pulmonary function tests before radiospirometry. For these patients, a longer rebreathing period (5–7 min) may be needed for equilibration to be reached. In some patients with severe lung disease equilibration of Xe-133 in the lung may never be reached. Further prolongation of rebreathing offers little benefit because xenon is lost progressively from the lungs as the gas is taken up in the pulmonary circulation or dissolved in the water seal and other parts of the spirometer.

Regardless of precautions, rebreathing measurements are affected by the regional distribution of ventilation whenever severe obstructive disease is present. This inability to equilibrate may have diagnostic value. In a patient with lung fields of nearly equal size on the chest roentgenogram, uneven distribution of aerated lung volume indicates severe regional trapping.[45]

Kr-81m Ventilation Studies

Patients are examined supine or sitting using a gamma camera equipped with a low-energy collimator. While the patient breathes normally, the Kr-81m-O_2 mixture eluted from the generator is added to the air in a plastic bag that is connected to a mask placed over his nose and mouth. In patients receiving mechanical ventilation, the Kr-81m-O_2 mixture is simply merged with the existing O_2 supply line. Scans in the posterior, anterior, lateral, and oblique projections are obtained routinely. Each image is recorded for about 300,000 counts with an individual imaging time of 0.5–2.0 min.

Paired ventilation and perfusion images can be obtained if the patient is injected with Tc-99m MAA in the same position (upright or supine) held for the Kr-81m ventilation study. These images are obtained by alternating the window settings in the camera between the 190-keV and 140-keV photopeaks for Kr-81m and Tc-99m, respectively. The patient is kept in the same position for each view, and elution of Kr-81m is halted while the perfusion images are taken.

Clinical Applications

Cystic Fibrosis

Cystic fibrosis is a hereditary disorder transmitted as an autosomal recessive trait. This disease causes most of the chronic progressive pulmonary disease

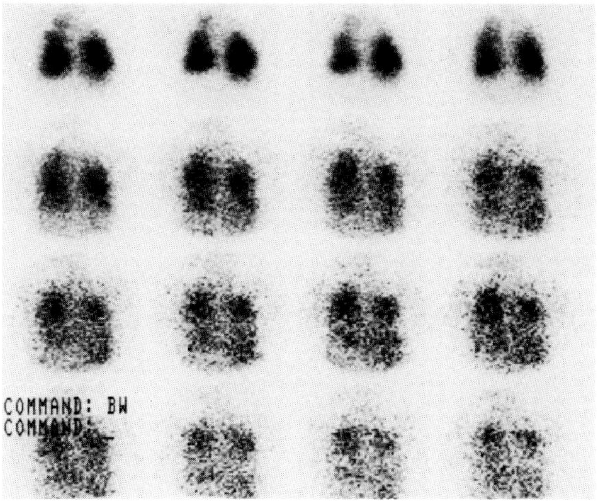

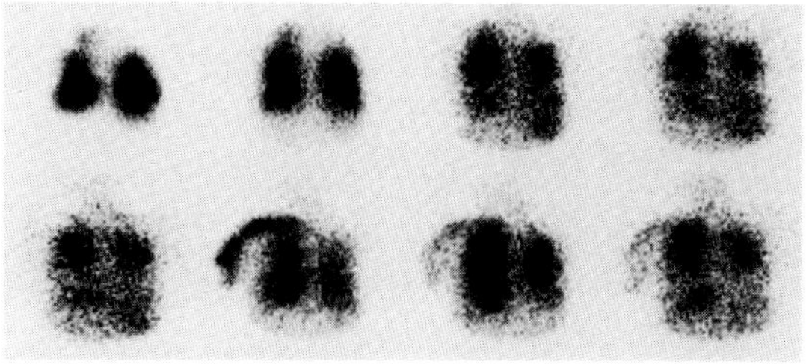

Figure 17-4. Cystic fibrosis. Diffuse involvement of both lungs, delayed Xe-133 washin and washout. Note significant systemic penetration of the tracer. *Left:* Ventilation. *Right:* Perfusion.

encountered in children. The incidence in the United States is 1:1600–2000 live Caucasian births. About 5% of the general population are carriers of the gene.[34,150]

Cystic fibrosis is a systemic disorder that involves almost all organ systems including the lungs, pancreas, liver, intestine, and genitalia. Over 99% of patients with cystic fibrosis have an elevated sweat electrolyte concentration.[34,123,150] During the past decade, there has been a significant improvement in the typical clinical course of cystic fibrosis. This is due to more accurate and earlier diagnosis, detection of mild involvement, better understanding of the pathophysiology of this disorder, and improved therapy.

In the lung, excessive mucus is produced that is very thick, and sticky. This mucus cannot be moved by the cilia and accumulates in the bronchi and bronchioles, causing obstruction. Stagnation of secretions favors the development of infection. *Staphylococcus aureus* and *Pseudomonas aeruginosa* are common pathogens found in the lungs of these patients. Obstruction and infection lead to hyperaeration or atelectasis depending on whether the obstruction is partial or total. Accumulation of thick mucus interferes with ventilation, mucociliary clearance, and the normal mechanism of cough, resulting in further accumulation of mucus.

The inflammatory reaction and infection destroy the ciliated epithelium. Bronchiectasis develops after the loss of integrity of the bronchial walls. Purulent secretions are accumulated in peribronchial pools. These regions become chronic sources of local infection and also seed infection to other parts of the lung. The course of the disease leads to complications such as abscess, hemoptysis, and spontaneous pneumothorax. As the disease progresses, it leads to respiratory insufficiency, cor pulmonale, and finally death.

Scintigraphic Appearance

In early, mild involvement Xe-133 studies reveal nearly normal distribution of inhaled gas and perfusion, with the only abnormality being diffuse, minimal to moderate delay of Xe-133 washout (trapping). In our laboratory, we have investigated the early pulmonary manifestations of cystic fibrosis in a group of young children with positive sweat chloride tests and good clinical condition. Xe-133 studies in these patients have detected early changes by demonstrating air trapping even in the presence of normal chest radiographs. In addition, some of these patients have shown evidence of high systemic penetration of Xe-133 both after inhalation of the gas and after its intravenous administration. The liver appears to concentrate relatively higher amounts of tracer than does the body background. This effect may be due to increased or altered permeability of the alveolar capillary membrane and/or pulmonary right-to-left shunting (Fig. 17-4). As the disease progresses, irregular abnormalities in regional ventilation and perfusion are seen along with more severe trapping of Xe-133. The lungs are involved globally, but the upper lung zones are usually more affected than the lower zones (Fig. 17-3).

In more advanced disease, distribution of Xe-

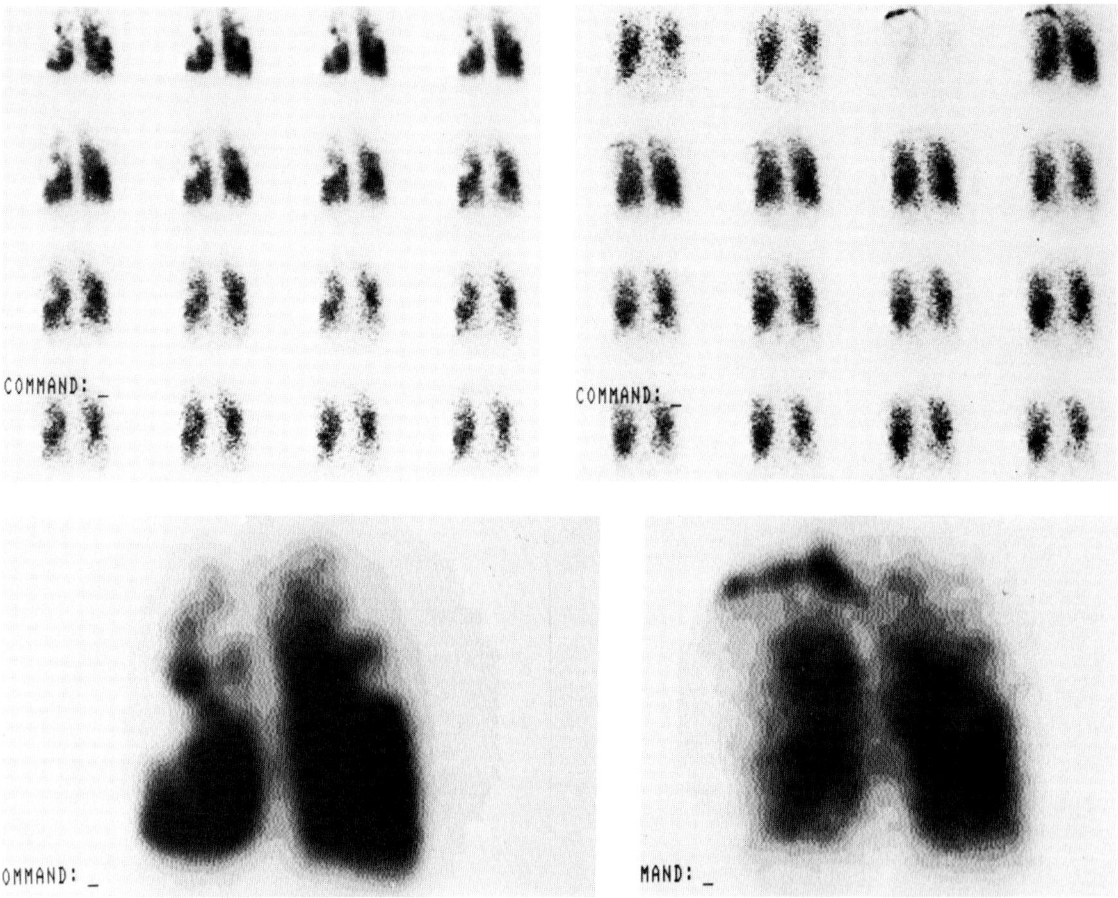

Figure 17-5. Cystic fibrosis. Xe-133 study. *Top left:* Distribution of Xe-133 during breathing shows bilateral involvement worse in the left lung and in both upper lung fields. There is delayed, irregular washin and trapping of the tracer diffusely within both lungs. *Top right:* Perfusion and washout of Xe-133. There is reduced blood flow to the left lung with irregular distribution in both lungs. In addition, severe diffuse trapping of radiotracer is seen in both lungs. *Bottom: left:* Image obtained during breathing of Xe-133. *Bottom right:* Image of perfusion after intravenous Xe-133. Distribution of blood flow appears more uniform than ventilation.

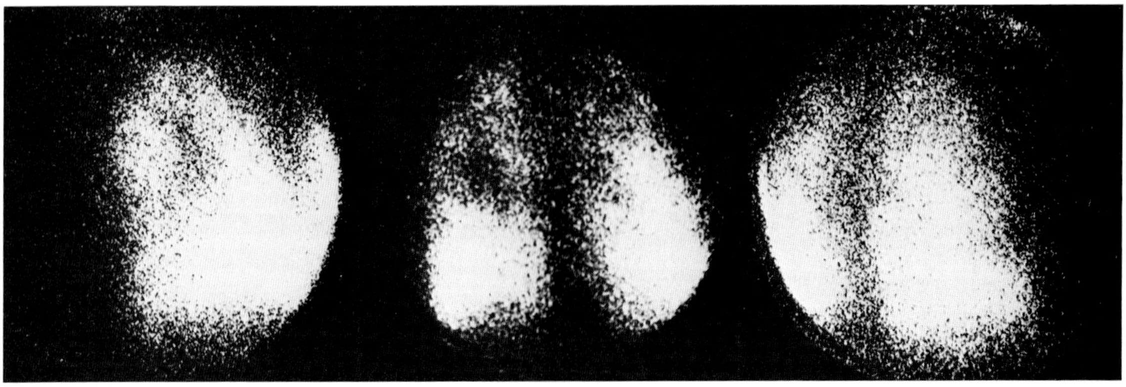

Figure 17-6. Cystic fibrosis. Images obtained during rebreathing of Kr-81m gas. Ventilation is severely impaired. Areas of decreased-to-absent ventilation are present in both upper lung fields.

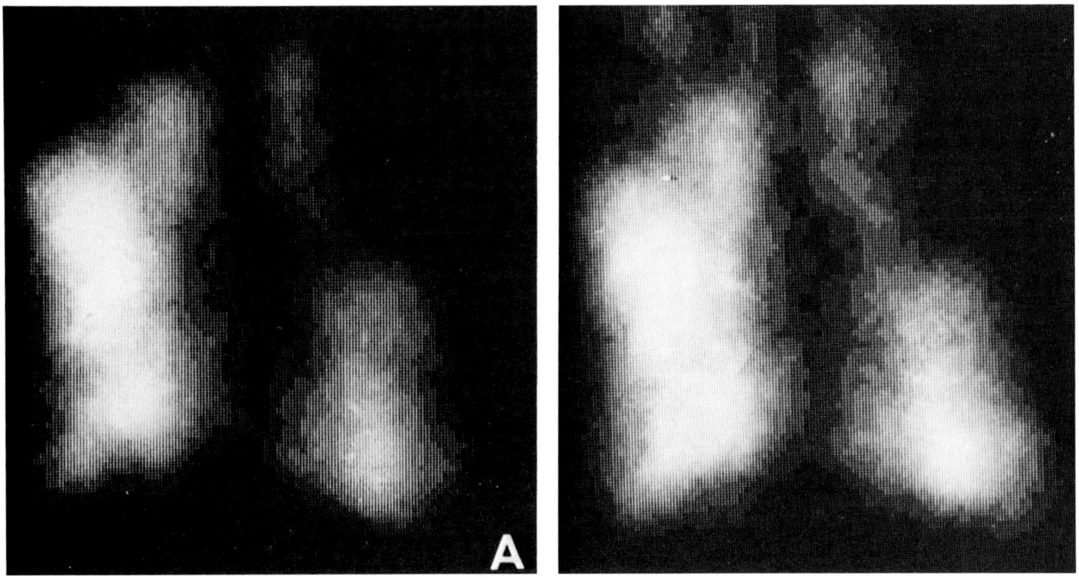

Figure 17-7. Cystic fibrosis. Effect of physical therapy of the chest on distribution of ventilation. Images obtained with Kr-81m before *(left)* and after *(right)* a session of physical therapy to the chest with postural drainage. There is an apparent improvement in the distribution of radiokrypton following therapy.

133 during inhalation is quite irregular throughout the lungs and it is difficult if not impossible to attain an equilibrium of Xe-133 in the lung during rebreathing. Some regions of the lung accumulate Xe-133, but the gas does not penetrate at all into obstructed air spaces. Generally, the distribution of pulmonary blood flow as assessed with Xe-133 in advanced stages of the disease matches well with the abnormal distribution of ventilation. In some cases, however, the distribution of pulmonary blood flow, although abnormal, appears more uniform than ventilation. Some regions of the lung that do not receive Xe-133 by inhalation are reached by some pulmonary blood flow. Marked air trapping is evident throughout the lung fields (Figs. 17-5 and 17-6).

In the remission phase, perfusion abnormalities correlate with the severity of disease. In the acute phase, striking transient alterations develop.[110] With hemoptysis, the region of the lung involved may show further reduction in ventilation with or without apparent reduction of regional blood flow. In cystic fibrosis, the ventilation/perfusion gradient is reversed from normal, and the regional ventilation-perfusion ratios are unevenly distributed.[4]

Gyepes et al. found good correlation between perfusion and ventilation abnormalities and the severity of disease in 18 children and young adults with cystic fibrosis. These authors also recognized the superior sensitivity of the perfusion lung scans (Tc-99m MAA) over roentgenograms of the chest in detecting the presence and extent of early pulmonary involvement.[61]

Radionuclide imaging has been used also to assess the effects of physical therapy of the chest on ciliary clearance and on ventilation. Bateman et al., using 5-μm polystyrene particles labelled with Tc-99m found that chest physiotherapy increases clearance of excessive bronchial secretions in patients with chronic airway obstruction.[11] Using Kr-81m, DeCesare et al. in our hospital evaluated the effect of bronchial drainage with percussion and vibration on peripheral ventilation in patients with cystic fibrosis. There were no changes in the distribution of ventilation in patients with mild disease. The ventilatory pattern in patients with moderate disease was variable and seemingly independent of treatment. The patients with severe lung disease exhibited an apparent improvement in regional aeration of the lungs (Fig. 17-7). As expected, there was a relationship between ventilatory changes and the amount of sputum produced. Because the distribution of regional ventilation in patients with cystic fibrosis is highly variable from time to time even without treatment, however, all changes in regional ventilation in these patients were not necessarily due to therapy.[32]

Xe-133 ventilation/perfusion studies in cystic fibrosis have been used to assess regional lung function before operation in order to ensure that removal of a lobe will not compromise further a patient with already severe pulmonary disease. In practice, most patients with cystic fibrosis referred for Xe-133 ventilation/perfusion studies are those with established and/or advanced lung disease.

Although early pulmonary involvement in cystic fibrosis can also be detected with Xe-133 studies (even in the presence of a normal chest radiograph and normal pulmonary function tests), radionuclide studies have not been utilized to make the diagnosis of early lung disease. Clinical assessment of lung disease is left to rather late changes appreciable by radiography of the chest and the stethoscope. Perhaps if lung involvement were identified earlier, earlier therapeutic intervention might improve further the clinical course of patients affected with cystic fibrosis.

Early radiologic manifestations include diffuse bronchial thickening, hyperinflation, and evidence of retained secretions. Later, there is peribronchial fibrosis, involvement of the hilar nodes, bronchiectasis, and enlargement of the pulmonary artery. Increased interstitial markings and/or cyst-like structures are apparent. Haziness of the bronchovascular shadows and irregular areas of hyperinflation are seen predominantly in the upper lobes. Interstitial markings tend to become more and more irregular and reticulonodular. A honeycomb appearance is produced when the walls of clustered, small cyst-like areas (ectatic bronchi or bronchioles on end) thicken and interstitial infiltration progresses. In advanced stages, a distorted picture suggesting swiss cheese is seen on the radiographs. Transient nodular densities are replaced by lucencies that may be due to endobronchial collections and peribronchial abscesses.

The appearance of bronchiectasis varies with the amount of secretion contained in the airways. In early involvement (mild disease) findings on radiographs of the chest do not correlate with radionuclide lung scans. Regions of the lung that may appear normal on radiographs of the chest may have ventilation/perfusion abnormalities. In advanced stages of lung disease, scintigraphic and radiographic findings correlate more closely.[4]

Pulmonary function tests may be normal in mild cystic fibrosis, but the Xe-133 studies are usually abnormal. As the disease progresses, small airway obstruction is followed by decreased vital capacity and expiratory flow rates, hyperinflation, and increased residual volume and total lung capacity.

Scintigraphy with Ga-67 citrate may help to identify regions of the lung with active inflammation (Fig. 17-8).

Hemoptysis

Scintigraphy of the lungs after intravenous injection of Tc-99m red blood cells or Tc-99m sulfur colloid may be useful in the localization of bleeding.[25,147] Due to their long residence time in the blood pool, *Tc-99m red blood cells* may increase the possibility of localizing intermittent bleeding because the observation period can be extended for several hours. One disadvantage of labelled red cells is that the bleeding-to-background ratio and the bleeding-to-cardiac blood pool ratio are lower than with Tc-99m sulfur colloid, preventing detection of small volumes of bleeding. Nevertheless, our limited experience with Tc-99m red blood cells suggests that the preparation has good potential for localizing pulmonary bleeding.

After intravenous injection, *Tc-99m sulfur colloid* is extracted rapidly from the blood by cells of the reticuloendothelial system. If bleeding occurs during its brief presence in the blood pool, the tracer will extravasate in the ara of active bleeding. Because of the high bleeding-to-background ratio with this tracer, theoretically small amounts of bleeding may be detected. In the gastrointestinal tract this technique has detected bleeding at rates as low as 0.1 ml/mm.[1,2] Bleeding rates of 0.1–0.2 ml/min have been detected in dogs, but in some of these animals significantly higher bleeding rates were not detected.[10]

A large source of error in detecting pulmonary bleeding in animals and in humans has been attributed to bleeding into a large bronchus and producing a diffuse distribution of the radiotracer.[10,99] Unfortunately, many patients have intermittent pulmonary bleeding, as in cystic fibrosis, and in our limited experience we have not been successful in localizing bleeding with Tc-99m sulfur colloid in these individuals. Presumably our failure occurred because bleeding did not coincide with the brief presence of radiocolloid in blood.

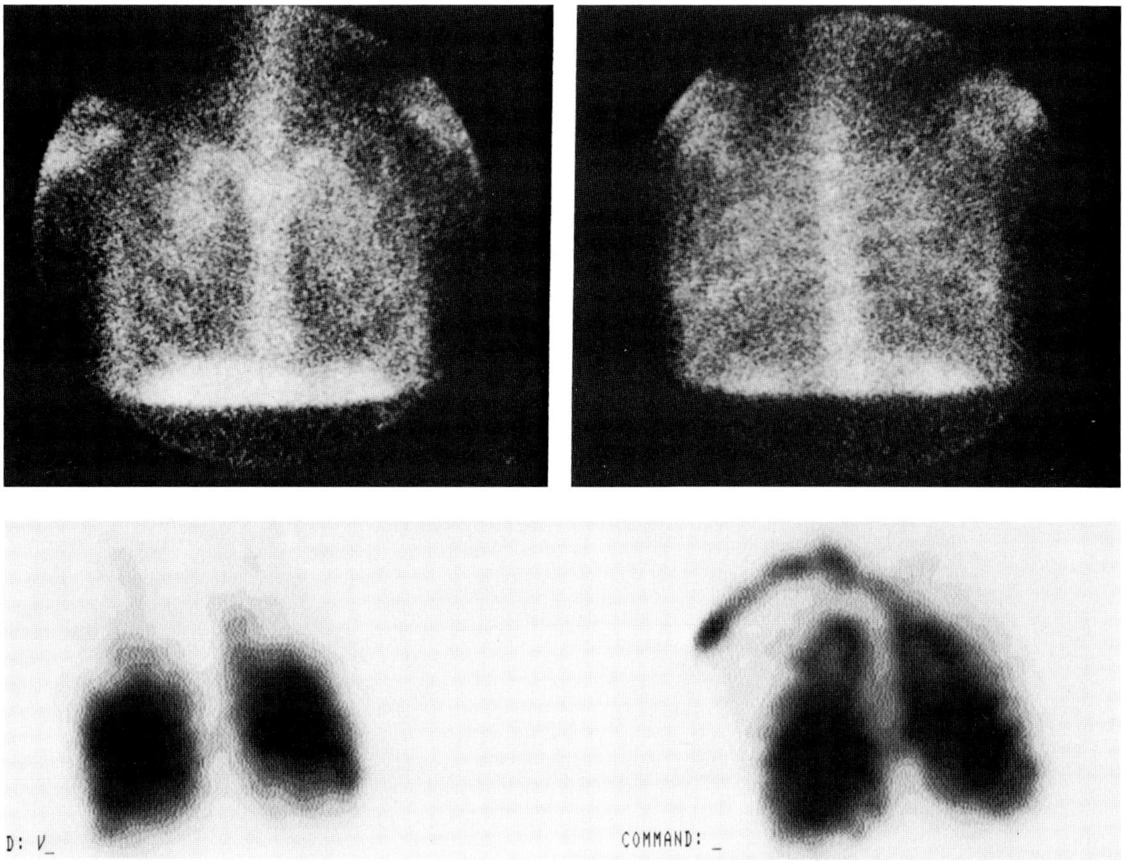

Figure 17-8. *Top:* Ga-67 scan of the chest from a patient with advanced cystic fibrosis and with severe bilateral compromise of his upper lobes. The right upper lobe contains high levels of radiogallium, indicating an active inflammatory process. There is in addition diffuse increase of Ga-67 uptake in the left lung. *Bottom:* Xe-133 ventilation *(left)*, and perfusion *(right)* study in the same patient showing diffuse disease and major compromise of the upper lung fields.

Congenital and Acquired Anomalies of Heart and Great Vessels

Pulmonary scintigraphy is helpful in the assessment of altered pulmonary dynamics in patients with congenital heart disease. In *valvular pulmonic stenosis*, pulmonary artery flow to the left lung is greater than to the right lung. The jet flow formed by the stenotic valve is directed preferentially to the left pulmonary artery[24,36] (Fig. 17-9).

Patients with *ventricular septal defect* tend to have decreased perfusion in the left lung due to enlargement of the left side of the heart compressing the left lung.[137] We have found increased pulmonary artery flow to the left lung after a *pulmonary artery band* has been placed in these patients. This band decreases the ventilation/perfusion ratio in the left lung and increases it in the right lung (Fig. 17-10). This imbalance in the distribution of pulmonary blood flow does not reverse in most patients after surgical removal of the band and repair of the ventricular septal defect.[117]

Decreased pulmonary artery flow may be observed after *palliative surgical shunts* such as the Blalock-Taussig (subclavian-pulmonary artery), the Waterston (ascending aorta-right pulmonary artery), and the Potts (descending aorta-left pulmonary artery) anastomoses. The decreased pulmonary flow to one lung is due to dilution by systemic blood arriving through the shunt.[51,101] In patent surgically created shunts, first-pass radionuclide angiography reveals a greater amount of early pulmonary recirculation of the tracer in the

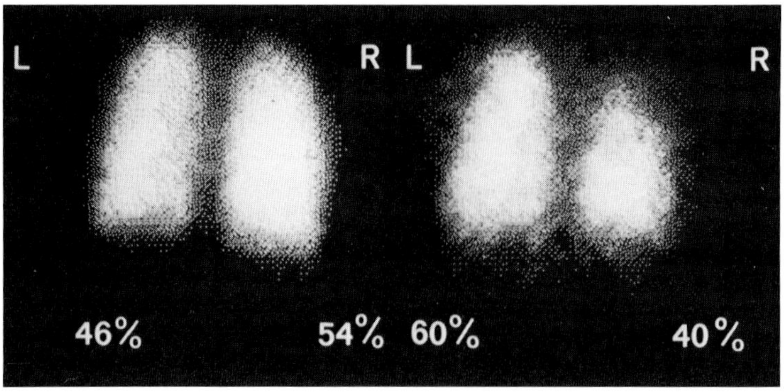

Figure 17-9. Pulmonary valve stenosis. Xe-133 study demonstrating a ventilation-perfusion imbalance. The flow to the left lung is 60% of the total pulmonary blood flow. *Left:* ventilation; *right:* perfusion.

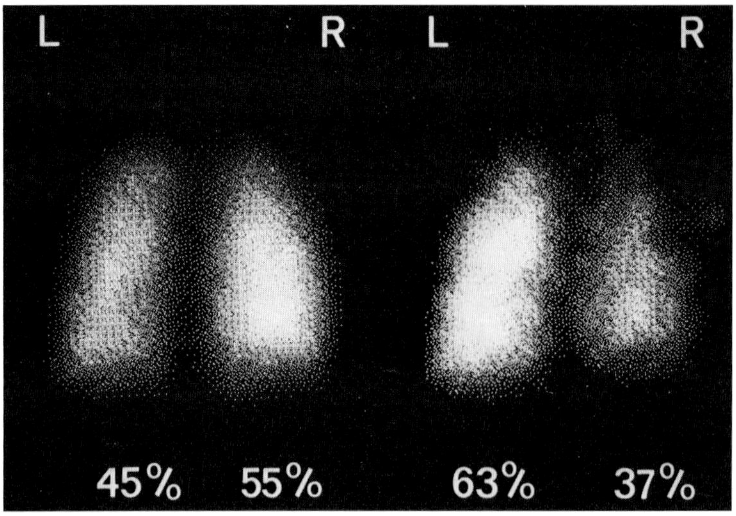

Figure 17-10. Pulmonary artery band and its effect on ventilation and perfusion. Xe-133 study. There is an increase in the pulmonary artery flow to the left lung (63% of the total pulmonary blood flow). *Left:* ventilation; *right:* perfusion.

lung receiving the shunt. A similar amount of early recirculation in both lungs indicates an occluded shunt.

Localization of MAA in the kidneys after its intravenous injection indicates the presence of a *right-to-left shunt* of at least 15% (Fig. 17-11).[101] Detection and quantitation of shunts with radionuclides were discussed in Chapter 16.

Normal children, even infants held in the erect position, have relatively more pulmonary perfusion in the lower lung fields than to the upper lung fields. The normal upper to lower lung pulmonary perfusion ratio is 0.5–0.6. Children with intracardiac *left-to-right shunts* have an abnormally higher fraction of pulmonary blood flow going to their upper lung fields with equal distribution between the right and left lungs. Infants with *pulmonic stenosis* have an abnormally higher proportion of pulmonary blood flow going to the left lung. In these patients the left lung also has relatively greater perfusion of the upper zone. Infants with pulmonic stenosis and left-to-right shunts have perfusion abnormalities in both lungs. There is increased flow to both upper zones and overperfusion of the left lung.

In older children with *atrial septal defect,* a greater than normal proportion of blood flows to the right lung. A factor invoked as cause for this include enlargement of the heart into the left hemithorax.[48]

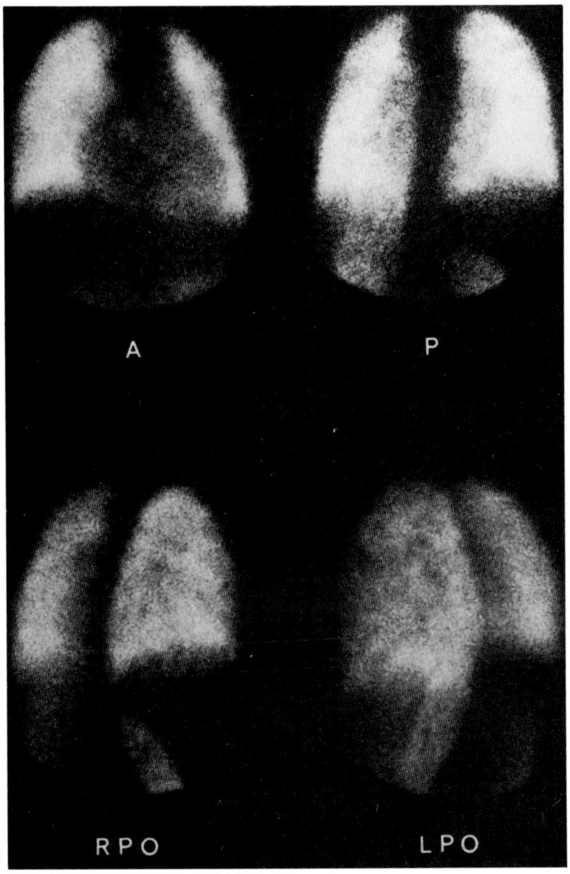

Figure 17-11. Right-to-left shunting. Images obtained after intravenous injection of Tc-99m macroaggregated albumin. This scintiscan was from a 16-year-old male with complex congenital heart disease and pulmonary vascular obstructive disease. Note the presence of radioactivity from particles in the kidneys and in the myocardium. Also his heart is enlarged, and there is irregular distribution of pulmonary blood flow.

In *partially anomalous pulmonary venous return* (PAPVR), one or more of the pulmonary veins enter the right atrium instead of the left atrium. This condition was found in about 0.7% of routine autopsies in one series.[68] The right lung is involved in some form of anomalous venous return almost twice as often as the left lung. A frequent association with right PAPVR is an atrial septal defect of the ostium secundum type.

The point of entry of the anomalous return to the right side of the heart, in order of frequency, is superior vena cava, inferior vena cava (scimitar syndrome), and right atrium.[74] The cresent shape (scimitar) of the anomalous right pulmonary vein draining into the inferior vena cava may be seen on a roentgenogram of the chest. In PAPVR from the left lung, the return is to the superior vena cava.[106] The clinical and physiologic features of PAPVR are similar to that of atrial septal defect with left-to-right shunting. The left-to-right shunt of PAPVR can be detected and quantified with first-pass radionuclide angiography. The results of surgery in *pulmonary artery sling* are variable. In some patients the neoanastomosis fails (Fig. 17-12), while in others pulmonary blood flow to the involved lung is maintained (Fig. 17-13).

Pulmonary arteriovenous malformations are congenital anomalies with direct connections between the pulmonary artery and vein. The abnormalities are usually cavernomatous and cause right-to-left shunting. These lesions can be solitary, multiple, diffuse (telangiectatic), or mixed. More than 60% are solitary and most occur in lower lobes. In about one-half of the patients there is associated familial relangiectasis and hemangiomas of the skin and mucus membranes. Clinical symptoms are secondary to abnormal oxygenation due to the right-to-left shunt (cyanosis, dyspnea, hemotysis, epistaxis, exercise intolerance) and secondary embolic pneumonia.

Physical examination of patients with pulmonary arteriovenous malformations may reveal conjunctival hemorrhages, digital clubbing, or murmur. Polycythemia or cerebrovascular accidents may occur. Radiographs of the chest show single or multiple lesions with linear, vascular shadows. Pulmonary angiography is diagnostic. Detection with radionuclide angiography depends on the size and location of the lesion. The appearance on radionuclide angiography is that of a distinct and localized blush of activity within a lung field immediately after appearance of the right side of the heart[66,105,135] (Fig. 17-14).

Patients with *mitral stenosis* (very rare in children), particularly those with high pulmonary pressures, may show a higher blood flow to the upper lung than to the lower lung.[31,35] This distribution of blood flow is the reverse of that found in normal subjects and is consistent with the radiologic and pathologic changes found in the lung in mitral stenosis.

Unilateral Hyperlucent Lung

Repeated airway infection in children causing bronchiolitis obliterans may result in a unilateral hyperlucent lung (Swyer-James-McLeod syn-

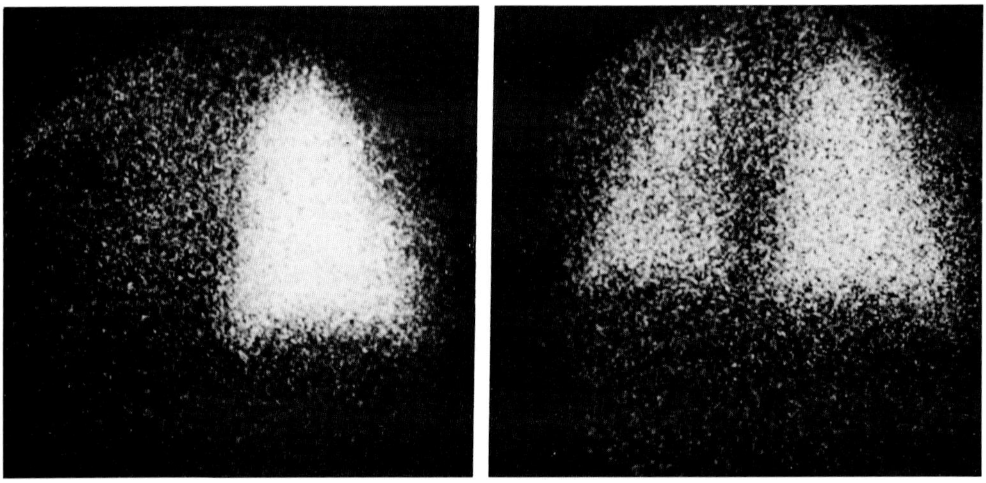

Figure 17-12

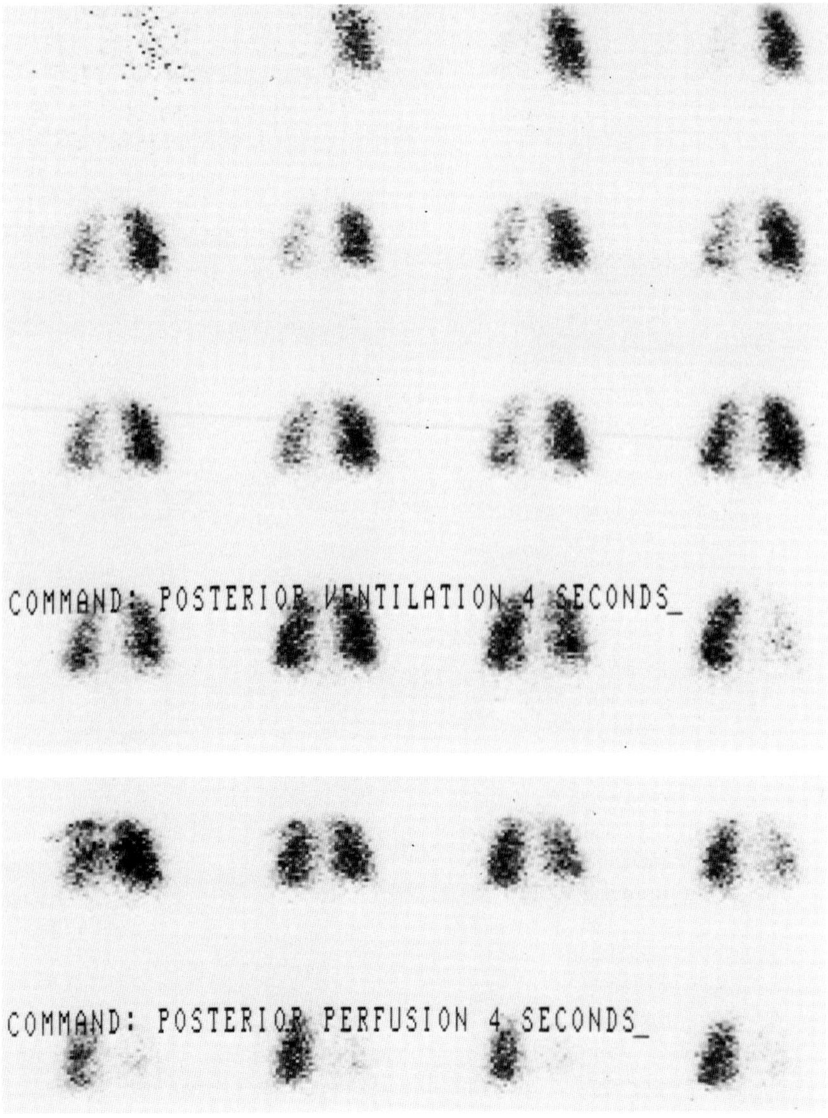

Figure 17-13

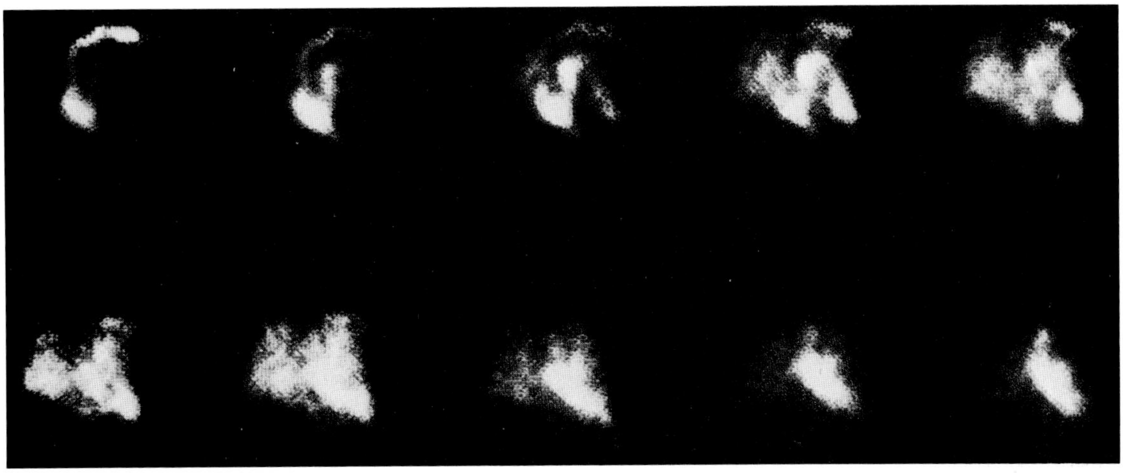

Figure 7-14

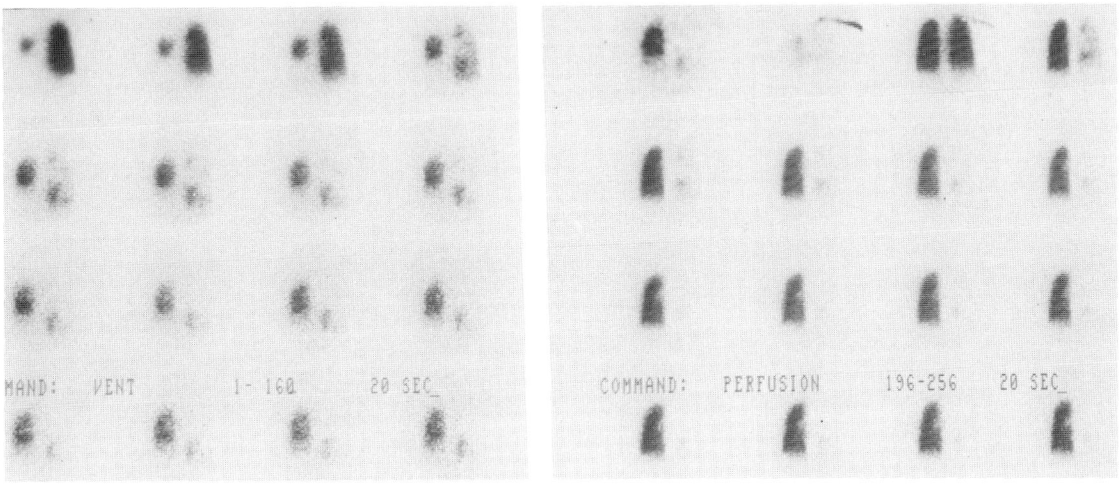

Figure 17-15

Figure 17-12. Pulmonary artery sling. Postoperative Xe-133 study from a 6-month-old female. There is lack of pulmonary blood flow to the entire left lung. Ventilation to the left lung is preserved but reduced. *Right:* perfusion; *left:* ventilation.

Figure 17-13. Pulmonary artery sling. Postoperative Xe-133 study from a 5.5-month-old female. Ventilation *(top)* is compromised in the left lung as evidenced by trapping of radioxenon indicating incomplete airway obstruction. Perfusion to the left lung is present *(bottom)*.

Figure 17-14. Pulmonary arteriovenous malformation. First-pass radionuclide angiocardiogram with Tc-99m NaO_4. Anterior view; each frame represents 1 sec. After the tracer appears within the right side of the heart and the pulmonary artery a large "blush" of activity is visualized in the left lower lung corresponding to an arteriovenous malformation. The activity within this lesion clears rapidly and is no longer visualized during the levophase of the angiogram.

Figure 17-15. Unilateral hyperlucent lung. The left lung of this child was hyperlucent on a radiograph of the chest. He had a history of repeated respiratory tract infections. On the series of 5-sec Xe-133 images *(left)* obtained during rebreathing of the tracer there is poor ventilation of the left lung with evidence of air trapping. The right lung functions better than the left one but shows some minor trapping of tracer. The series of 5-sec images obtained after intravenous injection of Xe-133 *(right)* reveal symmetric perfusion of both lungs with marked trapping of gas within the entire left lung. The right lung washes out normally. These findings are diagnostic of airway obstruction.

drome). This disorder most frequently follows pulmonary infection by adenovirus, but measles, pertussis, and tuberculosis have also been implicated.

The affected lung has usually a normal main bronchus with marked bronchiectatic changes in the more peripheral bronchi. Radiographs of the chest demonstrate diminished or normal lung volume and marked decrease in bronchovascular markings. Radionuclide studies using Xe-133 usually reveal markedly reduced perfusion and ventilation and trapping of air in the affected lung (Fig. 17-15). Pulmonary angiography shows a small ipsilateral pulmonary artery with thin branches and greatly reduced peripheral vascularity.[28,85,109,152]

Pulmonary Air Cysts

All thin-walled air-containing intrapulmonary spaces that are radiologically visible regardless of their pathogensis are called pulmonary air cysts. Their clinical significance varies widely. It is important to determine whether a cyst is solitary or part of generalized pulmonary disease. Functional implications of air cysts have been reviewed by Bates et al.[12]

An air cyst (bulla or bleb) is a space in the lung ranging from 1 cm in diameter to the volume of an entire hemithorax and possessing a smooth wall of minimal thickness. These lesions may be congenital or acquired. Congenital types include bronchogenic cysts whose fluid content have been expelled, and congenital cystic disease of the lung. Air cysts may also be part of congenital intrapulmonary sequestration. When acquired, the cysts may arise de novo or occur as part of other disorders, usually infectious, and are frequently associated with parenchymal damage.

Acquired cysts include blebs and bullae. Blebs are usually less than 1–2 cm in diameter and immediately subpleural. They have been invoked as a cause of spontaneous pneumothorax. Bullae, which are intrapulmonary, are usually attributable to excessive rupture of alveolar walls. Their walls are composed of compressed parenchymal tissue. The exact cause of this problem is not clear: obstruction, postinfection lung abscess (tuberculosis, staphylococcus), resolution of acute pneumonia, and trauma have been suggested.[52]

Most bronchogenic cysts are located near the trachea, stem bronchi, or carina although intrapulmonary and cervical locations have been found. The cysts are usually unilocular structures containing clear fluid, but mucoid, hemorrhagic, or purulent material may be present. The walls may contain bronchial elements (cartilage, fibrovascular connective tissue, pseudostratified columnar epithelium). Patients may be asymptomatic or may present with respiratory distress, cough and/or recurrent respiratory infections.

Radiographs of the chest usually reveal a rounded mass in proximity to the stem bronchi and the carina. Cysts may compress a major bronchus leading to air trapping and collapse. At fluoroscopy during expiration, the cysts appear to inflate while the rest of the lung deflates. Computed tomography can help differentiate cyst from tumor, lymph nodes, or other structures. Xe-133 studies may demonstrate lack of ventilation and perfusion within the cyst provided it is large enough to be detected. Alternatively, a cyst may cause air trapping (Figs. 17-16–17-18).

Airway Obstruction

Diffuse airway obstruction in children occurs in asthma, infection, cystic fibrosis, and α_1-antitrypsin deficiency. Local airway obstruction can be caused by mucous plugs, foreign objects, pneumonia, cystic fibrosis, and congenital lobar emphysema (Figs. 17-19 and 17-20).

Xe-133 studies characteristically show delayed washout of the tracer within the involved region of the lung. In airway obstruction no true equilibrium of Xe-133 within the lungs can be achieved. The pulmonary distribution of radioxenon depends on the degree and distribution of airway obstruction and on the length of the rebreathing period. Depending on penetration of the gas in the obstructed lung regions, the images may or may not reflect air trapping. Images after short periods of rebreathing Xe-133 may show one or several areas of reduced to absent accumulation of the tracer corresponding to lung regions supplied by obstructed airways. Longer periods of rebreathing result in greater penetration and even accumulation of the tracer in the obstructed lung tissue. Increased accumulation of gas in these obstructed lung regions represents decreased ventilation. Images obtained during the washout phase reveal the delayed clearance of radiotracer in areas of airway obstruction.

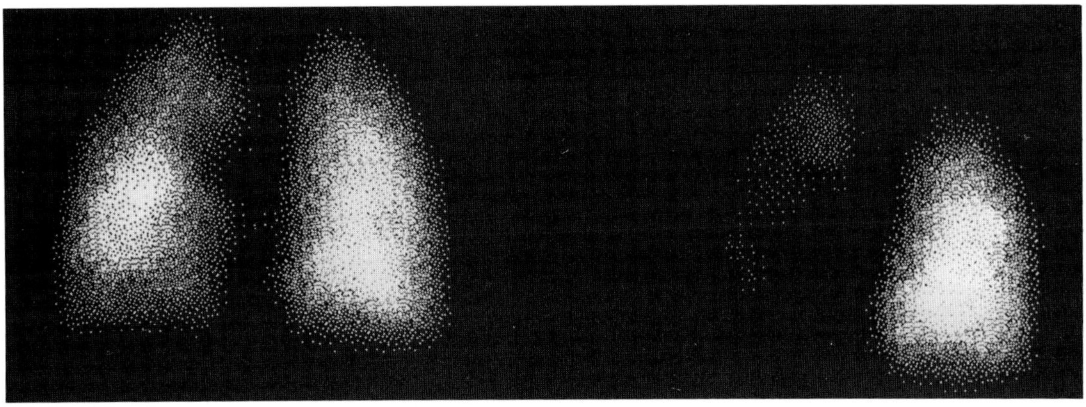

Figure 17-16. Large cyst in the left lung. The image on the *left* was obtained after a few minutes of rebreathing Xe-133. The distribution of radioxenon in the right lung is normal. The left lung shows an area of increased accumulation of gas in its midportion corresponding to a cystic lesion seen on the radiograph of the chest. The image on the *right* obtained after intravenous injection of Xe-133, shows severely reduced blood flow to most of the left lung also corresponding to the large air cyst. Perfusion of the right lung is normal.

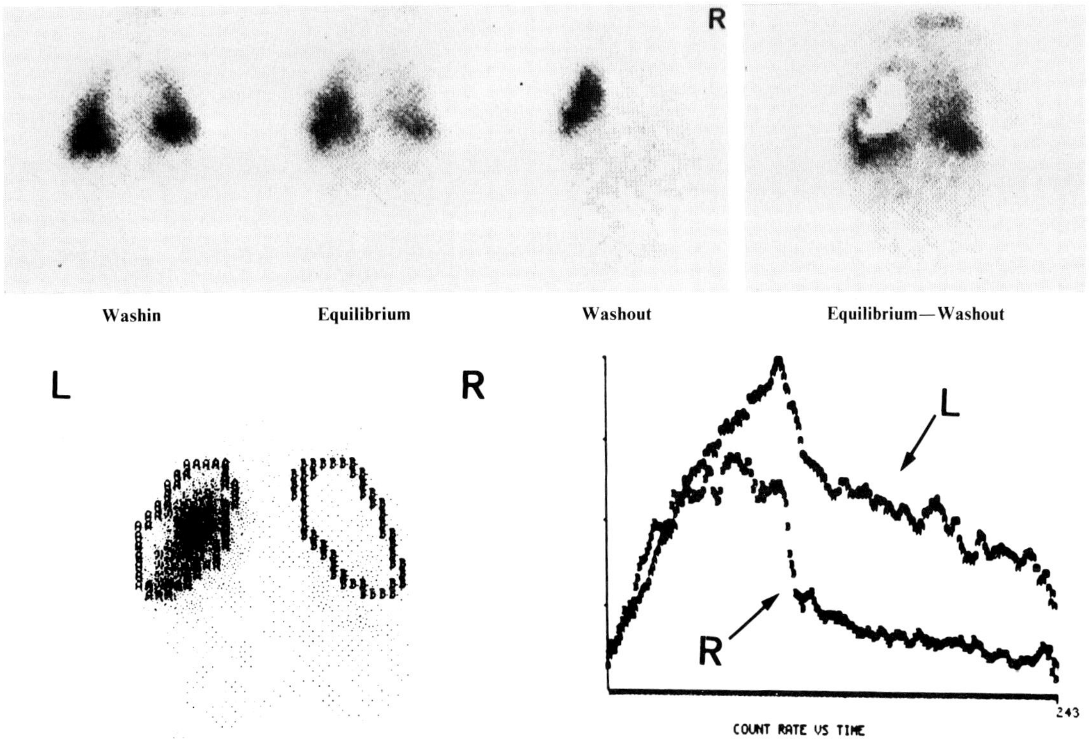

Figure 17-17. *Top:* Xe-133 images from a patient with an air cyst in the left mid-lung field. The initial image *(left)* which was obtained a few seconds during rebreathing of the gas shows irregular but symmetric distribution of Xe-133. After further rebreathing the left lung accumulates more radioxenon than the right lung, indicating the presence of a one-way valve system. The image during the washout phase reveals trapping of Xe-133 in the left lung corresponding to the cystic like lesion seen on the radiograph of the chest. *Bottom:* Time-activity curves in the same study from symmetric areas of the lungs. The curve corresponding to the right lung is normal. It shows a period of washin, a phase of equilibrium, and a phase of washout (R). The curve corresponding to the cystic lesion in the left lung reveals continuous tracer accumulation, never reaching equilibrium. Again this suggests a one-way valve mechanism. Washout is also prolonged.

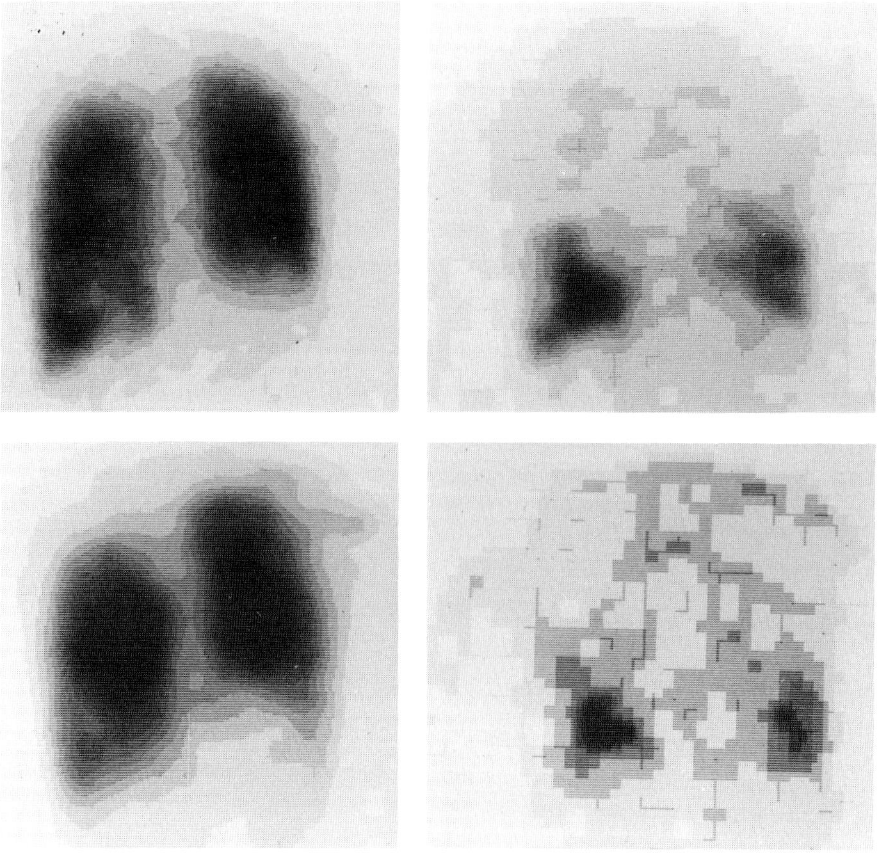

Figure 17-18. Large air blebs bilaterally in a 12-year-old female. *Top left:* Distribution of inhaled Xe-133 is irregular. There is a focal defect in the left lower lung field and another in the right lower lung field. *Top right:* Image 30 sec after rebreathing Xe-133 shows trapping of gas in both lower lung fields. *Bottom left:* Xe-133 perfusion image matches that of ventilation. *Bottom right:* Trapping in both lower lung fields.

When Xe-133 in saline is administered by intravenous injection, it will attain a more uniform distribution in the lung than that obtained with short rebreathing periods. Regions of airway obstruction may show perfusion with delayed washout. This pattern of delayed washin during inhalation and delayed washout after intravenous Xe-133 is characteristic of airway obstruction. In severe acute airway obstruction, trapping may be detected only after intravenous injection of Xe-133 because the inhaled gas may not reach the obstructed lung at all. Acute bronchial obstruction may be accompanied by pulmonary hypoperfusion, which is reversible. We have seen patients, however, in whom perfusion to the obstructed area is not affected (Fig. 17-19).

Mucous Plug

A mucous plug occluding a mainstem bronchus results in severe reduction of air flow to the lung involved (Fig. 17-20). Following removal of the mucous plug, ventilation usually returns to normal.[94,124] In addition, obstruction by a mucous plug results in secondary mild to severe reduction in regional blood flow. The mechanism by which abnormal ventilation causes diminished perfusion may be related to reduced oxygen in the alveoli rather than changes in air flow.[6] Xe-133 studies in mucous plug are similar to those found in aspiration of foreign objects. The involved region of lung typically shows reduced or absent ventilation during inhalation of Xe-133. Following intravenous Xe-

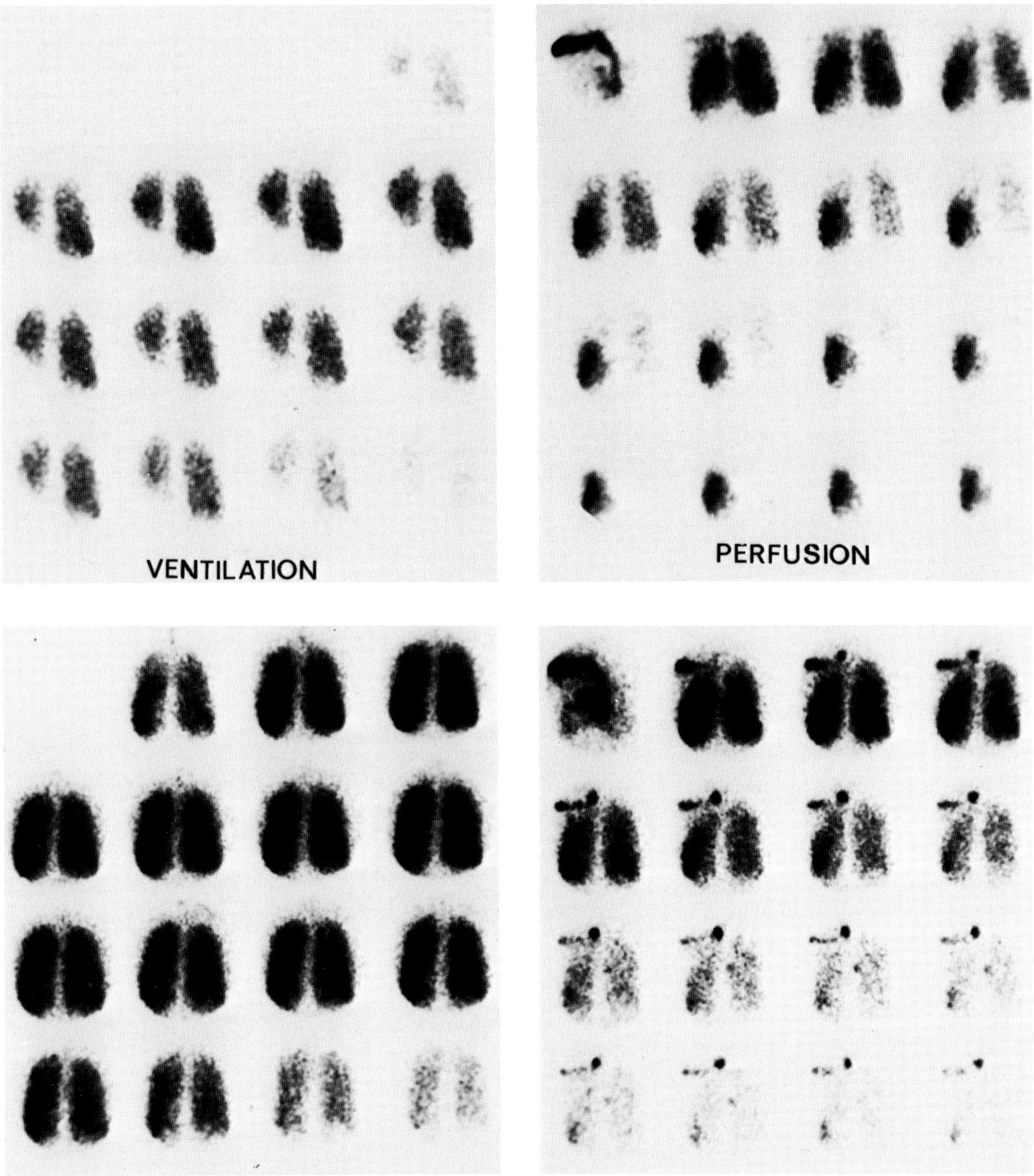

Figure 17-19. *Top:* Airway obstruction due to a foreign body. Xe-133 images during rebreathing of the tracer. Each image represents 5 sec. Ventilation is absent to the left lower lung field, probably the entire left lower lobe *(left)*. Perfusion, however, is normal in both lungs. Significant trapping of radioxenon is seen in the left lower lung field. This is diagnostic of airway obstruction *(right)*. *Bottom:* A followup study on the same patient 20 days later showing almost complete restoration of ventilation to the left lower lobe. Only minimal trapping of Xe-133 is present.

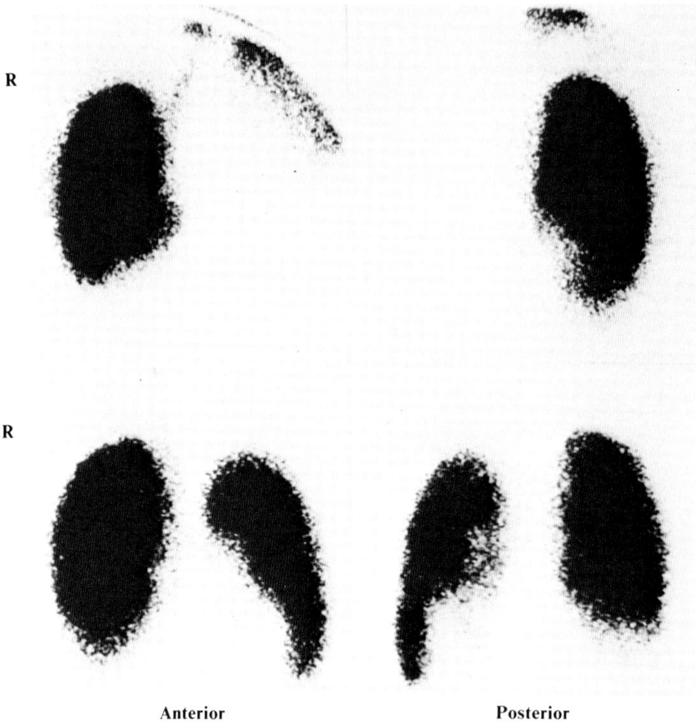

Figure 17-20. Complete airway obstruction to the left lung. Anterior view of a Kr-81m study showing no ventilation to the entire left lung. This was thought to be due to a mucus plug. A followup study 2 months later reveals restoration of ventilation to the left lung, with some alteration of ventilation of the right lower lung field. This patient had a history of repeated pulmonary infections. R, right.

133 in saline, the affected region of lung may reveal normal, reduced, or even absent pulmonary blood flow followed by air trapping in the same region.

Congenital Lobar Emphysema

Congenital lobar emphysema (congenital segmental lobar emphysema, emphysema of infancy, or congenital segmental bronchomalacia) exists in several forms and probably has several etiologies although the precise cause or causes are unknown. Patients with congenital lobar emphysema present with early onset of respiratory distress. About 80% have symptoms within the first 6 months of age, but the disorder has been discovered as late as 8 years of age.[126] Sometimes the abnormality is recognized incidentally on roentgenograms of the chest obtained for other reasons. Approximately 10–30% of the patients are found to have associated cardiovascular abnormalities such as ventricular septal defect or patent ductus arteriosus. The male-to-female ratio is 2:1.

Radiologically, overaeration of the lobe can be seen to cause compression of the adjacent lung, spreading of the ribs and mediastinal shift. The hyperlucent overdistended lobe may herniate across the midline. In the newborn infant, the overdistended lobe may be filled with fluid. Most commonly a single lobe is involved (50% left upper lobe, 25% right middle lobe, 20% right upper lobe, other lobes less frequently). Histologically there are overdistended alveoli with minimal or no interstitial involvement and an increased number of normal sized alveoli (polyalveolar lobe with emphysema).[67] Xe-133 studies show reduced or absent pulmonary blood flow and trapping of gas in the affected region of the lung (Fig. 17-21).

Pneumonia

In acute pneumonia, regional ventilation and perfusion may be affected. Ventilation is usually reduced to a greater degree than perfusion, resulting in a low ventilation perfusion ratio.

During recovery, residual trapping of Xe-133 is common in the areas previously affected even in the presence of a normal roentgenogram of the chest(Fig. 17-22).[80] With time, and providing there are no complications, normal regional lung function is eventually restored. Xe-133 studies are very sensitive to alterations in regional lung function due to infection.

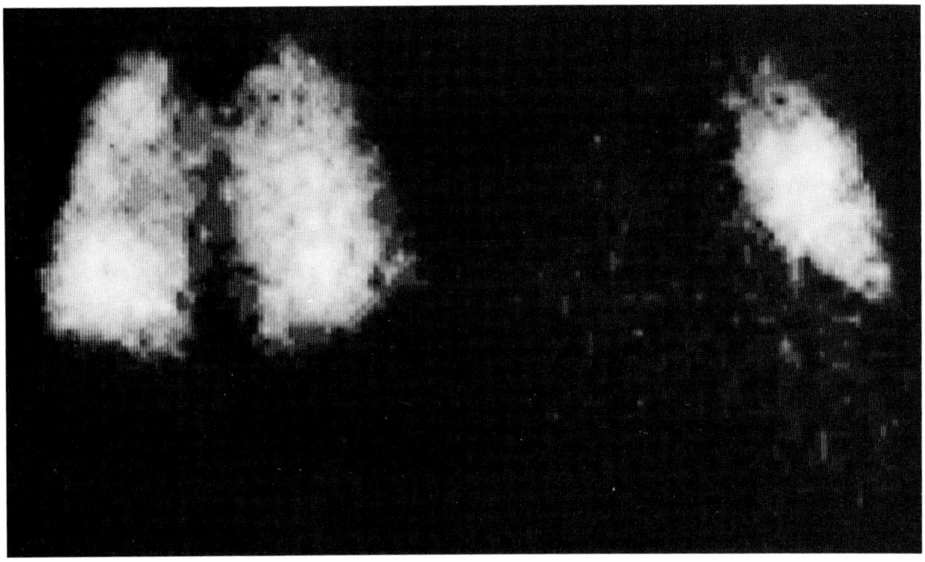

Figure 17-21. Congenital lobar emphysema. Image of perfusion *(left)* after intravenous administration of Xe-133 in saline showing apparent symmetric distribution of pulmonary blood flow. Thirty seconds after the arrival of Xe-133 in the lungs an area of marked trapping of the gas is seen. This corresponds to an hyperlucent right middle lobe which was seen on a radiograph of the chest.

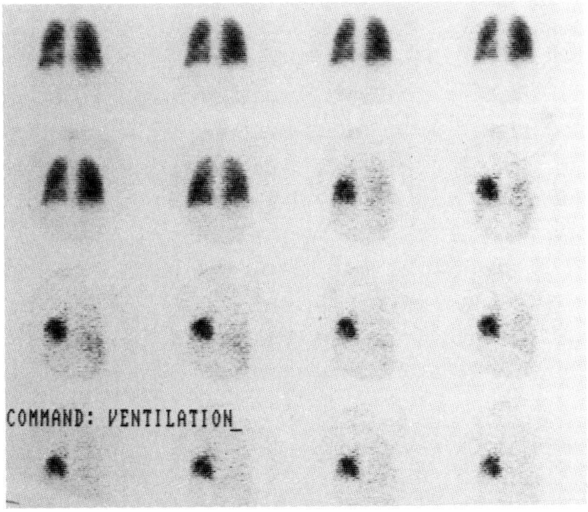

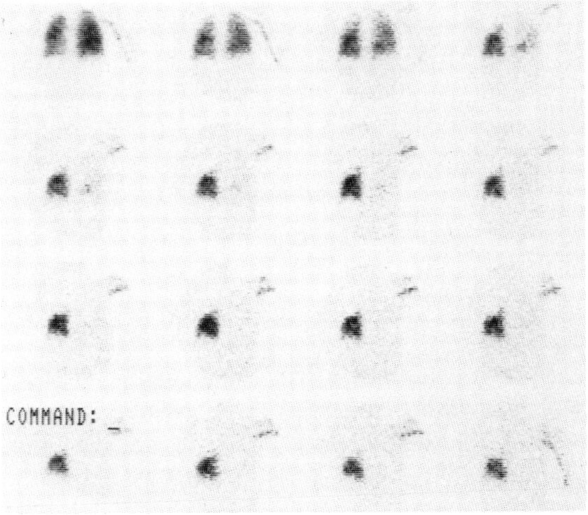

Figure 17-22. Residual trapping of air after pneumonia. Xe-133 study; each frame represents 5 sec. This is a study obtained on a 9 year-old female with a history of recurrent respiratory infections. At the time of this study the radiograph of the chest was normal. The ventilation phase of the study *(left)* shows reduced washin and washout of Xe-133 from the left lower lung field. The perfusion phase of the study, after intravenous injection of Xe-133 in saline *(right)*, reveals reduced perfusion to the left lower lung field with trapping of the radioxenon.

Pulmonary Embolism

In pulmonary emboli there is partial or total occlusion of the pulmonary vascular bed that may or may not be accompanied by pulmonary infarction. Arterial thrombi occur most frequently in association with a damaged vessel wall. Venous thrombi occur in association with reduced blood flow in the absence of a vascular lesion. Platelets are an important factor in arterial thrombosis while components of the intrinsic plasma clotting mechanism are involved in venous thrombosis.[23]

Pulmonary embolism remains one of the most common and difficult problems in medicine. It is more common in adults, with about 10% of all emboli occurring in the pediatric population.[72] Necropsy studies reveal that about 50% of patients who die of pulmonary embolism are not diagnosed before death.[54] The incidence of symptomatic pulmonary embolism in the United States is about 650,000 cases per year. Of these about 38% are fatal. The mortality is far greater in those patients in whom the diagnosis is not made.[13]

Emery[37] reported an incidence of pulmonary embolism in infants and toddlers of 1.25%. Jones and Sabiston[73] reported an incidence of pulmonary embolism at autopsy in children < 16 years of age of 0.70%. In another review of autopsies in children, Buck and coworkers found an incidence of pulmonary embolism of about 4.0% in patients from 0 to 19 years of age.[21] In that series, patients with known tumor emboli, fat emboli, or foreign material and those thought to have pulmonary thrombosis were not included.

Venous thromboses have been found in about 40% of patients with pulmonary emboli and were located, in order of frequency, in the heart, superior vena cava, mesenteric veins, brain, ileofemoral veins, inferior vena cava, and lower and upper extremities. In about 30% of these patients with pulmonary embolism it was thought to contribute to the patient's death.[21] In the remaining 70% of these patients, pulmonary embolism did not have a demonstrable effect on the clinical course, or was thought to be an incidental finding at autopsy.

Buck et al. state (and we agree) that pulmonary embolism in children is underdiagnosed and that an increased use of the perfusion lung scan should be encouraged.[21] Only about half (17 of 36) of their patients in whom pulmonary embolism was thought at autopsy to have had clinical importance had signs and symptoms usually attributable to pulmonary embolism. Pulmonary embolism was suspected clinically in only 5 of the 17 patients, and only two were on anticoagulant therapy at the time of death. There was no apparent age effect in the incidence of pulmonary embolism although infants made up 25% of the patients in this series. The risk of developing pulmonary embolism in children after operation was more than twice as great as in nonsurgical patients.

Pulmonary embolism has also been found as a complication of legally induced abortions.[79] Other causes include oral contraceptives, infected arteriovenous shunts, fat, and air.[55,122] Fat emboli may occur after bone fractures or after bone orthopedic procedures.[20,56,103] Central venous catheters used for hyperalimentation put a patient at risk of developing pulmonary emboli due to the chronic venous trauma and the thrombolic effect of the catheter.[47,107,141] Pulmonary embolism during cardiac catheterization may be caused by detachment of synthetic fibers from nondisposable catheters.[129] Heart disease is a major factor associated with pulmonary emboli in children and adults.[14,27] Victims of accidental trauma, especially those with fractures of the hip or pelvis, have a 15% incidence of pulmonary embolism.[118] Septic emboli may originate from any infectious focus. Young drug addicts may present with septic pulmonary emboli. In sickle-cell disease, microthrombosis frequently results in infarction of the lung, spleen, kidney, and bone, but medically important pulmonary embolism in these patients is rare. In polycythemia, increased blood viscosity and vascular stasis lead to thrombosis.[138] Pulmonary embolism may result from birth injury that dislodges cerebral or cerebellar tissue.[17,111,128]

Homocystinuria, an inborn error of metabolism, is characterized by the absence of cystathionine synthetase in several body tissues. In patients affected with this disorder, platelet abnormalities are believed to cause thrombosis. Also, homocystine may induce vascular endothelial damage that facilitates platelet plug formation and thrombosis.[63]

Pulmonary embolism may present acutely as an overwhelming catastrophic disease or insidiously as a chronic cardiopulmonary problem or a fever of unknown orign. It may occur in previously healthy individuals or those with a chronic or acute illness. The clinical presentation of pulmonary embolism varies. Commonly it suggests congestive heart failure or pneumonia, or less frequently myocardial infarction, chronic obstructive lung disease, or pleurisy. Hemoptysis and fever may be present in subacute cases. There is frequently tachypnea or dyspnea and elevation of jugular venous pressure.[14,41,119] Other signs and symptoms found in pulmonary embolism include cough, wheezing, rales, sweats, palpitations, nausea, vomiting, chills, syncope, tachycardia, phlebitis, edema, murmur, and cyanosis. A pleural friction rub is common. Hepatomegaly and occasionally splenomegaly may be present. None of these signs and symptoms are specific for or establish the diagnosis of pulmonary embolism.

Resolution of pulmonary embolism occurs principally by fibrinolysis. This mechanism can result in resolution within as little as 1 day. More commonly, restoration of pulmonary blood flow after pulmonary embolism takes a few days or even a few weeks. In young patients, resolution of pulmonary embolism is more rapid than in older patients.[95] Arterial blood oxygen is frequently but not always reduced in pulmonary embolism. Therefore, the presence of normal blood gases does not exclude the diagnosis of pulmonary embolism. Serum enzyme determinations (lactic dehydrogenase, LDH; aspartate aminotransferase, SGOT) are of limited or minimal value, and blood coagulation tests are not useful. Erythrocyte sedimentation rate is elevated in about 40% of the patients. The electrocardiogram may demonstrate right ventricular strain but the test has no specific value. The electrocardiogram is abnormal in the majority of patients with massive or submassive pulmonary embolism.

The signs of pulmonary embolism on radiographs of the chest are variable and nonspecific (elevated hemidiaphragm, pleural effusion, infiltrate or consolidation, atelectasis, changes in pulmonary vessels). Radiographs of the chest may show increased density in the area involved. Pleural effusion is found in most patients with pulmonary embolism. Many patients with proven pulmonary embolism have normal radiographs of the chest.[104]

Pulmonary function tests may be normal or abnormal and have limited value in the diagnosis of pulmonary embolism. Pulmonary emboli result in vasoconstriction and bronchoconstriction. These changes in turn lead to ventilation-perfusion abnormalities. Hemodynamic studies reveal a reduction in systemic pressure with an increase in pulmonary artery pressure, but such studies are usually done at the time of pulmonary angiography.

Pulmonary scintigraphy using Tc-99m MAA provides a simple, safe, sensitive, and precise method to evaluate pulmonary artery perfusion. Any disorder that affects pulmonary blood flow, including pulmonary embolism, will cause an abnormal perfusion scan.[76] In pulmonary embolism, perfusion defects may be single or multiple and follow a segmental or subsegmental distribution. An entire lobe of lung may be affected. In a patient suspected of acute pulmonary embolism with a perfusion defect on scintigraphy and a normal radiograph of the chest, the probability of pulmonary embolism is high (Figs. 17-23–17-26).

The addition of ventilation studies using radioactive gases in some cases assist further in the diagnosis of pulmonary embolism. In many patients with pulmonary embolism, ventilation will be preserved in the area of the lung affected. It is important to remember, however, that processes affecting the ventilatory areas first may affect the vascular network and produce a reduction in blood flow. Conversely lesions that affect the pulmonary vasculature first can compromise the ventilatory spaces. Atelectasis causes a defect in perfusion and ventilation. Emphysema, chronic obstructive lung disease, or bronchitis may compromise the vascular network of the lung and disrupt blood flow. Infectious diseases of the lung invade both ventilatory and vascular spaces. Although it is believed that pulmonary embolism is characterized by ventilation/perfusion mismatch, it can also cause ventilation/perfusion match.[39,77,89,96] Kim and DeLand[78] found V/Q mismatch in pulmonary embolism in two children with histoplasmosis.

Pulmonary angiography continues to be the most specific and precise test for the diagnosis of pulmonary embolism. With this method the hemodynamics and cardiac function can be measured simultaneously. Unfortunately, the procedure is invasive and expensive and carries a definite risk. The decision to perform arteriography is arrived at after careful analysis of the clinical situation, physical examination, radiography of the chest, radionuclide scan, and therapeutic considerations.

Pulmonary scintigraphy is a very useful method to determine the presence of lung disease and should be carried out every time a patient is suspected of having pulmonary embolism. A normal

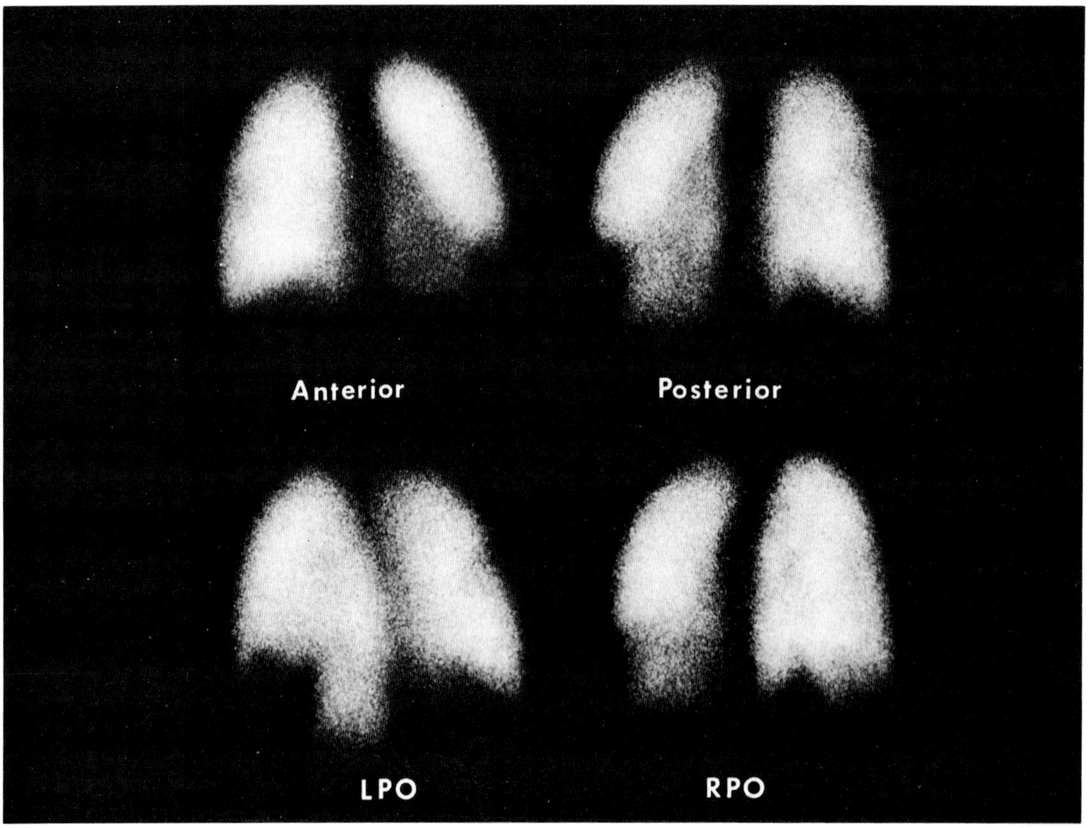

Figure 17-23. Pulmonary embolism. Tc-99m macroaggregated lung scan from a 10-year-old male who developed progressive pain in one of his legs for 1 day followed by respiratory distress. The scintiscan reveals a perfusion defect in the lateral posterior segment of the left lower lobe and another in the medial basal segment of the right lower lobe.

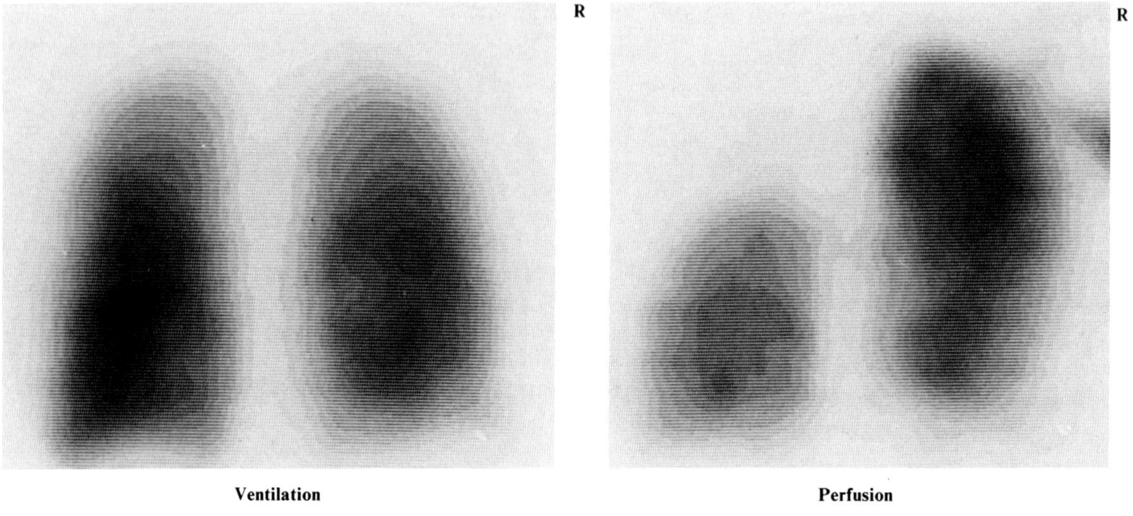

Figure 17-24. Pulmonary embolism. Massive perfusion defect in the left upper lung field with preserved ventilation. Selected images from a Xe-133 ventilation-perfusion study.

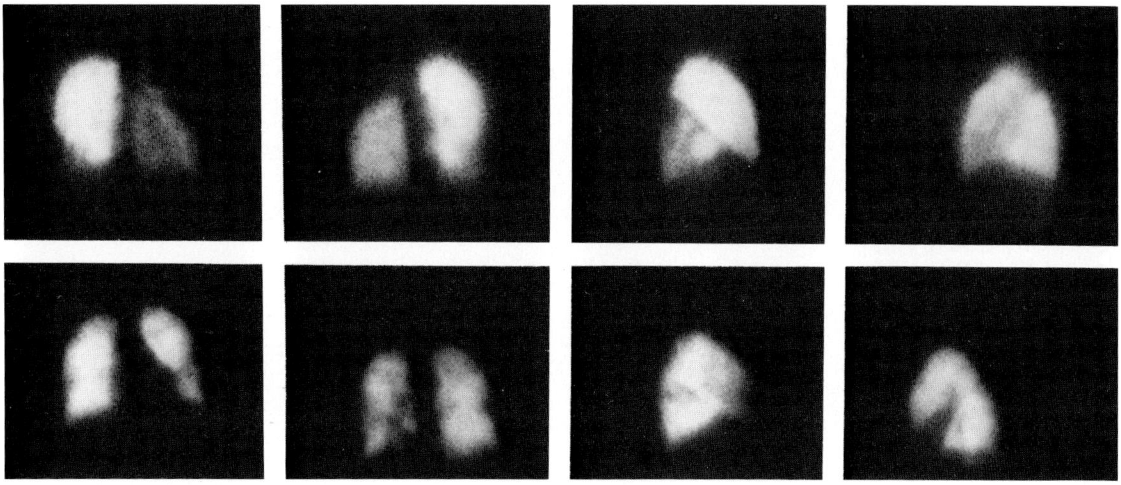

Figure 17-25. Pulmonary embolism. Tc-99m MAA lung scan. Large perfusion defects in various parts of both lungs. *Top:* Initial study (anterior, posterior, right and left lateral views). *Bottom:* Followup study 2 weeks later. One can observe partial recovery of the perfusion defects with time in this young patient who was treated with streptokinase.

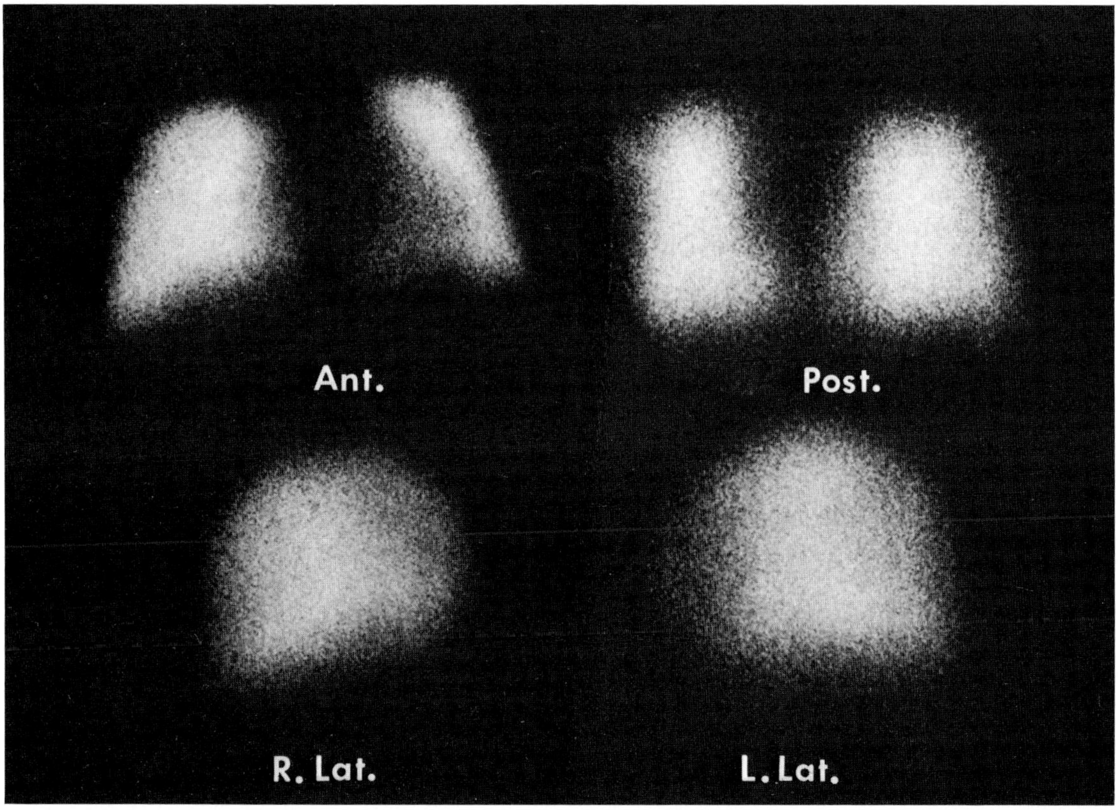

Figure 17-26. Fat embolism. Tc-99m macroaggregated albumin scan showing no evidence of perfusion defect(s) in spite of this patient having massive fat embolism which was the apparent cause of his death. The patient had severe scoliosis.

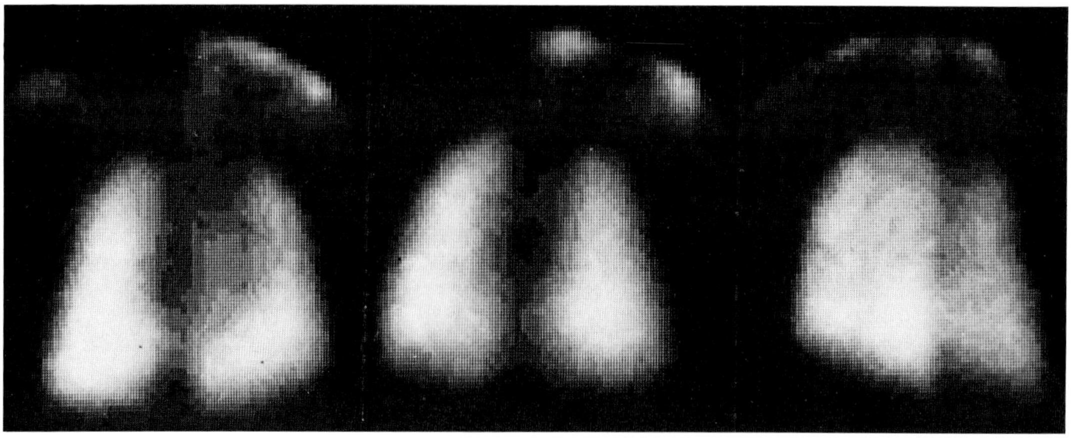

Figure 17-27. Asthma. Series of images of the lungs obtained during rebreathing of Kr-81m. There is irregular distribution of the tracer, seen particularly on the right and left posterior oblique projections. *Left:* left posterior oblique projection; *center:* posterior projection; *right:* right posterior oblique projection. This patient was wheezing during the examination.

lung scan essentially excludes pulmonary embolism. A lung scan with medium-to-low probability of pulmonary embolism is usually followed by a pulmonary angiogram. If perfusion lung scanning is highly suggetive of pulmonary embolism, pulmonary angiography is not indicated and the patient can be treated with heparin or given a thrombolytic agent. In some patients with significant preexisting pulmonary pathology, angiography should be done, perhaps without a prior radionuclide scan.

Asthma

In patients with bronchial asthma during remission, the MAA scans show normal or markedly improved perfusion.[102] Macroaggregated lung scanning during acute asthmatic attacks reveal focal perfusion abnormalities (Fig. 17-27). Regional ventilation becomes increasingly abnormal as symptoms increase but are reversible with treatment. Perfusion usually decreases in the area of decreased ventilation but the degree of change is not as great.[114,145]

Xe-133 distribution indices for ventilation and perfusion in asthmatic patients in remission generally agree with findings in normal subjects. In some asthmatic patients in remission, however, there are slight residual regional irregularities on the ventilation studies. Such ventilatory abnormalities do not seem to be accompanied by a significant alteration in perfusion.[15]

Bronchopulmonary Dysplasia

Bronchopulmonary dysplasia is a form of chronic lung diease that occurs in infants treated for prolonged periods of time with mechanical ventilation and oxygen. Bronchopulmonary dysplasia occurs most commonly in premature infants who require mechanical ventilation for hyaline membrane disease. It is rare in infants of advanced gestational age. In recent years, oxygen concentrations of more than 40% are frequently used for more than 4–6 days so that bronchopulmonary dysplasia is by far the most commonly encountered complication in these infants. Northway et al. divided bronchopulmonary dysplasia into four stages with distinct clinical, histologic, and radiographic findings.[108]

An infant is considered to have bronchopulmonary dysplasia when the following criteria are met: a requirement for ventilation with positive pressure during the first week of life and for a minimum of 3 days; clinical evidence of chronic respiratory disease (tachypnea, intercostal and subcostal retraction, and rales) persisting beyond 30 days of age; and arterial blood gas abnormalities for more than 30 days of age necessitating supplemental oxygen to maintain a PO_2 greater than 60 mm Hg or a PCO_2 greater than 45 mm Hg.

While the precise etiology of bronchopulmonary dysplasia is not known, it is likely that disease results from pulmonary immaturity combined with one or more of the following factors.

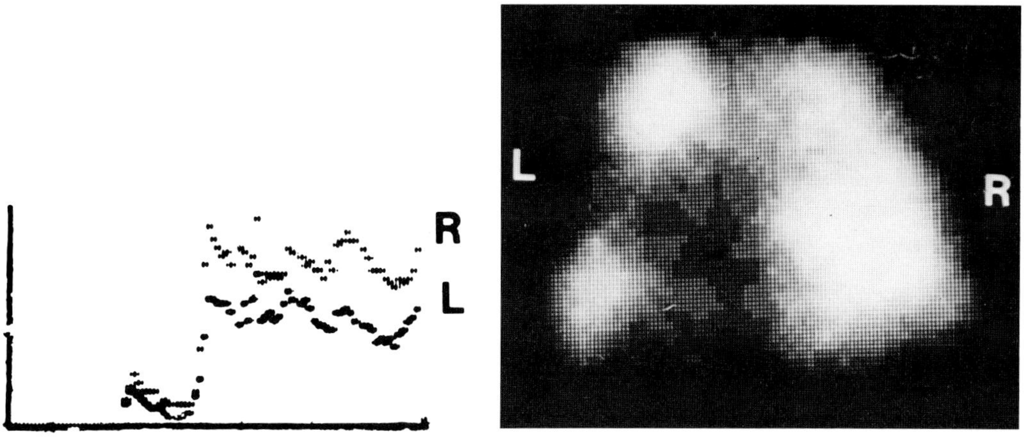

Figure 17-28. Bronchopulmonary dysplasia. Kr-81m study from a 1-month-old baby with pulmonary dysplasia. The right lung shows uniform ventilation; however, the left lung reveals decreased and irregular distribution of the tracer.

Oxygen

Breathing oxygen in high concentration is toxic to the lungs and causes edema and alveolar thickening. Prolonged exposure results in epithelial necrosis, hemorrhage and interstitial fibrosis.[33,75,113] The lack in premature infants of the antioxidant enzyme superoxidase dismutase may increase the patient's susceptibility to oxygen toxicity.[115]

Mechanical Ventilation

Ventilation with positive pressure is a likely contributor to the development of bronchopulmonary dysplasia.[127] The use of positive end-espiratory pressure results in pneumothorax and pulmonary interstitial emphysema during the acute course of hyaline membrane disease.[16]

Patent Ductus Arteriosus

Patent ductus arteriosus producing congestive heart failure increases the incidence of bronchopulmonary dysplasia.[18]

Fluid Overload

A high rate of intravenous fluid administration has been associated with development of bronchopulmonary dysplasia.[19]

Premature infants who require constant positive pressure with mechanical ventilation are at high risk for development of bronchopulmonary dysplasia. The patient exhibits tachypnea, interstitial retraction and rales. Congestive heart failure with hepatomegaly, and cyanosis are present.

Radiographs of the chest reveal various degrees of abnormality. Initially there is interstitial emphysema that appears as small radiolucent bubbles or streaks in an interstitial pattern. Later on, the radiologic appearance is one of white out lung with diffuse bilateral opacification. As the condition progresses, there is extensive disruption of pulmonary parenchyma with hyperinflation, bilateral cystic appearance and coarse interstitial markings. Left-to-right shunting and congestive heart failure result in cardiomegaly and hepatomegaly.

The electrocardiogram reveals right ventricular strain. Echocardiography helps in evaluating cardiac anomalies often associated with bronchopulmonary dysplasia or in demonstrating right and left ventricular hypertrophy.

Radionuclide angiocardiography assists in assessing the magnitude of left-to-right shunting through a patent ductus arteriosus.[134]

Xe-133 or Kr-81m studies in infants with bronchopulmonary dysplasia reveal diffuse or multifocal abnormal distribution of ventilation and perfusion (Fig. 17-28). Evidence of air trapping is common.

Long-term studies of patients with bronchopulmonary dysplasia between 1 and 5 years of age show persistent alterations of global and/or regional lung function[64] (Fig. 17-29).

In the case of the Wilson-Mikity lung, there is

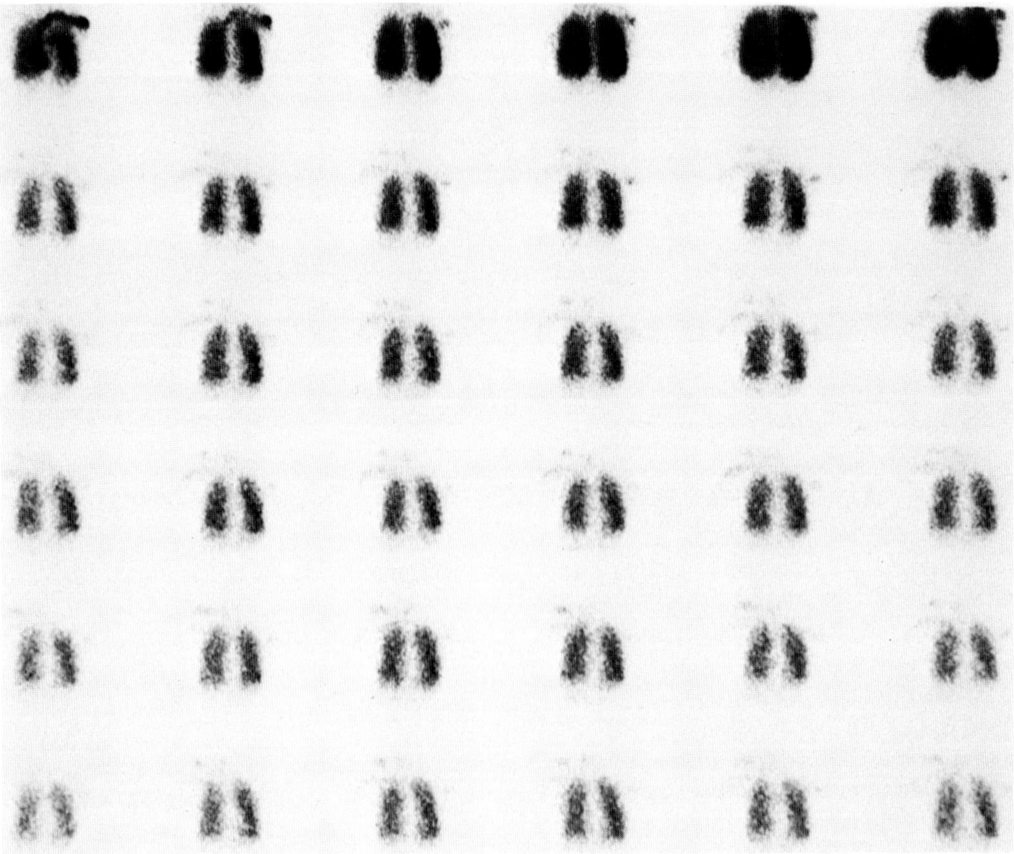

Figure 17-29. Bronchopulmonary dysplasia 5 years later. Series of 5-sec images after intravenous injection of Xe-133 in saline. There is irregular distribution of pulmonary blood flow and marked and diffuse trapping of gas.

fine collagenization and elastosis of structured portions of the lobule.[144] The areas of hyperaeration and atelectasis follow lobular or subsegmental patterns. These infants generally do not develop cor pulmonale although some minor hypertrophy of fetal arterioles may be present. This condition is not usually preceded by respiratory distress syndrome, and it appears after a longer interval of time than bronchopulmonary dysplasia (4–6 weeks of age).[7,59,144]

Neonatal Interstitial Emphysema

Intensive ventilatory treatment in premature infants with respiratory failure may become complicated by persistent interstitial emphysema involving one lobe or an entire lung. A suggested mechanism is alveolar rupture followed by dissection and entrapment of air in the pulmonary interstitium.[49,62,86,92,93,125] It is generally assumed that the overexpanded lobe has no functional value and that it compromises adjacent lung tissue causing alteration of respiratory function. Leonidas et al. found ventilation-perfusion scans useful in the assessment of neonatal emphysema.[86,87] The scintigraphic findings on Xe-133 studies are those of airway obstruction: reduced perfusion accompanied by trapping of gas in the affected lung region.

Bronchiectasis

Vandevivere et al. compared chest radiographs, Tc-99m MAA perfusion scans, and Kr-81m ventilation lung scans with bronchography in patients with bronchiectasis. They found a 73% sensitivity and 76% specificity for radiographs of the chest. For lung scintigraphy, the sensitivity was 92% and the specificity 60%. In this study, about 40% of the

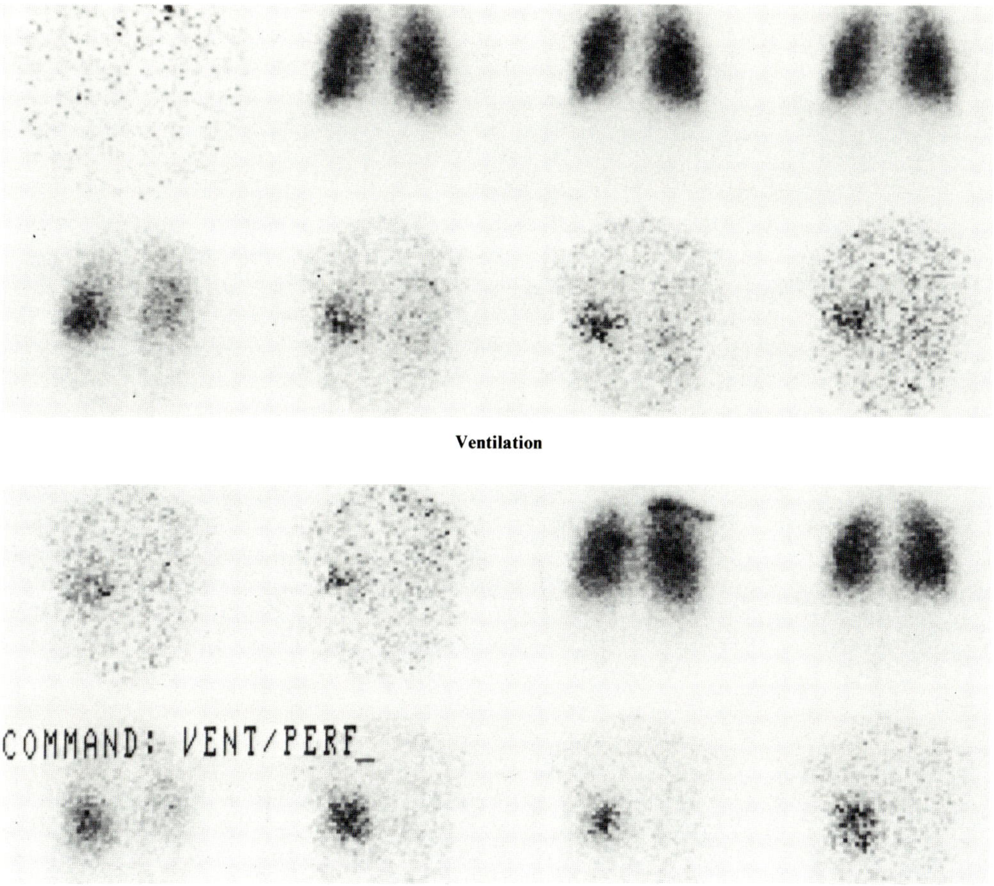

Perfusion

Figure 17-30. Bronchiectasis. Xe-133 study shows trapping of gas in the left lower lung field, both after inhalation *(top)* and perfusion *(bottom)* of the radiotracer. This patient had repeated respiratory infections and on the radiograph of the chest there was uncertainty whether or not there was bronchiectasis.

bronchograms performed might have been avoided on the basis of a normal chest radiograph and lung scintiscan.[136] The combination of pulmonary scintigraphy and chest radiography thus provides excellent screening when a decision on the advisability of bronchography is being made in children (Fig. 17-30).

Congenital Diaphragmatic Hernia

Herniation of intraabdominal organs through the diaphragm is much more common in the left hemidiaphragm (Bochdalek hernia). Diaphragmatic hernia results in hypoplasia of the ipsilateral lung with a reduction in the lung volume as well as in the number of airways and pulmonary arteries.

Wohl et al.[149] in our institution studied 19 patients after repair of congenital diaphragmatic hernia. Their total lung capacity and vital capacity averaged 99% of predicted value. Forced expiratory volume in one second averaged 89% of predicted. Maximum expiratory flow volumes were normal. Lung volume was equally distributed in the two lungs. Ventilation to the ipsilateral lung was reduced in two of nine patients. Blood flow to the affected lung was reduced on all patients studied. These findings are consistent with persistence of a reduced number of branches or generations of pulmonary arteries and bronchi on the side of the hernia. Since a substantial part of the vascular resistance resides in the peripheral vessels, this developmental abnormality influences the distribution of pulmonary blood flow even though it has little effect on tests reflecting airway resistance or the distribution of ventilation.[149]

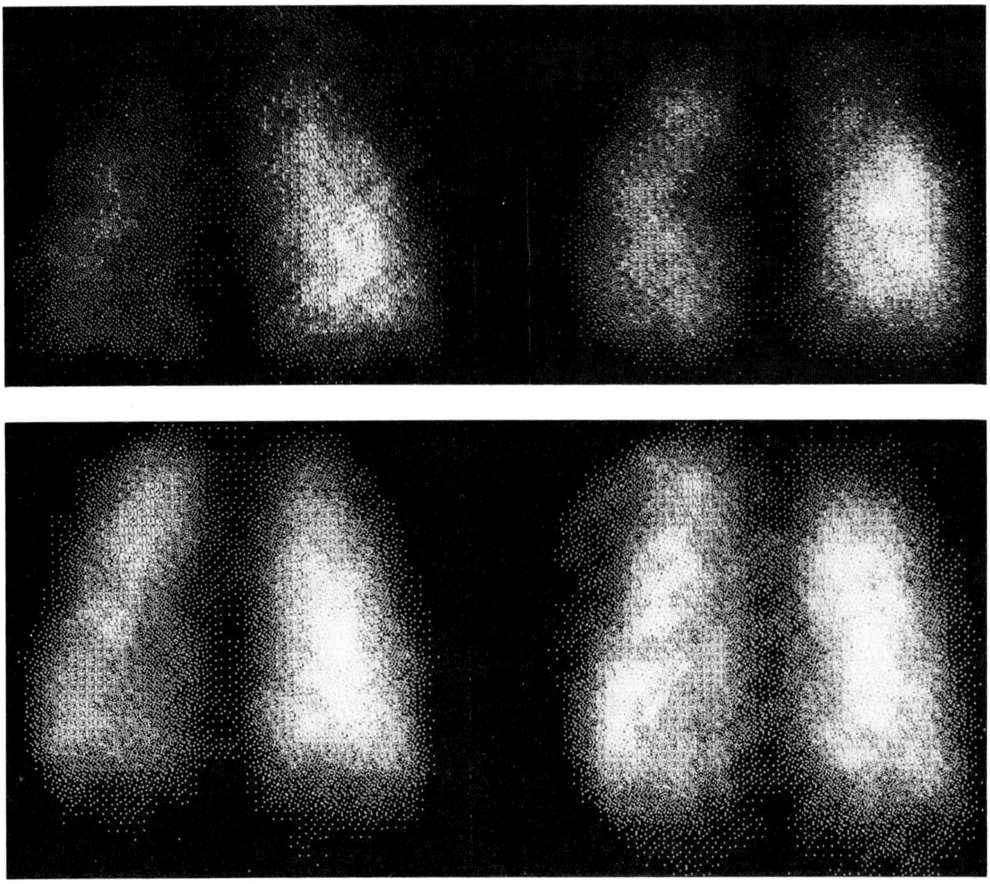

Figure 17-31. Pectus excavatum. Xe-133 pre- and postoperative studies from a 4-year-old female with pectus excavatum. *Top:* The preoperative study reveals imbalance in the distribution of ventilation *(left)* (left lung = 32%; right lung = 68%) and perfusion *(right)* (left lung = 44%; right lung = 56%). *Bottom:* The postoperative study reveals an improvement in the distribution of ventilation *(left)* (left lung = 44%; right lung = 56%) and perfusion (*right)* (right lung = 50%; left lung = 50%).

Pectus Excavatum

Patients with pectus excavatum frequently exhibit ventilation and perfusion imbalance between the right and left lungs. Most commonly, the left lung shows a reduction in ventilation and a greater reduction in perfusion. Commonly, ventilation/perfusion ratios in each lung are either high or low before surgery. Postoperative evaluation of these patients shows a tendency toward a more even distribution of lung function (Fig. 17-31). The effect of exercise on the ventilation/perfusion distribution in these patients has not been evaluated.

Scoliosis

Scoliosis may cause alveolar hypoventilation and hypoxemia followed by progressive cardiopulmonary failure. The distribution of perfusion and ventilation improves in the supine position when the spinal curvature is diminshed. Abnormal ventilation occurs primarily on the concave side of the spine.[121]

Bronchopulmonary Sequestration

Bronchopulmonary sequestration is part of a wide spectrum of bronchopulmonary developmental abnormalities resulting from abnormal bronchial vascular supply and drainage of normal, hypoplastic or dysplastic segments of the lung. This uncommon disorder enters in the differential diagnosis of certain intrathoracic masses. It is usually asymptomatic and is often discovered by chance when a chest radiograph is obtained for other reasons. When se-

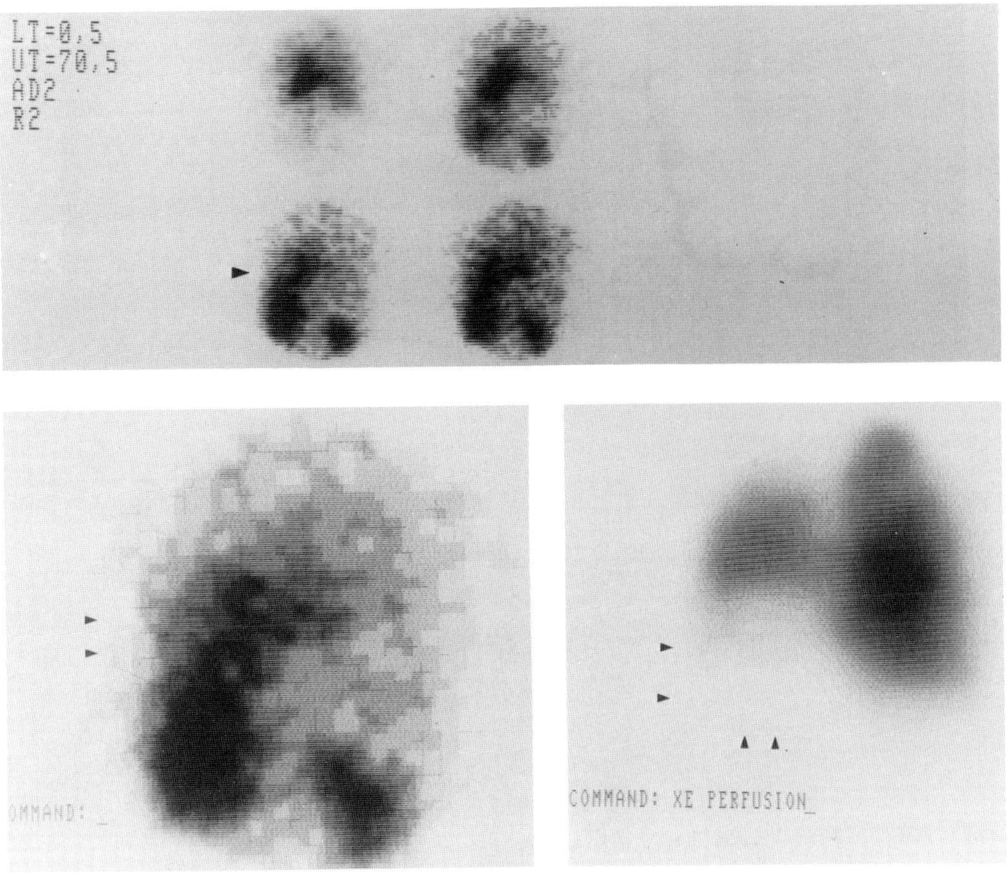

Figure 17-32. Bronchopulmonary sequestration. *Top:* Posterior Tc-99m radionuclide angiocardiogram. Selected images during the systemic phase. Each frame represents 1.5 sec. On the third image there is a faint blush of activity in the left lower lung *(arrow)*. *Bottom left:* The same image is magnified to demonstrate the systemic perfusion of the left lower lung field on the Tc-99m angiogram *(arrows)*. *Bottom right:* Posterior Xe-133 image of the pulmonary perfusion showing lack of pulmonary blood flow to the left lower lung field *(arrows)*.

questration is symptomatic, it manifests itself by repeated episodes of pneumonia or atelectasis. About two-thirds of the reported cases involve the left lower lobe. Systemic blood supply may arise from the descending thoracic aorta or the abdominal aorta in bronchopulmonary sequestration[46] (Fig. 17-32). In one report of the radionuclide angiographic findings in five patients with bronchopulmonary sequestration, the sequestered lobe did not perfuse during the pulmonary phase: it was supplied by the systemic circulation in all patients.[57]

Bronchopulmonary sequestration may be classified as intra or extralobar. The extralobar type involves an ectopic lobe of the lung situated above or below the diaphragm and enclosed in its own visceral pleura. The intralobar type involves malformation of a perfused, but often unventilated, lung segment sequestered within the normal lung without its own visceral pleura. In addition, the sequestered lobe or segment may not communicate with the tracheobronchial tree.

Radiation Therapy

After radiation therapy to the mediastinum or pulmonary parenchyma, there are marked alterations in regional lung function. Generally, perfusion seems to be more severely affected than ventilation in the areas of irradiated lung. Complications of radiation therapy to the chest include radiation pneumonitis, milder forms of restrictive lung disease, constrictive pericarditis, and growth retardation of the spine, ribs, sternum, and clavicle.

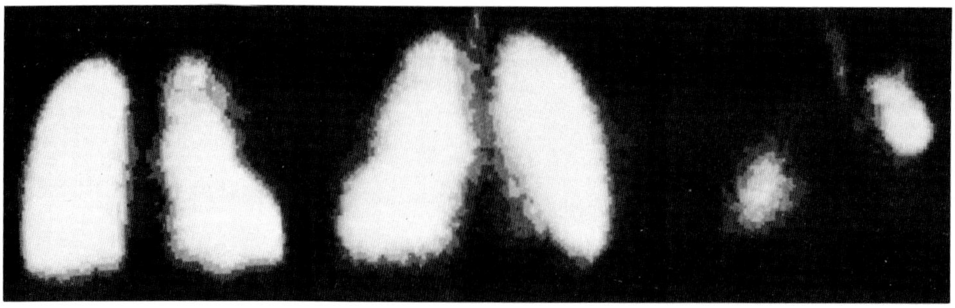

Figure 17-33. Changes in the distribution of air in the lung during normal and forced breathing. Kr-81m study from a girl with recurrent respiratory infections. She had a stridor during forced breathing. The image during tidal breathing reveals irregular distribution of gas within the lungs, particularly along the periphery of the left lung, but also in the lower and medial aspects of the right lower lung field *(center)*. The distribution of a forced, single deep inspiration is very anomalous showing preferential flow of air to two rather localized regions in each lung field *(right)*. Assessment of regional pulmonary blood flow also shows abnormal distribution, particularly along the periphery of the right lung field *(left)*.

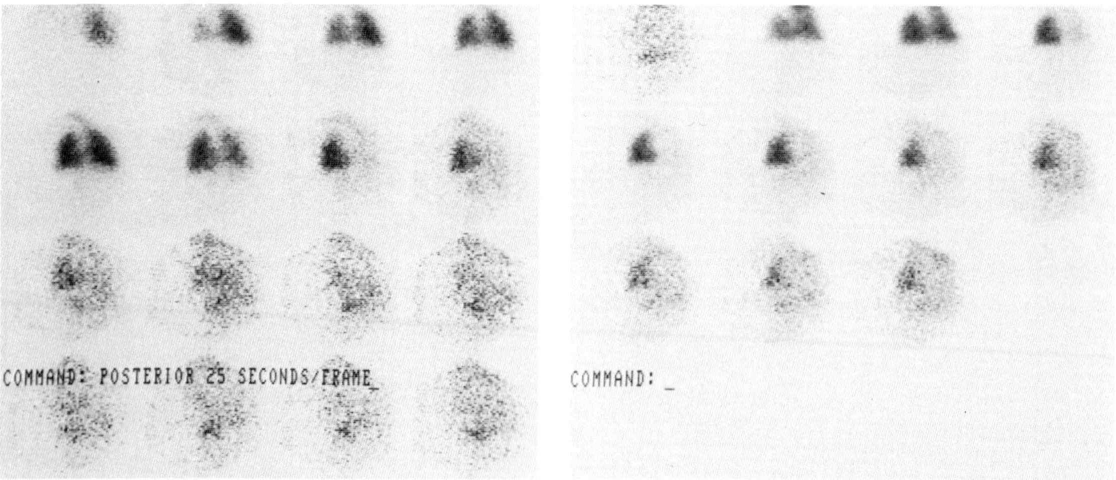

Figure 17-34. Thracheal compression due to a bronchogenic cyst in a 5-month-old male. This patient presented with wheezing. Xe-133 study; each frame represents 5 sec. There is decrease in ventilation *(left)* and perfusion *(right)* to the left lung field with trapping of radioxenon due to partial airway compression.

Irradiation given during rapid lung growth affects the parenchyma and results in smaller lungs and chest wall than predicted. There is also reduced lung volume and carbon monoxide diffusing capacity.[148]

Pulmonary Papillomatosis

Espinola et al.[40] studied three children with pulmonary papillomatosis using Xe-133 and Tc-99m microspheres. They observed different imaging patterns depending on the size, number, and distribution of the lesions. In early parenchymal involvement, a ventilation-perfusion imbalance was seen with relatively less perfusion than ventilation in the affected areas. Pulmonary scintigraphy in these patients was useful to evaluate ventilatory and perfusion impairment as well as the response to treatment.

Abnormalities of Airway Connective Tissues

When unexplained maldistribution of inhaled air in the lungs is present, one should consider disorders of the airways. Several disorders of the airways may cause air turbulence and secondary maldistri-

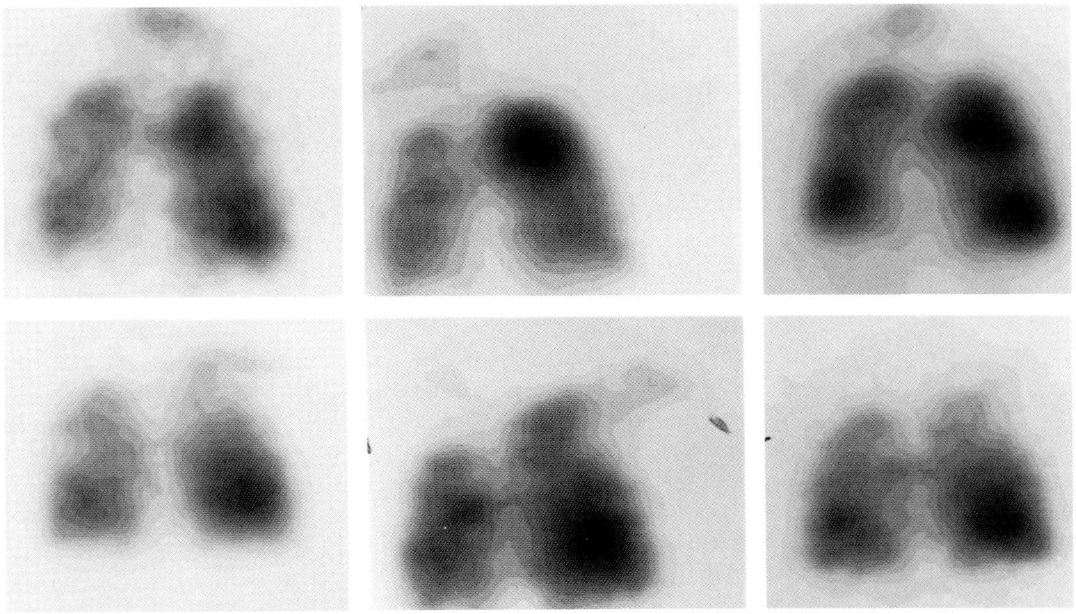

Figure 17-35. Pulmonary alveolar proteinosis. Three sequential Xe-133 ventilation *(top)* and perfusion *(bottom)* studies in a 2-year-old male with pulmonary alveolar proteinosis. The first study *(left)* obtained before bronchial lavage reveals gross maldistribution of ventilation and perfusion. The second study *(center)* shows changes in ventilation and perfusion 1 day following lavage. Finally the third study *(right)* shows further changes 1 month following lavage.

bution of radioactive gases within the lungs during tidal breathing and particularly during deep breathing (Fig. 17-33).

Tracheomalacia is caused by a weak or flaccid tracheal wall that allows excessive tracheal collapse during respiration. Tracheomalacia may be found after tracheostomy and prolonged use of endotracheal tubes, especially those with cuffed attachments. Other causes include mediastinal masses, vascular anomalies, tracheoesophageal fistula, and cutis laxa. Stridor is present in some of these patients (Fig. 17-34).

Children with laryngomalacia (infantile supraglottic hypermotility) often present with loud and stridorous breathing. During inspiration, the larynx collapses because the cartilages are not stiff enough to support the airway. Tracheal stenosis is a fixed narrowing of the trachea caused by external compression or intrinsic congenital or acquired lesions.

Pulmonary Alveolar Proteinosis

Pulmonary alveolar proteinosis is a syndrome of unknown etiology characterized by progressive dyspnea and cough. Most cases occur at older ages: the number of affected children and infants is small. The most striking histologic features are intraalveolar deposits of granular, eosinophilic, or proteinaceous material. On gross examination multiple, firm, gray or yellow nodules of various sizes are often located subpleurally throughout the lung. The bronchial tree appears normal, but there is evidence of alveolar wall damage.

The clinical picture is characterized by progressive dyspnea and cough. In children, productive cough with yellow sputum may be present. Cyanosis, fatigue, weight loss, and occasionally hemoptysis may be encountered. Chest radiographs show a fine, diffuse perihilar increase in lung density following a pattern similar to that of pulmonary edema without cardiac enlargement. The radiographic changes are due to the alveolar fluid. Occasionally, the pattern may be nodular in appearance.

The prognosis of pulmonary alveolar proteinosis is not favorable because the alveoli progressively fill and complicating infections are common. Variable changes in the distribution of ventilation and perfusion can be identified by Xe-133 pulmonary scintigraphy (Fig. 17-35).[29,91,112,116,146]

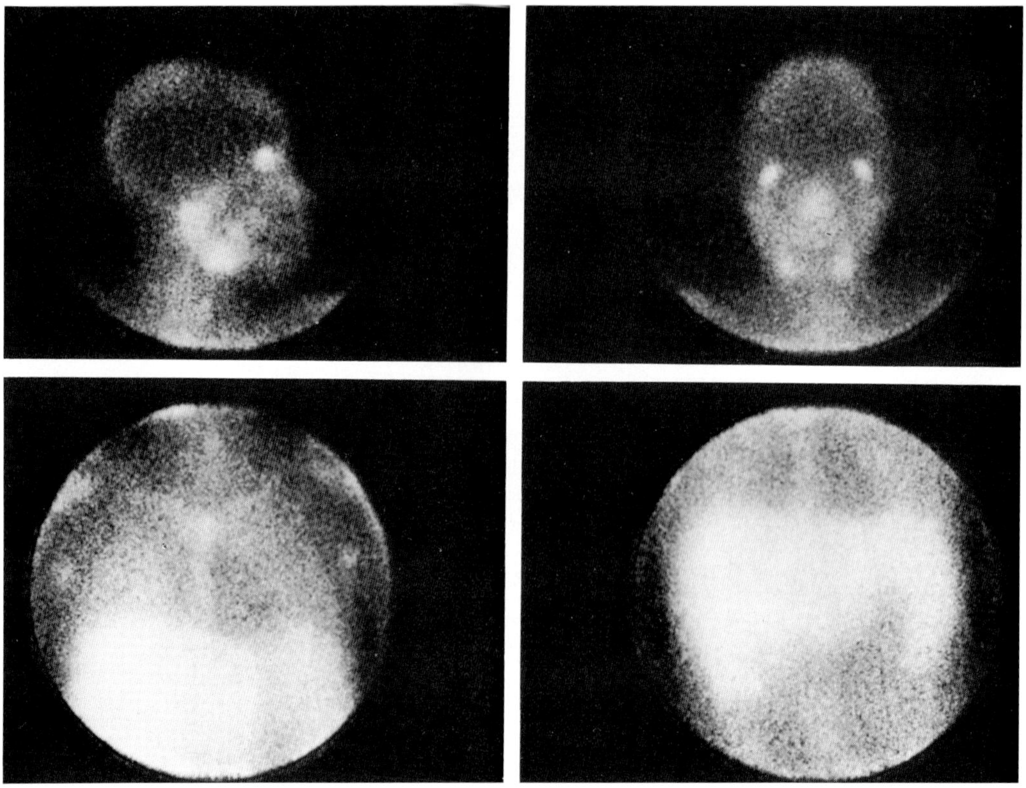

Figure 17-36. Sarcoidosis. Ga-67 scintiscan. There is increased uptake of the tracer diffusely in both lung fields. Other areas of increased uptake include the axillary lymph nodes, and salivary, and lacrimal glands.

Sarcoidosis

Sarcoidosis is a granulomatous disease of unknown origin that affects several systems in the body but most frequently affects the lungs, lymph nodes, eyes, skin, liver, and spleen. In sarcoidosis decreased and delayed hypersensitivity suggests impaired cell immunity as well as elevated or abnormal immunoglobulins. Histologically there is widespread noncaseating epitheloid granulomas in more than one organ. Dry cough, wheezing, pleuritic pain, and mild to moderate dyspnea are the symptoms of pulmonary sarcoidosis.

Most cases of sarcoidosis are found in adults between 20 and 40 years of age. The disease is occasionally seen in children, especially those between the ages of 9 and 15, and it has been described in infants as young as 2 months. Thoracic adenopathy has been found in most pediatric patients. Usually radiography of the chest reveals a mix of small irregular nodular shadows and fine linear densities diffusely scattered in the lungs. Rarely, sarcoidosis may exist with normal chest radiography.

About one-third of patients have discrete, painless lymphadenopathy. Uveitis, iritis, conjunctivitis, keratosis, retinitis, glaucoma, and involvement of the eyelids and lacrimal glands can be seen with this disease. Swelling of the parotid gland and induration can be seen also[26,71,97] (Fig. 17-36).

Gallium-67 citrate scintigraphy demonstrates areas of active sarcoidosis in the body and may be useful for assessing the extent and activity of the intrathoracic lesions. Serum lysozyme and angiotensin-converting enzyme measurements are usually helpful although normal values do not exclude activity and progression of pulmonary sarcoidosis.[3]

Klech et al. examined the value of several factors to assess activity in sarcoidosis. Ga-67 scintigraphy proved to be the most sensitive method (94%) followed by serum angiotensin-converting enzyme levels, chest radiograph, and lymphocyte assays. Despite poor specificity, negative Ga-67 scans together with normal angiotensin-converting enzyme have a high value for exclusion of active sarcoidosis. These authors found that in patients with pe-

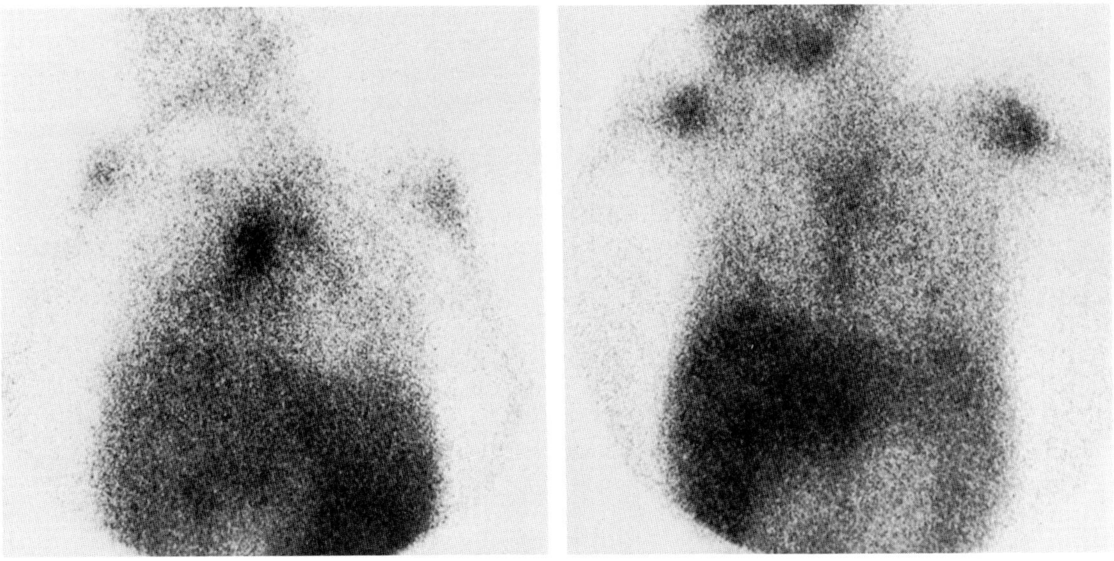

Figure 17-37. Ga-67 lung scans. Seven-year-old male with immunodeficiency, bilateral hilar infiltrates, and pulmonary granulomas. *Left:* Initial scan showing bilateral hilar uptake of radiogallium. *Right:* Followup scan shows disappearance of the abnormal hilar uptake of Ga-67 coinciding with patient's improvement.

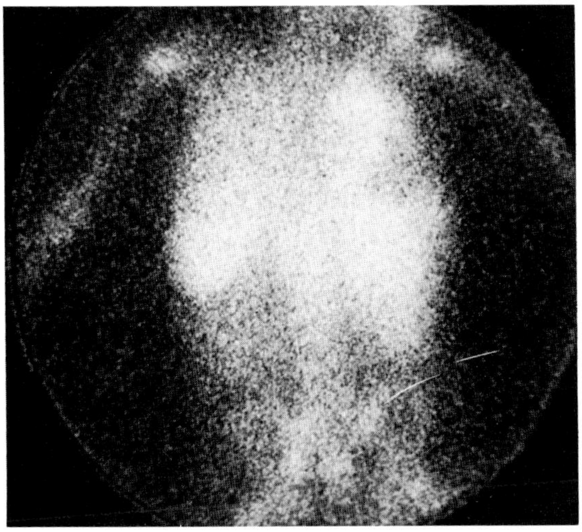

Figue 17-38. Pneumonitis. Ga-67 scan from a 3-year-old female with persistent fever. Posterior view showing intense radiotracer uptake within the right lung and less in the left lung, indicating an active inflammatory process.

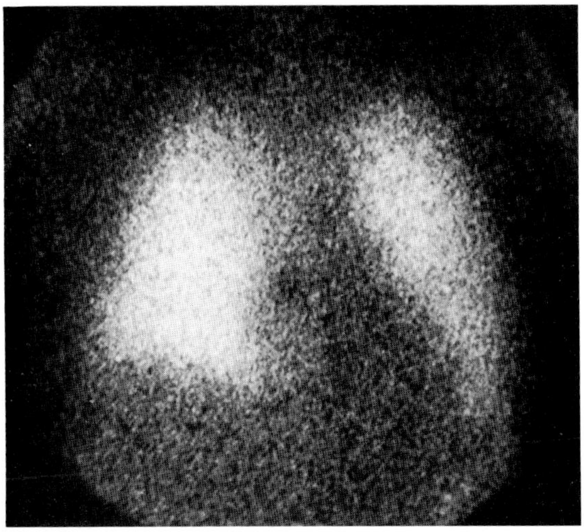

Figure 17-39. Ga-67 lung scan from a 16-year-old male with acute lymphocytic leukemia in remission. Findings of diffuse increased radiotracer uptake in the lungs may be secondary to chemotoxicity and/or oportunistic viral infection.

ripheral pulmonary lesions, chest radiographs have doubtful value for staging involvement and assessment of activity.[82] Ga-67 also may concentrate in sarcoid lesions of the heart.[50] Normal Ga-67 scans can be used to support clinical identification of inactive sarcoidosis.[60]

Inflammatory and Other Lesions Causing Uptake of Ga-67 in the Lungs

These include granulomatous lesions in immunodeficiency (Fig. 17-37), pneumonitis (Fig. 17-38), and chemotoxicity (Fig. 17-39).

α_1-Antitrypsin Deficiency

The pulmonary arterial bed in patients with α_1-antitrypsin deficiency seems to be involved early in the disease course. Altered distribution of regional pulmonary blood flow and loss of pulmonary perfusion gradients can be detected in these patients even before the development of obstructive lung disease.[88]

References

1. Alavi A. Scintigraphic demonstration of acute gastrointestinal bleeding. Gastrointest Radiol 1980; 5:205–8.
2. Alavi A, Dann RW, Baum S, Biery DN. Scintigraphic detection of acute gastrointestinal bleeding. Radiology 1977; 124:753–6.
3. Alberts C, Van Der Schoot JB, Van Datselaar JJ, Braat MCP, Roos CM. Ga-67 scintigraphy, serum lysozyme and angiotensin-converting enzyme in pulmonary sarcoidosis. Eur J Respir Dis 1983; 64:38–46.
4. Alderson PO, Secker-Walker RH, Strominger DB, McAlister WH, Hill RL, Markham J. Quantitative assessment of regional ventilation and perfusion in children with cystic fibrosis. Radiology 1974; 111:151–5.
5. Anderson T Jr, Mall JC, Hoffer PB, Tetalman MR, Hendrix RW. Efficacy of emergency radionuclide perfusion lung studies. Radiology 1976; 120:125–30.
6. Arborelius M Jr. Influence of moderate hypoxemia in one lung on the distribution of the pulmonary circulation and ventilation. Scand J Clin Lab Invest 1965; 17:257–9.
7. Baghdassarian OM, Avery ME, Neuhauser EBD. A form of pulmonary insufficiency in premature infants: pulmonary dysmaturity? AJR 1963; 89:1020–31.
8. Bajzer Z, Nosil J. A simple mathematical lung model for quantitative regional ventilation measurement using ^{81m}Kr. Phy Med Biol 1977; 22:975–80.
9. Ball WC Jr, Stewart PB, Newsham LGS, Bates DV. Regional pulmonary function studied with xenon-133. J Clin Invest 1962; 41:519–31.
10. Barry J, Alazraki NP, Heaphy JH. Scintigraphic detection of intrapulmonary bleeding using Tc-99m sulfur colloid. J Nucl Med 1981; 22:777–80.
11. Bateman JRM, Newman SP, Daunt KM, Pavia D, Clarke SW. Regional lung clearance of excessive bronchial secretions during chest physiotherapy in patients with stable chronic airways obstruction. Lancet 1979; i:294–7.
12. Bates DV, Macklem PT, Christie RV. Respiratory function in disease. An introduction to the integrated study of the lung, 2nd ed. Philadelphia: WB Saunders, 1971.
13. Bell WR, Simon TL. Current status of pulmonary thromboembolic disease: pathophysiology, diagnosis, prevention and treatment. Am Heart J 1982; 103:239–62.
14. Bell WR, Simon TL, DeMets DL. The clinical features of submassive and massive pulmonary emboli. Am J Med 1977; 62:355–60.
15. Bentivoglio LG, Beerel F, Bryan AC, Stewart PB, Rose B, Bates DV. Regional pulmonary function studied with xenon-133 in patients with bronchial asthma. J Clin Invest 1963; 42:1193–200.
16. Berg TJ, Pagtakhan RD, Reed MH, Langston C, Chernick V. Bronchopulmonary dysplasia and lung rupture in hyaline membrane disease: influence of continuous distending pressure. Pediatrics 1975; 55:51–4.
17. Bohm N, Keller KM, Kloke WD. Pulmonary and systemic cerebellar tissue embolism due to birth injury. Virchows Arch [Pathol Anat] 1982; 398:229–35.
18. Brown ER. Increased risk of BPD in infants with patent ductus arteriosus. J Pediatr 1979; 95:865–6.
19. Brown ER, Stark A, Sosenko I, Lawson EE, Avery ME. BPD: possible relationships to pulmonary edema. J Pediatr 1978; 92:982–4.
20. Buchanan D, Mason JK. Occurrence of pulmonary fat and bone marrow embolism. Am J Forensic Med Pathol 1982; 3:73–8.
21. Buck JR, Connors RH, Coon WW, Weintraub WH, Wesley JR, Coran AG. Pulmonary embolism in children. J Pediatr Surg 1981; 16:385–91.
22. Caride VJ, Pusi S, Slavin JD. The usefulness of posterior oblique views in perfusion lung imaging. Radiology 1976; 121:669–71.
23. Chandler AB. The anatomy of a thrombus. In: Sherry S, Brinkhous KM, Genton E, Stengle JM, eds. Thrombus. Washington: National Academy of Science, 1969.
24. Chen JTT, Robinson AE, Goodrich JK. Uneven distribution of pulmonary blood flow between left and right lungs in isolated valvular pulmonic stenosis. AJR 1969; 107:343–50.
25. Coel NM, Druger G. Radionuclide detection of the site of hemoptysis. Chest 1982; 81:242–3.
26. Cone RB. A review of Boeck's sarcoid with analysis of twelve cases occurring in children. J Pediatr 1948; 32:629–40.
27. Coon WW. Risk factors in pulmonary embolism in childhood. Surg Gynecol Obstet 1976; 143:385–90.
28. Cummings GR, MacPherson RI, Chernick V. Unilateral hyperlucent lung syndrome in children. J Pediatr 1971; 78:250–60.

29. Danigelis JA, Markarian B. Pulmonary alveolar proteinosis including pulmonary electron microscopy. Am J Dis Child 1969; 118:871–5.
30. Davies G, Reid L. Growth of the alveoli and pulmonary arteries in childhood. Thorax 1970; 25:669–81.
31. Dawson A, Kaneko K, McGregor M. Regional lung function in patients with mitral stenosis studied with Xe-133 during air and oxygen breathing. J Clin Invest 1965; 41:999–1008.
32. DeCesare JA, Babchyck BM, Colten HR, Treves S. Radionuclide assessment of the effects of chest physical therapy on ventilation in cystic fibrosis. Phys Ther 1982; 62:820–7.
33. deLemos R, Wolfsderf J, Nachman R, Block AJ, Leeley G, Wilkinsen HA, Allen T, Haller JA, Morgan W, Avery ME. Lung injury from oxygen in lambs: the role of artificial ventilation. Anesthesiology 1969; 30:609–18.
34. di Sant'Agnese PA, Davis PB. Research in cystic fibrosis. N Engl J Med 1976; 295:481–5; 534–41.
35. Dollery CT, West JB. Regional uptake of radioactive oxygen, carbon monoxide and carbon dioxide in the lungs of patients with mitral stenosis. Circ Res 1960; 8:765–71.
36. Dunne EF. Cardiac radiology. Philadelphia: Lea & Febiger, 1967:205–6.
37. Emery JL. Pulmonary embolism in children. Arch Dis Child 1962; 37:591–5.
38. Emery JL, Mithal A. The number of alveoli in the terminal respiratory unit of man during late intrauterine life and childhood. Arch Dis Child 1960; 35:544–7.
39. Epstein J, Taylor A, Alazraki N. Acute pulmonary embolus associated with transient ventilatory defect. J Nucl Med 1975; 16:1017–20.
40. Espinola D, Rupani H, Camargo EE, Wagner HN. Ventilation-perfusion imaging in pulmonary papillomatosis. J Nucl Med 1981; 22:975–77.
41. Esposito AL, Gleckman RA. A diagnostic approach to the adult with fever of unknown origin. Arch Intern Med 1979; 139:575–9.
42. Fazio F, Jones T. Assessment of regional ventilation by continuous inhalation of radioactive krypton-81m. Br Med J 1975; 3:673–6.
43. Fazio F, Solfanelli S, Santolicandro A, Palla A, Fornai E, Giuntini C. Imaging of pulmonary ventilation in asthma assessed with continuous inhalation of krypton-81m. In: Medical radionuclide imaging. Vienna: International Atomic Energy Agency, 1977.
44. Fazio F, Lavender JP, Steiner RE. ^{81m}Kr ventilation and ^{99m}Tc perfusion scans in chest disease: comparison with standard radiographs. AJR 1978; 130:421–8.
45. Featherby EA, Weng T-R, Crozier DN, Duic A, Reilly BJ, Levison H. Dynamic and static lung volumes, blood gas tensions and diffusing capacity in patients with cystic fibrosis. Am Rev Respir Dis 1970; 102:737–49.
46. Felson B. Chest roentgenology. Philadelphia: WB Saunders, 1973; 160–9; 425–528.
47. Firor HV. Pulmonary embolization complicating total intravenous alimentation. J Pediatr Surg 1972; 7:81.
48. Fleming HA. Differential lung function in atrial septal defect. Circulation 1959; 19:856–62.
49. Fletcher BD, Outerbridge EW, Youssef S, Bolande RP. Pulmonary interstitial emphysema in a newborn infant treated by lobectomy. Pediatrics 1974; 54:808–11.
50. Forman MB, Sandler MP, Sacks GA, Kronenberg MW, Powers TA. Radionuclide imaging in myocardial sarcoidosis. Demonstration of myocardial uptake of technetium-99m pyrophosphate and gallium. Chest 1983; 83:578–80.
51. Fragoyannis S, Kardalinos A. Congenital heart disease with pulmonary ischemia: a study of the pulmonary vascular lesions before and after systemic pulmonary anastomosis. Am Heart J 1962; 63:335–45.
52. Fraser RG, Pare JAP, eds. Diagnosis of diseases of the chest. Philadelphia: WB Saunders, 1977:561–8.
53. Freeman LM, Blaufox MD, eds. Physician desk reference for radiology and nuclear medicine. Oradell, NJ: Medical Economics, 1979:106.
54. Freiman DG, Sureymoto J, Wessler S. Frequency of pulmonary thromboembolism in man. N Engl J Med 1965; 272:1270.
55. Gandillo SB, Transwell AK, Mackie KW. Pulmonary vascular air embolism in hyaline membrane disease. J Can Assoc Radiol 1977; 28:294–6.
56. Gittman JE, Buchanan TA, Fisher BJ, Bergeson PS, Palmer PE. Fatal pulmonary embolism after spinal fusion for scoliosis. JAMA 1983; 249:779–81.
57. Gooneratne N, Conway JJ. Radionuclide angiographic diagnosis of bronchopulmonary sequestration. J Nucl Med 1976; 17:1035–7.
58. Goris ML, Daspit SG, Walter JP, McRae J, Lamb J. Applications of ventilation lung imaging with krypton-81m. Radiology 1977; 122:399–403.
59. Grossman H, Berdon WE, Mizrahi A, Baker DH. Neonatal focal hyperaeration of the lungs (Wilson-Mikity syndrome). Radiology 1965; 85:409–17.
60. Gupta RG, Beckerman C, Sicilian L, Oparil S, Pinsky SM, Szidon JP. Gallium-67 citrate scanning and serum angiotensin converting enzyme levels in sarcoidosis. Radiology 1982; 144:895–9.
61. Gyepes MT, Bennett LR, Hassakis PC. Regional pulmonary blood flow in cystic fibrosis. AJR 1969; 106:567–75.
62. Hall RT, Rhodes PG. Pneumothorax and pneu-

momediastinum in infants with idiopathic respiratory distress syndrome receiving continuous positive airway pressure. Pediatrics 1975; 55:493–6.
63. Harker LA, Slichter SJ, Scott CR, Ross R. Homocystinemia. Vascular injury and arterial thrombosis. N Engl J Med 1974; 291:537–43.
64. Harrod JR, L'Heureux P, Wagenstun OD, Hunt CE. Long-term followup of severe respiratory distress syndrome treated with IPPB. J Pediatr 1974; 84:277–85.
65. Heyman S. Toxicity and safety factors associated with lung perfusion studies with radiolabeled particles (letter to the editor). J Nucl Med 1979; 20:1098–9.
66. Higgins CB, Wexler L. Clinical and angiographic features of pulmonary arterovenous fistulas in children. Radiology 1976; 119:171–5.
67. Hislop A, Reid L. New pathological findings in emphysema of childhood: 1. Polyalveolar lobe with emphysema. Thorax 1970; 25:682–90.
68. Hughes CW, Rumore PC. Anomalous pulmonary veins. Arch Pathol 1944; 37:364–6.
69. Hughes JMB, Glazier JB, Maloney JE, West JB. Effect of interstitial pressure on pulmonary blood flow. Lancet 1967; i:192–3.
70. Hughes JMB, Glazier JB, Maloney JE, West JB. Effect of lung volume on the distribution of pulmonary blood flow in man. Respir Physiol 1968; 4:58–72.
71. James DG, Turiaf J, Hosoda Y, Williams WJ, Israel HL, Douglas AC, Siltzbach LE. Description of sarcoidosis: report of the subcommittee on classification and definition. Seventh International Conference on Sarcoidosis and Other Granulomatous Disorders. Ann NY Acad Sci 1976; 278:742.
72. Jones DRB, MacIntyre IMC. Venous thromboembolism in infancy and childhood. Arch Dis Child 1975; 50:153–5.
73. Jones RH, Sabiston DC. Pulmonary embolism in childhood. Monogr Surg Sci 1966; 3:35–51.
74. Jue KL, Amplatz K, Adams P Jr, Anderson RC. Anomalies of great vessels associated with lung hypoplasia. The scimitar syndrome. Am J Dis Child 1966; 111:35–44.
75. Kaplan HP, Robinson FR, Kapance Y, Weibel ER. Pathogenesis and reversibility of the pulmonary lesions of oxygen toxicity in monkeys. I. Clinical and light microscopic studies. Lab Invest 1969; 20:94–100.
76. Kelley MJ, Elliott LP. The radiologic evaluation of the patient with suspected pulmonary thromboembolic disease. Med Clin North Am 1975; 59:3–36.
77. Kessler RM, McNeil BJ. Impaired ventilation in a patient with angiographically demonstrated pulmonary emboli. Radiology 1975; 114:111–2.
78. Kim EE, DeLand FH. V/Q mismatch without pulmonary embolism in children with histoplasmosis. Clin Nucl Med 1978; 3:328–30.
79. Kimball AM, Hallum AV, Cates W. Deaths caused by pulmonary thromboembolism after legally induced abortion. Am J Obstet Gynecol 1978; 239:948–50.
80. Kjellman B. Regional lung function studied with Xe-133 in children with pneumonia. Acta Paediatr Scand 1967; 56:467–76.
81. Kjellman B. Regional lung function studied with Xe-133 external detectors (radiospirometry) in children without cardiopulmonary disease. Acta Paediatr Scand 1968; 57:527–33.
82. Klech H, Kohn H, Kummer F, Mostbeck A. Assessment of activity in sarcoidosis. Sensitivity and specificity of Ga-67 scintigraphy, serum ACE levels, chest roentgenography and blood lymphocyte subpopulations. Chest 1982; 82:732–8.
83. Knipping HW, Bolt W, Venrath H, Valentin H, Ludes H, Indler P. A new method for regional lung function with radioactive Xe-133 gas. Dtsch Med Wochenschr 1955; 80:1146–7.
84. Lassen NA. Assessment of tissue radiation dose in clinical use of radioactive inert gases with examples of absorbed dose from H^3, Kr^{85}, and Xe^{133}. Radioakt Isot Klin Fortschr 1965; 6:37–47.
85. Lee HK, Granada M. Swyer-James syndrome: diagnostic application of combined radionuclide ventilation and perfusion scanning. Clin Nucl Med 1977; 2:100–2.
86. Leonidas JC, Hall RT, Rhodes PG. Conservative management of unilateral pulmonary emphysema under tension. J Pediatr 1975; 87:776–8.
87. Leonidas JC, Moylan FM, Kahn PC, Ramenofsky ML. Ventilation-perfusion scans in neonatal regional pulmonary emphysema complicating ventilatory assistance. AJR 1978; 131:243–6.
88. Levine BW, Talamo RC, Shannon DC, Kazemi H. Alteration in distribution of pulmonary blood flow. An early manifestation of alpha-1-antitrypsin deficiency. Ann Intern Med 1970; 79:397–401.
89. Li DL, Seltzer SE, McNeil BJ. V/Q mismatches unassociated with pulmonary embolism: case report and review of the literature. J Nucl Med 1978; 19:1331–3.
90. Li DK, Treves S, Heyman S, Kirkpatrick JA, Lambrecht RM, Ruth TJ, Wolf AP. Krypton-81m: a better radiopharmaceutical for the assessment of regional lung function in children. Radiology 1979; 130:741–7.
91. Liebow AA, Steer A, Billingsley JG. Desquamative interstitial pneumonia. Am J Med 1965; 39:369–404.
92. Macklin MT, Macklin CC. Malignant interstitial emphysema of the lungs and mediastinum as an

important occult complication in many respiratory diseases and other conditions: an interpretation of the clinical literature in the light of laboratory experiment. Medicine 1944; 23:281–358.

93. Magilner AD, Capitanio MA, Wertheimer I, Burko H. Persistent localized intrapulmonary interstitial emphysema: an observation in three infants. Radiology 1974; 111:379–84.
94. Makler PT, Malmud LS, Charkes ND. Diminished perfusion to an entire lung due to mucus plug. Clin Nucl Med 1977; 2:160–2.
95. McGoldrick PJ, Rudd TG, Figley MM, Wilheim JP. What becomes of pulmonary infarcts? AJR 1979; 133:1039–45.
96. Medina JR, L'Heureux P, Lillehei JP, Loken MK. Regional ventilation in the differential diagnosis of pulmonary embolism. Circulation 1969; 39:831–5.
97. Merten DF, Kirks DR, Grossman H. Pulmonary sarcoidosis in childhood. AJR 1980; 135:673–9.
98. Milic-Emili J, Henderson JAM, Dolovich MB, Trop D, Kaneko K. Regional distribution of inspired gas in the lung. J Appl Physiol 1966; 21:749–59.
99. Miller T, Tanaka T. Nuclear scan of pulmonary hemorrhage in idiopathic pulmonary hemosiderosis. AJR 1979; 132:120–1.
100. Miorner G. ^{133}Xe-radiospirometry. A clinical method for studying regional lung function. Scand J Respir Dis Suppl 1968; 64:1–84.
101. Mishkin F, Knote J. Radioisotope scanning of the lungs in patients with systemic-pulmonary anastomosis. AJR 1968; 102:267–73.
102. Mishkin F, Wagner HN. Regional abnormalities in pulmonary arterial blood flow during acute asthmatic attacks. Radiology 1967; 88:142–4.
103. Moore P, James O, Saltos N. Fat embolism syndrome: incidence, significance and early features. Aust NZ J Surg 1981; 51:546–51.
104. Moses DC, Silver TM, Bookstein JT. The complementary roles of chest radiography, lung scanning, and selective pulmonary angiography in the diagnosis of pulmonary embolism. Circulation 1974; 49:179–88.
105. Moyer JH, Glantz G, Brest AN. Pulmonary arteriovenous fistulas: physiologic and clinical considerations. Am J Med 1962; 32:417–35.
106. Nadas AS, Fyler DC. Pediatric cardiology. Philadelphia: WB Saunders, 1972:653–5.
107. Nichols MM, Tyson KR. Saddle embolus occluding pulmonary arteries. Am J Dis Child 1978; 132:926.
108. Northway WH, Rosan RC, Porter DY. Pulmonary disease following respiratory therapy of hyaline-membrane disease. N Engl J Med 1967; 276:357–68.
109. O'Dell CW Jr, Taylor A, Higgins CB, Ashburn WL, Schillaci RF, Alazraki NP. Ventilation-perfusion lung images in the Swyer-James syndrome. Radiology 1976; 121:423–6.
110. Piepsz A, Decostre P, Baran D. Scintigraphic study of pulmonary blood flow distribution in cystic fibrosis. J Nucl Med 1978; 14:326–30.
111. Pillay SV. Pulmonary embolism of cerebral tissue in a neonate: a case report. S Afr Med J 1980; 20:498.
112. Plenck HP, Swift SA, Chambers WL, Peltzer WE. Pulmonary alveolar proteinosis. A new disease? Radiology 1960; 74:928–38.
113. Pratt PC. Pulmonary capillary proliferation induced by oxygen inhalation. Am J Pathol 1958; 34:1033.
114. Rao M, Steiner P, Victoria MS, Solomon, Kassner EG, Co C, De Graff M. Regional lung functions in children with astham. J Asthma Res 1977; 14:107–10.
115. Roberts RJ. Employment of pulmonary superoxide dismutase, catalase, and glutathione peroxidose activity as criteria for assessing suitable animal models for studies of BPD. J Pediatr 1979; 95:904–10.
116. Rosen SH, Castleman B, Liebow AA. Pulmonary alveolar proteinosis. N Engl J Med 1958; 258:1123–42.
117. Sade RM, Williams RG, Castaneda AR, Treves S. Abnormalities of regional lung function associated with ventricular septal defect and pulmonary artery band. J Thorac Cardiovasc Surg 1976; 71:572–80.
118. Salzman EW, Harris WH, DeSanctis RW. Anticoagulation for prevention of thromboembolism following fracture of the hip. N Engl J Med 1966; 275:122–30.
119. Sasahara AA, Cannilia JE, Morse RL, Sidd JJ, Tremblay GM. Clinical and physiologic studies in pulmonary thromboembolism. Am J Cardiol 1967; 20:10–20.
120. Schor RA, Shames DM, Weber PM, DosRemedios LV. Regional ventilation studies with Kr-81m and Xe-133; a comparative analysis. J Nucl Med 1978; 19:348–53.
121. Shannon DC, Riseborough EJ, Valenca LM, Kazemi H. The distribution of abnormal lung function in kyphoscoliosis. J Bone Joint Surg (Am) 1970; 52A:131–44.
122. Shook DR, Cram KB, Williams HJ. Pulmonary venous air embolism in hyaline membrane disease. AJR 1975; 125:538–42.
123. Shwachman H, Kulczych LL, Khan KT. A report of 65 patients over 16 years of age. Pediatrics 1965; 36:689–99.
124. Stinnett RG, Hietala S, Fratkin MJ. Reversible

unilateral pulmonary hypoperfusion secondary to mucus plugs. Clin Nucl Med 1977; 2:157–9.
125. Stocker JT, Madewell JE. Persistent interstitial pulmonary emphysema: another complication of the respiratory distress syndrome. Pediatrics 1977; 59:847–57.
126. Stocker JT, Drake RM, Madewell JE. Cystic and congenital lung disease in the newborn. Perspect Pediatr Pathol 1978; 4:93–154.
127. Taghizadeh A, Reynolds EOR. Pathogenesis of BPD following hyaline membrane disease. Am J Pathol 1976; 82:241–64.
128. Tan KL, Hwang WS. Neonatal brain tissue embolism in the lung. Aust NZ J Med 1976; 76:146–9.
129. Tang TT, Chambers CH, Gallen WJ, McCready SR. Pulmonary fiber embolism and granuloma. JAMA 1978; 239:948–50.
130. Taplin GV, McDonald NS. Radiochemistry of macroaggregated albumin and newer lung scanning agents. Semin Nucl Med 1971; 1:132–52.
131. Thurlbeck WM. Postnatal growth and development of the lung. In: Murray JF, ed. Lung disease. State of the art (1974–1975). New York: American Lung Association, 1976.
132. Treves S, Strieder DJ, Adelstein SJ. Scintillation camera radiospirometry. Prog Nucl Med 1973; 3:149–65.
133. Treves S, Ahnberg DS, Laguarda R, Strieder DJ. Radionuclide evaluation of regional lung function in children. J Nucl Med 1974; 15:582–7.
134. Treves S, Fogel R, Lang P. Radionuclide angiography in congenital heart disease. Am J Cardiol 1980; 46:1247–55.
135. Utzon F, Bradrup F. Pulmonary arteriovenous fistulas in children. A review with special reference to the disperse telangiectatic type. Acta Paediatr Scand 1973; 62:422–32.
136. Vandevivere J, Spehl M, Dab J, Baran D, Piepsz A. Bronchiectasis in childhood. Comparison of chest roentgenograms, bronchography and lung scintigraphy. Pediatr Radiol 1980; 9:193–8.
137. Wagner HN Jr, Sabiston DC, Iio M, McAfee JG, Meyer JK, Langan JK. Regional pulmonary blood flow in man by radioisotope scanning. JAMA 1964; 187:601–3.
138. Walker BK, Ballas SK, Burka ER. The diagnosis of pulmonary thromboembolism in sickle cell disease. Am J Hematol 1979; 7:219–32.
139. Wartak J, Overton TR, Friedenberg LW, Sproule BJ. Computer-aided evaluation of regional pulmonary function. Comput Biomed Res 1972; 5:429–39.
140. Wellman HN, Mack JF, Saenger EL. Clinical experience with oblique views in pulmonary perfusion scintiphotography in normal and pathological anatomy (abstract). J Nucl Med 1968; 9:374.
141. Wesley JR, Keens TG, Miller SW, Platzker AC. Pulmonary embolism in the neonate: occurrence during the course of total parenteral nutrition. J Pediatr 1978; 93:113–5.
142. West JB. Pulmonary function studies with radioactive gases. Annu Rev Med 1967; 18:459–70.
143. West JB. Ventilation, blood flow and gas exchange, 2nd ed. London: Blackwell, 1970.
144. Wilson MG, Mikity VG. A new form of respiratory disease in premature infants. Am J Dis Child 1960; 99:489–99.
145. Wilson AF, Surprenant EL, Beall GN, Siegel SC, Simmons DH, Bennett LR. The significance of regional pulmonary function changes in bronchial asthma. Am J Med 1970; 48:416–23.
146. Wilkinson RH, Blanc WA, Hagstrom JWC. Pulmonary alveolar proteinosis in three infants. Pediatrics 1968; 41:510–5.
147. Winzelberg GG, Wholey MH, Sachs M. Scintigraphic localization of pulmonary bleeding using Tc-99m sulfur colloid: a preliminary report. Radiology 1982; 143:757–62.
148. Wohl MEB, Griscom NT, Traggis DG, Jaffe N. Effects of therapeutic irradiation delivered in early childhood upon subsequent lung function. Pediatrics 1975; 55:507–16.
149. Wohl MEB, Griscom NT, Strieder DJ, Schuster SR, Treves S, Zwerdling RG. The lung following repair of congenital diaphragmatic hernia. J Pediatr 1977; 90:405–14.
150. Wood RE, Boat TF, Doershuk CF. Cystic fibrosis. Am Rev Respir Dis 1976; 113:833–78.
151. Yano Y, McRae J, Anger HO. Lung function studies using short-lived Kr-81m and the scintillation camera. J Nucl Med 1970; 11:674–9.
152. Zeiger LS, Moss EG. Ventilation and perfusion imaging in the Swyer-James syndrome. Clin Nucl Med 1977; 2:103–5.

Index

Abdominal scintigraphy (Meckel's diverticulum)
abnormal uptake in, 184, 187
accuracy of, 187
clinical applications of, 182–187
examination technique, 181–182
images, 181–182
patient preparation, 181
false-negative studies, 187
Meckel's diverticulum and, 183–184
normal scan, 182–183
Abscess, splenic, 153
Activator therapy, for facial growth, results of, 56
Acute renal failure, 95
Acute tubular necrosis, 90
Adolescent, hepatobiliary scintigraphy in, indications for, 157
Adrenal hemorrhage, renal scintigraphy of, in newborn, 75, 77
Air cyst, pulmonary, 306
Airway connective tissue, abnormalitics of, 322–323
Airway obstruction, Xe-133 studies in, 306, 308
Albright's syndrome, 24
α_1-antitrypsin deficiency, 326
Angiography
first-pass radionuclide, 245–267
gated blood pool, 268–272
Anuria, radionucleic studies in, 77
Appendix testis torsion, 122
scintigraphy of, 125–126
Arnold-Chiari malformation, 221
Arteriovenous malformation, 219–220
Arthritis, septic, *see* Septic arthritis
Ascites, in newborn, 75
Aseptic necrosis, 17–18
differential diagnosis of, 17–18
radiographic images of, 17
scintigraphic images of, 17
Asplenia, 150
functional, 152–153
reversible functional, 152
Asthma, 316
Atresia, biliary, *see* Biliary atresia
Atrial septal defect, 264
pulmonary blood flow in, 303

Barrett's esophagus, 187
Biliary scan, with Tc-99m HIDA, 158
Biliary atresia
clinical characteristics of, 160
differential diagnosis of, 161, 164
etiology of, 161
vs. neonatal hepatitis, 160–164
Biliary leak, 168
Biliary obstruction, 164–165
Bilirubin levels, Tc-99m hepatobiliary agents and, 158–159
Bladder capacity, 111–113
Bladder emptying, 117–118
Bladder volume, residual, 118
Bone, 1–43
eosinophilic granuloma of, 37
Bone marrow scintigraphy, clinical applications, 59–61
Bone marrow scintigraphy, 59–61
Bone-seeking pharmaceuticals, extaosseous uptake of, 40–43
Brain, 205–221
radionuclide studies of, indications for, 205
static scintigraphy of, 205, *see also* Cerebral scintigraphy
radiopharmaceuticals for, 205–206
Brain death
clinical examination for, 213
determination of, 212
Brain stem unresponsiveness, 213
Bronchiectiasis, 318–319
Bronchopulmonary dysplasia, 316–318
factors affecting, 317–318
Bronchopulmonary sequestration, 320–321
Budd-Chiari syndrome, 137

Caffey's disease, 24–25
Candisiasis, of spleen, 153
Carcinoma, thyroid, 201–202, *see also* Thyroid carcinoma
Cardiac output, calculation of, 256–257
Cardiomyopathy, TI-201, 278–279
Cardiopulmonary death, determination of, 212
Cardiovascular surgery, postoperative assessment of, 265–267
Cardiovascular system
first-pass radionuclide angiography of, 245–267

Cardiovascular system (*cont.*)
radionuclide study of, 245–282
Caroli's disease, 168
diagnosis of, 168
Cerebral death, 211–213
determination of, 212
Cerebral radionuclide angiography, 205
examination technique, 206
radiopharmaceuticals for, 205–206
Cerebral scintigraphy
clinical applications of, 206–221
headache and, 219
of infectious diseases, 217
normal study, 206, 208
seizure disorders and, 217, 219
stroke and, 219
subdural hematoma and, 211
trauma and, 208, 211
tumor detection by, 208
Cerebral unresponsiveness, 213
Cerebrospinal fluid, 223–230
blocked flow of, radionuclide cisternography in, 228
circulation of, 223
leakage of, evaluation of, 225
loculations of, radionuclide cisternography in, 226
production rate of, 223
Cerebrospinal fluid liquorrhea, radionuclide cisternography in, 226
Cerebrospinal fluid shunt, 228–230
clinical applications of, 230
examination technique, 228–230
Tc-99m sodium pertechnetate and, 228
Cervical metastases, thyroid carcinoma and, 201
Chest, radiation therapy to, complications of, 321–322
Childhood malignancy, radiotracers in, 61
Cholecystitis, diagnosis of, 164–165
Choledochal cyst, types of, 167
Cholescintigraphy, hepatobiliary agents for, 157–160
Cimetidine, before abdominal scintigraphy, 181
Cisternography, radionuclide, 223–228, *see also* Radionuclide cisternography
Coma, irreversibility of, 212–213
Computed tomography, of hepatic lesions, 129
Congenital abnormality
of liver, 132
of spleen, 132
Congenital diaphragmatic hernia, 319
Congenital heart disease, cerebral complications of, 213, 217
Congenital lobar emphysema, Xe-133 studies in, 130
Coronary artery, anomalous, TI-201 scintiscan in, 274
Cyanosis, radionuclide angiocardiography and, 262
Cystic fibrosis, 296–300
incidence of, 296
pathogens of, 297
scintigraphic appearance of, 297–300
X9-133 imaging in, 297–299
Cystography, radionuclide, *see* Radionuclide cystography
Cysts, skeletal scintigraphy of, 23

Dacryocystography
case histories, 236–243
clinical application of, 236–243
method of, 235–236
Dacryoscintigraphy, 233–243
Dandy-Walker malformation, 221
Death, determination of, 212–213
Deconvolution analysis, 69
Dental disorders, scintigraphic abnormalities and, 25
Diplococcus penumoniae, splenic infection and, 145
Dosimetry, 1–5
radionuclide cystography and, 118–119
Ductus arteriosis, patent, left-to-right shunting and, 261
respiratory distress syndrome and, 260–261
Dysplasia
bronchopulmonary, 316–318
factors affecting, 317–318
fibrous, scintigraphy of, 23–24

Ectopic calcification, in paraplegic patient, 41–42
Ectopic kidney-solitary kidney, 93
Ectopic thyroid, 194
Effective renal plasma flow (ERPF), estimatation of, 72
Ejection fraction, ventricular, estimation of, 258–259
Embolism, pulmonary, 312–316, *see also* Pulmonary embolism
Emphysema
congenital lobar, Xe-133 studies in, 310
interstitial, neonatal, 318
Encephalitis, herpes, 217
Enterocolitis in neonate, 42–43
Eosinophilic granuloma, of bone, 37
Epididymitis, 122
Epididymoorchitis, 125
Epiphora, 233
Escherichia coli, urinary infection with, 118
Ethane-1-hydroxyl-1, 1-diphosphonate (EHDP), 1
Euthyroid goiter, 201
Ewing's sarcoma, 30–32
survival rates, 32
Extrarenal activity, detection of, 68–69
Extravaginal torsion, 122

Facial growth
activator therapy for, results of, 56
evaluation of, 49
Females, radionuclide cystography in, 106
Fibroma, nonossifying, 25
Fibrosarcoma, 38
Fibrous dysplasia, scintigraphy of, 23–24
First-pass radionuclide angiography
advantages of, 245
of cardiovascular system, 245–267
clinical applications of, 249–267
data display, 249
data recording of, 249
equipment for, 246
imaging in, 248–249
injection technique in, 247–248
Ir-191m for, 246–247
left-to-right shunting in, 250–252
limitations of, 245
normal, 249–250
patient preparation for, 246
radiopharmaceuticals for, 246–247
right-to-left shunting in, 255–256

Tc-99m sodium pertechnetate for, 246
Flank masses, in newborn, 73–74
Fluid overload, bronchopulmonary dysplasia and, 317–318
Forward stroke volume, calculation of, 260
Fraconi's anemia, Tc-99m sulfur colloid scan for, 59
Furosemide (Lasix), 80–81
Furosemide stimulation test, 80–81

Gallium-67 citrate (Ga-67), 2–3
administered dose of, 2–3
estimated absorbed radiation dose from, 2–3
imaging technique, 3
liver abscess and, 136
mechanism of uptake, 2
in pyelonephritis diagnosis, 84–85
sarcoidosis and, 324–325
Gamma variate analysis, of left-to-right shunting, 253–254
Ganglioneuroblastoma, 34
Ganglioneuroma, 34
Gastric emptying, 172
determination of, 174
patterns of, 176
and percent gastric residual, 174
relationship between GER and, 176
Gastroesophageal reflex (GER), 171–176
complications of, 171
definition of, 171
diagnosis and quantitation of, 171–172
natural history of, 171
symptoms of, 171
Gastroesophageal scintigraphy
clinical applications of, 174–176
interpretation of, 174–176
examination technique, 172, 174
radiopharmaceuticals for, 172
Gated blood pool angiography, 268–272
analysis of, 270
clinical applications of, 271–272
data recording of, 269–270
instrumentation for, 269
quality control, 270
radiopharmaceuticals for, 268
Gaucher's disease, 18
Glomerular filtration rate (GFR), 70–72
Goiter
euthyroid, 201
hypothyroidism with, 200
neoplastic causes of, 201
Graves' disease, 200
Great vessels, congenital and acquired anomalies of, pulmonary scintigraphy for, 300–306
Haemophilus influenzae
meningitis due to, 217
septic arthritis due to, 15
splenic infection due to, 145
Hand-Schuller-Christian disease, 37
Hashimoto's thyroiditis, 201
Head, irradiation of, 201
Headache, radionuclide brain scan and, 219
Heart, 245–282
congenital and acquired anomalies of, pulmonary scintigraphy for, 301–306
Heinz bodies, 150
Hematoma, subdural, scintigraphic detection of, 211
Hemologic disorders, In-111 imaging for, 59–61
Hemotysis, pulmonary scintigram in, 300
Hemorrhage, adrenal, in newborn, 75, 77
Henoch-Schonlein purpura, 122
Hepatic lesions
computed tomography of, 129
ultrasonography of, 129
Hepatic scintigraphy, 129
clinical applications of, 131–139
imaging technique, 130–131
in leukemia, 138–139
in lymphoma, 138
normal variants of, 132
radiopharmaceuticals for, 129–130
Hepatic visualization, with Tc-99m BIDA, 159
Hepatitis, neonatal, *see* Neonatal hepatitis
Hepatobiliary scintigraphy, 157–168
clinical applications of, 160–168
I-131 rose bengal for, 157
indications for, 157
method of, 160
radiopharmaceuticals for, 157–160
Tc-99m PIPIDA, 159
Tc-99m PRIDA, 159
Hernia
congenital diaphragmatic, 319
splenic, 154
Herpes encephalitis, 217
Heterotaxia syndrome, 132, 150
Histiocytosis, 37–38
bone scans for, 38
Homocystinuria, 312
Horseshoe-shaped kidney, 93
Howell-Jolly bodies, 150
Hydrocele, scintigraphic patterns of, 126
Hydrocephalus, radionuclide cisternography in, 225–226
Hydronephrosis, Tc-99m DTPA study in, 77–80
Hyperemia, peripheral, rim sign of, in testicular torsion, 124
Hyperostosis, cortical, infantile, 24–25
Hypertension, 86–89
incidence of, 86
IVP imaging in, 87
pulmonary vascular, with shunts, 264–265
Tc-99m compounds in evaluation of, 89
Hyperthyroidism, 200
Hypothyroidism, 200–201
neonatal, 200–201

IDA agents
biokinetics of, 159–160
chemical characteristics of, 158
Ileal diverticulum, *see* Meckel's diverticulum
Imaging
abdominal, 181–182, *see also* Abdominal scintigraphy
for hematologic disorders, with In-111, 59–61
hepatobiliary, method of, 160
methods of, 1–5
Imaging techniques, splenic
with Tc-99m heat-denatured red blood cells, 141
with Tc-99m MDP, 143
with Tc-99m sulfur colloid, 141
Iminodiacetic acid, *see* IDA agents
Indium-111 chloride
administered dose of, 4
estimated absorbed radiation dose from, 4–5
imaging technique, 5
mechanism of uptake, 4

Indium-111 DTPA, for radionuclide cisternography, 224
Indium-111 imaging, for hematologic disorders, 59–61
Infantile cortical hyperostosis, 24–25
Infarction
detection of, with Tc-99m DMSA, 93
scintigraphic diagnosis of, 14
Infectious diseases, radionuclide scanning in, 217
Interstitial emphysema, neonatal, 318
Intrathoracic splenosis, radiocolloid uptake and, 147
Intravenous urography (IVP), in hypertension, 87
Intravesical pressure
ranges of, 113
recording, 113–117
Iodine-123, for thyroid scintigraphy, 191–192
Iodine-123 orthoiodohippurate (OIH)
ERPF measurement with, 72
renal scintigraphy with, 66
Iodine-125, for thyroid scintigraphy, 192
Iodine-125 orthoiodohippurate (OIH), ERPF measurement with, 72
Iodine-131, for thyroid scintigraphy, 192
Iodine-131 orthoiodohippurate (OIH)
in acute tubular necrosis, 90
ERPF measurement with, 72
renal scintigraphy with, 65–66
Iodine-131 rose bengal, hepatobiliary scintigraphy with, 157
Iridium-191m, first-pass radionuclide angiography with, 246–247
Irradiation, of head and neck, 201
Irrevesibility, of coma, determination of, 212–213

Juxtacortical osteosarcoma, 30

Kawasaki disease, 279
Kidney, 63–99
imaging of, effects of contrast agents on, 66
MTTT through, formula for, 70
multicystic dysplastic, in newborn, 75
obstructed
furosemide stimulation test in, 80–81
Tc-99m DMSA study in, 81
radiotherapy effects on, 97
unit impulse response (UIR) of, 69
Kr-81m, for pulmonary scintigraphy, 292
Kr-81m ventilation studies, technique of, 296
Kupffer cells, Tc-99m sulfur colloid uptake by, 129

Lacrimal drainage, assessment of, 234–235
Lasix (furosemide), 80–81
Legg-Calvé-Perthes disease, 17, *see also* Aseptic necrosis
Letterer-Siwe disease, 37
Leukemia
bone scans for, 38
hepatic scintigraphy in, 138–139
Ligandis, 158
Liver, 129–139
congenital abnormality of, 132
scan size of, 131
trauma to, 136
Liver abscess, Ga-67 scintiscan of, 136
Liver disease, diffuse, 132–133
focal, 133–139
Lungs, 289–326
scintigraphy of, 289
Lymphoma, 38
hepatic scintigraphy in, 138

Males, radionuclide cystography in, catheterization for, 106
Malignancy, childhood, radiotracers in, 61
Mandible, examination and analysis of, 50–57
Mandibular asymmetry
assessment of, 52–56
surgical therapy for, 55–56
results of, 56
Mandibular growth
assessment of, 49–57
skeletal maturation and, 51–56
skeletal scintigraphy for, clinical applications, 50–56
Mean tubular transit time (MTTT), through kidney, formula for, 70
Mechanical ventilation, bronchopulmonary dysplasia and, 317
Meckel's diverticulum, 179–187
abdominal scintigraphic survey of, 183–184
diagnosis of, 179
indications of, 180
radiopharmaceuticals for, 180–181
symptoms of, 179
Meningitis, due to *Haemophilus influenzae,* 217
radionuclide scanning for, 217
Meningoencephalitis, radionuclide scanning for, 217
Mental retardation, cerebral scintigraphy and, 219
Metastases
osseous, early diagnosis of, 27–28
pulmonary, confirmation of, 28
Methylene diphosphonate (MDP), 1
Micturition, delayed onset of, 77
Mitral stenosis, 303
Mucocutaneous lymph node syndrome, TI-201 scintigram in, 279–282
Mucous plug, Xe-133 studies in, 308, 310
Multicystic dysplastic kidney, in newborn, 75
Myocardial perfusion scintigraphy, 273–282
clinical applications of, 274–282
imaging technique, 274
radiopharmaceuticals for, 273
Myocardial wall motion abnormalities, blood pool angiogram of, 271–272

Nasolacrimal apparatus
anatomy of, 234
physiology of, 234
Neck, irradiation of, 201
Neck nodules, thyroid gland and, 194–200
Necrosis, aseptic, *see* Aseptic necrosis
Necrotizing enterocolitis, in neonate, 42–43
Neisseria meningitidis, splenic infection due to, 145

Neonatal hepatitis
vs. biliary atresia, 160–164
clinical characteristics of, 160
differential diagnosis of, 164
etiology of, 161
Nephrotic syndrome, 95–96
Neuroblastoma, 34–37
clinical evaluation of, 34
scanning with Tc-99m MDP, 34–37
scanning with Tc-99m sulfur colloid, 37
stages of, 34
Neurologic disease, degenerative, diagnosis of, 220–221
Newborn
adrenal hemorrhage in, renal scintiscan of, 75, 77
ascites in, 75
flank masses in, radionuclide studies of, 73–74
hepatobiliary scintigraphy in, indications for, 157
hypothyroidism in, 200–201
interstitial emphysema in, 318
multicystic dysplastic kidney in, 75
necrotizing enterocolitis in, 42–43
polycystic renal disease in, 74
radionuclide angiograms in, evaluation of, 260–263
renal vein thrombosis in, 77
Tc-99m DTPA study in, 72
Nonossifying fibroma, 25

Osseous metastasis, early diagnosis of, 27–28
Osteochondritis dissecans, 22–23
Osteoma, osteoid, 32–33
Osteomyelitis, 5–14
biopsy of, 12
case material, 13–14
clinical features of, 12
differential diagnosis of, 13
follow-up scintigraphy of, 13
hematogenous, pathology of, 12
due to *Staphylococcus aureus,* 12
radiologic appearance of, 12
scintigraphic diagnosis of, 12–13
Osteosarcoma, 26–30
chemotherapy for, 29
detection of, 26–27
juxtacortrical, 30
parosteal, 30
survival rates, 29
Oxygen, toxicity of, 317

Panencephalitis, sclerosing, 217
Papillomatosis, pulmonary, 322
Para-amonohippuric acid (PAH), ERPF measurement with, 65
Paraplegic patient, ectopic calcification in, 41–42
Parosteal osteosarcoma, 30
Partially anomalous pulmonary venous return (PAPVR), 302–303
Patent ductus arteriosis, bronchopulmonary dysplasia and, 317
Patient preparation
for abdominal scintigraphy, 181
for first-pass radionuclide angiography, 246
for radionuclide cystography, 106
Pectus excavatum, 320
Pentagastrin, before abdominal scintigraphy, 181
Periosteal lucency, 30
Pharmaceuticals, bone-seeking, extaosseous uptake of, 40–43
Phenobarbital therapy, for biliary atresia, 164
Pneumonia, Xe-133 studies in, 310, 312
Polycystic renal disease, 93
in newborn, 74
Polysplenia, 150, 152
Porencephalic cyst, 226
Postnatal period, renal abnormalities in, 77–99
Potassium perchlorate, 123
Premature infant, radionuclide angiograms in, evaluation of, 260–263
Proteinosis, pulmonary alveolar, 323
Prune belly syndrome, 97–98
Tc-99m DMSA imaging in, 98
Tc-99m DTPA imaging in, 97
Pseudocyst, splenic, 145
Pseudomonas aeruginosa, in cystic fibrosis, 297
Pseudoneurologic syndrome, 171
Pulmonary air cyst, 306
Pulmonary alveolar proteinosis, 323
Pulmonary arteriovenous malformation, 303
Pulmonary artery band, 301
Pulmonary artery flow, decreased, surgical shunts and, 302
Pulmonary artery sling, 303
Pulmonary blood flow
in atrial septal defect, 302
in pulmonic stenosis, 301–302
Pulmonary blood volume, calculation of, 260
Pulmonary embolism, 312–316
angiography for, 313
clinical presentation of, 313
incidence of, 312
resolution of, 313
scintigraphy for, 313, 316
Tc-99m MAA scintiscan in, 313
Pulmonary metastases
confirmation of, 28
thyroid carcinoma and, 201–202
Pulmonary papillomatosis, 322
Pulmonary scintigraphy
clinical applications of, 296–326
examination techniques in, 292–296
indictions for, 289
radiopharmaceuticals for, 289–292
Pulmonary time-activity curve
in left-to-right shunt, 250–252
of normal radionuclide angiogram, 250
in right-to-left shunt, 256
sequential components of, 253
Pulmonary vascular hypertension, with shunts, 264–265
Pulmonary vascular resistance, radionuclide angiogram of, 261–262
Pulmonic stenosis, 264
pulmonary blood flow in, 301–302
valvular, pulmonary scintigraphy in, 301
Pyelonephritis, 82–85
Ga-67 citrate in diagnosis of, 84–85
symptoms of, 82
Tc-99m DMSA imaging in, 85
Pyogenic meningitis, 217

Radiation dose, absorbed
from Ga-67, 2–2
from In-111, 4–5
from Tc-99m MDP, 1

Radiation dose, absorbed (*cont.*)
from Tc-99m sulfur colloid, 4
Radiation therapy, to chest, complications of, 321–322
Radionuclide angiography, 66
first-pass, of cardiovascular system, 245–267
Radionuclide cisternography, 223–228
clinical applications of, 225–228
examination technique, 224–225
normal, 225
radiopharmaceuticals for, 224
Radionuclide cystography
analysis of, 107–108
catheterization for, 106–107
dosimetry and, 118–119
equipment for, 106
filling and voiding during, 107
indications for, 106
interpretation of, 108–118
method, 106–107
patient preparation for, 106
radiologic grading, 108–109
radiopharmaceuticals used in, 106
recording, 107
urine cultures and, 118
Radionuclide studies
of acute renal failure, 95
in anuria, 77
of ectopic kidneys, 93
of horseshoe-shaped kidney, 93
of nephrotic syndrome, 95–96
of renal abnormality, in neonatal period, 72–77
of renal vein thrombosis, in newborn, 77
of solitary kidney, 93
of ureter duplication, 93
Radionuclide voiding cystography, 105–119
Radiopharmaceuticals, 1–5, *see also specific types*
for cerebal radionuclide angiography, 205–206
in diagnosis, of renal disorders, 64–66
for first-pass radionuclide angiography, 246–247
for cystography, 106
for gastric esophagel scintigraphy, 172
for gated blood pool angiography, 268
for hepatic scintigraphy, 129–130
for hepatobiliary scintigraphy, 157–160
inulin-like, renal time-activity curve from, 70
mandibular examination with, 50–57
for Meckel's diverticulum, 180–181
for myocardial perfusion scintigraphy, 273
PAH-like, renal time-activity curve from, 70
for pulmonary scintigraphy, 289–292
for radionuclide cisternography, 224
in renal disorders, clinical applications, 72–99
for scrotal scintigraphy, 123
for splenic scintigraphy, 141
for static scintigraphy of brain, 205–206
for thyroid scintigraphy, 191–193
Radiotherapy, effect of, in kidney, 97
Radiotracer clearance, from plasma, GFR estimation by, 70–71
Radiotracer delivery, correction for, 254
Radiotracer uptake, by kidney, GFR estimation by, 71–72
Rapid-sequence urography, in renal vascular disease, 88
Ratio of uptake (RU)
measurement of, 51–52
of radiopharmaceuticals, formula for, 50
Rectal bleeding, differential diagnosis of, 180, *see also* Meckel's diverticulum
Reflux, vesicoureteric, *see* Vesicoureteric reflux
Renal abnormality, radionuclide studies of
in neonatal period, 72–77
in postnatal period, 77–99
Renal disorders, diagnosis of, 63
Renal failure, acute, 95
Renal function, immaturity of, 72–73
Renal infarction, 86
Renal pelvis, duplication of, 93
Renal scintigraphy
of adrenal hemorrhage, in newborn, 75, 77
clinical applications, 72–99
examination technique, 66–72
of flank masses, in newborn, 73–74
with I-123 OIH, 66
with I-131 OIH, 65–66
methods of, 64–66
of multicystic dysplastic kidney, in newborn, 75
of polycystic renal disease, 74
renal transplantation and, 89, 89–93
with Tc-99m DMSA, 64
with Tc-99m DTPA, 64
with Tc-99m glucoheptonate, 65
of transplant rejection, 89–90
Renal time-activity curve (Rc(t))
formula for, 69
from inulin-like radiotracer, 70
from PAH-like radiotracer, 70
Renal transplantation, 89–93
acute tubular necrosis, 84, 90
from cadaver, 90
from living donor, 89
rejection in, 89–90
Renal UIR, interpretation of, 69–70
Renal vascular disease, rapid-sequence urography in, 88
Renal vein thrombosis, 85–86
detection of, 86
in newborn, 77
Respiratory distress syndrome, patent ductus arteriosis and, 260–261
Reticuloendothelial scintigraphy, 129
in diagnosis of liver trauma, 136
Rhabdomyosarcoma, 38

Sarcoidosis, 324–325
Ga-67 citrate scans for, 324–325
Sarcoma, Ewing's, 30–32
survival rates, 32
Scintigraphy, *see Specific types*
Scoliosis, 320
Scrotal scintigraphy, 121–127
clinical applications of, 123–126
examination technique, 123
general considerations, 121
normal appearance of, 123
phases of, 123
radiopharmaceuticals for, 123
Seizure disorders, radionuclide scanning of, 217, 219
Septal defect

atrial, 264
ventricular, 264
Septic arthritis, 14–17
clinical appearance of, 15
due to *Hemophilus influenzae,* 15
due to *Staphylococcus aureus,* 15
scintographic findings in, 15–17
Septicemia, following splenectomy, 145
Shunts
left-to-right
in first-pass radionuclide angiography, 250–252
gamma variate analysis in, 253–254
patent ductus arteriosis and, 261
pulmonary artery flow and, 301
pulmonary vascular hypertension with, 264–265
right-to-left, in first-pass radionuclide angiography, 255–256
Sickle-cell disease, Tc-99m sulfur colloid scan for, 59
Skeletal maturation, mandibular growth and, 51–56
Skeletal scintigraphy, 1–43
clinical applications of, 5–43
for neuroblastoma, 34–37
for mandibular growth assessment, 49–57
Skull, diseases of, 221
Spermatic cord, torsion of, 121
Spleen, 141–154
accessory, 147
candisiasis of, 153
congenital abnormality of, 132
focal defects of, 143
herniation of, 154
nonvisualization of, 152
normal size of, 143
radiopharmaceuticals for, 141
scan size of, 131
Tc-99m sulphur colloid uptake of, 143
torsion of, 147, 150
trauma to, 145
wandering, 150
Splenectomy, infection following, 145
Splenic abscess, 153
Splenic artery ligation, 154
Splenic infarction, 154
Splenic pseudocyst, 145
Splenic scintigraphy
clinical applications of, 143–154
injury diagnosis with, 145
normal variants of, 132
Tc-99m MDP for, 141
Tc-99m sulfur colloid for, 141
Splenomegaly, 143
Splenosis, 147
radiocolloid uptake and, 147
Staphylococcus aureus
cystic fibrosis and, 297
hematogenous osteomyelitis and, 12
septic arthritis and, 15
Stenosis
mitral, 303
pulmonic, 264
pulmonary blood flow in, 302
valvular, 301
Streptococcus fecalis, urinary infection with, 118
Stress fracture, 19–21
Stress fracture: stress reaction, 19–21
Stress reaction, in bone, 21
Stroke, cerebral radionuclide angiography for, 219
Subdural space, diseases of, 217
Sudden infant death syndrome, 171
Swyer-James-McLeod syndrome, 303
Synovitis, toxic, 18

Tc-99m BIDA, hepatic visualization with, 159
Tc-99m DEIDA, in biliary atresia diagnosis, 164
Tc-99m DISIDA, in biliary atresia diagnosis, 164
Tc-99m DMSA
in hypertension diagnosis, 89
in infarction detection, 93
in obstructed kidney, 81
in prune belly syndrome, 98
in pyelonephritis, 85
renal scintigraphy with, 64
study of, 67–68
Tc-99m DTPA
in acute tubular necrosis diagnosis, 90
for gastric esophageal scintigraphy, 172
in hydronephrosis, 77–80
in hypertension diagnosis, 89
in newborn, 72
in prune belly syndrome, 97
for radionuclide cisternography, 224
renal scintigraphy with, 64
study of, 66
Tc-99m glucoheptonate, renal scintigraphy with, 65
Tc-99m heat-denatured red blood cells, splenic imaging with, 141
Tc-99m hepatobiliary agents
bilirubin levels and, 158–159
characteristics of, 157–160
Tc-99m HIDA, 158–159
biliary vision with, 158
Tc-99m MAA
in pulmonary embolism, 313
for pulmonary scintigraphy, 289–291
Tc-99m MAA perfusion studies, technique of, 292
Tc-99m MDP
absorbed radiation dose from, 1
mandible imaging with, 50
in neuroblastoma, 34–37
splenic imaging with, 141, 143
in Wilm's tumor, 96–97
Tc-99m microspheres, for pulmonary scintigraphy, 290
Tc-99m phosphate compound
absorbed radiation dose from, 1
administered dose of, 1
for hypertension, 89
imaging technique, 1–2
mechanism of uptake, 1
Tc-99m PIPIDA
in biliary atresia diagnosis, 164
hepatobiliary visualization with, 159
Tc-99m PRIDA, hepatobiliary visualization with, 159
Tc-99m red blood cells, for gated blood pool angiography, 268
Tc-99m sodium pertechnetate
for brain scans, 206
cerebrospinal fluid shunt and, 228
in diagnosis of Meckel's diverticulum, 180, 180–181
for first-pass radionuclide angiography, 246
for thyroid scintigraphy, 192
Tc-99m sulfur colloid
absorbed radiation dose from, 4
administered dose of, 4
bone metastases and, 37

Vesicoureteric reflux (*cont.*)
Franconi's anemia and, 59
for gastric esophageal scintigraphy, 172
for hepatic scintigraphy, 129
imaging technique, 4
Kupffer cells uptake of, 129
mechanism of uptake, 3–4
sickle-cell diseases and, 59
for splenic scintigraphy, 141
splenic uptake of, 143
Technetium-99m dimercaptosuccinic acid, *see* Tc-99m DMSA
Technetium-99m methylene diphosphonate, *see* Tc-99m MDP
Technetium-99m N(2,6)-dimethylphenylcarbamolmethyl-IDA, *see* Tc-99m HIDA
Technetium-99m p-bityl-IDA, *see* Tc-99m BIDA
Technetium-99m p-isopropyl IDA. *see* Tc-99m PIPIDA
Technetium-99m stannous diethylenetriamine pentacetic acid, *see* Tc-99m DTPA
Testes, anatomy of, 121
Testicular torsion, 121–122
acute, 123
anatomic anomalalies associated with, 122
missed, 123–124
scintigraphy of, 123–125
symptoms of, 122
Testicular tumors, scintigraphic patterns of, 126
Thallium–201
in anomalous coronary artery, 274
in cardiomyopathy, 278–279
in mucocutaneous lyumph node syndrome, 279–282
for myocardial perfusion scintigraphy, 273
in right ventricular hypertrophy, 274–278
Thrombosis, renal vein, *see* Renal vein thrombosis
Thyroid carcinoma, 201–202
anaplastic, 202
and cervical metastases, 201
follicular, 202
medullary, 202
metastases and, 201
occurrence of, 202
pulmonary metastases and, 201–202
treatment of, 202
Thyroid gland, 191–202
ectopic, 194
and neck nodules, 194–200
normal study of, 193–194
scintigraphy of
clinical applications of, 193–202
examination technique, 192–193
indications for, 191
radiopharmaceuticals, 191–193
TSH stimulation test, 193
TSH suppression test (T3), 193
Thyroid nodules
classification of, 194, 199
solitary, 200
Thyroiditis, 201
chronic lymphocytic, 201
subacute, 201
Tissue attenuation, correction for, 69
Transplantation, renal, *see* Renal transplantation
Trauma
cerebral, scintigraphic detection of, 208, 211
radiopharmaceutical uptake, 18–19
TSH stimulation test, of thyroid gland, 193
TSH suppression test (T3), of thyroid gland, 193
Tubular necrosis, acute, radionuclide angiogram of, 90
Tumor
cerebral, scintigraphic detection of, 208
renal scintigraphy of, 96–97

Ultrasonography, of hepatic lesions, 129
Unilateral hyperlucent lung, 306
Unit impulse response (UIR), of kidney, 69
interpreation of, 69–70
Ureter, duplication of, 93
Ureterovesical junction, maturation of, 115
Urinary leakage, scintigraphy detection of, 90
Urine cultures, 118
radionuclide cystography and, 118
Urinoma, 90–91

Valvular regurgitation, measurement of, 272
Ventricle, end-diastolic volume of, calculation of, 260
Ventricular hypertrophy, right, Tl-201 imaging in, 274–278
Ventricular septal defect, 264
pulmonary scintigraphy in, 300–301
Ventriculo-atrial shunt, 230
Ventriculo-peritoneal shunt, 230
Vesicoureteric reflux, 109–111
bilateral, 109
classification of, 109
grading of, 108–109
incidence of, 105, 109
longterm consequence of, 105
management of, 105
patterns of, 110–111
unilateral, 109
Voiding flow rate, 117–118

Wilms' tumor, 38
Tc-99m MDP imaging of, 96–97
treatment of, liver changes and, 139
Wilson-Mikity lung, 317–318

Xenon-133 camera radiospirometry
analysis of, 295
normal distribution of, 295–296
regional volume of, 296
technique of, 294–295
Xenon-133 studies
in airway obstruction, 306, 308
in congenital lobar emphysema, 310
in cystic fibrosis, 297–299
of mucous plug, 308, 310
in pneumonia, 310, 312
in pulmonary evaluation, 291–292
in small child, 292–294
in uncooperative patient, 292–294
Xenon-133 ventilation-perfusion studies, 292